Complex and Revision Problems in Shoulder Instability

Emilio Calvo • Giovanni Di Giacomo
Augustus D. Mazzocca
Editors

Complex and Revision Problems in Shoulder Instability

Springer

ISAKOS
International Society of Arthroscopy, Knee Surgery and Orthopaedic Sports Medicine

Editors
Emilio Calvo
Department of Orthopedic Surgery and Traumatology
Hospital Universitario Fundacion Jimenez, Universidad Autonoma
Madrid, Spain

Giovanni Di Giacomo
Department of Orthopaedics & Trauma
Concordia Hospital
Rome, Italy

Augustus D. Mazzocca
Harvard Medical School, Sports Medicine
Massachusetts General Brigham
Boston, MA, USA

ISBN 978-3-031-81388-7 ISBN 978-3-031-81389-4 (eBook)
https://doi.org/10.1007/978-3-031-81389-4

This Springer imprint is published by the registered company Springer Nature Switzerland AG
The registered company address is: Gewerbestrasse 11, 6330 Cham, Switzerland

Preface

Shoulder instability remains one of the most challenging conditions in orthopedic and sports medicine. While many cases can be effectively treated with standard surgical or conservative approaches, complex and revision cases present a unique set of difficulties. Recurrent instability, poor soft tissue quality, bone loss, failed surgical repairs, and patient-specific factors demand a deeper understanding of advanced diagnostic techniques and surgical strategies.

This book is dedicated to addressing the intricacies of complex and revision shoulder instability. It explores key issues such as glenoid and humeral bone defects, soft tissue insufficiency, failed previous stabilization procedures, and the biomechanical principles underlying recurrent instability. Special emphasis is placed on patient selection criteria and surgical techniques, including bone augmentation procedures and arthroscopic and open revision strategies.

Through a combination of evidence-based research and clinical experience, the ISAKOS Shoulder Committee aims to provide orthopedic surgeons, sports medicine specialists, and rehabilitation professionals with the knowledge necessary to navigate these difficult cases. By integrating the latest innovations and surgical techniques, our goal is to optimize patient outcomes and improve long-term joint stability.

We extend our appreciation to the members of the ISAKOS Shoulder Committee as well as to the experts who have contributed to the evolution of complex shoulder instability treatment. Their dedication continues to drive progress in this demanding field, ultimately improving the lives of patients worldwide.

Madrid, Spain — Emilio Calvo
Rome, Italy — Giovanni di Giacomo
Boston, MA, USA — Augustus D. Mazzocca

Contents

Part V Complications After Shoulder Stabilization

Part I

Bone Defects in Anterior Shoulder Instability

The Glenoid Track Concept

1

Giovanni Di Giacomo, Andrea De Vita,
and Gianmarco Marcello

1.1 Bipolar Bone Loss

Glenohumeral stability is a complex issue, reliant on a multitude of static and dynamic factors. Static factors include intrinsic stability depending on the glenoid concavity and the congruency of the glenoid and labrum with the humeral head, the capsuloligamentous structures and negative intra-articular pressure. Dynamic factors include rotator cuff muscles, as well as other muscles to a lesser degree, which create a joint reaction force compressing the humeral head in the concave glenoid fossa (concavity-compression effect), proprioception and scapular stabilizers which allow a dynamic coupled motion of scapulothoracic and glenohumeral joints [1, 2].

At the end-range of movement, a part of the shoulder capsule is tight, which prevents a translation of the humeral head on the glenoid socket, so the capsuloligamentous structures are the main stabilizers with the arm at the end-range of movement. On the other hand, the shoulder capsule is lax in the mid-range of movement, and negative intra-articular pressure and concavity-compression effect are the main stabilizers with the arm in the mid-range of movement [3].

An anterior shoulder dislocation can cause damage to several structures in the joint. However, bone loss is an essential factor. Bone loss is quite common in shoulder instability. 41% of glenoid bone loss following a first dislocation and 86% following recurrent dislocations were documented by Griffith et al. [4]. This is consistent with the findings of Piasecki's et al. study [5], which showed that in patients with recurrent instability glenoid bone loss ranged from 49% to 89% and humeral bone loss from 70% to 100%. Similarly, Widjaja et al. discovered simultaneous defects following traumatic anterior shoulder dislocations in 54% of patients [6]. On the glenoid side, bone loss can manifest as erosion-type (more common in chronic instability) or fragment-type (also known as bony Bankart). On the humeral side, the anterior glenoid rim causes a compression fracture of the posterior humeral head when the shoulder dislocates, resulting in the Hill-Sachs lesion (HSL). Bipolar bone loss is the term used to describe these coupled glenoid and humeral head abnormalities.

G. Di Giacomo (✉) · A. De Vita
Orthopaedics and Traumatology Unit, Concordia Hospital, Rome, Italy
e-mail: concordia@iol.it

G. Marcello
Fondazione Policlinico Universitario Campus Bio-Medico, Via Alvaro del Portillo, Rome, Italy

Research Unit of Orthopaedic and Trauma Surgery, Department of Medicine and Surgery, Università Campus Bio-Medico di Roma, Via Alvaro del Portillo, Rome, Italy

Orthopaedics and Traumatology Unit, Ospedale dei Castelli, Via Nettunense, Ariccia, Italy
e-mail: gianmarco.marcello@aslroma6.it

E. Calvo et al. (eds.), *Complex and Revision Problems in Shoulder Instability*,
https://doi.org/10.1007/978-3-031-81389-4_1

The intrinsic stability is modified in a variety of ways by anterior labrum detachment and anterior glenoid rim bone loss. Glenoid bone loss implicates a decrease in the glenoid depth, arc length, articular curvature, and articular surface that maintains contact with the humeral head [7]. The mean contact pressures in the posterosuperior quadrant decrease with increasing glenoid bone loss, while the forces in the anteroinferior quadrant increase [8]. According to Greis et al., a 20% glenoid defect increases the mean contact pressure by more than 40% throughout the glenoid and more than 200% of normal in the anteroinferior quadrant [9]. Additionally, as the size of the glenoid defect increases, the maximal force needed to dislocate the shoulder drops proportionately [10].

Since in the mid-range the glenoid bone is an important contributor to shoulder stability and the Hill-Sachs lesion is away from the glenoid, the glenoid bone loss alone causes instability in the mid-range of movement, and consequently the risk of instability related to the glenoid bone loss can be evaluated by the size of the glenoid defect alone, independently of the Hill-Sachs lesion. The effect of the Hill-Sachs lesion, instead, can be seen when the arm comes close to the end-range of movement, because the glenoid comes close to the posterolateral portion of the humeral head. At this point, if the Hill-Sachs lesion is out of the glenoid coverage, it can engage the anterior rim of the glenoid. A Hill-Sachs lesion which doesn't cause instability with a preserved glenoid may cause instability if a glenoid bone loss is present. So, the risk related to the Hill-Sachs lesion does not correspond to the size of the HSL alone, it is dependent on the entity of glenoid bone loss and is related to the end-range of movement [3].

1.2 How to Measure the Instability Risk Related to Bone Loss: The On-/Off-Track Concept

The glenoid bone defect can be evaluated using a variety of techniques, including radiography [11–13], CT [14], 3D CT [15], MRI [16], and arthroscopy [17]. Presently, the "en face" view of the glenoid obtained with 3D CT is the gold standard, because it allows the most precise evaluation of the glenoid bone deformity [18–22].

In order to measure the bone defect, we first need to estimate the original glenoid dimension. There are two methods to do so: the best-fit circle method and the contralateral glenoid method. The lower half of the glenoid closely approximates a circular shape. Consequently, the first method involves positioning a circle over the inferior portion of the glenoid in the sagittal view, using the outer cortex as a reference landmark. This circle is aligned with the posterior and inferior curvature of the glenoid, and the absent segment of the circle represents the extent of the bone defect (Fig. 1.1) [16].

The circle method is widely used, but it is not so simple to manually determine the best-fit circle, and as a result there is variability of the calculated bone loss among observers using this method. The reliability of this method is a major concern. Also, the normal glenoid may not present a perfect circle, thus overestimating the amount of bone loss [23].

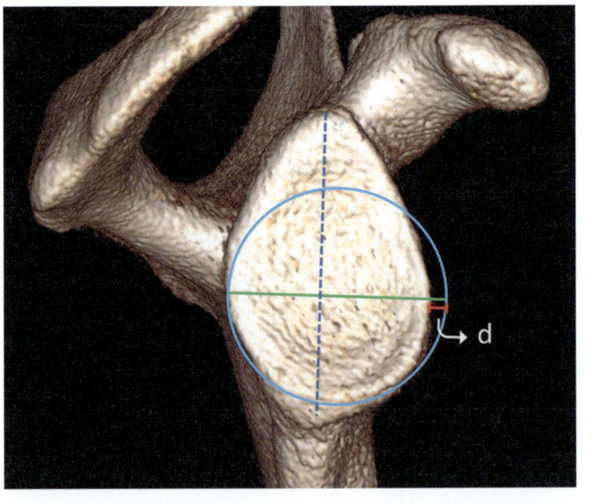

Fig. 1.1 Linear measurement of the glenoid bone defect with the perfect circle method. First, the vertical axis of the glenoid, which goes from the supraglenoid tubercle to the inferior margin of the glenoid, is identified (dotted line). Then, a best-fit circle drawn in the inferior part of the glenoid allows to estimate the native width of the glenoid (undotted line), which corresponds to the diameter of the circle perpendicular to the vertical axis. At this point, it is possible to measure the defect width (d) and, consequently, the remaining glenoid track width

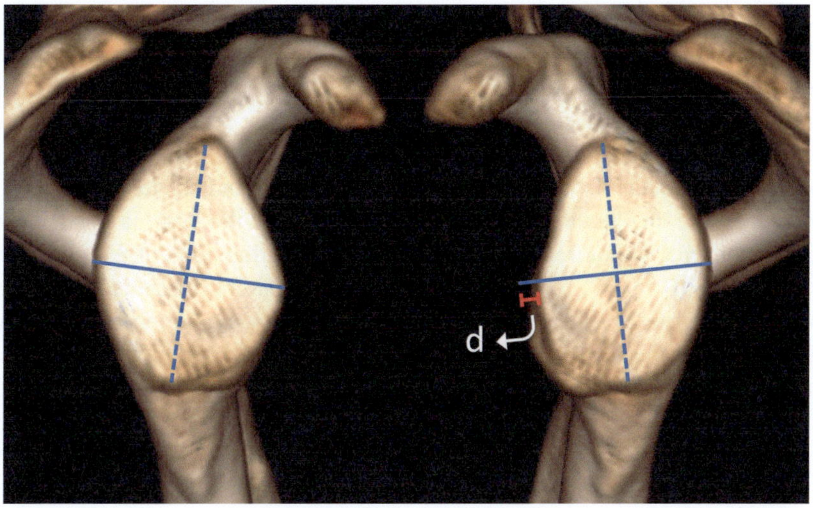

Fig. 1.2 Linear measurement of the glenoid bone defect with the contralateral method. The glenoid width (undotted line) is first measured on the contralateral side (if not involved in shoulder instability). It corresponds to a line perpendicular to the vertical axis of the glenoid (dotted line) at the point of its maximum anteroposterior length (left side image). The measured width is then reported on the affected shoulder, using the vertical axis as reference for its positioning (right side image). The difference between the native width and the actual width corresponds to the glenoid bone defect (d) [3, 15]

Using the contralateral method, instead, we can precisely estimate the original shape of the glenoid. Since the side-to-side difference is <1% of the length and width [24], the contralateral method considers the shape of the contralateral shoulder (which can be included in the same CT scan) as reference, unless it is also involved in shoulder instability (Fig. 1.2) [15].

Because of these reasons, it is recommended to use the contralateral method [3].

The second step is choosing how to estimate the size of the glenoid bone defect. One of the best indicators of glenoid bone loss was the width of the glenoid and the width-to-length ratio of the glenoid [16]. Area description is a little arduous; it requires a software to calculate it [14]. Instead, using the linear description through the measurement of the width of the glenoid, it is possible to express the bone loss easily with no special software (Figs. 1.1 and 1.2). Thus, the linear description of the glenoid width is recommended. The defect width is divided by the native glenoid width and multiplied by 100% to obtain the percentage value of the glenoid bone loss.

In order to evaluate the risk of instability caused by the HSL, it is critical to know if it can engage the glenoid rim, and this depends not only on the size and location of the HSL itself but also on the glenoid bone loss.

There are two methods to assess the risk of HSL. One method is dynamic examination during shoulder arthroscopy to distinguish between HSLs that engage with the glenoid rim at the end-range of movement (engaging HSLs) and HSLs that do not (nonengaging HSLs) [25–27]. This examination should be performed after a Bankart repair has been done, otherwise engagement would be easily produced with the humeral head not centered in the glenoid cavity, leading to an overdiagnosis of engaging HSLs [28]. Thus, the dynamic examination before the Bankart repair makes no sense: it is not important if engagement is present before the Bankart repair, we are interested in determining whether there is a residual risk of engagement after the repair has been performed, in order to indicate further treatments like the *remplissage* procedure [3]. However, the problem of a dynamic examination performed after the Bankart repair is that it poses a risk of damaging the repair [3]. Plus, it would be difficult to perform *remplissage* after a Bankart repair has been performed. For these reasons, the dynamic examination method is useless.

That is why the second method, the glenoid track method, was introduced. This method allows to overcome the inadequate engaging/nonengaging concept with the more appropriate on-/off-track concept [29].

The glenoid track is the track, the contact area, created by the glenoid on the humeral head during the posterior end-range of motion. If the HSL stays within this track, the shoulder is stable as engagement is not produced. The width of the glenoid track is relevant for this evaluation, and it is defined as the distance between the medial margin of the glenoid track and the medial margin of the footprint of the rotator cuff. This width is not equal to the glenoid width because the posterior glenoid rim overrides the footprint of the rotator cuff at the posterior end-range of motion. This width was found to correspond on average to 84% of the glenoid width in cadaveric shoulders [30] and to 83% of the glenoid width in live shoulders with the arm at 90° of abduction [31].

This percentage is an average value, in fact it was noted that the width of the glenoid track varies with the range of shoulder motion [32], and the strongest correlation was found to be with the active horizontal extension angle in the sitting position, which we can measure on the contralateral shoulder [33]. According to this relation, it is possible to more precisely estimate the glenoid track width. The following equation can be used to obtain for each patient an adjusted percentage value that better defines the glenoid track width: glenoid track width (%) = 90 – (0.49 * horizontal extension angle) [34].

However, the value of 83% of the glenoid width is commonly used to define the glenoid track width.

In case of anterior glenoid bone loss, the real glenoid track width is determined by subtracting the bone loss width from the previously calculated value. We then report this resulting width on the posterior view of the humeral head. If the medial margin of the HSL is located inside the glenoid track, it poses no risk of engagement with the anterior glenoid rim and we define it an on-track HSL. That is because in such case the HSL does not reach the glenoid rim, which corresponds to the medial margin of the glenoid track, at the end-range of motion. Engagement may occur if the HSL is located more medially over the medial edge of the glenoid track; in this case, the lesion is classified as off-track.

To express this mathematically, we can measure the Hill-Sachs interval (HSI), defined as the distance from the medial margin of the HSL to the medial margin of the footprint of the rotator cuff. If the Hill-Sachs interval is lower than the glenoid track width, we have an on-track HSL, otherwise we have to deal with an off-track HSL [29].

The HSI should be measured on a plane perpendicular to the footprint of the rotator cuff. It is possible to do this measurement with the 3D CT, which is the considered the most accurate method for evaluating bone loss and the glenoid track [20].

To achieve the right 3D view of the humeral head in which the measure of the HSI is taken, it is possible to start from the cranial view of the head with the lesser tuberosity oriented anteriorly and the articular cartilage positioned medially. From this position, the head is moved 90° in order to have a point of view exactly posterior to the head [35, 36]. Now a line is drawn following the medial margin of the footprint of the rotator cuff, and a second line parallel to the first one is drawn more medially. The distance between these two lines is equal to the previously calculated value of the glenoid track width. At this point, the HSI can be measured drawing a line starting from the most medial margin of the HSL and going perpendicular to the footprint of the rotator cuff, up to the medial margin of the footprint (Fig. 1.3).

Sometimes it is not easy to identify the medial margin of footprint of the rotator cuff because it has been involved in the HSL. In these cases, it is possible to draw a curved line which starts from the contact point between the inferior margin of the cartilage and the medial margin of the footprint of the teres minor, and arrives to the medial

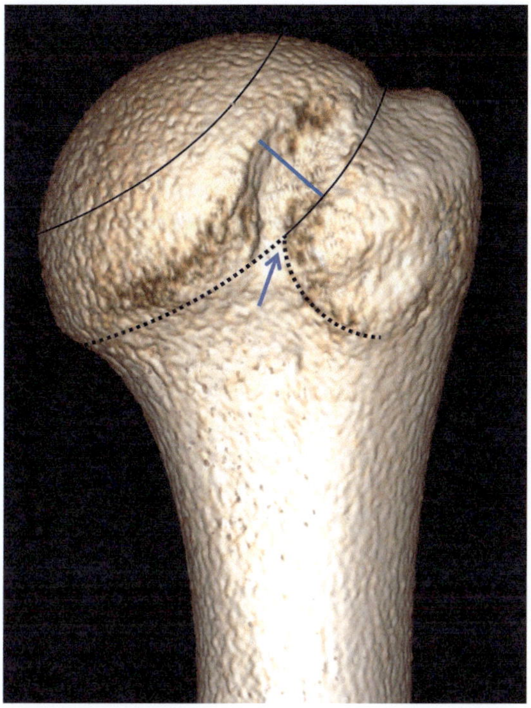

Fig. 1.3 Measuring the Hill-Sachs interval on the posterior view of the humeral head with 3D CT. The undotted curved lines represent the medial margin of the glenoid track (on the left) and the medial margin of the rotator cuff footprint or lateral margin of the glenoid track (on the right). If the medial margin of the footprint it not clearly identifiable because of the presence of the HSL, as in this case, it is possible to draw a curved line which follows the curvature of the articular cartilage, passes on the imaginary contact point (arrow) between the inferior margin of the cartilage and the medial margin of the footprint of the teres minor (dotted lines), and arrives to the medial margin of the supraspinatus footprint [35]. The Hill-Sachs interval is then obtained measuring the distance perpendicular to the undotted curved lines from the most medial point of the HSL to the lateral margin of the glenoid track (straight line)

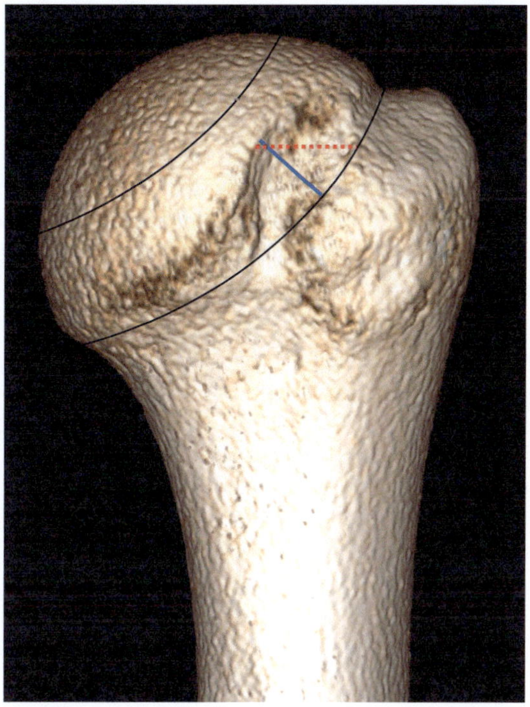

Fig. 1.4 Difference between the HSI measurements obtained with CT and with MR. CT measurement is made perpendicular to the lateral margin of the glenoid track (undotted line), while in MR the HSI is measured on axial images, thus overestimating the real value (dotted line) [35]

margin of the supraspinatus footprint. This curved line follows the curvature of the inferior margin of the articular cartilage and can be used as reference for the medial margin of the rotator cuff footprint (Fig. 1.3) [35].

However, the CT method has the disadvantage of radiation exposure, so in the last period the MRI method is gaining popularity [37–39]. This method consists of measuring the HSI in the axial plane in which the HSL shows the highest width [37]. Although it is a simple method, the MRI method is probably less accurate because this method uses the axial images so the HSI is not measured perpendicular to the footprint as in 3D CT, but rather oblique to it, therefore bringing the risk of overdiagnosing off-track HSLs by obtaining HSIs bigger than the real ones (Fig. 1.4) [35]. Nevertheless, it can be easily used to classify HSLs in the first place. In case an off-track HSL is found, one can then use the 3D CT method to accurately confirm the result [35].

1.3 Clinical Applications

After first-time instability episodes, nonsurgical management may be an effective therapeutic option for low-demand patients, while surgery is frequently recommended for high-risk patients [40]. The patient's age and the degree of glenoid and humeral bone loss are the two main factors impacting the probability of recurrence of anterior shoulder instability, although there are many risk factors for persistent instability, such as male gender, hyperlaxity, and participation in contact or overhead sport activities [41–47]. Another important determinant of redislocation rate is the number of instability episodes [48–52]. Absolute indications for surgical treatment are off-track HSL or critical glenoid bone loss, which is defined as a bone loss ≥25% of the glenoid width [35]. Accurate assessment of the bipolar bone loss is crucial for managing shoulder instability because it has a critical role in predicting outcomes [41]. Since it is a method to analyze bipolar bone loss and predict the possibility of engagement of Hill-Sachs lesions, we can use the glenoid track concept to better determine when to recommend surgical treatment and which surgical procedure is best for each patient suffering from anterior shoulder instability with bone loss [53].

To choose the correct treatment, we must consider at the same time the extent of the glenoid bone loss and the risk related to the Hill Sachs lesion, given that both contribute to instability (bipolar bone loss).

In the past, critical glenoid bone loss was considered the limit beyond which the Bankart repair was contraindicated, making it necessary to perform a bone graft to reconstruct the glenoid bone, being the bone loss responsible of a high risk of postoperative recurrence in these cases. However, more recently, a gray area has been identified between the safe zone of insignificant bone loss and the critical zone, ranging from 13.5–17.5% to 20–25% [35, 54–57]: this area has been defined as subcritical glenoid bone loss. Patients with subcritical glenoid bone loss undergoing Bankart repair have not shown a high rate of postoperative recurrence, but an unjustified decrease in quality of life, to the point that now the Bankart repair is usually indicated in case of glenoid bone loss <15%, while glenoid bone grafting is normally indicated when the glenoid bone loss ≥15% [55].

When we consider the risk of the HSL, we first distinguish between on-track and off-track lesions, with the previous explained methods. We know that the Bankart repair alone is contraindicated with off-track HSLs: these lesions necessitate to be converted into on-track, so they require an added procedure like *remplissage* or can alternatively be treated with glenoid bone grafting, as these techniques are able to convert the HSL from off-track to on-track.

Nevertheless, it is important to accurately analyze on-track Hill-Sachs lesions as well, because the ones close to be off-track are linked to worse outcomes. According to Yamamoto et al., patients treated with the Bankart repair with a Hill-Sachs occupancy ratio (ratio between the HSI and the glenoid track width) ≥ 75% (peripheral-track Hill-Sachs lesion) had a significantly worse WOSI score [58]. A Hill–Sachs interval to glenoid track width ratio > 0.7 was found to be a significant predictor of increased risk for recurrent instability in another investigation by Yang et al. [38]. Recurrence is also more frequent in near-track lesions, defined as those with a distance to dislocation (distance between the medial margin of the glenoid track and the medial margin of an on-track HSL) ≤ 8 mm [59]. All these patients, provided that glenoid bone loss does not reach the threshold of subcritical, can be treated with Bankart repair plus *remplissage*, which increases stability and results in considerably lower recurrence rates and better WOSI scores [60–62].

However, one must consider that the distance to dislocation threshold is not a percentage value. With a glenoid width of 25 mm, for example, the glenoid track would be 20.75 mm. According to the peripheral–/central-track concept, in this case remplissage would be performed with an HSI ≥ 15.56 mm. Instead, using the distance to dislocation concept, an HSI equal to 12.75 mm would be enough to indicate remplissage. Thus, the use of the latter would overestimate the risk of recurrence [35]. Also, it must be noted that the G/T ratio was based on an MRI study.

It is preferable to utilize the peripheral–/central-track concept, which was based on the most accurate 3DCT measurement, to determine whether an augmentation treatment such as remplissage is necessary [35].

1.4 ISI and GTIM Scores

The Instability Severity Index Score (ISIS) was developed to assist in differentiating individuals who require soft tissue repair from those who will benefit from an open bone reconstruction [63]. Using this score, patients are ranked on a 10-point scale based on preoperative risk factors. According to the authors, individuals who score more than 6 have a 70% chance of experiencing recurrent instability after arthroscopic Bankart repair; as a result, the Latarjet procedure is suitable for these patients, while patients who score ≤ 6 can be treated with the Bankart repair. Afterwards, it has been proposed to lower this threshold to 4 [64] or 3 [65, 66].

A drawback of this scoring system is that simple x-rays are used to evaluate bone abnormalities, which is a straightforward but inaccurate procedure.

Di Giacomo et al. integrated the glenoid track concept in the ISI score, introducing the Glenoid Track Instability Management Score (GTIMS) [67]. This score uses the on−/off-track concept to assess the risk associated with bone loss while taking into account the same risk factors not related to bone loss as the ISI score (age at surgery, sport type, degree of competition in sport, and shoulder hyperlaxity). A possible total score of 10 is reached by attributing a specific score to each factor.

Patients with a GTIMS <4 can be treated with a soft tissue procedure like the Bankart repair [67]. In some cases the Bankart repair may not be enough to properly stabilize the shoulder. In these cases a Bankart plus procedure may be performed (Bankart repair plus remplissage or ASA or bone block) depending on characteristics of the patient or the entity of the bone loss: remplissage can be indicated in recurrent instability [68] or peripheral-track HSL [58], the ASA procedure is useful in constitutional hyperlaxity [69, 70] and bone block is suitable for subcritical glenoid bone loss [71, 72].

Patients with GTIMS ≥4 should be treated with the Latarjet procedure [67], a surgical technique usually reserved for high-risk patients [73], severe bone loss [74], deficient capsular tissue [75], or revision of surgical failures [76], since it is a reliable treatment with successful results [77, 78] and high return to sport rates [79, 80].

A considerable number of patients did not undergo the Latarjet operation when GTIMS was applied instead of ISIS to indicate treatment ($p < 0.001$) [67]. Even though more clinical research is needed to verify the hypothesis, the literature now available on the glenoid track suggests that GTIMS may more reliably predict failure after arthroscopic soft tissue repair and, therefore, more accurately identify patients who require the Latarjet procedure [54, 81, 82].

However, patients with GTIMS ≥4 receive different surgical treatments worldwide, with an approach varying from surgeon to surgeon. These patients, in fact, can be distinguished into two groups: patients who score ≥ 4 because of a severe bone loss (off-track HSLs) and patients with high risk factors but not related to bone loss, yet scoring ≥4 [35].

Patients with GTIMS ≥4 and off-track HSLs are usually treated with the Latarjet procedure [74]; alternatively, their bone loss is addressed with a capsulolabral repair associated to a bone block plus remplissage, restoring translation and stiffness closer to the native glenohumeral joint [83] and reserving the Latarjet procedure for a revision setting [35].

Whether the Latarjet technique can turn every off-track HSL into an on-track lesion is a matter of concern. It is advised to measure the glenoid track and coracoid process size before surgery since a Hill-Sachs interval wider than the glenoid track in a value larger than 7.45 mm has been found to be a risk factor for a residual postoperative off-track HSL [84]. In these rare cases, bone grafting of the HSL or remplissage may be added to the Latarjet technique [85, 86], or, as an alternative, larger free bone block procedures (iliac crest bone graft [71], distal tibial allograft [87], and Eden-Hybbinette procedure [88]) can be performed, instead of the Latarjet [84]. However, these larger bone graft procedures are typically carried out in the context of a revision of a glenoid reconstruction [89].

The treatment of patients with GTIMS ≥4 without severe bipolar bone loss is controversial. Many techniques may be suitable for them since in these cases the bone loss may be minimal or absent. Treatment is determined based on the specific characteristics and risk factors of each individual, and it varies with the surgeon's preference [35].

Merrill Jr. and Arciero perform an open Bankart repair in the following cases: collision male athletes less than 20 years old, 10–20% of glenoid bone loss, more than five dislocations, deficient capsulolabral tissue, revision of well-performed arthroscopic procedure with minor bone loss, instability episodes occurring during daily living activities or sleep [90].

Depending on whether bone loss is predominant on the glenoid or humeral side, other surgeons perform a bone block in conjunction with Bankart repair or Bankart repair plus remplissage because, in certain cases, these procedures can yield clinical outcomes comparable to Latarjet with less postoperative complications [91–93].

In patients with 10–20% of glenoid bone loss, first dislocation ≤3 years earlier and ≤5 dislocations, Taverna et al. do an arthroscopic bone block with Bankart repair. For cases with more than five dislocations or first dislocation more than 3 years earlier, they use the Latarjet procedure [94].

Since the Latarjet procedure is a technique with low failure rates, which enables contact athletes to return to competition more quickly than soft tissue repair [80], some other surgeons still resort to it even in the absence of bone loss.

1.5 Limitations

The glenoid track concept allows to evaluate the risk of the HSL together with the glenoid bone loss, but it has some limitations. There is variability in the method used to measure the glenoid bone loss and the HSI, leading to different results. Also, it can be difficult to identify the medial margin of the footprint of the rotator cuff, and the measure may vary depending on variability of the insertion of the rotator cuff.

Furthermore, there are still controversies worldwide on how to manage subcritical glenoid or humeral bone loss. GTIMS is a tool for guiding treatment, and we provided indications for common clinical scenarios in anterior shoulder instability. However, treatment must be tailored to each patient, as the complexity of variables makes a universal algorithm impractical [35].

References

1. Di Giacomo G, Piscitelli L, Pugliese M. The role of bone in glenohumeral stability. EFORT Open Rev. 2018;3(12):632–40.
2. Di Giacomo G, de Gasperis N, Scarso P. Bipolar bone defect in the shoulder anterior dislocation. Knee Surg Sports Traumatol Arthrosc. 2015;24(2):479–88.
3. Itoi E. "On-track" and "off-track" shoulder lesions. EFORT Open Rev. 2017;2(8):343–51.
4. Griffith JF, Antonio GE, Yung PSH, Wong EMC, Yu AB, Ahuja AT, et al. Prevalence, pattern, and spectrum of glenoid bone loss in anterior shoulder dislocation: CT analysis of 218 patients. Am J Roentgenol. 2008;190(5):1247–5.
5. Piasecki DP, Verma NN, Romeo AA, Levine WN, Bach BR, Provencher MT. Glenoid bone deficiency in recurrent anterior shoulder instability: diagnosis and management. J Am Acad Orthop Surg. 2009;17(8):482–93.
6. Widjaja AB, Tran A, Bailey M, Proper S. Correlation between Bankart and Hill-Sachs lesions in anterior shoulder dislocation. ANZ J Surg. 2006;76(6):436–8.
7. Yamamoto N, Muraki T, Sperling JW, Steinmann SP, Cofield RH, Itoi E, et al. Stabilizing mechanism in bone-grafting of a large glenoid defect. J Bone Joint Surg. 2010;92(11):2059–66.
8. Yamamoto A, Massimini DF, DiStefano J, Higgins LD. Glenohumeral contact pressure with simulated anterior labral and osseous defects in cadaveric shoulders before and after soft tissue repair. Am J Sports Med. 2014;42(8):1947–54.
9. Greis PE, Scuderi MG, Mohr A, Bachus KN, Burks RT. Glenohumeral articular contact areas and pressures following labral and osseous injury to the anteroinferior quadrant of the glenoid. J Shoulder Elbow Surg. 2002;11(5):442–51.
10. Shin SJ, Ko YW, Scott J, McGarry MH, Lee TQ. The effect of defect orientation and size on glenohumeral instability: a biomechanical analysis. Knee Surg Sports Traumatol Arthrosc. 2015;24(2):533–9.
11. Rokous JR, Feagin JA, Abbott HG. Modified axillary roentgenogram. a useful adjunct in the diagnosis of recurrent instability of the shoulder. Clin Orthop Relat Res. 1972;82:84–6.
12. Bernageau J, Patte D, Debeyre J, Ferrane J. Value of the glenoid profil in recurrent luxations of the shoulder. Rev Chir Orthop Reparatrice Appar Mot. 1976;62(2 Suppl):142–7.
13. Garth WP, Slappey CE, Ochs CW. Roentgenographic demonstration of instability of the shoulder: the apical oblique projection. A technical note. J Bone Joint Surg Am. 1984;66(9):1450–3.

14. Baudi P, Righi P, Bolognesi D, Rivetta S, Rossi Urtoler E, Guicciardi N, et al. How to identify and calculate glenoid bone deficit. Chir Organi Mov. 2005;90(2):145–52.
15. Griffith JF, Antonio GE, Tong CWC, Ming CK. Anterior shoulder dislocation:quantification of glenoid bone loss with CT. AJR Am J Roentgenol. 2003;180(5):1423–30.
16. Huijsmans PE, Haen PS, Kidd M, Dhert WJ, van der Hulst VPM, Willems WJ. Quantification of a glenoid defect with three-dimensional computed tomography and magnetic resonance imaging: a cadaveric study. J Shoulder Elbow Surg. 2007;16(6):803–9.
17. Burkhart SS, DeBeer JF, Tehrany AM, Parten PM. Quantifying glenoid bone loss arthroscopically in shoulder instability. Arthroscopy. 2002;18(5):488–91.
18. Provencher CMT, Bhatia S, Ghodadra NS, Grumet RC, Bach BR, Dewing LCB, et al. Recurrent shoulder instability: current concepts for evaluation and management of glenoid bone loss. J Bone Joint Surg. 2010;92(Suppl_2):133–51.
19. Bishop JY, Jones GL, Rerko MA, Donaldson C. 3-D CT is the most reliable imaging modality when quantifying glenoid bone loss. Clin Orthop Relat Res. 2012;471(4):1251–6.
20. Weber AE, Bolia IK, Horn A, Villacis D, Omid R, Tibone JE, et al. Glenoid bone loss in shoulder instability: superiority of three-dimensional computed tomography over two-dimensional magnetic resonance imaging using established methodology. Clin Orthop Surg. 2021;13(2):223–8.
21. Rossi LA, Frank RM, Wilke D, Provencher M, Millet PJ, Chahla J. Bone loss in the setting of glenohumeral instability: an expert consensus statement using the modified delphi technique. Arthroscopy. 2021;37(6):1719–28.
22. Sugaya H. Techniques to evaluate glenoid bone loss. Curr Rev Musculoskeletal Med. 2014;7(1):1–5.
23. Do WS, Kim JH, Lim JR, Yoon TH, Chun YM. Disagreement between the accepted best-fit circle method to calculate bone loss between injured and uninjured shoulders. Am J Sports Med. 2023;51(4):885–92.
24. Shi L, Griffith JF, Huang J, Wang D. Excellent side-to-side symmetry in glenoid size and shape. Skeletal Radiol. 2013;42(12):1711–5.
25. Cho SH, Cho NS, Rhee YG. Preoperative analysis of the Hill-Sachs lesion in anterior shoulder instability. Am J Sports Med. 2011;39(11):2389–95.
26. Haviv B, Mayo L, Biggs D. Outcomes of arthroscopic "remplissage": capsulotenodesis of the engaging large Hill-Sachs lesion. J Orthop Surg Res. 2011;6(1):29.
27. Zhu YM, Lu Y, Zhang J, Shen JW, Jiang CY. Arthroscopic Bankart repair combined with remplissage technique for the treatment of anterior shoulder instability with engaging Hill-Sachs lesion. Am J Sports Med. 2011;39(8):1640–8.
28. Hwang ST, Horinek JL, Ardebol J, Menendez ME, Denard PJ. Arthroscopic remplissage for the treatment of anterior shoulder instability. JBJS Rev. 2022;10(11):e22.00151. https://doi.org/10.2106/JBJS.RVW.22.00151.
29. Di Giacomo G, Itoi E, Burkhart SS. Evolving concept of bipolar bone loss and the Hill-Sachs lesion: from "engaging/non-engaging" lesion to "on-track/off-track" lesion. Arthroscopy. 2014;30(1):90–8.
30. Yamamoto N, Itoi E, Abe H, Minagawa H, Seki N, Shimada Y, et al. Contact between the glenoid and the humeral head in abduction, external rotation, and horizontal extension: a new concept of glenoid track. J Shoulder Elbow Surg. 2007;16(5):649–56.
31. Omori Y, Yamamoto N, Koishi H, Futai K, Goto A, Sugamoto K, et al. Measurement of the glenoid track in vivo as investigated by 3-dimensional motion analysis using open MRI. Am J Sports Med. 2014;42(6):1290–5.
32. Yamamoto N, Kawakami J, Nagamoto H, Shiota Y, Itoi E. The relationship between the glenoid track and the range of shoulder motion: a cadaver study. Orthop Traumatol Surg Res. 2018;104(6):793–6. https://doi.org/10.1016/j.otsr.2017.12.006.
33. Kawakami J, Yamamoto N, Etoh T, Hatta T, Mineta M, Itoi E, et al. In vivo glenoid track width can be better predicted with the use of shoulder horizontal extension angle. Am J Sports Med. 2019;47(4):922–7. https://doi.org/10.1177/0363546519825629.
34. Itoi E. Shoulderology. Springer; 2023.
35. Itoi E, Yamamoto N, Di Giacomo G, Marcello G. Glenoid track revisited. J Shoulder Elbow Surg. 2024;33(12):2791–9.
36. Itoi E, Yamamoto N. Shoulder instability. Curr Orthop Pract. 2012;23(6):609–15.
37. Gyftopoulos S, Beltran LS, Bookman J, Rokito A. MRI evaluation of bipolar bone loss using the on-track off-track method: a feasibility study. AJR Am J Roentgenol. 2015;205(4):848–52.
38. Yang TC, Chen KH, Chiang ER, Chang MC, Ma HL. Using the "Hill-Sachs interval to glenoid track width ratio" for prediction of recurrent instability after arthroscopic Bankart repair. Orthop Traumatol Surg Res. 2018;104(6):797–801. https://doi.org/10.1016/j.otsr.2018.02.
39. Vopat ML, Hermanns CA, Midtgaard KS, Baker J, Coda RG, Cheema SG, et al. Imaging modalities for the glenoid track in recurrent shoulder instability: a systematic review. Orthop J Sports Med. 2021;9(6):23259671211006750.
40. Rose GD, Borroni M, Castagna A. The role of arthroscopic capsulo-labral repair in unidirectional post-traumatic shoulder instability in adolescent athletes participating in overhead or contact sports. Joints. 2024;1(3):108.
41. Schwihla I, Wieser K, Grubhofer F, Zimmermann SM. Long-Term recurrence rate in anterior shoulder instability after Bankart repair based on the on—and off-track-concept. J Shoulder Elbow Surg. 2022;32(2):269–75.
42. Carlson Strother CR, McLaughlin RJ, Krych AJ, Sanchez-Sotelo J, Camp CL. Open shoulder stabiliza-

tion for instability: anterior labral repair with capsular shift. Arthrosc Tech. 2019;8(7):e749–54.
43. Chan AG, Kilcoyne KG, Chan S, Dickens JF, Waterman BR. Evaluation of the instability severity index score in predicting failure following arthroscopic Bankart surgery in an active military population. J Shoulder Elbow Surg. 2019;28(5):e156–63.
44. Lobo FL. Arthroscopic treatment of anterior shoulder dislocation using knotted and knotless anchors. clinicaltrials.gov. 2021.
45. Tokish JM, Lafosse L, Giacomo GD, Arciero R. Patients in whom arthroscopic Bankart repair is not enough: evaluation and management of complex anterior glenohumeral instability. Instr Course Lect. 2017;66:79.
46. Calvo E, Granizo JJ, Fernández-Yruegas D. Criteria for arthroscopic treatment of anterior instability of the shoulder: a prospective study. J Bone Joint Surg Br. 2005;87(5):677–83.
47. Vermeulen AE, Landman EBM, Veen EJD, Nienhuis S, Koorevaar CT. Long-term clinical outcome of arthroscopic Bankart repair with suture anchors. J Shoulder Elbow Surg. 2019;28(5):e137–43.
48. Wasserstein D, Dwyer T, Veillette C, Gandhi R, Chahal J, Mahomed NN, et al. Predictors of dislocation and revision after shoulder stabilization in Ontario, Canada, from 2003 to 2008. Am J Sports Med. 2013;41(9):2034–40.
49. Gasparini G, De Benedetto M, Cundari A, De Gori M, Orlando N, McFarland EG, et al. Predictors of functional outcomes and recurrent shoulder instability after arthroscopic anterior stabilization. Knee Surg Sports Traumatol Arthrosc. 2016;24(2):406–13.
50. Shin SJ, Ko YW, Lee J. Intra-articular lesions and their relation to arthroscopic stabilization failure in young patients with first-time and recurrent shoulder dislocations. J Shoulder Elbow Surg. 2016;25(11):1756–63.
51. Fox MA, Drain NP, Rai A, Zheng A, Carlos NB, Serrano Riera R, et al. Increased failure rates after arthroscopic Bankart repair after second dislocation compared to primary dislocation with comparable clinical outcomes. Arthroscopy. 2023;39(3):682–8.
52. Cordasco FA, Lin B, Heller M, Asaro LA, Ling D, Calcei JG. Arthroscopic shoulder stabilization in the young athlete: return to sport and revision stabilization rates. J Shoulder Elbow Surg. 2020;29(5):946–53.
53. Provencher MT, Midtgaard KS, Owens BD, Tokish JM. Diagnosis and management of traumatic anterior shoulder instability. J Am Acad Orthop Surg. 2020;29(2):e51–61.
54. Shaha JS, Cook JB, Rowles DJ, Bottoni CR, Shaha SH, Tokish JM. Clinical validation of the glenoid track concept in anterior glenohumeral instability. J Bone Joint Surg Am. 2016;98(22):1918–23.
55. Shaha JS, Cook JB, Song DJ, Rowles DJ, Bottoni CR, Shaha SH, et al. Redefining "critical" bone loss in shoulder instability: functional outcomes worsen with "subcritical" bone loss. Am J Sports Med. 2015;43(7):1719–25.
56. Shin SJ, Kim RG, Jeon YS, Kwon TH. Critical value of anterior glenoid bone loss that leads to recurrent glenohumeral instability after arthroscopic Bankart repair. Am J Sports Med. 2017;45(9):1975–81.
57. Yamamoto N, Kawakami J, Hatta T, Itoi E. Effect of subcritical glenoid bone loss on activities of daily living in patients with anterior shoulder instability. Orthop Traumatol Surg Res. 2019;105(8):1467–70.
58. Yamamoto N, Shinagawa K, Hatta T, Itoi E. Peripheral-track and central-track Hill-Sachs lesions: a new concept of assessing an on-track lesion. Am J Sports Med. 2020;48(1):33–8.
59. Li RT, Kane G, Drummond M, Golan E, Wilson K, Lesniak BP, et al. On-track lesions with a small distance to dislocation are associated with failure after arthroscopic anterior shoulder stabilization. J Bone Joint Surg Am. 2021;103(11):961–7.
60. Mirzayan R, Itoi E, Karpyshyn J, Wong IH, Giacomo GD. Controversies in surgical management of anterior shoulder instability. J ISAKOS. 2023;9(2):168–83.
61. Lin A, Barrow AE, Charles S, et al. Remplissage reduces recurrent instability in high-risk patients with on-track Hill-Sachs lesions. J Shoulder Elbow Surg. 2023;32(6S):S99–S105.
62. Liu JN, Gowd AK, Garcia GH, Cvetanovich GL, Cabarcas BC, Verma NN. Recurrence rate of instability after remplissage for treatment of traumatic anterior shoulder instability: a systematic review in treatment of subcritical glenoid bone loss. Arthroscopy. 2018;34(10):2894–907.e2.
63. Balg F, Boileau P. The instability severity index score. A simple pre-operative score to select patients for arthroscopic or open shoulder stabilisation. J Bone Joint Surg Br. 2007;89(11):1470–7.
64. Thomazeau H, Courage O, Barth J, Pelegri C, Charousset C, Lespagnol F, et al. Can we improve the indication for Bankart arthroscopic repair? A preliminary clinical study using the ISIS score. Orthop Traumatol Surg Res. 2010;96(8 Suppl):S77–83.
65. Boughebri O, Maqdes A, Moraiti C, Dib C, Leclère FM, Valenti P. Results of 45 arthroscopic Bankart procedures: does the ISIS remain a reliable prognostic assessment after 5 years? Eur J Orthop Surg Traumatol. 2015;25(4):709–16. https://doi.org/10.1007/s00590-014-1562-.
66. Phadnis J, Arnold C, Elmorsy A, Flannery M. Utility of the instability severity index score in predicting failure after arthroscopic anterior stabilization of the shoulder. Am J Sports Med. 2015;43(8):1983–8.
67. Di Giacomo G, Peebles LA, Pugliese M, Dekker TJ, Golijanin P, Sanchez A, et al. Glenoid track instability management score: radiographic modification of the instability severity index score. Arthroscopy. 2020;36(1):56–67.
68. Leroux T, Bhatti A, Khoshbin A, Wasserstein D, Henry P, Marks P, et al. Combined arthroscopic Bankart repair and remplissage for recurrent shoulder instability. Arthroscopy. 2013;29(10):1693–701.
69. Maiotti M, Massoni C, Russo R, Schroter S, Zanini A, Bianchedi D. Arthroscopic subscapularis augmen-

tation of Bankart repair in chronic anterior shoulder instability with bone loss less than 25% and capsular deficiency: clinical multicenter study. Arthroscopy. 2017;33(5):902–9.
70. Maiotti M, Russo R, Zanini A, Castricini R, Castellarin G, Schröter S, et al. Bankart repair with subscapularis augmentation in athletes with shoulder hyperlaxity. Arthroscopy. 2021;37(7):2055–62.
71. Malahias MA, Chytas D, Raoulis V, Chronopoulos E, Brila-kis E, Antonogiannakis E. Iliac crest bone grafting for the management of anterior shoulder instability in patients with glenoid bone loss: a systematic review of contemporary literature. Sports Med Open. 2020;6(1):12.
72. Anderl W, Pauzenberger L, Laky B, Kriegleder B, Heuberer PR. Arthroscopic implant-free bone grafting for shoulder instability with glenoid bone loss. Am J Sports Med. 2016;44(5):1137–45.
73. Yang JC, Mehran N, Mazzocca AD, Pearl ML, Chen VC-H, Arciero RA. Remplissage versus modified Latarjet for off-track Hill-Sachs lesions with subcritical glenoid bone loss. Am J Sports Med. 2017;46(8):1885–91.
74. Brandariz RN, Gorodischer TD, Pasqualini I, Rossi LA, Tanoira I, Ranalletta M. The Latarjet procedure without remplissage is effective to restore stability in athletes with glenoid bone defects greater than 25% and off-track Hill-Sachs lesions. Arthroscopy. 2021;37(8):2455–61.
75. Russo R, Maiotti M, Taverna E. Arthroscopic bone graft procedure combined with arthroscopic subscapularis augmentation (ASA) for recurrent anterior instability with glenoid bone defect: a cadaver study. J Exp Orthop. 2018;5:5.
76. Russo A, Grasso A, Arrighi A, Pistorio A, Molfetta L. Accuracy of coracoid bone graft placement: open versus arthroscopic Latarjet. Joints. 2017;5(2):85–8.
77. Hurley ET, Jamal MS, Ali ZS, Montgomery C, Pauzenberger L, Mullett H. Long-term outcomes of the Latarjet procedure for anterior shoulder instability: a systematic review of studies at 10-year follow-up. J Shoulder Elbow Surg. 2019;28(2):e33–9.
78. Gupta A, Delaney R, Petkin K, Lafosse L. Complications of the Latarjet procedure. Curr Rev Musculoskeletal Med. 2015;8(1):59–66.
79. Rossi LA, Gorodischer T, Brandariz R, Tanoira I, Pasqualini I, Ranalletta M. High rate of return to sports and low recurrences with the Latarjet procedure in high-risk competitive athletes with glenohumeral instability and a glenoid bone loss <20%. Arthrosc Sports Med Rehabil. 2020;2(6):e735–42.
80. Joshi MA, Young AA, Balestro JC, Walch G. The Latarjet-Patte procedure for recurrent anterior shoulder instability in contact athletes. Orthop Clin North Am. 2015;46(1):105–11.
81. Burkhart SS, De Beer JF. Traumatic glenohumeral bone defects and their relationship to failure of arthroscopic Bankart repairs. Arthroscopy. 2000;16(7):677–94.
82. Trivedi S, Pomerantz ML, Gross D, Golijanan P, Provencher MT. Shoulder instability in the setting of bipolar (glenoid and humeral head) bone loss: the glenoid track concept. Clin Orthop Relat Res. 2014;472(8):2352–62.
83. Callegari JJ, McGarry M, Crook L, Adamson NA, Fraipont GM, Provencher M, et al. The addition of remplissage to free bone block restores translation and stiffness compared to bone block alone or Latarjet in a bipolar bone loss model. Arthroscopy. 2022;38(9):2609–17.
84. Calvo E, Delgado C. Management of off-track Hill-Sachs lesions in anterior glenohumeral instability. J Exp Orthop. 2023;10(1):30.
85. Katthagen JC, Anavian J, Tahal DS, Millett PJ. Arthroscopic remplissage and open Latarjet procedure for the treatment of anterior glenohumeral instability with severe bipolar bone loss. Arthrosc Tech. 2016;5(5):e1135–41.
86. Saliken D, Lavoué V, Trojani C, Gonzalez JF, Boileau P. Combined all-arthroscopic Hill-Sachs Remplissage, Latarjet, and Bankart repair in patients with bipolar glenohumeral bone loss. Arthrosc Tech. 2017;6(5):e2031–7.
87. Provencher MT, Frank RM, Golijanin P, et al. Distal tibia allograft glenoid reconstruction in recurrent anterior shoulder instability: clinical and radiographic outcomes. Arthroscopy. 2017;33(5):891–7.
88. Villatte G, Spurr S, Broden C, Martins A, Emery R, Reilly P. The Eden-Hybbinette procedure is one hundred years old! A historical view of the concept and its evolutions. Int Orthop. 2018;42(10):2491–5.
89. Tytherleigh-Strong GM, Morrissey DI. Failed Latarjet procedure treated with a revision bone block stabilization using a suture-button fixation. J Shoulder Elb Surg. 2017;26(4):e102–7.
90. Merrill CA, Arciero R. Open Bankart repair: a reproducible technique. Oper Tech Sports Med. 2019;27(1):42–8.
91. Gilat R, Haunschild ED, Lavoie-Gagne OZ, Tauro TM, Knapik DM, Fu MC, et al. Outcomes of the Latarjet procedure versus free bone block procedures for anterior shoulder instability: a systematic review and meta-analysis. Am J Sports Med. 2020;49(3):805–16.
92. Moroder P, Schulz E, Wierer G, Auffarth A, Habermeyer P, Resch H, et al. Neer award 2019: Latarjet procedure vs. iliac crest bone graft transfer for treatment of anterior shoulder instability with glenoid bone loss: a prospective randomized trial. J Shoulder Elbow Surg. 2019;28(7):1298–307.
93. Haroun HK, Sobhy MH, Abdelrahman AA. Arthroscopic Bankart repair with remplissage versus Latarjet procedure for management of engaging Hill-Sachs lesions with subcritical glenoid bone loss in traumatic anterior shoulder instability: a systematic review and meta-analysis. J Shoulder Elbow Surg. 2020;29(10):2163–74.
94. Taverna E, D'Ambrosi R, Perfetti C, Garavaglia G. Arthroscopic bone graft procedure for anterior inferior glenohumeral instability. Arthrosc Tech. 2014;3(6):e653–60.

Bankart-Remplissage

2

Tammy R. Hoffman, Lisa A. Galasso,
Matthew B. Noble, Pablo A. Narbona,
and Patrick J. Denard

2.1 Introduction

Anterior shoulder dislocations represent the most common form of glenohumeral instability, comprising up to 97% of shoulder dislocations [1]. Dislocation often occurs when forceful contact is made while the shoulder is externally rotated and abducted [2]. The mechanism of anterior shoulder dislocation leads to tearing of anteroinferior labral tissue known as a Bankart lesion, stretching or tearing of the capsule, and possibly bipolar bony injury from impaction of the humeral head on the glenoid rim. This defect on the posterolateral humeral head is referred to as a Hill-Sachs lesion (HSL).

Certain activities and patient characteristics place an individual at increased risk for shoulder instability, as previously described by Balg and Boileau [3]. Sports that require repetitive overhead movements (e.g., baseball, volleyball, basketball, and swimming) place additional stress and laxity on the joint leading to significant microtrauma over time [4]. Further, contact sports such as rugby and football increase the risk of a traumatic dislocation [3, 4]. A prospective analysis of individuals attending the United States Military Academy reported a rate of 15.4% in dislocation events and an average of 84.6% subluxations, with 43.6% of instability events being a result of contact injuries [5].

Individuals whose first dislocation occurs at a younger age are more likely to experience recurrent instability. A 25-year follow-up study of patients with anterior shoulder instability managed with nonsurgical intervention reported a recurrence rate of 72% in patients between the ages of 12–22 years, 56% in patients between 23 and 29 years, and 27% in patients 30 years or older [6].

Remplissage was first described in 2008 by Purchase et al. as an adjustment to the Connolly procedure [7]. As the French term "remplissage" translates to "filling," this technique aims to prevent engagement of an off-track lesion as well as providing posterior restraint in the setting of anterior translation. Supplementing the Bankart repair with remplissage, thus performing a Bankart-remplissage, serves to address the anatomical risks of recurrent instability following operative intervention. This chapter reviews the background anatomy, indications, surgical technique, and clinical outcomes for Bankart-remplissage.

T. R. Hoffman · L. A. Galasso · M. B. Noble · P. J. Denard (✉)
Oregon Shoulder Institute, Medford, OR, USA

P. A. Narbona
Department of Shoulder Surgery, Arthoscopy of Sanatorio Allende, Córdoba, Argentina

E. Calvo et al. (eds.), *Complex and Revision Problems in Shoulder Instability*,
https://doi.org/10.1007/978-3-031-81389-4_2

2.2 Background

In the United States, Bankart repair in isolation has historically been the standard for addressing anterior shoulder instability; however, recurrent instability rates range from 9.4% to 35.5% [8–12]. Burkhart and De Beer first called attention to glenoid bone loss and engaging HSLs as risk factors for recurrence after isolated arthroscopic Bankart repair [9]. Subsequently, the glenoid track concept was developed to quantify the bipolar bone loss relationship and guidelines emerged for considering remplissage with off-track HSLs. A full description of the glenoid track concept is described in detail in the previous chapter. An off-track lesion has been clinically shown to have a high risk of recurrence with arthroscopic Bankart repair in isolation [13]. While the glenoid track concept is a useful technique for conceptualizing bipolar bone loss and quantifying higher risk, it has several limitations. First, it does not account for patient characteristics such as soft tissue laxity or patient activity. Second, it assumes a perfect surgical technique. Each of these factors contribute to what is an unacceptably high recurrence rate of isolated Bankart repair in many patients with on-track and near-track lesions. Within the past decade, the surgical techniques for remplissage have improved, resulting in many surgeons adding remplissage to Bankart repairs for patients with on-track and near-track lesions with encouraging early outcomes.

2.3 Anatomy

When anterior shoulder instability occurs, there is often impaction of the humeral head on the anterior glenoid resulting in soft tissue injury at the anteroinferior labral rim involving the labrum and capsular tissue [14], otherwise known as a Bankart lesion. At times the Bankart lesion may include a portion of the glenoid bone that has avulsed, at which point it is referred to as a bony Bankart lesion [14]. The impaction of the humeral head on the glenoid rim creates a defect in the posterolateral humeral head referred to as the HSL. The size of the HSL often increases with recurrent dislocations when the soft, cancellous bone of the posterolateral humeral head engages on the hard, cortical bone of the anterior glenoid rim. Subsequent dislocations can also wear away the glenoid rim creating further damage to the anterior labrum and capsular tissue, compounding the risk for recurrence [15]. An example of a Bankart tear and a large HSL is seen in Fig. 2.1. Due to this process, we know that even patients with on-track or near-track lesions, but with con-

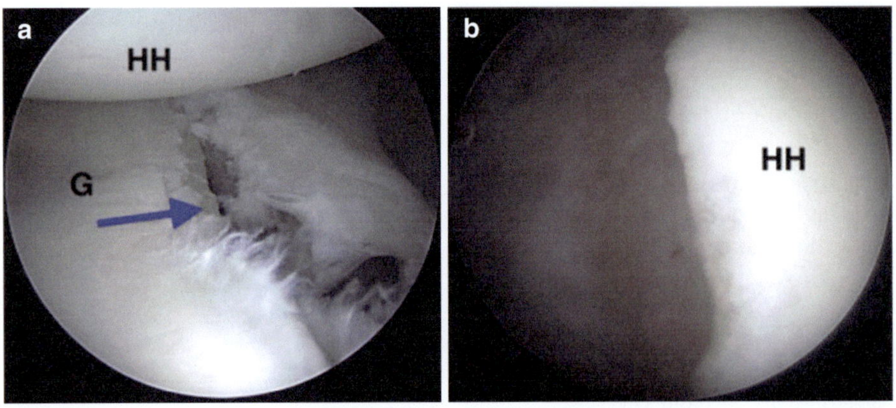

Fig. 2.1 Arthroscopic view of a left shoulder from the posterior viewing portal with the patient in lateral decubitus position. (**a**) Arrow pointing to a Bankart tear. (**b**) Large Hill-Sachs lesion (*G* glenoid, *HH* humeral head). (Reprinted from Arthroscopy Techniques, Volume 10, Authors: Jonathan J. Callegari, DO; Cameron J. Phillips, MD; Patrick J. Denard MD, All-Inside Knotless Remplissage Technique, Pages E1479-E1484, Copyright (2021), with permission from Elsevier)

current capsuloligamentous laxity, are at high risk for recurrent instability [15].

A solution to this is the utilization of the remplissage technique. Historically, remplissage was described as a capsulotenodesis of the infraspinatus tendon alone [7, 16]. Previous cadaveric studies have shown that modern-day remplissage techniques result in the capsulomyodesis of the infraspinatus and teres minor rather than capsulotenodesis of the infraspinatus alone [17]. This alteration in the anatomy of the posterior rotator cuff not only fills the bony defect but also adds a posterior restraint to a shoulder which naturally wants to translate anteriorly. The addition of remplissage was found to increase the amount of force necessary to cause anterior translation of the humeral head by providing posterior restraint [18]. Additionally, another biomechanical study by Yoshida et al. demonstrated the decreased force necessary for subsequent dislocation, suggesting that early operative intervention for high-risk patients may be warranted [19]. However, the nonanatomical changes have raised concern such as loss of external rotation and the risk of long-term arthritis.

2.4 Indications

Original indications for arthroscopic Bankart-remplissage were an engaging HSL and associated glenoid bone loss less than 25% in patients who were suffering from recurrent anterior shoulder instability [20]. A systematic review supported this, noting agreement across multiple clinical studies, concluding that the presence of a HSL with <25% glenoid bone loss was an indication for arthroscopic Bankart-remplissage [21]. However, interpretation of this criteria is at risk for variations as HSL engagement is based on contact with the glenoid when the shoulder is positioned in 90° abduction and 90° external rotation at the time of arthroscopy, where laxity may be influenced by the effects of anesthesia [22]. In response to this, the glenoid track concept (Fig. 2.2) was developed to quantify the

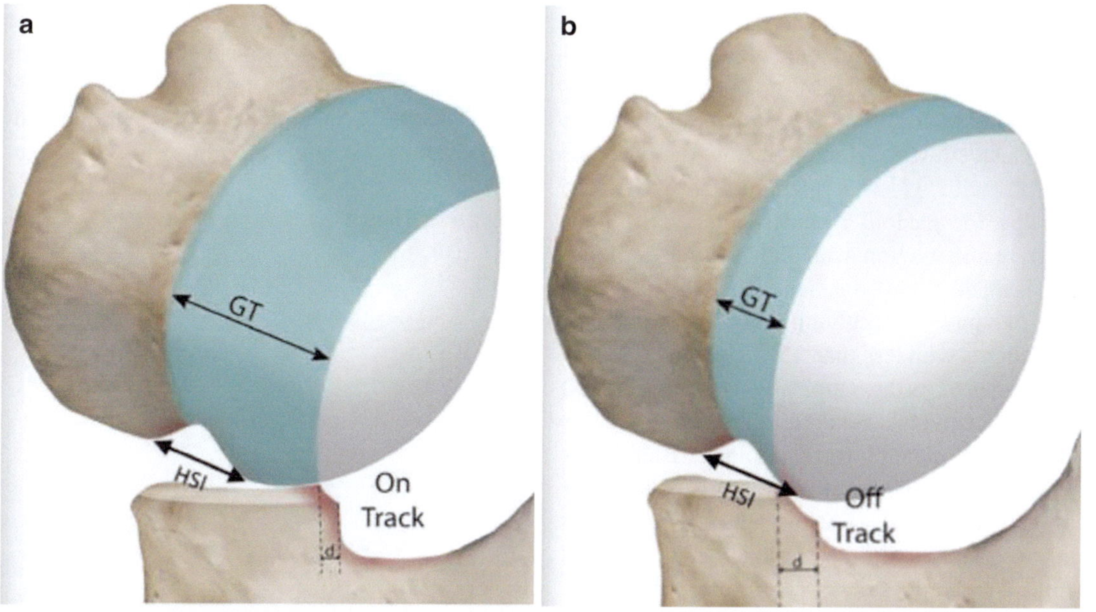

Fig. 2.2 (**a**) An on-track (non-engaging) Hill-Sachs lesion has the glenoid track (GT) width larger than the Hill-Sachs interval (HSI). (**b**) Since glenoid bone loss (d) is larger in the off-track scenario, the GT width is now smaller than the HSI allowing engagement. (Reprinted from Operative Techniques in Sports Medicine, Volume 27, Authors: Robert U. Hartzler, MD, MS; Patrick J. Denard MD, The Glenoid Track and How It Can Guide Management, Pages 12–17, Copyright (2019), with permission from Elsevier)

bipolar bone loss relationship and guidelines emerged for considering remplissage with off-track HSLs. Hartzler et al. supported the glenoid track concept for incorporation of remplissage in a bipolar bone loss biomechanical model. They found that isolated Bankart repair restored stability in on-track lesions, but for off-track lesions remplissage was required. Supplementing the Bankart repair with remplissage prevented HSL engagement in 100% of cadaveric specimens, whereas Bankart repair alone was able to prevent engagement only in up to 67% of specimens at mid-range rotation and 0% of specimens at the end-of-range of rotation [18].

As surgical techniques have improved, the indications for remplissage have expanded to include cases of patients with on-track HSLs and a high potential for recurrence [23, 24]. In fact, there is consideration for the addition of remplissage to Bankart repair in nearly all patients with subcritical bone loss due to decreased risk for recurrent instability when compared to isolated Bankart repair, with a low complication rate [18, 19]. The senior author's primary decision making for the addition of remplissage is based on patient characteristics (age and activity level), and glenoid bone loss more than the glenoid track paradigm described by Di Giacomo et al. [20]. Nearly all patients with 25% or greater glenoid bone loss are managed with glenoid reconstruction. For patients with 15–25% glenoid bone loss, the decision for glenoid reconstruction versus soft tissue reconstruction with Bankart and remplissage is made based on patient characteristics with high-risk patients receiving bony reconstruction. All patients with less than 15% glenoid bone loss are managed arthroscopically with nearly all patients receiving a Bankart remplissage, regardless of the glenoid track. Isolated Bankart is reserved primarily for first-time dislocations in low-risk individuals (i.e., over the age of 25). As our experience with remplissage has grown and surgical techniques have been refined, the indications for remplissage have broadened to include patients with borderline off-track lesions or patients with a high risk of recurrence despite having on-track lesions [25]. Further, there are rare cases in which large amounts of bipolar bone loss are observed, in which remplissage may be considered in addition to glenoid reconstruction. For instance, a biomechanical study performed by Callegari et al. demonstrated that remplissage with a free bone block resulted in improved translation and stiffness closer to the intact glenohumeral joint state compared with the bone block alone [25].

2.5 Surgical Technique

The author's preferred technique is performed in lateral decubitus position with the operative arm placed in a sterile arm holder. A low posterior portal is created parallel to the glenoid and a diagnostic examination is performed. Standard portals for instability repair are established utilizing working cannula, consisting of an anterior portal just above the subscapularis tendon, as well as an anterosuperolateral (ASL) portal (Fig. 2.3). Time is taken to carefully plan our anterior working portals with a spinal needle to ensure our angle of approach is appropriate. The anterior portal enters just above the subscapularis tendon and typically angles superior so that the cannula can be used to push the subscapularis down and obtain access to the inferior glenoid rim. The ASL portal enters the joint over the mid-biceps with a 45° angle of approach to the supe-

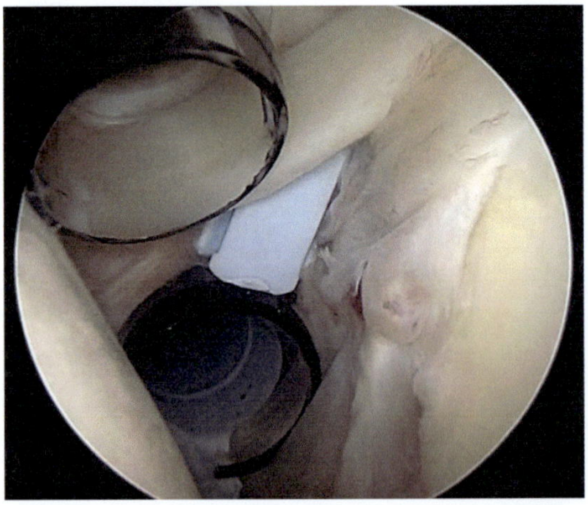

Fig. 2.3 Arthroscopic view from the posterior viewing portal demonstrating the placement of the ASL portal (superior) and anterior portal (inferior)

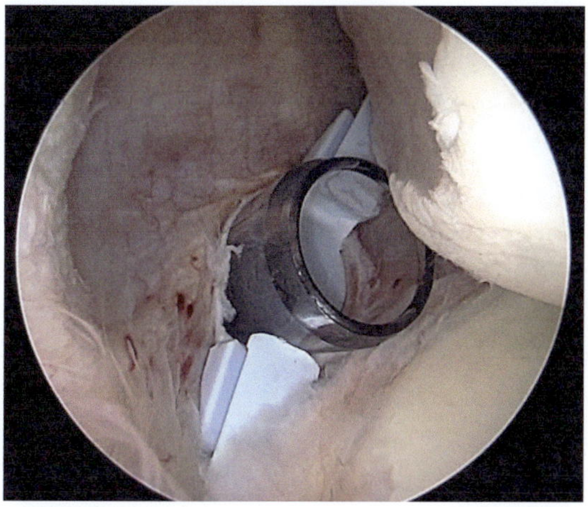

Fig. 2.4 Posterior working portal and cannula placement while viewing from the ASL portal. Noted HSL of the posterior humeral head

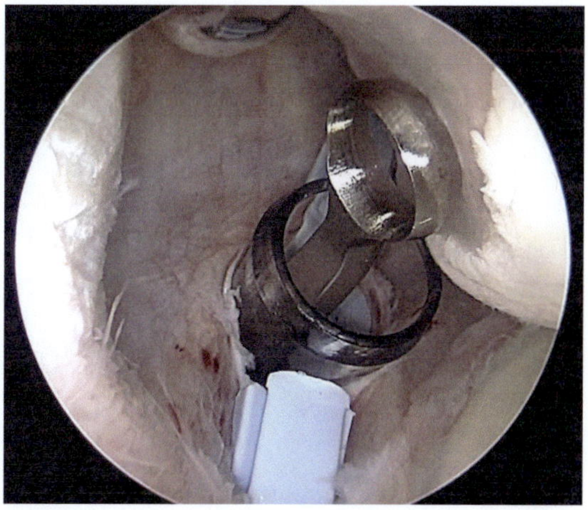

Fig. 2.5 HSL prep with ring curette through the posterior portal

rior glenoid. Once the presence of a Bankart lesions and HSL are identified, the arthroscope is moved to the anterosuperolateral portal to obtain an en-face view of the lesions. A posterior cannula is placed at the previously established posterior portal (Fig. 2.4). Glenoid bone loss and the HSL width are estimated with a calibrated probe. A dynamic examination can also be performed while visualizing through this portal.

Following diagnostic arthroscopic exam, the HSL is prepared for anchors to be placed for remplissage. The humeral head defect is prepared with an angled ring curette through the posterior cannula (Fig. 2.5). Next, a spinal needle is used to triangulate the center of the HSL defect. Care is taken to enter perpendicular to the HLS with the arm in neutral rotation to avoid over- or under tension on the posterior tissue. Next, a switching stick is inserted until it can be seen to indent the capsule without advancing through (Fig. 2.6). An additional 7 mm threaded cannula is then inserted, taking care to not allow penetration of the capsule. This maneuver places the cannula through the posterior deltoid down to the posterior capsule and tendon (Fig. 2.7), which is then rotated to clear the subacromial space. This will allow for knotless fixation of the remplissage without having to enter the subacromial space.

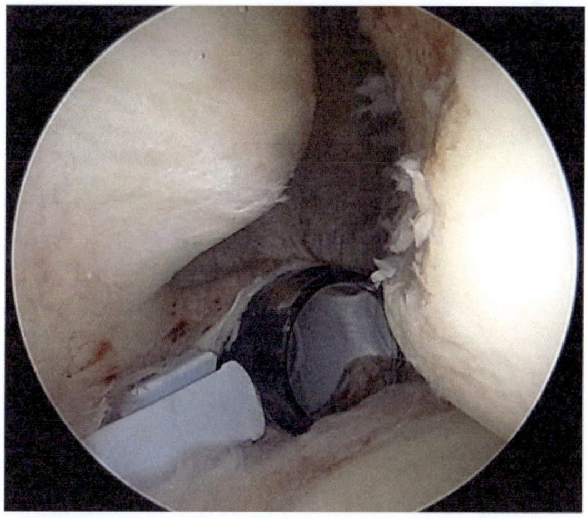

Fig. 2.6 While viewing from the ASL portal a switching stick (seen indenting the posterior capsule) is used to clear off posterior capsule prior to placement of second posterior cannula

Next, the remplissage is performed with a knotless anchor technique. One superior and one inferior anchor are placed through the cannula. A guide is placed within the cannula and a knotless 1.8 mm knotless anchor is passed through the capsule (1.8 mm Knotless FiberTak; Arthrex Inc. Naples, FL). Arm rotation be adjusted prior to advancement through the capsule to apply the correct amount of tension. First, the inferior remplissage anchor is placed

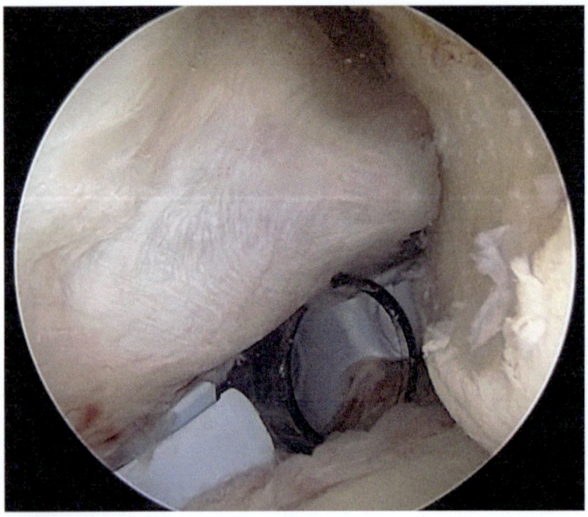

Fig. 2.7 While making sure not to penetrate the posterior capsule with the cannula, the first Fibertak anchor is placed into inferior aspect of HSL

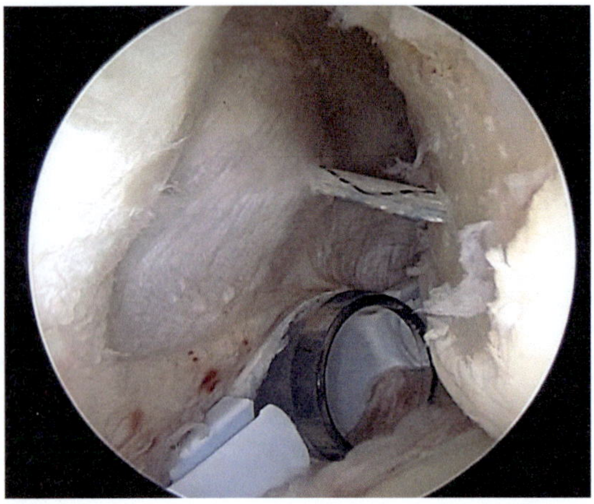

Fig. 2.8 First Fibertak anchor placed into inferior aspect of HSL

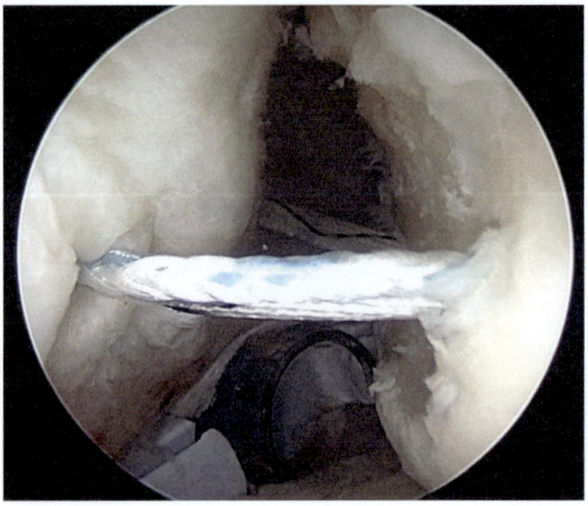

Fig. 2.9 Both Fibertak anchors are placed within the HSL noting separate entry points through the posterior capsule

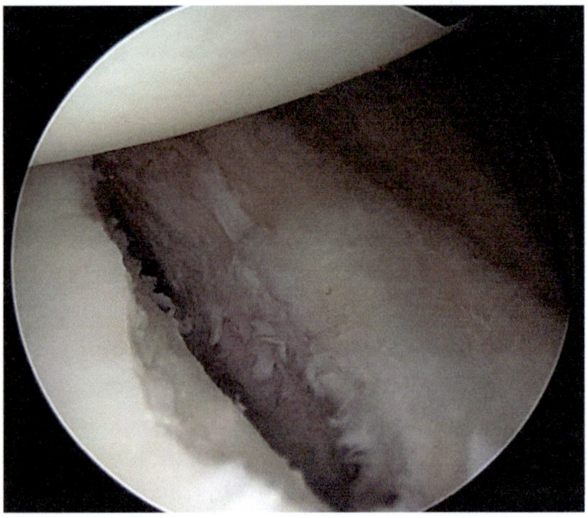

Fig. 2.10 Bankart lesion and completed preparation of anterior glenoid rim

at the more inferior aspect of the defect (Fig. 2.8). This is because once the superior remplissage anchor is placed, it restricts visualization of inferior anchor placement. While the cannula remains superficial to the capsule, the guide is retracted and reinserted more superiorly at the top of the defect (Fig. 2.9). While both anchors have been passed through the capsule, they are not linked at this time as this would function to close the glenohumeral joint down and risks limiting visualization of the Bankart repair. To assist with proper identification later, a hemostat is applied to the sutures.

Following this, attention is brought to the Bankart repair. The labrum is prepared in standard fashion (Fig. 2.10) and a knotless technique (using 3–4 1.8 mm Knotless FiberTak anchors; Arthrex) is utilized to place the anchors from inferior to superior. A large bump is used with an assistant pushing it into the patient's axilla to help provide some joint distraction (Fig. 2.11). A curved guide may be used as needed to place the inferior anchors through the anterior portal. A mattress configuration is preferred for these sutures.

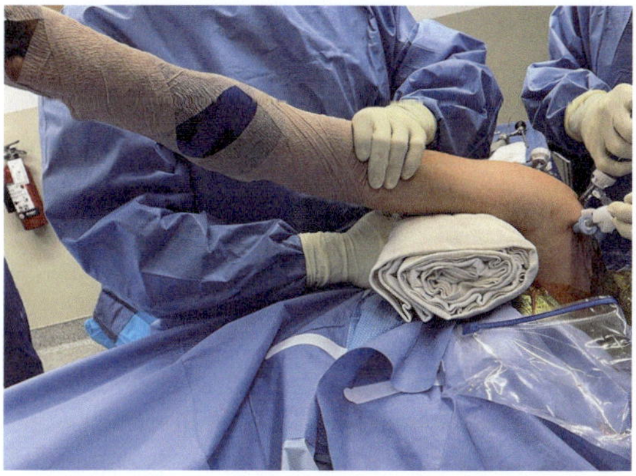

Fig. 2.11 A large bump is used with an assistant pushing it into the patient's axilla while simultaneously pulling traction on arm to help provide some joint distraction

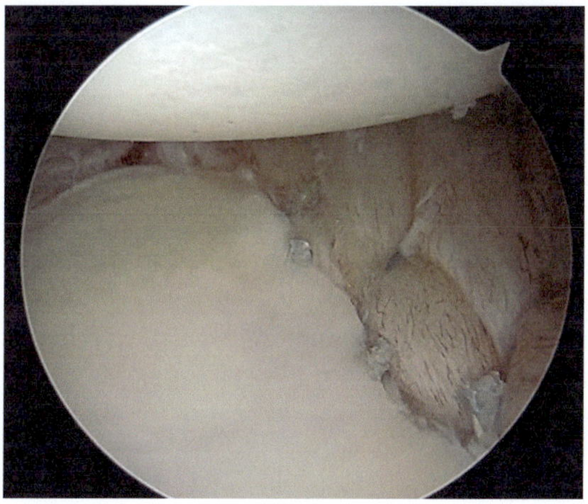

Fig. 2.12 Final Bankart repair

Once Bankart repair is completed (Fig. 2.12), the remplissage anchors are linked to complete the remplissage with a knotless double-mattress suture configuration. The inferior anchor repair suture is shuttled into the body of the superior anchor and vice versa. The sutures are then tightened until the posterior capsule and tendon are compressed into the HSL defect and cut with a closed knot cutter, completing the Bankart-remplissage (Fig. 2.13).

Patients are then placed in a sling with abduction pillow for 6 weeks. For the first 6 weeks patients will focus on exercises of hand, wrist, and elbow with the arm at their side. We also encourage isometric scapular retraction exercises during the period. Patients will begin ROM and strengthening at 6 weeks postoperatively. ROM should be focused on passive elevation and external rotation (ER). Our goal for ER is half that of the opposite arm until 12 weeks postoperative. At 3 months postoperatively, patients may return to the gym with avoidance of activities requiring rapid acceleration such as throwing. Patients may return to contact sports at 6 months after surgery.

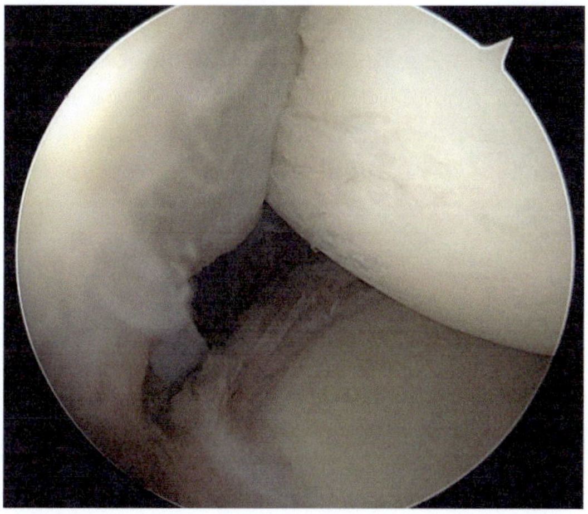

Fig. 2.13 Completed remplissage after final tightening

2.6 Outcomes

In the appropriate patient, outcomes for Bankart-remplissage are good, consisting of low complication rate, decreased recurrent instability, promising healing rates, return to sport, and acceptable short- to mid-term outcomes.

Studies comparing Bankart-remplissage and Latarjet report increased risk of postoperative complications (e.g., fibrotic unions, impingement of screws, development of osteoarthritis, and suprascapular nerve irritation) with the latter [26–29]. A systematic review of 185 open Latarjet patients and 194 remplissage patients performed by Hurley et al. supports these findings, reporting a postoperative complication rate of 8.6% following Latarjet (complications consisting of deep wound infection, painful/loose hardware, malunion, nonunion, suprascapular nerve palsy, and postoperative stiffness), and 0.5% following Bankart-remplissage (consisting of deep wound infection) [26]. Lastly, a multicenter retrospective analysis of 258 patients at a minimum 2-year follow-up determined rate of complication was found to be 5.9% in primary Latarjet, and 0% in primary Bankart-remplissage [29]. Overall, the data supports less risk of postoperative complications with Bankart-remplissage; however, one of the main considerations lies within the risk of recurrent shoulder instability.

Regarding the comparison of failure rates, those following isolated Bankart repair vary from 9.4% to 35.3%, whereas the failure rates following Bankart-remplissage are reported as low as 4% [8, 11, 12, 15, 21, 30]. In a series of patients with less than 15% glenoid bone loss, Horinek et al. reported a lower rate of recurrence with the addition of remplissage (2.1% vs. 9.3%); however, the differences did not meet statistical significance [29]. Lin et al. performed a multicenter retrospective analysis of patients with on-track HSLs who underwent arthroscopic repair versus repair with remplissage [31]. They reported 11% rate of recurrent dislocation in the former group, and a 1.8% rate of recurrence in the group of patients who underwent repair with remplissage. Another study reported recurrence of shoulder dislocation following Bankart-remplissage as 5% at the 26-month follow-up point, compared with a 30% recurrence rate following individuals who underwent Bankart repair alone [32]. Additional support is provided by Hughes et al. who performed a Level III cohort study on individuals who underwent Bankart repair and Bankart repair with remplissage, and reported 47% recurrent instability with the former group, and 13% in the latter group [10].

While some studies have reported a loss of ER following Bankart-remplissage, ranging from 8° to 14° [8, 32–34], the average loss in ER averages at 11° with the Latarjet and 14° with an isolated Bankart repair [32, 34]. Further, Hurley et al. performed a systematic review and concluded that there were no statistically significant losses in ROM between individuals who underwent each of these three procedures [26]. A recent systematic review and meta-analysis performed by Gonzales-Morgado et al. compared ER loss between patient's who underwent Bankart repair, Bankart with remplissage, and Latarjet [35]. They found no statistically significant ER loss between groups, a lower rate of recurrent instability with Bankart-remplissage, and an increased incidence of complications within the Latarjet group. Additional studies have also reported that the ER loss which was found was not significant enough to affect quality of life or ability to return to preoperative activities [8, 21].

When evaluating healing of remplissage, previous studies utilizing CT or MRI to assess capsulotenodesis healing demonstrated an 85–100% healing rate at the 2-to-3-year follow-up [8, 21, 36]. On the shorter term, Ko et al. reported a 91.7% healing rate at 6-month clinical follow-up [32]. Magnetic resonance imaging used by Randelli et al. following remplissage at the 3-year follow-up point demonstrated minimal fatty infiltration of the infraspinatus and overall satisfactory healing of the repair [36]. This finding is promising as it demonstrates positive tissue response, supporting the safety of remplissage regarding the lack of potential for long-term pathological changes in the structures involved.

Regarding returning to sport, a large-scale retrospective study comparing primary Bankart-remplissage and primary Latarjet reported a 91.5% return to contact sport rate following Bankart-remplissage, and 72.7% following Latarjet. Additional analysis of their data demonstrated a 65.5% return to throwing sports [29]. A retrospective study from 2007 to 2017 analyzed a total of 70 patients found that 100% of patients who underwent Bankart-remplissage were able to return to their sports at any level of performance compared to 84.2% for those who underwent isolated Bankart repair [37]. Further, this same study reported that 77.8% of Bankart-remplissage patients were able to return to their previous level of performance compared to 50% for those who underwent Bankart repair alone. Merrola et al. specifically reported an ability to return to preoperative sports, with their study including professional and contact athletes [33]. In terms of patient satisfaction following Bankart-remplissage, Garcia et al. performed a retrospective case series on patients with off-track HSLs and reported a 90% satisfaction rate, with 70% of patients reporting that the procedure improved their overall quality of life at an average of 60.7 months follow-up [38].

There remains concern regarding the long-term impact of remplissage as it is not yet well-defined. A theoretical concern is that tightening the posterior soft tissue may lead to the development of arthritis as has been reported for open Bankart repair by Fabre et al. in a 26-year follow-up of open Bankart repair [39]. Nonetheless, a handful of mid-term studies have been performed on Bankart-remplissage. At the 5-year postoperative point, there was 16% rate of failure (recurrent shoulder instability), with minimal development of osteoarthritis [40]. Univariate analysis of this data revealed that those who experienced recurrent instability had deeper HSLs and were younger than their average population. Further along, Brilakis et al. reported a 5.6% incidence of recurrent dislocation at the 8-year follow-up point. Their study also indicated 94.4% satisfaction, 71% of maintained sport involvement following the operation, and insignificant losses in postoperative motion, indicating that the Bankart-remplissage is a safe and effective treatment option for treating HSLs [41]. In contrast, a 10-year follow-up study including 79 patients compared functional outcomes of patients who underwent Bankart repair in isolation versus patients who underwent Bankart-remplissage reported significantly improved outcomes in terms of mobility and stability in the latter group [42]. Specifically, the average Rowe score improved from 54.3 to 83.8, with no shoulder instability recurrence and no apprehension on physical exam in any of their Bankart-remplissage patients. In addition, this study concluded that the issues reported in studies investigating Bankart-remplissage outcomes at the shorter-term follow-up seem to be not present at the 10-year point [42].

2.7 Conclusion

Bankart-remplissage has been associated with a reduction in recurrent instability when compared to the Bankart repair in isolation. Stability is achieved through preventing engagement of an off-track HSL with the glenoid rim. Additional resistance to anterior translation of the humeral head is obtained via the tightening of the posterior soft tissue. Patients with less than 25% glenoid bone loss should be considered for Bankart-remplissage. Additional patient characteristics including HSL size, age, number of dislocations, sport, and previous surgery should also be considered when choosing the appropriate surgical plan. A thorough discussion of expected outcomes including rate of recurrent instability, healing, return to sport, and loss of ER should be held with every patient. Patients should also be informed currently, there are studies which report mid-term outcomes, but there remain limitations in understanding the longer-term outcomes of Bankart-remplissage. This poses a need for additional studies focused on outcomes resulting from the anatomic alterations induced by the procedure. Further, the use of the track model in operative planning focuses solely on bony anatomy and does not consider surrounding soft tissues or other factors that may place an individual at increased risk for recurrent instability.

Key Points

- Anterior shoulder dislocation leads to a Bankart lesion and a Hill Sachs lesion (HSL).
- With each repeated dislocation, the HSL continues to engage with the anterior glenoid rim, causing the HSL to enlarge, compounding the risk for additional dislocation events.
- When Bankart repair is supplemented with remplissage (Bankart-remplissage), it results in decreased risk of recurrent instability.

(continued)

- Although some independent studies have reported a loss in external rotation (ER) after Bankart-remplissage, systemic meta-analyses have indicated that this is not the case.
- Overall, Bankart-remplissage patients report an ability to return to their usual activities and a restoration of quality of life with low risk of recurrent instability and postoperative complications.

References

1. Abrams R. Shoulder dislocations overview. StatPearls; 2023. https://www.ncbi.nlm.nih.gov/books/NBK459125/. Accessed 24 Feb 2024.
2. Hughes JD, Vaswani R, Paras TM, Lin A. Treatment algorithm for recurrent anterior shoulder instability: putting it all together. Oper Tech Orthop. 2021;31:100862. https://doi.org/10.1016/j.oto.2021.100862.
3. Balg F, Boileau P. The instability severity index score. J Bone Joint Surg Br. 2007;89-B:1470–7. https://doi.org/10.1302/0301-620x.89b11.18962.
4. Alkaduhimi H, van der Linde JA, Willigenburg NW, et al. Redislocation risk after an arthroscopic Bankart procedure in collision athletes: a systematic review. J Shoulder Elb Surg. 2016;25:1549–58. https://doi.org/10.1016/j.jse.2016.05.002.
5. Owens BD, Duffey ML, Nelson BJ, et al. The incidence and characteristics of shoulder instability at the United States military academy. Am J Sports Med. 2007;35:1168–73. https://doi.org/10.1177/0363546506295179.
6. Hovelius L, Olofsson A, Sandström B, et al. Nonoperative treatment of primary anterior shoulder dislocation in patients forty years of age and younger. J Bone Joint Surg Am. 2008;90:945–52. https://doi.org/10.2106/jbjs.g.00070.
7. Connolly J. Humeral head defects associated with shoulder dislocation: their diagnostic and surgical significance. Instr Course Lect. 1972;2:210–8.
8. Boileau P, O'Shea K, Vargas P, et al. Anatomical and functional results after arthroscopic Hill-Sachs remplissage. J Bone Joint Surg. 2012;94:618–26. https://doi.org/10.2106/jbjs.k.00101.
9. Burkhart SS, De Beer JF. Traumatic glenohumeral bone defects and their relationship to failure of arthroscopic Bankart repairs. Arthroscopy. 2000;16:677–94. https://doi.org/10.1053/jars.2000.17715.
10. Hughes JL, Bastrom T, Pennock AT, Edmonds EW. Arthroscopic Bankart repairs with and without remplissage in recurrent adolescent anterior shoulder instability with Hill-Sachs deformity. Orthop J Sports Med. 2018;6:232596711881398. https://doi.org/10.1177/2325967118813981.
11. Liu JN, Gowd AK, Garcia GH, et al. Recurrence rate of instability after remplissage for treatment of traumatic anterior shoulder instability: a systematic review in treatment of subcritical glenoid bone loss. Arthroscopy. 2018;34(10):2894–2907.e2. https://doi.org/10.1016/j.arthro.2018.05.031.
12. Ono Y, Dávalos Herrera DA, Woodmass JM, et al. Long-term outcomes following isolated arthroscopic Bankart repair: a 9- to 12-year follow-up. JSES Open Access. 2019;3:189–93. https://doi.org/10.1016/j.jses.2019.05.002.
13. Boden SA, Charles S, Hughes JD, et al. Recurrent instability after arthroscopic Bankart repair in patients with hyperlaxity and near-track lesions. Orthop J Sports Med. 2023;11:23259671231200231. https://doi.org/10.1177/23259671231200231.
14. Bankart AS. The pathology and treatment of recurrent dislocation of the shoulder-joint. Br J Surg. 1938;26:23–9. https://doi.org/10.1002/bjs.18002610104.
15. Omi R, Hooke AW, Zhao KD, et al. The effect of the remplissage procedure on shoulder range of motion: a cadaveric study. Arthroscopy. 2014;30:178–87. https://doi.org/10.1016/j.arthro.2013.11.003.
16. Purchase RJ, Wolf EM, Hobgood ER, et al. Hill-Sachs "remplissage": an arthroscopic solution for the engaging Hill-Sachs lesion. Arthroscopy. 2008;24:723–6. https://doi.org/10.1016/j.arthro.2008.03.015.
17. Lädermann A, Arrigoni P, Barth J, et al. Is arthroscopic remplissage a tenodesis or capsulomyodesis? An anatomic study. Knee Surg Sports Traumatol Arthrosc. 2015;24:573–7. https://doi.org/10.1007/s00167-015-3756-8.
18. Hartzler RU, Bui CNH, Jeong WK, et al. Remplissage of an off-track Hill-Sachs lesion is necessary to restore biomechanical glenohumeral joint stability in a bipolar bone loss model. J Shoulder Elb Surg. 2016;25:e325. https://doi.org/10.1016/j.jse.2016.07.051.
19. Yoshida M, Takenaga T, Chan CK, et al. Altered shoulder kinematics using a new model for multiple dislocations-induced Bankart lesions. Clin Biomech. 2019;70:131–6. https://doi.org/10.1016/j.clinbiomech.2019.08.014.
20. Di Giacomo G, Itoi E, Burkhart SS. Evolving concept of bipolar bone loss and the Hill-Sachs lesion: from "engaging/non-engaging" lesion to "on-track/off-track" lesion. Arthroscopy. 2014;30:90–8. https://doi.org/10.1016/j.arthro.2013.10.004.
21. Buza JA, Iyengar JJ, Anakwenze OA, et al. Arthroscopic hill-sachs remplissage. J Bone Joint Surg. 2014;96:549–55. https://doi.org/10.2106/jbjs.l.01760.
22. Faber KJ, Homa K, Hawkins RJ. Translation of the glenohumeral joint in patients with anterior instability: awake ewamination versus examination with the patient under anesthesia. J Shoulder Elb Surg. 1999;8:320–3. https://doi.org/10.1016/s1058-2746(99)90153-2.

23. Horinek JL, Menendez ME, Callegari JJ, et al. Consideration may be given to lowering the threshold for the addition of remplissage in patients with subcritical glenoid bone loss undergoing arthroscopic Bankart repair. Arthrosc Sports Med Rehabil. 2022;4:e1283. https://doi.org/10.1016/j.asmr.2022.04.004.
24. Callegari JJ, McGarry M, Crook L, et al. The addition of remplissage to free bone block restores translation and stiffness compared to bone block alone or Latarjet in a bipolar bone loss model. Arthroscopy. 2022;38:2609–17. https://doi.org/10.1016/j.arthro.2022.03.018.
25. Callegari JJ, Phillips CJ, Denard PJ. All-inside knotless remplissage technique. Arthrosc Tech. 2021;10:e1479. https://doi.org/10.1016/j.eats.2021.02.014.
26. Hurley ET, Toale JP, Davey MS, et al. Remplissage for anterior shoulder instability with Hill-Sachs lesions: a systematic review and meta-analysis. J Shoulder Elb Surg. 2020;29:2487–94. https://doi.org/10.1016/j.jse.2020.06.021.
27. Haroun HK, Sobhy MH, Abdelrahman AA. Arthroscopic Bankart repair with remplissage versus Latarjet procedure for management of engaging Hill-Sachs lesions with subcritical glenoid bone loss in traumatic anterior shoulder instability: a systematic review and meta-analysis. J Shoulder Elb Surg. 2020;29:2163–74. https://doi.org/10.1016/j.jse.2020.04.032.
28. Cho NS, Yoo JH, Rhee YG. Management of an engaging Hill–Sachs lesion: arthroscopic remplissage with Bankart repair versus Latarjet procedure. Knee Surg Sports Traumatol Arthrosc. 2015;24:3793–800. https://doi.org/10.1007/s00167-015-3666-9.
29. Horinek JL, Menendez ME, Narbona P, et al. Remplissage yields similar 2-year outcomes, fewer complications, and low recurrence compared to Latarjet across a wide range of preoperative glenoid bone loss. Arthroscopy. 2022;38:2798–805. https://doi.org/10.1016/j.arthro.2022.03.031.
30. Martinez-Catalan N, Kazum E, Zampeli F, et al. Long-term outcomes of arthroscopic Bankart repair and Hill-Sachs remplissage for bipolar bone defects. Eur J Orthop Surg Traumatol. 2022;33:947–53. https://doi.org/10.1007/s00590-022-03237-8.
31. Lin A, Barrow AE, Charles S, et al. Remplissage reduces recurrent instability in high-risk patients with on-track Hill-Sachs lesions. J Shoulder Elb Surg. 2023;32:S99. https://doi.org/10.1016/j.jse.2023.02.011.
32. Ko S-H, Cha J-R, Lee C-C, et al. The influence of arthroscopic remplissage for engaging Hill-Sachs lesions combined with Bankart repair on redislocation and shoulder function compared with Bankart repair alone. Clin Orthop Surg. 2016;8:428. https://doi.org/10.4055/cios.2016.8.4.428.
33. Merolla G, Paladini P, Di Napoli G, et al. Outcomes of arthroscopic Hill-Sachs remplissage and anterior Bankart repair. Am J Sports Med. 2014;43:407–14. https://doi.org/10.1177/0363546514559706.
34. Lazarides AL, Duchman KR, Ledbetter L, et al. Arthroscopic remplissage for anterior shoulder instability: a systematic review of clinical and biomechanical studies. Arthroscopy. 2019;35:617–28. https://doi.org/10.1016/j.arthro.2018.09.029.
35. Gonzales-Morgado D, Ardebol J, et al. No difference in external rotation loss following isolated Bankart repair, Remplissage, or Latarjet. A systemic review and meta-analysis. Am J Sports Med 2025;53(2):493–500. https://doi.org/10.1177/03635465241241825. Epub 2025 Jan 11.
36. Randelli PS, Compagnoni R, Radaelli S, et al. Arthroscopic remplissage is safe and effective: clinical and magnetic resonance results at a minimum 3 years of follow-up. J Orthop Traumatol. 2022;23:5. https://doi.org/10.1186/s10195-021-00624-5.
37. Feng S, Chen M, Chen J, et al. Patient outcomes and fear of returning to sports after arthroscopic Bankart repair with remplissage. Orthop J Sports Med. 2021;9:232596712110017. https://doi.org/10.1177/23259671211001775.
38. Garcia GH, Wu H-H, Liu JN, et al. Outcomes of the remplissage procedure and its effects on return to sports. Am J Sports Med. 2016;44:1124–30. https://doi.org/10.1177/0363546515626199.
39. Fabre T, Abi-Chahla ML, Billaud A, et al. Long-term results with Bankart procedure: a 26-year follow-up study of 50 cases. J Shoulder Elb Surg. 2010;19:318–23. https://doi.org/10.1016/j.jse.2009.06.010.
40. Brejuin A, Girard M, Barret H, et al. Long-term results of arthroscopic Bankart repair with Hill-Sachs remplissage. JSES Int. 2022;6:723–9. https://doi.org/10.1016/j.jseint.2022.06.005.
41. Brilakis E, Avramidis G, Malahias M-A, et al. Long-term outcome of arthroscopic remplissage in addition to the classic Bankart repair for the management of recurrent anterior shoulder instability with engaging Hill–Sachs lesions. Knee Surg Sports Traumatol Arthrosc. 2018;27:305–13. https://doi.org/10.1007/s00167-018-5261-3.
42. Bastard C, Herisson O, Gaillard J, Nourissat G. Impact of remplissage on global shoulder outcome: a long-term comparative study. Arthroscopy. 2019;35:1362–7. https://doi.org/10.1016/j.arthro.2019.01.013.

3 Grafting for Humeral Bone Loss

Christian Cruz, Ioanna K. Bolia, and Raffy Mirzayan

3.1 Introduction

The glenohumeral joint is the most commonly dislocated joint in the body [1]. Anterior dislocation may result in bony defects of the glenoid and/or posterosuperior aspect of the humeral head [2]. Osseous defects have a direct impact on recurrent instability by altering joint contact area, congruency, and function of the static restraints [3–5]. Flower was the first to describe the bony lesions found on the humeral head in 1861, with many subsequent investigators reporting on these bony defects [6]. In 1940, two radiologists, Hill and Sachs, reported that these defects were actually compression fractures produced when the posterolateral humeral head impacted against the anterior rim of the glenoid [4]. Hill-Sachs lesions are associated with approximately 40–90% of initial anterior glenohumeral dislocations [7]. The management of Hill-Sachs lesions depends mainly on the size of the lesion and whether it engages with the glenoid or if it renders the joint "off-track" [2]. Most lesions are small and have minimal impact on recurrent instability [8]. However, smaller lesions that are clinically relevant are treated with procedures aimed to filling the bony defect with grafts including a remplissage or by performing a Latarjet which makes the lesion "on-track" thereby preventing engagement of the lesion with the anterior glenoid [6, 9]. For larger humeral head defects, humeral head reconstruction is required which is the focus of this chapter [10].

C. Cruz · I. K. Bolia
Department of Orthopaedic Surgery, USC Keck School of Medicine, Los Angeles, CA, USA

R. Mirzayan (✉)
Department of Orthopaedic Surgery, Kaiser Permanente Southern California, Baldwin Park, CA, USA
e-mail: Raffy.mirzayan@kp.org

3.2 Pathogenesis

The most common mechanism responsible for a traumatic anterior shoulder dislocation occurs when an indirect force is applied to an abducted and externally rotated arm. Burkhart and De Beer described an "engaging" Hill-Sachs lesion as one that encounters the anterior glenoid rim with the arm at 90° of abduction and external rotation from 0° to 135° [2, 11]. These humeral head defects are parallel to the surface of the anterior glenoid when the arm is abducted and externally rotated [8]. The latter has been termed an articular arc deficit as there is disruption of the arc of the glenohumeral articulation when the Hill-Sachs lesion rotates over the anterior glenoid rim [5]. Lesions that are not parallel to the glenoid rim in the "active" or "athletic" position do not engage and are termed nonengaging lesions [2, 11]. The Hill-Sachs defect passes diagonally across the anterior glenoid with external rotation;

E. Calvo et al. (eds.), *Complex and Revision Problems in Shoulder Instability*,
https://doi.org/10.1007/978-3-031-81389-4_3

therefore, there is continual contact of the articulating surfaces and no engagement of the Hill-Sachs lesion by the anterior glenoid [6]. As stated above, Itoi and Yamamoto developed the concept of the glenoid track based on these previous works [12]. Cho et al. [1] looked at three-dimensional (3-D) computed tomography (CT) scans of 107 shoulders undergoing surgery for recurrent anterior instability to preoperatively predict engagement of a Hill-Sachs lesion; the mean width was 52% (range, 27–66%) and depth was 14% (range, 8–20%) of the humeral head diameter on axial images [1].

Hill-Sachs lesions typically are accompanied with other pathology including soft tissue and/or bony Bankart lesions as well as anterior glenohumeral ligament disruption. Optimal surgical management requires addressing these lesions with or without management of the Hill-Sachs lesion. Multiple options exist to address Hill-Sachs defects in anterior glenohumeral instability, including humeroplasty, remplissage, allograft reconstruction (osteochondral plugs vs. size-matched bulk allograft), partial resurfacing, and total resurfacing/arthroplasty [9, 13–16]. Furthermore, a large Hill-Sachs defect can be addressed by a Latarjet or similar procedure where the glenoid track is widened and therefore changes an off-track defect to an on-track defect [9].

Treatment of the Hill-Sachs defect is based on size of the defect and accompanying glenoid bone loss. In large Hill-Sachs defects with accompanying glenoid bone loss, the authors' preferred technique is an anatomic allograft reconstruction of the humeral head using a size-matched humeral head osteoarticular allograft that eliminates the structural pathology while allowing maintenance of the range of motion of the glenohumeral joint.

3.3 Imaging and Other Diagnostic Studies

Preoperative imaging includes a comprehensive radiographic evaluation with anteroposterior (AP), true AP, axillary, and Stryker notch views of the involved shoulder. Patients with shoulder instability should first undergo a magnetic resonance imaging (MRI) scan to evaluate labrum, capsule, rotator cuff, and the bony morphology of the glenoid and humeral head. CT and MRI to evaluate glenoid bone loss has been compared in multiple studies, Yanke et al. found MRI allowed for accurate evaluation of a bony Bankart [17, 18]. MRI also allows better characterization of the rotator cuff insertion, which is a key component of determining whether the defect is on track or off track [17].

A preoperative CT is obtained by a majority of shoulder surgeons to clearly understand the bony architecture of the glenoid and humeral head. A 3D reconstruction can be useful to more clearly define the size and location of the defect and to estimate the amount of the articular surface involved. The humeral head and glenoid can be subtracted from the reconstructed image to allow complete visualization. The plane of the Hill-Sachs defect is oblique to the plane of the axial image, therefore, the size of these defects, and even occurrence, is often underestimated with standard axial imaging.

3.4 Nonoperative Management

The focus of this chapter is on Hill-Sachs lesions with reconstruction, therefore there is minimal role for nonoperative management in these patients. A monitored rehabilitation program focusing on strengthening the dynamic stabilizers (deltoid, rotator cuff, and periscapular muscles) of the shoulder should be started after an initial brief period of immobilization. Patients should avoid the position of instability initially while they rehabilitate the shoulder. Prolonged immobilization is not recommended as this can lead to issues with stiffness [19].

3.5 Surgical Management

3.5.1 Surgical Options

Rotational proximal humeral osteotomies internally rotate the proximal humerus, increasing humeral retroversion and minimizing the potential for the defect to engage the anterior glenoid on external rotation. This technique is essentially of historic interest given the risk of complications and more successful alternatives [2].

Open anterior procedures can be performed including an east–west plication, shifting the glenoid track medially and superiorly to limit external rotation and preventing the humeral head defect from engaging [2, 11]. However, these soft tissue–only techniques may not be adequate in the setting of a large humeral head defect; furthermore, concerns with restricted motion in young patients may prevent return to function and cause late arthrosis.

Remplissage is the tenodesis of the infraspinatus tendon and posterior capsule into the defect to render the lesion essentially extra-articular [8, 20]. Recently, several publications have shown the combination of remplissage and Bankart repair to be highly effective in preventing re-dislocations, in patients with critical glenoid bone loss [11, 21].

3.6 Anatomic Allograft Reconstruction

The indications for anatomic allograft reconstruction of the humeral head include a large engaging Hill-Sachs lesion that lesion involves more than 25–30% of the articular surface [6], bipolar bony lesions of both the glenoid and humeral head, ongoing symptomatic anterior glenohumeral instability or painful clicking, catching, or popping in patients with a large engaging Hill-Sachs lesion who have failed to respond to previous soft tissue stabilization procedures. Contact athletes may be considered for lower thresholds of bone loss as these athletes are at very high risk for recurrent instability. Contraindications to this procedure include routine medical comorbidities precluding an elective surgical procedure with general anesthetic, existing infection, or presence of a non-engaging or functionally nonengaging Hill-Sachs lesion.

3.6.1 Preoperative Planning

A fresh (not fresh-frozen), humeral head osteochondral allograft is obtained from a certified tissue bank. It is important to obtain a side- and size-matched graft as this allows for an optimal recreation of the radius of curvature of the humeral head. If a humeral head is not available, a lateral femoral condyle (Fig. 3.1) osteochondral allograft can be used as well, with meticulous attention to detail paid to matching the patient's anatomy. Furthermore, a talus can be used for smaller defects [22]. Proper allograft sizing of the humeral head requires the patient's imaging to be sent to the chosen bone bank for measurement. CT or MRI imaging of the proximal humerus allows for direct sizing as magnification is accounted for in the scan. The match from the tissue bank should have a side and size match within ±2 mm. It is important to understand and disclose the details of allograft use as it may have direct implications to your patient.

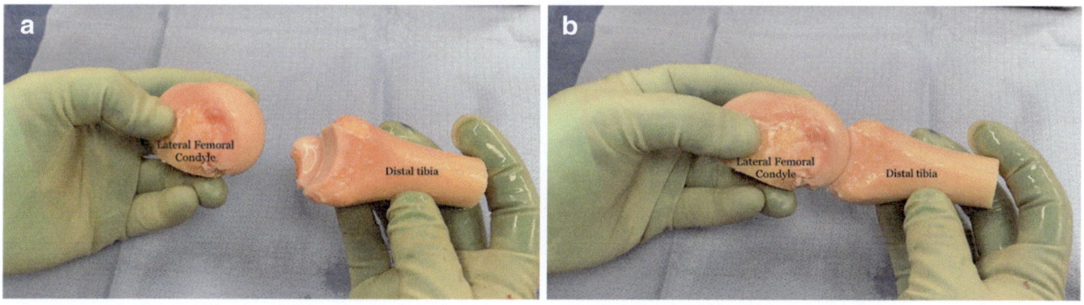

Fig. 3.1 (**a, b**) Showing the articulation of a lateral femoral condyle with a distal tibial allograft

3.6.2 Positioning

The patient is positioned in a modified beach-chair position, inclined about 45°, with the upper extremity draped free similar to positioning in a total shoulder arthroplasty.

3.7 Exposure of the Hill-Sachs Lesion

There are two ways to approach the Hill-Sachs lesion. The approach chosen is based on whether anterior glenoid (labral or distal tibial allograft) work needs to be performed. If no anterior glenoid work needs to be performed, a posterior muscle splitting approach is typically chosen [23]. A deltoid splitting approach is used without detachment from the scapular spine which gives access to the interval between the infraspinatus and teres minor tendons. These tendons are split as well without take down, giving adequate exposure to the Hill-Sachs defect. If anterior glenoid work needs to be accomplished, then an anterior axillary incision and deltopectoral approach is used. The cephalic vein is retracted laterally with the deltoid. The lateral border of the conjoined tendon is identified and gently retracted medially to expose the underlying subscapularis tendon. There are multiple ways to treat the subscapularis in this procedure including a tenotomy or a peel. The senior author (RM) prefers tenotomy as most patients undergoing this procedure are young and have excellent tendon quality with very low risk of re-tear. The subscapularis tendon is transected vertically approximately 0.5 cm medial to its insertion onto the lesser tuberosity. Great care is taken to ensure tendon is left on both the medial and lateral side of the tenotomy to allow for repair. High-tensile sutures are placed in the lateral aspect of the subscapularis tendon as it is released from the lesser tuberosity. The interval between the subscapularis and the anterior capsule is then carefully developed using sharp dissection, continuing medially to the neck of the glenoid. The inferior capsule is then further isolated using careful blunt dissection. A laterally based capsulotomy is made with the vertical limb in line with the subscapularis incision and continuing superiorly. The anteroinferior capsule is then released off the surgical neck of the humerus with intra-articular dissection using a periosteal elevator. The humeral head retractor is withdrawn, and the humerus is brought into maximal external rotation to expose the Hill-Sachs lesion. A flat narrow retractor (e.g., Darrach) is then placed over the reflected undersurface of the subscapularis tendon and behind the neck of the humerus on the posterior rotator cuff to lever out the humeral head.

3.8 Fresh Osteochondral Allograft

Several grafting options exist including osteochondral cylindrical plugs (Fig. 3.2) and a single oval-shaped plug [3] (Fig. 3.3), which are press-fit and do not require fixation. Another option is a shell graft, shaped like a lemon wedge which requires screw fixation (Fig. 3.4).

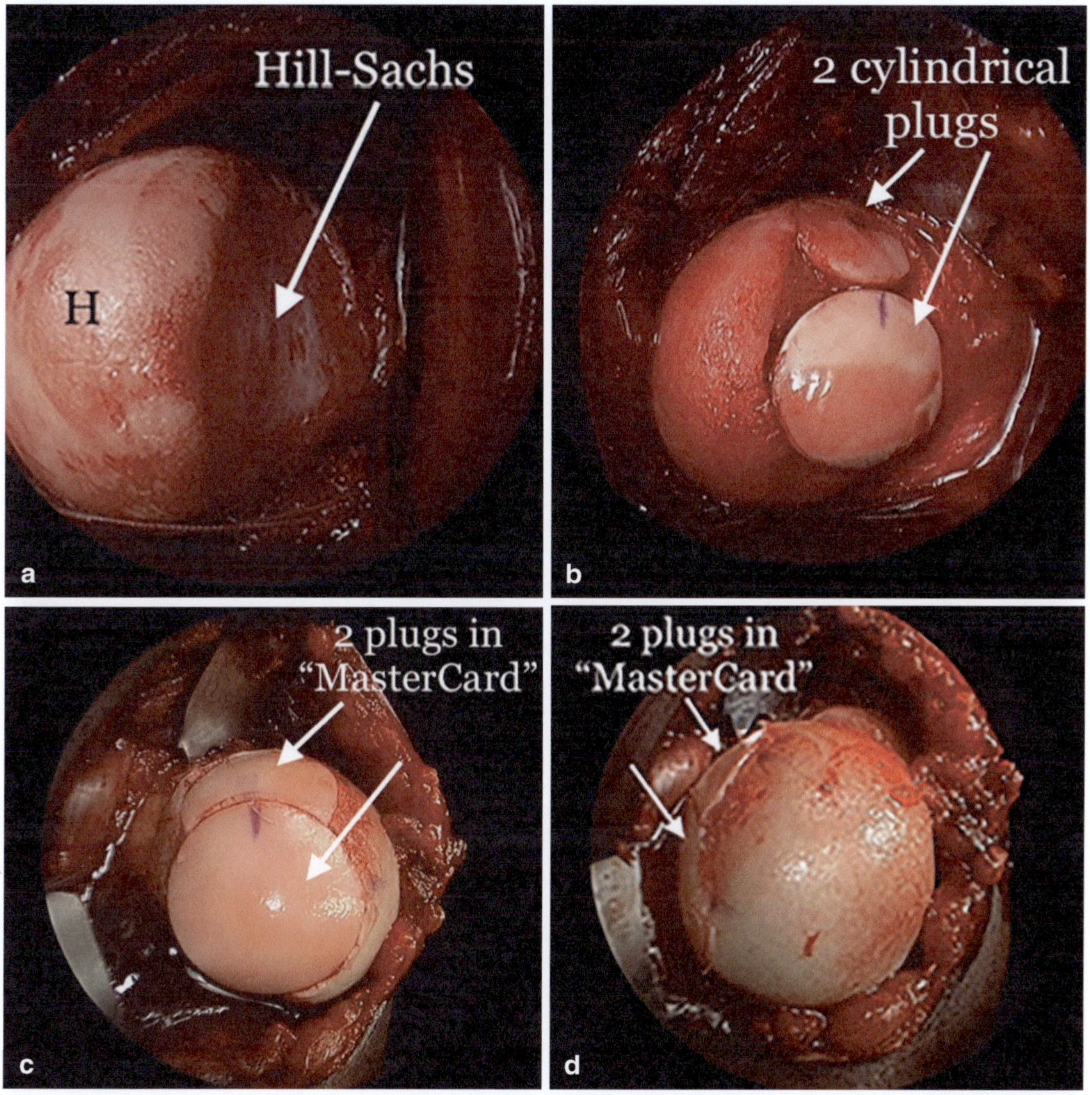

Fig. 3.2 (**a**) A Hill-Sachs defect is seen. (**b**) The defect is filled with two press-fit cylindrical plugs. (**c**) Another example of two large cylindrical fresh osteochondral grafts obtained from a lateral femoral condyle placed in a "MasterCard" fashion. (**d**) The same grafts with arm rotated demonstrating matching of radius of curvature with the humeral head

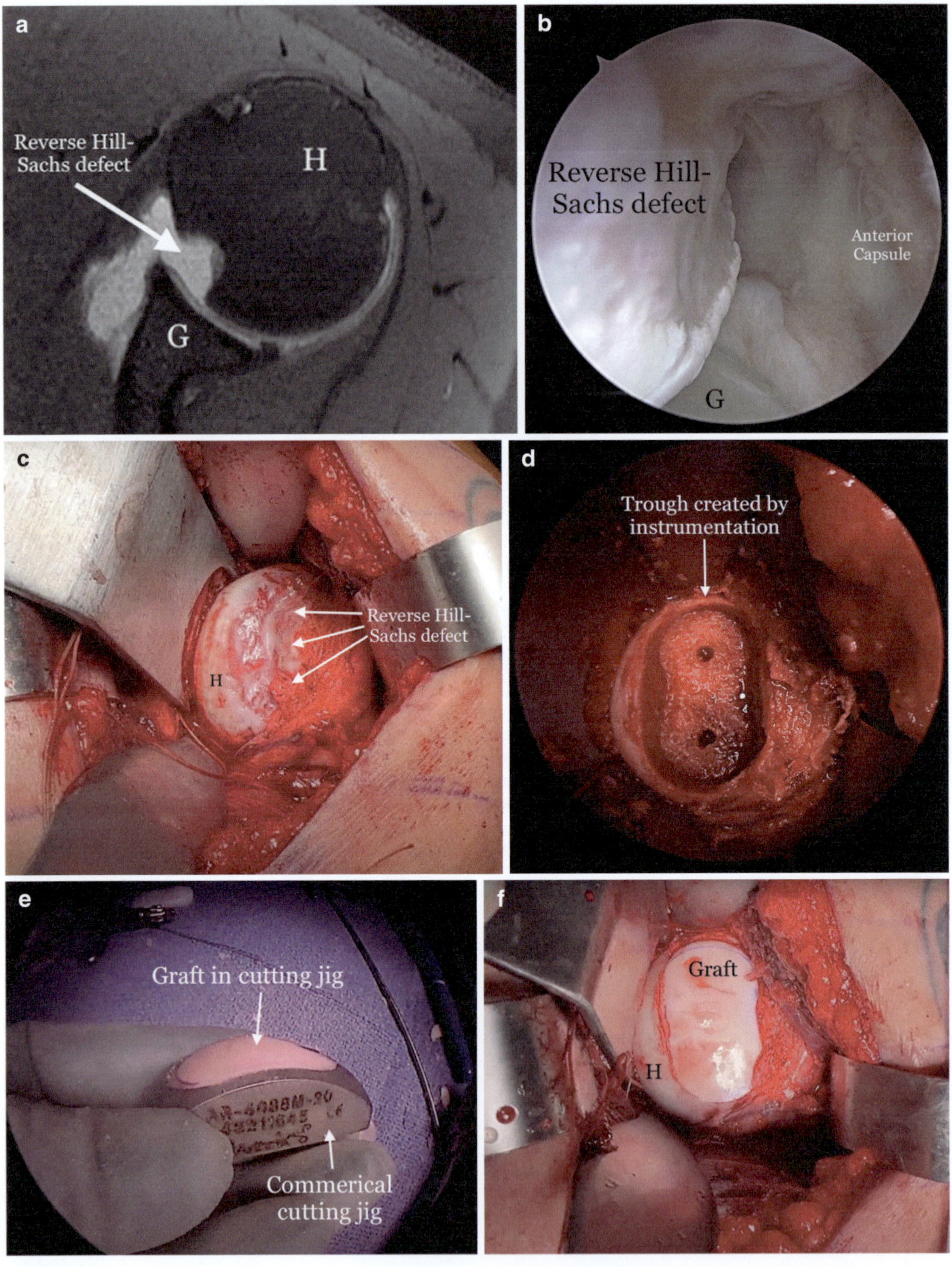

Fig. 3.3 (**a**) Axial MRI demonstrating a large reverse Hill-Sachs lesion in an 18-year-old patient with a posterior dislocation. (**b**) Arthroscopic view of the reverse Hill-Sachs from the superior anterior portal. (**c**) Open exposure of the defect after subscapularis tenotomy. (**d**) Trough created into the defect with commercially available instrumentation (BioUni, Arthrex, Naples, FL). (**e**) The fresh osteochondral allograft harvested from a humeral head is cut and placed into cutting jig to ensure it will fit into the trough. (**f**) Final press-fit fixation of the graft into the defect

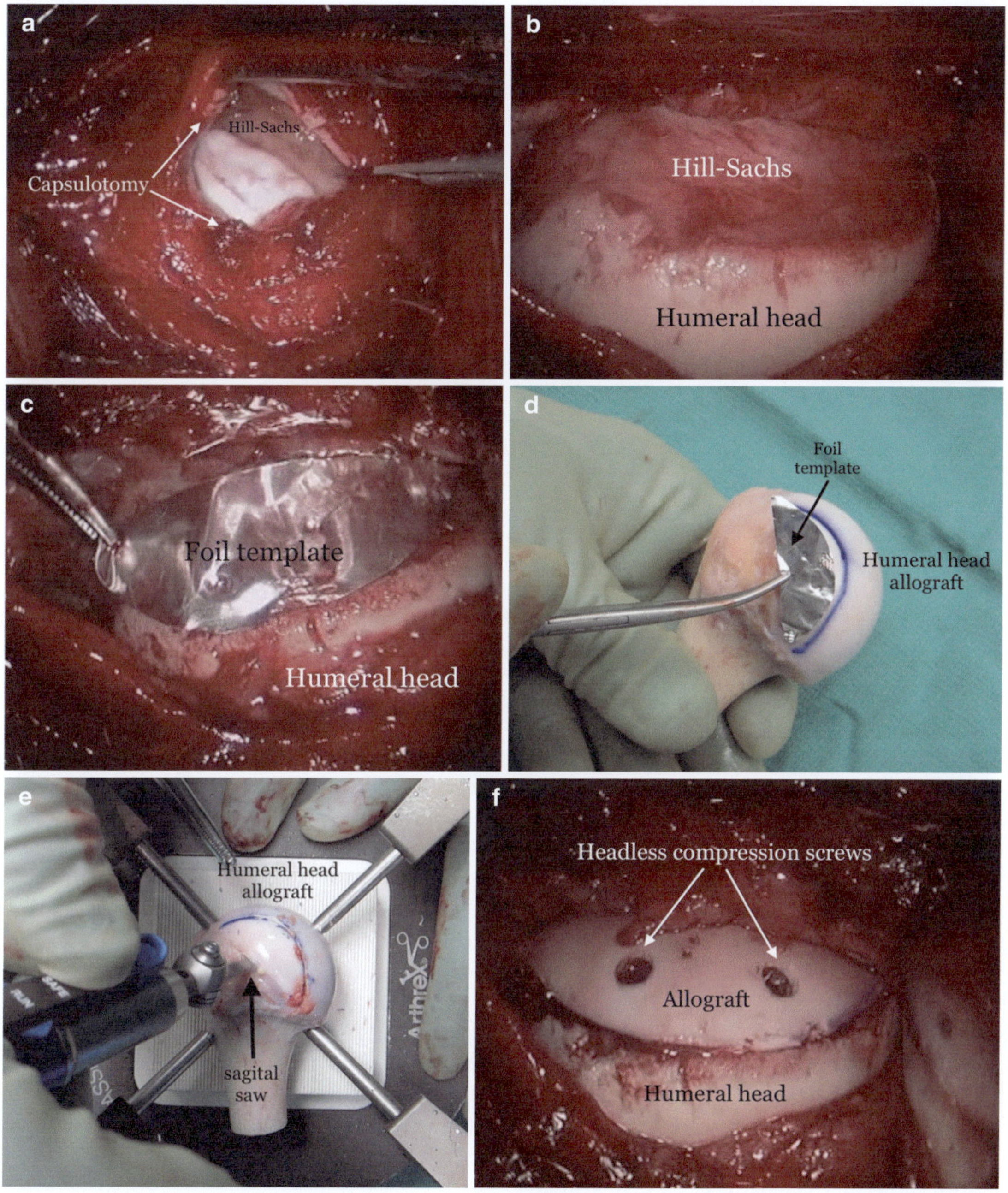

Fig. 3.4 (**a**) Posterior deltoid-splitting approach to an isolated Hill-Sachs defect with capsulotomy. (**b**) After capsulotomy is completed, the Hill-Sachs defect is exposed. (**c**) A piece of foil from suture wrapping is used to template the defect. (**d**) The foil template is placed over the posterior aspect of humeral head allograft. (**e**) A sagittal saw is used to make a "lemon wedge"-shaped graft. (**f**) The graft is fixated with low-profile (headless) screws. (**g**) Postoperative radiograph demonstrating fixation of the graft with two screws

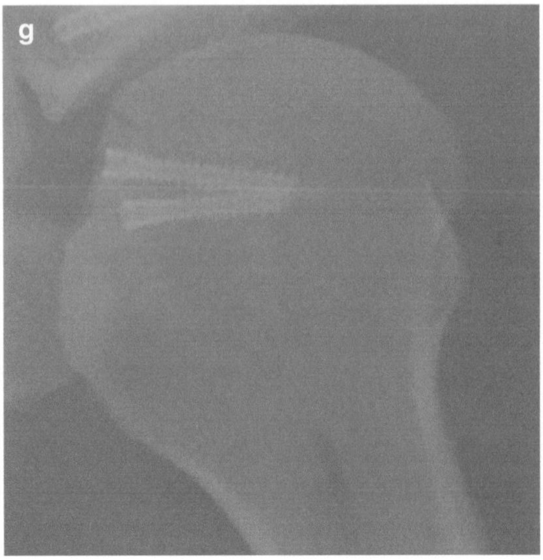

Fig. 3.4 (continued)

3.9 Humeral Head Preparation for Cylindrical and Oval Plugs

The defect must be shaped to accommodate the allograft. Standard instrumentation (Arthrex, Naples, FL) is used by placing a cannulated sizing guide over the lesion. A central guide pin is inserted through the guide. The appropriately sized triple reamer is used to create a socket for the plug. Depth measurements are made at 12, 3, 6, and 9 o'clock of the socket and recorded.

3.10 Preparation of the Humeral Head Allograft

Typically, a size-matched humeral head is used; however, recently Ganokroj et al. demonstrated that reconstructing the humeral head with osteochondral bone plugs from the talus provided excellent fit and restoration of the Hill-Sachs defect, but it is typically used in small defects [22]. The matched humeral head or lateral femoral condyle allograft is secured to a workstation. The same sizing guide used on the native humeral head is used through an aimer that places the guide perpendicular to the articular surface of the graft. A Coring reamer is then used to harvest the osteochondral cylindrical plug. The plug is slightly larger in diameter to the socket created in the patient; therefore, it is secured in the socket by press-fit fixation. Thus, the graft does not have to be bottomed out into the socket for fixation. No screws, bolts, or pins are required for fixation. The graft height is measured at the same locations of the socket and the base of the graft is cut at least 1 mm shorter than what is measured in the socket. For example, if the depth of the socket is 8 mm at 12 o'clock position, the graft is cut to 7 mm at the 12 o'clock position. This is done to ensure that the plug will not be left too proud. The remaining graft is placed back in sterile saline to keep the cartilage hydrated in case this is needed later in the case.

3.11 Wedges (Shell Graft)

3.11.1 Humeral Head Preparation

The defect must be shaped to accommodate the allograft. How the defect is shaped is based on the amount of bone loss, etc. A chevron type osteotomy using a micro-sagittal saw can be performed in cases with more significant bone loss, whereas a burr can be used to shape the defect into lemon peel in cases with less severe bone loss. The piece of matching allograft humeral head is then inserted into the created wedge-shaped defect. The base and side of the defect can then be further smoothed using a hand rasp to achieve precise, flat surfaces.

3.11.2 Preparation of the Humeral Head Allograft

A corresponding piece is cut from the matched humeral head allograft that is 2–3 mm larger in all dimensions than the measured defect. Various techniques can be used to template the defect size. The senior author (RM) prefers to use a piece of foil to measure the defect and plan the size of the allograft. The allograft is secured via commercial graft holders. The humeral head is then marked based on the foil template and cut using a sagittal saw. The graft can be fine-tuned based on size match with a saw or rasp. The remaining graft is placed back in sterile saline to keep the cartilage hydrated in case this is needed later in the case. The allograft segment is then provisionally placed into the Hill-Sachs defect and resized in all three planes. Excess graft is then carefully trimmed with a burr or micro-sagittal saw and is reshaped in the other two planes as well. Fine-tuning of graft size is then continued in one plane at a time until a perfect size match is achieved in all planes.

3.11.3 Fixation of the Humeral Head Allograft

The allograft segment is placed into the defect and aligned to achieve a congruent articular surface. The allograft should have a near press fit feel when inserted into the native humeral head. The graft is then provisionally secured in place with two or three smooth 0.045-inch Kirschner wires. The wires are then sequentially replaced with either headless compression screws or 3.5-mm fully threaded cortical or 4.0-mm cancellous screws placed in a lag fashion. It is essential to ensure that the screw heads are countersunk so that they are below the level of the articular surface. This is imperative to avoid chondral damage to the glenoid. The joint is irrigated and taken through a range of motion to ensure that the reconstructed humeral head provides a smooth congruent articulating surface.

3.11.4 Anterior Labral Inspection and Bankart Reconstruction

A standard humeral head retractor (Fukuda) is placed into the glenohumeral joint, allowing inspection of the glenoid and anteroinferior capsulolabral structures for any pathology. If a Bankart lesion is encountered, it is noted for later repair. Repairing the Bankart lesion before reconstructing the humeral head can make exposure of the humeral head challenging. Similarly, if a concomitant distal tibial allograft is planned, the humeral head allograft is placed first to allow for easier exposure.

3.12 Labral and Subscapularis Repair

If a bony augmentation procedure to the glenoid is planned, this is now performed. If an isolated soft tissue Bankart is present, this is repaired using multiple suture anchors in either a knotted or knotless fashion. The capsulotomy is closed with absorbable suture. Check the stability of the shoulder before repairing the capsule. If the shoulder is very stable, the capsule should not be overtightened. One finger should fit in the axillary pouch of the shoulder when the repair is secured down, so check this tension by pulling on the sutures before securing them down. The subscapularis tendon is then reapproximated to its stump anatomically, without shortening, using suture anchors or a soft tissue repair with nonabsorbable suture. Allow the conjoined tendon, deltoid, and pectoralis major muscles to return to their normal anatomic positions. A routine subcutaneous and skin closure is then performed. Sterile dressing is applied. The arm is placed into a shoulder immobilizer.

3.13 Postoperative Care

After surgery, patients are given a sling for comfort and allowed to begin pendulum exercises at 1 week. Elbow, hand, and wrist motion is immediately allowed. The subscapularis repair is protected for the first 6 weeks. No active internal rotation or shoulder extension is allowed for the first 6 weeks. External rotation at the side is limited to 20° for 2 weeks and progresses to 40° by 4–6 weeks. After the initial 6-week period, patients are allowed to progress to full range of motion. Strengthening is begun once full range of motion is obtained. The shoulders are imaged with repeat radiographs at 6 weeks and 6 months and with CT scans at 6 months to assess for consolidation and incorporation of the graft.

3.14 Outcomes

Successful outcomes have been reported following osteochondral allograft transplantation for the management of large Hill Sachs lesion with the majority of studies reporting no episodes of recurrent shoulder instability [24]. Riff et al. [25] reported the results of 18 patients with an average age of 24.8 years who underwent osteochondral allograft transplantations to the humeral head at an average of 67 months follow-up. The authors found 89% of the allografts incorporated. Significant improvements were seen in all clinical outcome scores. Four of the patients underwent subsequent shoulder arthroplasty at an average of 25 months secondary to chondrolysis from postoperative pain pumps. A systematic review by Saltzman et al. [10] found 12 studies that reported outcomes of osteochondral allograft transplantation to the humeral head for large Hill-Sachs defects. Thirty-five patients (77% male) were included with an average age of 35.4 years. The authors found significant improvements in range of motion and clinical outcome scores. Interestingly, on radiographic follow-up, 8.7% of patients experienced osteonecrosis of the graft, 36.2% saw allograft resorption, and 35.7% had osteoarthritic changes to the glenoid. The reoperation rate was 26%, whereas the complication rate varied between 20% and 30%. Miniaci et al. [6] reported the results of 18 patients who underwent osteochondral allograft transplantation to the humeral head for failed previous attempts at surgical stabilization with an average follow-up of 50 months (range 24–96 months). All patients had posterolateral humeral head defects (Hill-Sachs lesions) that represented greater than about 25–30% of the humeral head. There were no episodes of recurrent instability. Sixteen of eighteen (89%) patients returned to work. Significant improvements were seen in clinical outcome scores. Diklic et al. [26] treated 13 patients with fresh frozen femoral head allograft reconstructions for Hill-Sachs lesions between 25% and 50% of the humeral head. At an average of 54 months postoperatively, the mean Constant score for the cohort was 86.8. Twelve patients had stable shoulders, and one patient had evidence of osteonecrosis. No episodes of recurrent shoulder subluxation were noted in a small group of patients reported by DiPaola et al. who received humeral head bone graft with acceptable functional outcomes, despite slight decrease in shoulder FF as well as internal and external rotation [27].

3.15 Complications

Allograft reconstruction of the humeral head is a technically demanding procedure and complications do occur [10]. Miniaci et al. [6] reported partial graft collapse in 2 of 18 patients, early evidence of osteoarthritis in three patients (marginal osteophytes), and one mild subluxation (posterior). They also reported screw penetrance in two patients who complained of pain with extreme external rotation. Both required screw removal. Use of headless screws can potentially mitigate this complication One must weigh the risks of continued shoulder dysfunction versus the risk associated with the use of fresh osteoarticular allografts [10]. A metallic partial resurfacing arthroplasty is an option that allows for reestablishment of the humeral articular surface without the use of allograft.

References

1. Cho SH, Cho NS, Rhee YG. Preoperative analysis of the Hill-Sachs lesion in anterior shoulder instability: how to predict engagement of the lesion. Am J Sports Med. 2011;39(11):2389–95.
2. Burkhart SS, Danaceau SM. Articular arc length mismatch as a cause of failed Bankart repair. Arthroscopy. 2000;16(7):740–4.
3. Bryant JD, Caldwell PE III, Pearson SE. The "BioHumi" humeral head osteochondral allograft transplantation for reverse Hill-Sachs lesion of the shoulder. Arthrosc Tech. 2023;12(1):e107–e14.
4. Hill HA, Sachs MD. The grooved defect of the humeral head: a frequently unrecognized complication of dislocations of the shoulder joint. Radiology. 1940;35(6):690–700.
5. Matsen FA III, Chebli C, Lippitt S. Principles for the evaluation and management of shoulder instability. JBJS. 2006;88(3):647–59.
6. Miniaci A, Gish MW. Management of anterior glenohumeral instability associated with large Hill–Sachs defects. Tech Should Elbow Surg. 2004;5(3):170–5.
7. Taylor DC, Arciero RA. Pathologic changes associated with shoulder dislocations: arthroscopic and physical examination findings in first-time, traumatic anterior dislocations. Am J Sports Med. 1997;25(3):306–11.
8. Armitage MS, Faber KJ, Drosdowech DS, Litchfield RB, Athwal GS. Humeral head bone defects: remplissage, allograft, and arthroplasty. Orthop Clin North Am. 2010;41(3):417–25.
9. Provencher MT, Frank RM, LeClere LE, Metzger PD, Ryu J, Bernhardson A, et al. The Hill-Sachs lesion: diagnosis, classification, and management. J Am Acad Orthop Surg. 2012;20(4):242–52.
10. Saltzman BM, Riboh JC, Cole BJ, Yanke AB. Humeral head reconstruction with osteochondral allograft transplantation. Arthroscopy. 2015;31(9):1827–34.
11. Burkhart SS, De Beer JF. Traumatic glenohumeral bone defects and their relationship to failure of arthroscopic Bankart repairs: significance of the inverted-pear glenoid and the humeral engaging Hill-Sachs lesion. Arthroscopy. 2000;16(7):677–94.
12. Yamamoto N, Itoi E, Abe H, Minagawa H, Seki N, Shimada Y, et al. Contact between the glenoid and the humeral head in abduction, external rotation, and horizontal extension: a new concept of glenoid track. J Shoulder Elb Surg. 2007;16(5):649–56.
13. Kralinger FS, Golser K, Wischatta R, Wambacher M, Sperner G. Predicting recurrence after primary anterior shoulder dislocation. Am J Sports Med. 2002;30(1):116–20.
14. Park MJ, Garcia G, Malhotra A, Major N, Tjoumakaris FP, Kelly JD IV. The evaluation of arthroscopic remplissage by high-resolution magnetic resonance imaging. Am J Sports Med. 2012;40(10):2331–6.
15. Chen AL, Hunt SA, Hawkins RJ, Zuckerman JD. Management of bone loss associated with recurrent anterior glenohumeral instability. Am J Sports Med. 2005;33(6):912–25.
16. Connolly J. Humeral head defects associated with shoulder dislocation: their diagnostic and surgical significance. Instr Course Lect. 1972;2:210–8.
17. Lansdown DA, Cvetanovich GL, Verma NN, Cole BJ, Bach BR, Nicholson G, et al. Automated 3-dimensional magnetic resonance imaging allows for accurate evaluation of glenoid bone loss compared with 3-dimensional computed tomography. Arthroscopy. 2019;35(3):734–40.
18. Yanke AB, Shin JJ, Pearson I, Bach BR Jr, Romeo AA, Cole BJ, et al. Three-dimensional magnetic resonance imaging quantification of glenoid bone loss is equivalent to 3-dimensional computed tomography quantification: cadaveric study. Arthroscopy. 2017;33(4):709–15.
19. Hovelius L, Olofsson A, Sandström B, Augustini B-G, Krantz L, Fredin H, et al. Nonoperative treatment of primary anterior shoulder dislocation in patients forty years of age and younger: a prospective twenty-five-year follow-up. JBJS. 2008;90(5):945–52.
20. Boileau P, O'Shea K, Vargas P, Pinedo M, Old J, Zumstein M. Anatomical and functional results after arthroscopic Hill-Sachs remplissage. JBJS. 2012;94(7):618–26.
21. Leroux T, Bhatti A, Khoshbin A, Wasserstein D, Henry P, Marks P, et al. Combined arthroscopic Bankart repair and remplissage for recurrent shoulder instability. Arthroscopy. 2013;29(10):1693–701.
22. Ganokroj P, Hollenbeck J, Peebles AM, Brown JR, Hanson JA, Whalen RJ, et al. Humeral head reconstruction with osteochondral allograft: bone plug optimization for Hill-Sachs lesions using CT-based computer modeling analysis. Orthop J Sports Med. 2023;11(9):23259671231193768.
23. Wirth MA, Butters KP, Rockwood CA Jr. The posterior deltoid-splitting approach to the shoulder. Clin Orthop Relat Res (1976–2007). 1993;296:92–8.
24. Piasecki DP, Verma NN, Romeo AA, Levine WN, Bach BR Jr, Provencher MT. Glenoid bone deficiency in recurrent anterior shoulder instability: diagnosis and management. J Am Acad Orthop Surg. 2009;17(8):482–93.
25. Riff AJ, Yanke AB, Shin JJ, Romeo AA, Cole BJ. Midterm results of osteochondral allograft transplantation to the humeral head. J Shoulder Elb Surg. 2017;26(7):e207–e15.
26. Diklic I, Ganic Z, Blagojevic Z, Nho S, Romeo A. Treatment of locked chronic posterior dislocation of the shoulder by reconstruction of the defect in the humeral head with an allograft. J Bone Joint Surg Br Vol. 2010;92(1):71–6.
27. DiPaola MJ, Jazrawi LM, Rokito AS, Kwon YW, Patel L, Pahk B, et al. Management of humeral and glenoid bone loss—associated with glenohumeral instability. Bull NYU Hosp Jt Dis. 2010;68(4):245–50.

4 Open Latarjet Procedure

Paulo José Llinás Hernández
and Gustavo Antonio Gil Noriega

4.1 History

The Latarjet procedure represents an advancement in the surgical management of anterior shoulder instability, especially for patients experiencing glenoid bone loss or those with failed soft tissue stabilization surgeries. Pioneered by the French surgeon Michel Latarjet [1], the procedure aimed to restore stability to the shoulder by transferring the coracoid process to the anterior border of the glenoid. This innovative approach not only augmented the glenoid articular surface but also described the sling effect created by the conjoint tendon passing anteroinferior to the humeral head in the position where the arm is at risk of dislocating, marking an important landmark in the treatment of complex shoulder instability conditions.

Historically, the development of the Latarjet procedure follows the evolution in understanding and addressing shoulder instability. Prior to Latarjet's innovation, treatment options for recurrent shoulder dislocations, particularly in the context of bone loss, were limited and often led to suboptimal results. By introducing a method that provided a biomechanical solution to a challenging clinical problem, Latarjet set a new standard in the field.

Over the decades, the technique has seen numerous modifications aimed at enhancing its efficacy and minimizing the risk of complications. The original method described by Latarjet has seen changes, with improvements in surgical techniques, fixation methods, and graft positioning contributing significantly to the procedure's success in reducing dislocation recurrence and improving patient outcomes [2, 3].

New horizons have been developed with the advent of arthroscopic surgery [4], which has favored a more precise assessment of the glenohumeral joint and corrected associated pathologies under arthroscopic vision, but it wasn't until 2007 that Lafosse et al. published the first series of the arthroscopic Latarjet procedure. However, the learning curve is long, and the cost-benefit must be assessed very carefully (Fig. 4.1).

P. J. Llinás Hernández (✉)
Clínica Fundación Valle de Lili/ICESI University, Cali, Colombia
e-mail: paulo.llinas@fvl.org.co

G. A. Gil Noriega
Clínica Fundación Valle de Lili, Cali, Colombia
e-mail: gustavo.gil@fvl.org.co

E. Calvo et al. (eds.), *Complex and Revision Problems in Shoulder Instability*,
https://doi.org/10.1007/978-3-031-81389-4_4

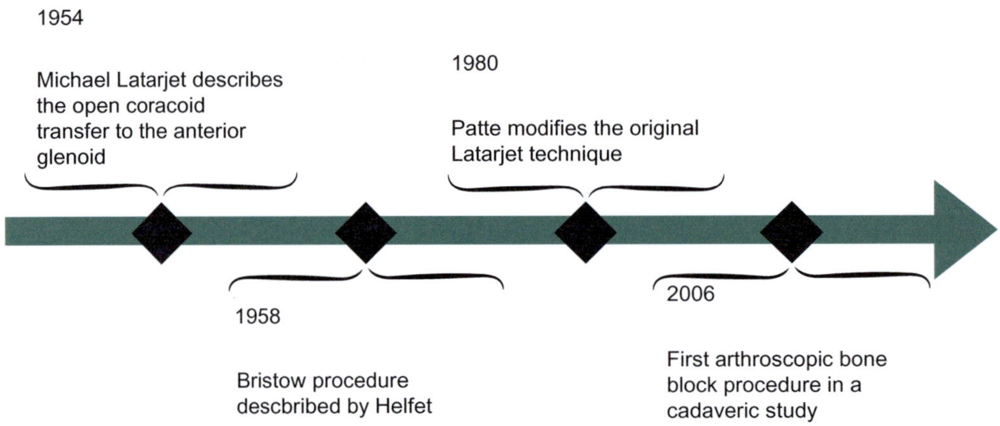

Fig. 4.1 Timeline of the evolution of the Latarjet surgery since its inception and the new modifications of the technique

4.2 Biomechanics

The inception of the Latarjet surgery initially included a double effect, with the coracoid graft functioning as an augmentation of the glenoid surface and the conjoint tendon working as a sling with the arm in its maximum abduction and external rotation. However, it wasn't until the modifications performed by Patte et al. [5] that a third effect of controlling anterior glenohumeral instability was identified [5].

This triple effect consists, firstly, of a bone block effect, that is the coracoid graft, positioned in the anterior border of the glenoid in continuity with the articular surface, this allows for recovery of the lost glenoid track described by Itoi et al. [6] and converts bipolar off-track defects in on-track defects with lower risk of recurrence. Secondly, the coracoid tendon transfer reroutes the conjoint tendon and lowers the inferior portion of the subscapularis tendon, so when the arm is positioned at 90° abduction and maximal external rotation, this complex functions as a hammock that provides dynamic stability. Lastly, the capsular reinsertion to the coracoid graft, specifically to a previously prepared stump of the coracoacromial ligament, complements the blocking function in the outstretched position of the arm.

The Latarjet surgery works biomechanically differently depending on the ranges of motion. In mid-ranges, the restoration of the glenoid surface with the addition of the bone block is the most significant effect (38–49%), while in maximal ranges, the sling effect of the conjoint tendon is the most important (76–77%), with capsular reinsertion supporting the remainder (24–25%) [7]. The positioning and fixation of the graft are key to ensuring biology and biomechanics. The most vascularized part of the coracoid is the distal portion near the tendon insertion; hence, it has the best biological integration and the least osteolysis. The placement should be in the anteroinferior quadrant of the glenoid to ensure optimal consolidation and biomechanics that allow graft remodeling according to Wolff's law [8]. Additionally, the restoration of the glenoid width should aim for at least 100% of the native glenoid width, as lesser coverage leads to unacceptable stress on the coracoid that can predispose the procedure to failure [9].

In an effort to maximize the reconstruction of the articular geometry of the glenoid and improve outcomes, Burkhart et al. [10] introduced some modifications to what we will call the traditional Latarjet surgery. They described what they call the "Congruent Arc Latarjet" (CAL). In this technique, after performing an osteotomy of the distal coracoid process to the coracoclavicular ligaments, the graft is rotated 90° so that the concave inferior surface of the coracoid process aligns with the glenoid fossa and the medial edge of the coracoid comes into

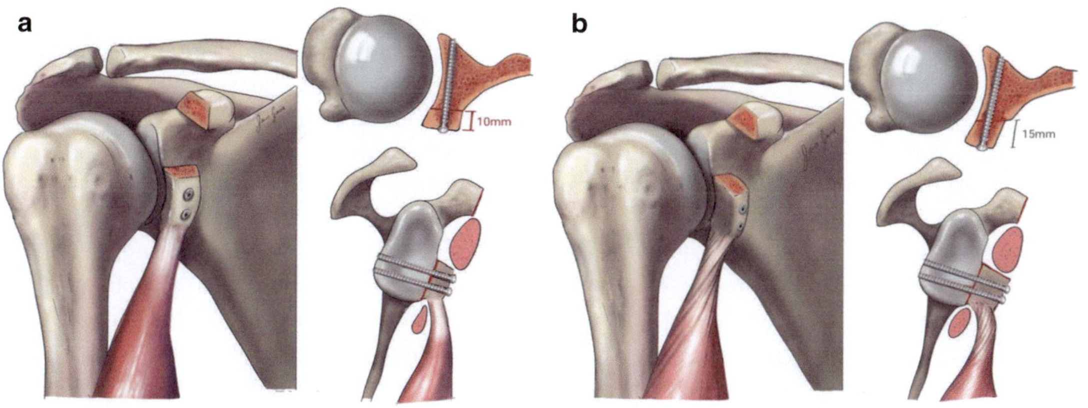

Fig. 4.2 (**a**) Classical Latarjet procedure in the coronal, axial, and sagittal plane. (**b**) Congruent arc Latarjet in the coronal, axial, and sagittal plane. Notice the effect of the track augmentation in the axial plane done by the congruent arc, with the disadvantage of having the graft with lower contact on the bone surface

contact with the anterior surface of the glenoid (Fig. 4.2).

4.3 Indications

Classically, Latarjet surgery is indicated in patients with anterior shoulder instability and bone loss greater than 25% [11]. However, there is increasing evidence of the use of Latarjet in minor defects, especially in high-risk patients due to their activity, sport, or competitiveness [12–15]. A study by Rossi [16] demonstrates the procedure's effectiveness in competitive athletes with bone defects smaller than 20%, suggesting a broader applicability beyond the conventional criteria. This study highlights that even with less extensive bone loss, the Latarjet procedure facilitates a high rate of return to sports, indicating its robustness in restoring shoulder stability. Brandariz [17] further elucidates the procedure's efficacy in converting off-track Hill-Sachs lesions to on-track, reinforcing its value even in cases with less severe bone loss. This adaptability speaks to the procedure's dual mechanism of action: not only does it compensate for the glenoid bone deficit but also leverages the conjoint tendon's sling effect for additional stability. Additionally, Gowd et al. [18] demonstrated that return to sports with the same level of pre-injury competition is good, which increases the indications in collision, contact sports, and throwing athletes.

The ISIS (Index Severity Instability Score) and the GTIMS (Glenoid Track Instability Management Score) are scoring systems used to predict the likelihood of failure in soft tissue surgeries. The ISIS, proposed by Balg and Boileau [19], considers factors such as the patient's age, sports participation, competence level, hyperlaxity, and bone loss to assess the risk of postsurgical redislocation after Bankart surgery and determine the need for Latarjet surgery. On the other hand, the GTIMS, a modification introduced by Di Giacomo et al. [20], enhances the ISIS by incorporating tomographic assessment and on-track/off-track concepts, enabling a more comprehensive evaluation of glenoid anatomy and offering additional insights for decision-making on soft tissue/bone block surgeries. Recently, in a concept review by DiGiacomo on shoulder instability, a guide was provided with current evidence on decision-making, offering recommendations that encompass all factors, not just bone loss, and taking the suggested value of glenoid bone loss to as low as 13.5% [21].

4.4 Surgical Technique

4.4.1 Anesthesia

We typically opt for general anesthesia to promote relaxation of the muscles in the surgical region. Local anesthetic is administered at the surgical approach site, and a suprascapular nerve block is also utilized for effective pain control postsurgery, providing relief for 4–6 h [22].

4.4.2 Patient Positioning

An examination is carried out under anesthesia to assess anterior glenohumeral translation. Arthroscopic evaluation is not conducted prior to the open Latarjet surgical procedure. The patient is positioned on a surgical table inclined at 30–35°, with the upper extremity completely draped to allow full mobilization during the surgery (Fig. 4.3).

4.4.3 Surgical Approach

Careful attention to anatomical landmarks and preferably marking, focusing our attention on the position of the coracoid process. An incision of approximately 5–7 cm in length is made, starting 1 cm proximal to the coracoid process towards the axillary fold, prior infiltration with local anesthesia with epinephrine. The surgical approach progresses up to the deltopectoral interval, with care taken to protect and laterally mobilize the cephalic vein. The clavi-pectoral fascia is visualized, along with the superior aspect of the coracoid process, the pectoralis minor medially, the coracoacromial ligament laterally, and the conjoint tendon anteriorly (comprising the short head of the biceps and the coracobrachialis). Anatomical studies have highlighted the variability of the musculocutaneous nerve and its proximity to the coracoid process, typically situated distally at 4.7 cm. The musculocutaneous nerve is absent in 3.7% of cases and communicates with other terminal branches of the brachial plexus in 19.7% [23].

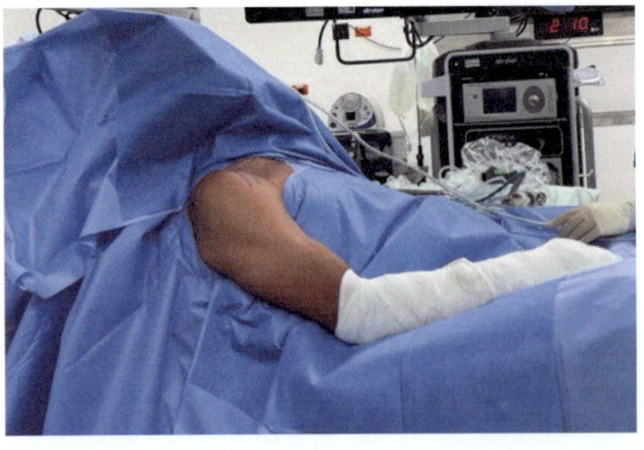

Fig. 4.3 Patient positioning

4.5 Coracoid Process Graft Preparation

After identifying the superior aspect of the coracoid process, the pectoralis minor is released, while preserving the insertion of the conjoint tendon. Additionally, the coracoacromial ligament is transected 1 cm laterally to the coracoid to facilitate the graft preparation (Fig. 4.4).

Subsequently, the superior aspect of the coracoid process is palpated, and the length and site of the osteotomy 2 cm proximal to the tip of the coracoid process is measured, preserving the coracoid neck and coracoclavicular ligaments. Anatomical studies have described the vascular supply of the coracoid process in which the irrigation in its superior horizontal aspect comes from the axillary artery, while in its vertical and posterior portion comes from the suprascapular artery (Fig. 4.5) [24].

The osteotomy is then performed with a coracoid process cut with a 90° oscillating saw, subsequently the coracoid process is released and mobilized. For the classic Latarjet procedure, as depicted in this section, the graft's inferior aspect is decorticated using an oscillating saw to achieve bleeding and optimize the consolidation of this bone block.

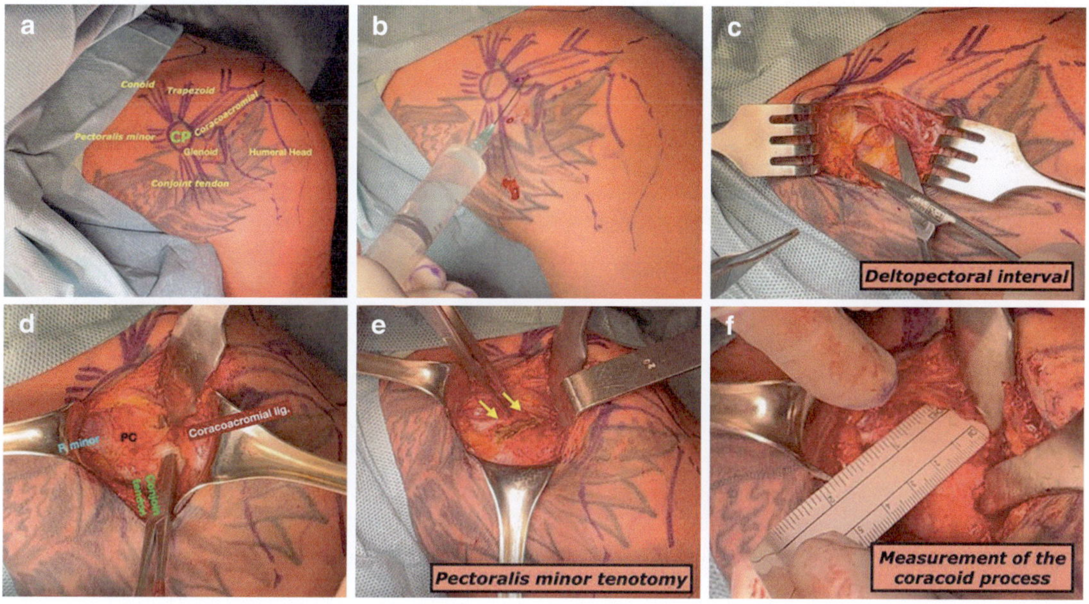

Fig. 4.4 Description of the surgical approach and coracoid process exposure. (**a**) Landmark marking. (**b**) Local anesthetic infiltration. (**c**) Limited deltopectoral approach. (**d**) Deep structure identification. (**e**) Pectoralis minor tenotomy. (**f**) Measurement of the coracoid process. *CP* coracoid process. *Pi minor* pectoralis minor, *Lig* ligament

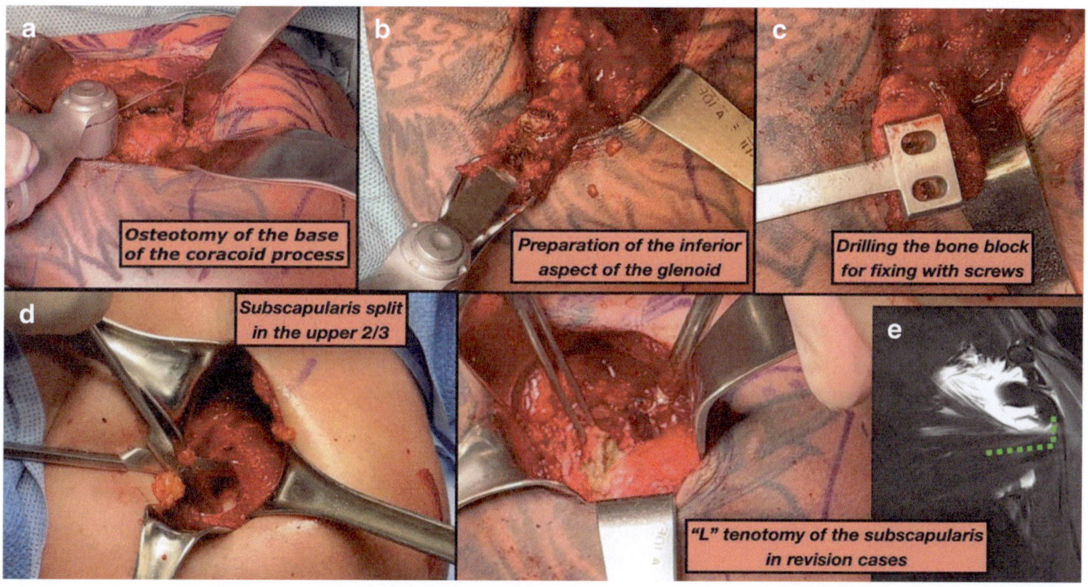

Fig. 4.5 Coracoid osteotomy and graft preparation. (**a**) Coracoid osteotomy. (**b**) Coracoid graft preparation. (**c**) Graft drilling. (**d**) Subscapularis split. (**e**) "L"-shaped subscapular tenotomy

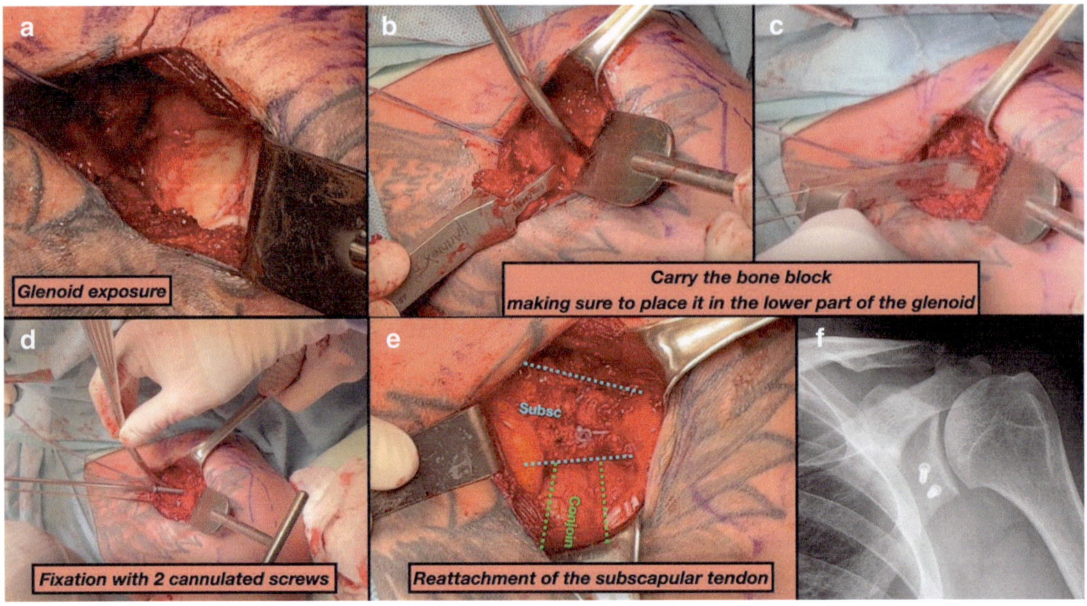

Fig. 4.6 Graft fixation. (**a**) Glenoid exposure. (**b**) Graft positioning in the drilling guide. (**c**) Placement of the bone block. (**d**) Placement of the cannulated screws. (**e**) Subscapular tendon reattachment after "L" tenotomy. (**f**) Postoperative x-rays. *Subsc* subscapularis tendon, *Conjoin* Conjoint tendon

4.6 Exposure and Preparation of the Glenoid

Identification of the rotator interval and insertion of the subscapularis tendon on the lesser tuberosity distal and lateral to the coracoid process. In cases of primary surgery, a standard subscapularis tendon split is made in the direction of its fibers between the inferior 2/3 and the superior 1/3. This will allow proper exposure while protecting the anterior humeral circumflex artery and its two venous companions, also called the "three sisters" [25]. However, in revision cases of capsulolabral repairs, fibrosis in the anterior capsule may difficult the exposure via a tendon split, that is why our preference in these cases is to access the glenohumeral joint with an inverted L-shaped incision until the upper third of the subscapularis is released. The anterior bone defect of the glenoid is assessed, decortication and exposure of the subchondral bone is performed to improve healing in the recipient area for the coracoid graft (Fig. 4.6).

4.7 Coracoid Fixation

Fixation following the standard technique is recommended, with the undersurface of the coracoid graft heading the anterior border of the glenoid using two 3.5 mm cannulated screws. Using a guide that allows allocation of the bone graft parallel to the articular surface in the anterior aspect of the glenoid rim and thus restoring the glenoid track.

4.8 Capsular Reinsertion

It is important to note that when the coracoid is being prepared for the osteotomy, after the pectoralis minor tenotomy is made, the coracoacromial ligament must be transected leaving a 1 cm stump attached to the coracoid. This will allow the visualization of the stump after the graft is fixed to the anterior glenoid border. The previously made capsulotomy used to visualize the intraarticular structures must be closed and sutured with an absorbable suture to the coracoacromial ligament stump, with care taken to position the arm with 50° of external rotation to avoid limitation of this specific range of motion.

4.9 Outcomes

The Latarjet procedure aims primarily to provide patients with a full range of motion postoperatively, no pain, and no recurrence of dislocation. In this section, the most important outcomes will be discussed and compared with similar procedures published in the literature.

4.10 Recurrence

The Latarjet procedure has proved its potential in maintaining the long-term stability of the shoulder. Despite its effectiveness, the recurrence of the instability is still a concerning point over the evolution of the patients and has been proved to be influenced by several factors. Studies where the medium- and long-term outcomes after the Latarjet procedure were evaluated, the proportion of patients with instability recurrence with a minimum follow-up of 5 years was 4%, while in those with a minimum follow-up of 10 years it was 11% [26]. However, studies like the one published by Young, Walch et al. [2], in a series of more than 2000 patients, show a 1% recurrence rate of shoulder instability. Griesser et al. [27] found in their systematic review of complications after the Latarjet procedure that 73% of recurrences occurred in the first year. Zimmerman et al. [28] reported in their study, which analyzed patients with 10 years of follow-up, that all recurrences occurred within the first 2 years after the Latarjet procedure. This contrasts with the arthroscopic Bankart repair, where they found that the functional outcome decreased over time with higher rate of recurrence. A systematic review conducted by Hurley et al. [29] revealed a recurrence rate of instability of 8.5% during a minimum follow-up of 10 years, demonstrating the lasting efficacy of the procedure. Moreover, a study conducted by Scanlon et al. [30] reported the absence of recurrent instability within a postoperative window of 90 days in a high-volume center, suggesting the rarity of early recurrence when performed by experienced surgeons. On the contrary, Frank et al. [31] documented an overall recurrence rate of 1.5% within the first 90 days, indicating that early recurrence, although infrequent, occurs.

These findings collectively indicate that the Latarjet procedure effectively mitigates the risk of recurrent shoulder instability. However, there is a recurrence rate, highlighting the need for meticulous patient selection, appropriate surgical technique, and dedicated postoperative care to maximize the success rate of the intervention.

4.11 Return to Sports

A key postoperative outcome of interest is athletes' ability to return to sport, a crucial factor for their career and quality of life. Recent systematic reviews and cohort studies have provided valuable insights into the success rates and factors influencing return to sport after the Latarjet procedure. Kee et al. [32] highlighted a distinction in return levels between collision and non-collision athletes, with a notably higher success rate observed in non-collision athletes, where 96.4% of patients returned to sports activity, albeit at different levels of participation. Similarly, Sridharan et al. [33] reported a substantial rate of return to competitive play among young contact athletes, with high rates of satisfaction despite some cases of unresolved postoperative pain or stiffness.

Further analysis by Hurley et al. [34] through a systematic review found an overall return to play rate of 88.8%, with a significant number returning to the same level of play. These findings underscore the efficacy of the procedure in restoring shoulder stability and function, allowing athletes to resume competitive sports. Gowd et al. [18] contributed to this understanding by identifying factors such as body mass index (BMI), gender, and the volume of preoperative humeral bone loss as predictors of a successful return to sport.

4.12 Residual Postoperative Pain

Postoperative pain after Latarjet surgery is a concern for both patients and physicians, given its potential impact on recovery, rehabilitation, and ultimately, the functional outcomes of the surgery. It's noteworthy that pain is a multifactorial process as concomitant pathologies can also influence it. Despite the high satisfaction rate, some studies have found a certain degree of residual pain in a significant number of patients. This relatively high rate of residual pain could be related to progressive degenerative changes in the joint. Läderman et al. [35] found that instability arthropathy was related to lower patient satisfaction, supporting this theory. In terms of functional outcomes and potential predictors of postoperative pain, Mook et al. [36] investigated clinical and anatomical characteristics, including the glenoid track, as predictors of outcomes after the Latarjet procedure. They found that patients with moderate or higher preoperative pain scores had a negative correlation with postoperative scores, suggesting that preoperative pain levels could be an important consideration in managing patient expectations and outcomes.

Lastly, a study focused on functional recovery, conducted by Nourissat et al. [37] found that arthroscopic Latarjet procedures generated less immediate postoperative pain compared to open procedures. This perception supports the idea that less-invasive techniques could expedite functional recovery by minimizing early postoperative discomfort. These studies collectively underline the importance of surgical technique selection and preoperative planning in managing postoperative pain after Latarjet surgery. They also highlight the need for further research on pain predictors and functional recovery to optimize patient outcomes.

4.13 Comparative Studies of Bankart Versus Latarjet Procedures

Choosing between Latarjet and Bankart surgeries involves careful consideration of patient-specific factors and anticipated outcomes, which will affect the efficacy, complication rates, and functional outcomes associated with each procedure. After arthroscopic Bankart repairs, recurrence rates of instability have been observed to range from 0% to 37.5%, whereas recurrence rates after the open Latarjet procedure have been reported in a range of 1.7–14.2%. Thus, the latter is considered to better restore stability compared to the arthroscopic Bankart repair, according to medium-term studies [28].

In a 10-year follow-up study where an open Latarjet procedure was performed in one group and an arthroscopic Bankart repair in the second group, instability or apprehension persisted or recurred after 11% of the Latarjet procedures and after 41.7% of Bankart surgeries. Redislocation occurred in 13% of Bankart surgeries and 1% of Latarjet procedures. It was observed that the arthroscopic Bankart procedure was less effective than the open Latarjet procedure for repairing recurrent anterior shoulder dislocation [28].

A systematic review and meta-analysis conducted by An et al. [38] highlighted the superiority of the Latarjet procedure over Bankart repair in reducing recurrence and redislocation rates, with patients undergoing Latarjet also reporting higher Rowe scores and less loss of external rotation. These findings suggest that the Latarjet procedure may offer improved stability for patients with recurrent traumatic anterior shoulder instability. Werthel et al. [39] focused on the outcomes of the Latarjet procedure when performed as a revision surgery after a failed arthroscopic Bankart repair versus as a primary operation. Their study revealed that functional outcomes and postoperative pain were significantly worse for revision cases, highlighting the importance of initial surgical success. On the contrary, Calvo et al. reported similar outcomes after primary arthroscopic Latarjet compared to arthroscopic Latyarjet performed as a revision surgery. However, a decreased level of sports participation should be expected in the revision cases [40]. Kukkonen et al. [41] conducted a randomized controlled trial comparing arthroscopic Bankart repair and open Latarjet procedures in young men, finding a significantly higher rate of redislocation in the Bankart group. This underlines the effectiveness of the Latarjet procedure in pre-

Table 4.1 Tabulation of the results comparing Latarjet vs. Bankart surgery in multiple studies

References	Latarjet vs Bankart	% Recurrence (%)	% Satisfaction	% Return to sports	% Apprehension
Zimmermann [44]	Latarjet	1	77%	Higher in Latarjet	29%
	Bankart	13	48%		9%
An [45]	Latarjet	11	85 Rowe score	Not quantified	Not evaluated
	Bankart	21	79 Rowe score		
Kukkone [41]	Latarjet	2	No difference	56%	16%
	Bankart	21		9%	33%
Ernstbrunner [43]	Latarjet	0	100%	Not evaluated	13%
	Bankart	17	97%		8%

venting recurrent instability. Flinkkilä et al. [42] identified a previous arthroscopic Bankart repair as an independent risk factor for an inferior outcome after Latarjet surgery, highlighting the challenges associated with revision surgeries. Finally, Ernstbrunner et al. [43] compared the long-term outcomes of arthroscopic Bankart repair versus open Latarjet procedure in patients over 40 years of age. Both procedures provided reliable pain relief and patient satisfaction; however, the Latarjet procedure was notably more effective in restoring stability.

These studies collectively emphasize the precise decision-making required when choosing between Latarjet and Bankart procedures, considering the patient's age, activity level, and percentage of glenoid bone loss, to optimize outcomes for patients with anterior shoulder instability.

Table 4.1 describes some of the expected outcomes for Latarjet and Bankart surgery in studies where they were performed comparatively.

4.14 Open Versus Arthroscopic Latarjet Surgery

The debate between open and arthroscopic Latarjet surgery remains a key point of discussion among shoulder surgery experts. Recent literature provides valuable insights into the effectiveness, clinical outcomes, and procedural costs of these two surgical techniques. Nourissat et al. [37] conducted a multicenter study that provided evidence of lower levels of immediate postoperative pain in patients undergoing arthroscopic Latarjet procedures compared to the open procedure, although both techniques showed similar functional outcomes after 1 year. Similarly, Ali et al. [46] compared the two methods and found minor differences in the loss of internal rotation favoring the open procedure and in the scores of the WOMAC (Western Ontario and MacMaster Universities Ostearthritis Index) favoring the arthroscopic procedure. Randelli et al. [47] performed a cost analysis along with a comparison of clinical outcomes between open and arthroscopic Latarjet surgeries. Although both techniques had excellent clinical outcomes, the arthroscopic procedure was significantly more expensive, raising questions about the cost-benefit of the procedure. Zhu et al. [48], in their prospective study, did not observe significant differences in clinical outcomes between the two groups operated with arthroscopic or open surgery. However, they highlighted that the open group had more precisely positioned coracoid grafts, while the arthroscopic group showed less graft resorption at 1 year postoperatively.

In addition to the studies described, multiple articles have been published in the literature comparing both techniques, in which, in general terms, no significant difference has been found in rates of recurrence and postoperative pain.

Table 4.2 shows some of the studies with the outcomes evaluated comparing open Latarjet surgery versus the arthroscopic procedure.

Table 4.2 Tabulation of the results comparing open versus arthroscopic Latarjet in multiple studies

References	Open versus arthroscopic	Surgical time (Minutes)	% Recurrence	Postoperative pain	Arthritis
Deng [49]	Open	93.3	No difference	No difference	No difference
	Arthroscopic	112.3			
Randelli [47]	Open	Not evaluated	3.30%	No difference	0–70%
	Arthroscopic	85	0.30%		9–32%
Cunningham [50]	Open	81	Not present	No difference	Not evaluated
	Arthroscopic	146			
Zhu [48]	Open	89.3	Not present	No difference	Not evaluated
	Arthroscopic	122.8			
Honrner [51]	Open	93.3	1.40%	No difference	Not evaluated
	Arthroscopic	112.2	1.90%		
Hurley [52]	Open	Not evaluated	No difference	No difference	Not evaluated
	Arthroscopic				

4.15 Complications

4.15.1 Nerve Lesions

Although rare, nerve lesions may arise due to the mobilization of the coracoid and its conjoint tendon attachment. To reduce this risk, it is advised against performing extensive dissection around the coracoid without exposing the medial edge of the conjoint tendon, and the surgeon should always remain lateral to this tendon [53]. Generally, there is no need to routinely explore or locate the musculocutaneous or axillary nerves. The management of nerve injuries is expectant, with regular follow-ups and appropriate investigations, referring if there are no improvements.

4.15.2 Musculocutaneous Nerve

Southam et al. [54] reported a case of transient musculocutaneous nerve (MCN) paralysis occurring 13 months after the initial Latarjet procedure. The author theorized that the paralysis resulted from the relative elongation of the MCN due to the Latarjet procedure and a recent history of strenuous mechanical work.

The anatomical changes in the position of the MCN following the Latarjet procedure are well documented. Freehill et al. [55], in their cadaveric study, demonstrated that the MCN was displaced medially and inferiorly relative to its original location.

4.15.3 Suprascapular Nerve

Transient paralysis of the suprascapular nerve (SSN) is well documented [56]. Special attention must be paid to the direction of the superior screw. The average distance from the exit site of the superior screw to the SSN (at the base of the scapular spine) has been shown to be 4 mm. Misdirected screws (towards the scapular spine) can lead to compression of the infraspinous branch of the SSN [57].

Shishido et al. [58] estimated a safe drilling zone from the anterior glenoid rim. An angle of <28° of medial inclination in the axial plane and <29° of inclination in the caudocranial direction (coronal plane) were safe to avoid inadvertent SSN injuries.

In the event of noticing a suprascapular nerve injury within the first 2 weeks of postoperative follow-up, this is managed with an urgent computed tomography (CT) scan to assess the position of the screws. If the superior screw is long and incorrectly positioned, then the patient is scheduled for urgent removal of this screw and insertion of another screw in a more caudal direction. If the CT scan shows that the screw is correctly placed, then the patient is monitored for clinical recovery [57].

4.16 Glenohumeral Arthritis

A long-term potential consequence of the Latarjet procedure is glenohumeral arthritis. Domos et al. [59] reported that the rate of arthritis development after the open Latarjet procedure was 20% at 20 years. In the same study, it was observed that among patients who had preexisting arthritis related to shoulder instability events, 50% of them showed progression of arthrosis. With a multivariate logistic regression analysis, older age at the time of the final follow-up, participation in high-demand sports, and lateral overhang of the coracoid graft were significantly associated with postoperative arthritis. In a radiological and clinical follow-up after an open Latarjet procedure, Gordins et al. [60] found mild arthropathy in 27% of the patients, moderate in 23% and severe in 11%, after 33 years of follow-up, according to the Samilson and Prieto classification system. The most significant predictor of arthropathy was being 23 years or older at the first dislocation. Longo et al. [60], in a systematic review, found no significant difference between the rates of osteoarthritis after bone block procedures and Bankart repairs (Fig. 4.7).

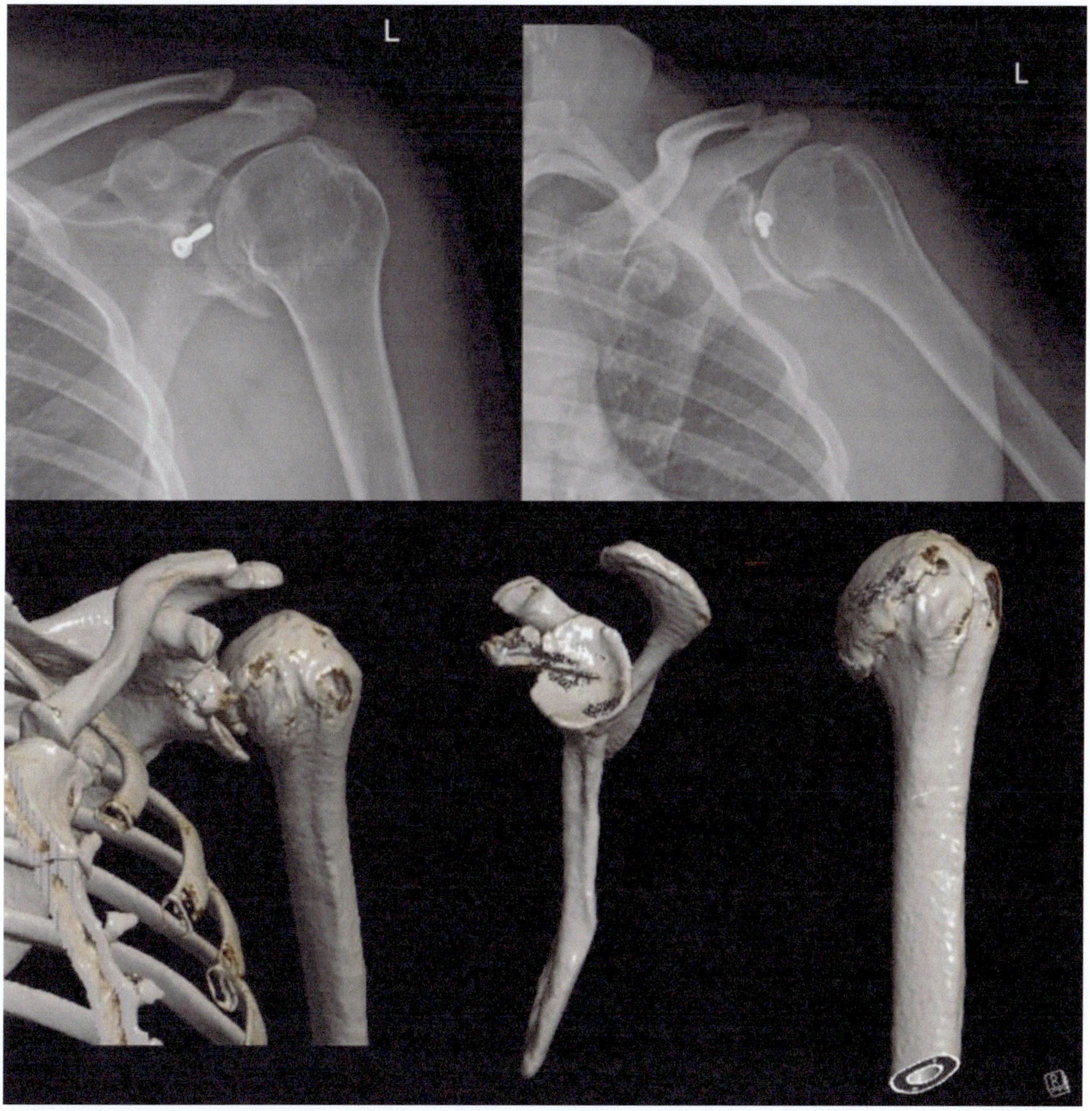

Fig. 4.7 X-rays and CT scans of a 10-year follow-up of a complication after Latarjet surgery. Note the intraarticular position of the screw and clear changes of glenohumeral arthritis

The main limitation of any study attempting to quantify arthropathy after the Latarjet procedure, whether open or arthroscopic, is that it is very difficult to distinguish the natural evolution of posttraumatic arthropathy from dislocation-related arthropathy associated with the surgical procedure [61].

Technical errors, such as lateral overhang of the coracoid process, are also a cause of postoperative arthritis. It is recommended to verify the final position of the coracoid by visualization and palpation. If there is overhang, the graft's position should be adjusted, or the surface of the bone block should be trimmed with a high-speed burr. Additionally, it's important to avoid the intraarticular placement of screws and screw washers in relation to reducing the risk of degenerative changes later [61].

4.17 Conclusion

The Latarjet procedure and its evolution reflect directly on the knowledge and treatment of anterior shoulder instability. Armed biomechanically with a triple effect, it provides stability by augmenting the glenoid track to restore mid-range stability, adds the conjoint tendon as a sling to the anterior capsular structures and recreates the capsular closure to ensure maximum-range shoulder stability. It has withstood the time and follow-up in high volume studies, with a recurrence rate as low as 1% and proved low rate of complications. However, the procedure has an important learning curve to allow proper coracoid exposure and graft preparation, as well as to avoid misplacement of the graft at the moment of fixation.

With the advent of new technologies and better understanding of the surgical process, the Latarjet procedure has proved its value in well indicated patients with anterior shoulder instability and with or without glenoid bone loss. New horizons open with the relatively new arthroscopic-assisted technique and studies focusing on its effectiveness and safety in patients with no glenoid bone loss.

References

1. Latarjet M. A propos du traitement des luxations récidivantes de l'épaule. Lyon Chir. 1954;49(8):994–7.
2. Young AA, Maia R, Berhouet J, Walch G. Open Latarjet procedure for management of bone loss in anterior instability of the glenohumeral joint. J Shoulder Elbow Surg. 2011;20:S61–9.
3. Giles JW, Boons HW, Elkinson I, Faber KJ, Ferreira LM, Johnson JA, et al. Does the dynamic sling effect of the Latarjet procedure improve shoulder stability? A biomechanical evaluation. J Shoulder Elb Surg. 2013;22(6):821–7.
4. Lafosse L, Boyle S. Arthroscopic Latarjet procedure. J Shoulder Elbow Surg. 2010;19:2–12.
5. Joshi MA, Young AA, Balestro JC, Walch G. The Latarjet-Patte procedure for recurrent anterior shoulder instability in contact athletes, vol. 46. Orthop Clin N Am; 2015. p. 105–11.
6. Itoi E. "On-track" and "off-track" shoulder lesions. EFORT Open Rev. 2017;2(8):343–51.
7. Yamamoto N, Muraki T, An KN, Sperling JW, Cofield RH, Itoi E, et al. The stabilizing mechanism of the latarjet procedure: a cadaveric study. J Bone Joint Surg. 2013;95(15):1390–7.
8. Di Giacomo G, Costantini A, De Gasperis N, De Vita A, Lin BKH, Francone M, et al. Coracoid graft osteolysis after the Latarjet procedure for anteroinferior shoulder instability: a computed tomography scan study of twenty-six patients. J Shoulder Elb Surg. 2011;20(6):989–95.
9. Rauck RC, Brusalis CM, Jahandar A, Lamplot JD, Dines DM, Warren RF, et al. Complete restoration of native glenoid width improves Glenohumeral biomechanics after simulated Latarjet. Am J Sports Med. 2023;51(8):2023–9.
10. Burkhart SS, De Beer JF, Barth JRH, Criswell T, Roberts C, Richards DP. Results of modified Latarjet reconstruction in patients with anteroinferior instability and significant bone loss. Arthroscopy. 2007;23(10):1033–41.
11. Di Giacomo G, Itoi E, Burkhart SS. Evolving concept of bipolar bone loss and the hill-sachs lesion: from "engaging/non-engaging" lesion to "on-track/off-track" lesion. Arthroscopy. 2014;30(1):90–8.
12. Dickens JF, Owens BD, Cameron KL, DeBerardino TM, Masini BD, Peck KY, et al. The effect of subcritical bone loss and exposure on recurrent instability after arthroscopic Bankart repair in intercollegiate American football. Am J Sports Med. 2017;45(8):1769–75.
13. Shin SJ, Kim RG, Jeon YS, Kwon TH. Critical value of anterior glenoid bone loss that leads to recurrent Glenohumeral instability after arthroscopic Bankart repair. Am J Sports Med. 2017;45(9):1975–81.
14. Burkhart SS, De Beer JF. Traumatic glenohumeral bone defects and their relationship to failure of

arthroscopic Bankart repairs: significance of the inverted-pear glenoid and the humeral engaging Hill-Sachs lesion. Arthroscopy. 2000;16(7):677–94.
15. Walch G. What I've learned? J Shoulder Elbow Surg. 2019;28:1214–6.
16. Rossi LA, Tanoira I, Gorodischer T, Pasqualini I, Ranalletta M. Recurrence and revision rates with arthroscopic Bankart repair compared with the Latarjet procedure in competitive Rugby players with glenohumeral instability and a glenoid bone loss <20%. Am J Sports Med. 2021;49(4):866–72.
17. Brandariz RN, Gorodischer TD, Pasqualini I, Rossi LA, Tanoira I, Ranalletta M. The Latarjet procedure without Remplissage is effective to restore stability in athletes with glenoid bone defects greater than 25% and off-Track Hill-Sachs lesions. Arthroscopy. 2021;37(8):2455–61.
18. Gowd AK, Liu JN, Polce EM, Agarwalla A, Garcia GH, Nicholson GP, et al. Return to sport following Latarjet glenoid reconstruction for anterior shoulder instability. J Shoulder Elb Surg. 2021;30(11):2549–59.
19. Balg F, Boileau P. The instability severity index score: a simple pre-operative score to select patients for arthroscopic or open shoulder stabilisation. J Bone Joint Surgery Ser B. 2007;89(11):1470–7.
20. Di Giacomo G, Peebles LA, Pugliese M, Dekker TJ, Golijanin P, Sanchez A, et al. Glenoid track instability management score: radiographic modification of the instability severity index score. Arthroscopy. 2020;36(1):56–67.
21. Di Giacomo G, Pugliese M, Lie DTT, Chou ACC, Chen J, Rosenberg N, et al. How to handle minor and major bone loss in the shoulder? Current concepts. J ISAKOS. 2020;5(3):117–22.
22. Kay J, Memon M, Hu T, Simunovic N, Duong A, Paul J, et al. Suprascapular nerve blockade for postoperative pain control after arthroscopic shoulder surgery: a systematic review and meta-analysis. Orthop J Sports Med. 2018;6:2325967118815859.
23. Quintero ID, Buitrago ER, Ballesteros LE. The innervation of the biceps brachii and brachialis muscles in specimens with a high incidence of an accessory biceps head. J Hand Surg Eur Vol. 2022;47(7):761–5.
24. Hamel A, Hamel O, Ploteau S, Robert R, Rogez JM, Malinge M. The arterial supply of the coracoid process. Surg Radiol Anat. 2012;34(7):599.
25. Birmingham P, Sperling JW, Craig E. Glenoid exposure in shoulder arthroplasty. Tech Shoulder Elbow Surg. 2010;11:92.
26. Gilat R, Lavoie-Gagne O, Haunschild ED, Knapik DM, Parvaresh KC, Fu MC, et al. Outcomes of the Latarjet procedure with minimum 5- and 10-year follow-up: a systematic review. Shoulder Elbow. 2020;12(5):315.
27. Griesser MJ, Harris JD, McCoy BW, Hussain WM, Jones MH, Bishop JY, et al. Complications and re-operations after Bristow-Latarjet shoulder stabilization: a systematic review. J Shoulder Elb Surg. 2013;22:286–92.
28. Zimmermann SM, Scheyerer MJ, Farshad M, Catanzaro S, Rahm S, Gerber C. Long-term restoration of anterior shoulder stability: a retrospective analysis of arthroscopic Bankart repair versus open Latarjet procedure. J Bone Joint Surg Am Vol. 2016;98:1954–61.
29. Hurley ET, Shazil Jamal M, Ali ZS, Montgomery C, Pauzenberger L, Mullett H. Long-term outcomes of the Latarjet procedure for anterior shoulder instability: a systematic review of studies at 10-year follow-up. J Shoulder Elb Surg. 2018;28:e33–9. https://doi.org/10.1016/j.jse.2018.08.028.
30. Scanlon JP, Hurley ET, Davey MS, Gaafar M, Pauzenberger L, Moran CJ, et al. 90-day complication rate after the Latarjet procedure in a high-volume center. Am J Sports Med. 2020;48(14):3467–71.
31. Frank RM, Gregory B, O'Brien M, Bernardoni E, Verma NN, Cole BJ, et al. Ninety-day complications following the Latarjet procedure. J Shoulder Elb Surg. 2019;28(1):88–94.
32. Kee YM, Kim JY, Kim HJ, Lim CT, Rhee YG. Return to sports after the latarjet procedure: high return level of non-collision athletes. Knee Surg Sports Traumatol Arthrosc. 2018;26(3):919–25.
33. Sridharan M, Patel A, Swinehart S, Rauck R, Cvetanovich G, Bishop J. Paper 10: return-to-play following Latarjet procedure in young contact athletes. Orthop J Sports Med. 2023;11(3_Suppl 2):2325967123S0001.
34. Hurley ET, Lunn K, Bethell M, Levin J, Pasqualini I, Frangiamore S, et al. Return to play following operative management of anterior shoulder instability in overhead athletes—a systematic review, vol. 16; 2024. p. 15.
35. Lädermann A, Lubbeke A, Stern R, Cunningham G, Bellotti V, Gazielly DF. Risk factors for dislocation arthropathy after Latarjet procedure: a long-term study. Int Orthop. 2013;37(6):1093–8.
36. Mook WR, Petri M, Greenspoon JA, Horan MP, Dornan GJ, Millett PJ. Clinical and anatomic predictors of outcomes after the latarjet procedure for the treatment of anterior glenohumeral instability with combined glenoid and humeral bone defects. Am J Sports Med. 2016;44(6):1407–16.
37. Nourissat G, Neyton L, Metais P, Clavert P, Villain B, Haeni D, et al. Functional outcomes after open versus arthroscopic Latarjet procedure: a prospective comparative study. Orthop Traumatol Surg Res. 2016;102(8):S277–9.
38. An VVG, Sivakumar BS, Phan K, Trantalis J. A systematic review and meta-analysis of clinical and patient-reported outcomes following two procedures for recurrent traumatic anterior instability of the shoulder: Latarjet procedure vs. Bankart repair. J Shoulder Elbow Surg. 2016;25(5):853–63.
39. Werthel JD, Sabatier V, Schoch B, Amsallem L, Nourissat G, Valenti P, et al. Outcomes of the Latarjet procedure for the treatment of chronic

anterior shoulder instability: patients with prior arthroscopic Bankart repair versus primary cases. Am J Sports Med. 2020;48(1):27–32.
40. Calvo E, Dzidzishvili L, Valencia M, Calvo C. Outcomes of arthroscopic Latarjet as a revision surgery after failed arthroscopic Bankart repair. A case-control study. Am J Sports Med. 2024;52(1):190–200.
41. Kukkonen J, Elamo S, Flinkkilä T, Paloneva J, Mäntysaari M, Joukainen A, et al. Arthroscopic Bankart versus open Latarjet as a primary operative treatment for traumatic anteroinferior instability in young males: a randomised controlled trial with 2-year follow-up. Br J Sports Med. 2022;56(6):327–33.
42. Flinkkilä T, Knape R, Nevalainen M, Sirniö K, Ohtonen P, Leppilahti J. Previous arthroscopic Bankart repair is an independent risk factor for an inferior outcome after Latarjet procedure. Orthop Traumatol Surg Res. 2019;105:1481–5. https://doi.org/10.1016/j.otsr.2019.06.020.
43. Ernstbrunner L, De Nard B, Olthof M, Beeler S, Bouaicha S, Gerber C, et al. Long-term results of the arthroscopic Bankart repair for recurrent anterior shoulder instability in patients older than 40 years: a comparison with the open Latarjet procedure. Am J Sports Med. 2020;48(9):2090–6.
44. Zimmermann SM, Scheyerer MJ, Farshad M, Catanzaro S, Rahm S, Gerber C. Long-term restoration of anterior shoulder stability: a retrospective analysis of arthroscopic Bankart repair versus open Latarjet procedure. J Bone Joint Surg Am. 2016;98:1954–61.
45. An VV, Sivakumar BS, Phan K, Trantalis J. A systematic review and meta-analysis of clinical and patient-reported outcomes following two procedures for recurrent traumatic anterior instability of the shoulder: Latarjet procedure vs. Bankart repair. J Shoulder Elbow Surg. 2016;25(5):853–63. https://doi.org/10.1016/j.jse.2015.11.001. Epub 2016 Jan 19. PMID: 26809355.
46. Ali J, Altintas B, Pulatkan A, Boykin RE, Aksoy DO, Bilsel K. Open versus arthroscopic Latarjet procedure for the treatment of chronic anterior Glenohumeral instability with glenoid bone loss. Arthroscopy. 2020;36(4):940–9.
47. Randelli P, Fossati C, Stoppani C, Evola FR, De Girolamo L. Open Latarjet versus arthroscopic Latarjet: clinical results and cost analysis. Knee Surg Sports Traumatol Arthrosc. 2016;24(2):526–32.
48. Zhu Y, Jiang C, Song G. Arthroscopic versus open Latarjet in the treatment of recurrent anterior shoulder dislocation with marked glenoid bone loss: a prospective comparative study. Am J Sports Med. 2017;45(7):1645–53.
49. Deng Z, Zheng Y, Su J, Chen S, Deng Z, Zhu W, Li Y, Lu W. Open versus arthroscopic Latarjet for recurrent anterior shoulder instability: a systematic review and meta-analysis. Orthop J Sports Med. 2023;11(5):23259671231174476. https://doi.org/10.1177/23259671231174476. PMID: 37346777; PMCID: PMC10280521.
50. Cunningham G, Benchouk S, Kherad O, Lädermann A. Comparison of arthroscopic and open Latarjet with a learning curve analysis. Knee Surg Sports Traumatol Arthrosc. 2016;24(2):540–5. Available from: https://pubmed.ncbi.nlm.nih.gov/26658571/
51. Horner NS, Moroz PA, Bhullar R, Habib A, Simunovic N, Wong I, et al. Open versus arthroscopic Latarjet procedures for the treatment of shoulder instability: a systematic review of comparative studies. BMC Musculoskelet Disord. 2018;19(1) Available from: https://pubmed.ncbi.nlm.nih.gov/30045745/
52. Hurley ET, Davey MS, Montgomery C, O'Doherty R, Gaafar M, Pauzenberger L, Mullett H. Arthroscopic Bankart repair versus open Latarjet for first-time dislocators in athletes. Orthop J Sports Med. 2021;9(8):23259671211023803. https://doi.org/10.1177/23259671211023803. PMID: 34485583; PMCID: PMC8414621.
53. LaPrade CM, Bernhardson AS, Aman ZS, Moatshe G, Chahla J, Dornan GJ, et al. Changes in the neurovascular anatomy of the shoulder after an open Latarjet procedure: defining a surgical safe zone. Am J Sports Med. 2018;46(9):2185–91.
54. Southam JD, Greis PE. Delayed, transient musculocutaneous nerve palsy after the Latarjet procedure. J Shoulder Elb Surg. 2012;21(5):e8.
55. Freehill MT, Srikumaran U, Archer KR, McFarland EG, Petersen SA. The Latarjet coracoid process transfer procedure: alterations in the neurovascular structures. J Shoulder Elb Surg. 2013;22(5):695–700.
56. Sastre S, Peidro L, Méndez A, Calvo E. Suprascapular nerve palsy after arthroscopic Latarjet procedure: a case report and review of literature. Knee Surg Sports Traumatol Arthroscop. 2016;24:601–3.
57. Gupta A, Delaney R, Petkin K, Lafosse L. Complications of the Latarjet procedure. Curr Rev Musculoskelet Med. 2015;8:59–66.
58. Shishido H, Kikuchi S. Injury of the suprascapular nerve in shoulder surgery: an anatomic study. J Shoulder Elb Surg. 2001;10(4):372–6.
59. Domos P, Lunini E, Walch G. Contraindications and complications of the Latarjet procedure. Shoulder Elbow. 2018;10:15–24.
60. Gordins V, Hovelius L, Sandström B, Rahme H, Bergström U. Risk of arthropathy after the Bristow-Latarjet repair: A radiologic and clinical thirty-three to thirty-five years of follow-up of thirty-one shoulders. J Shoulder Elb Surg. 2015;24(5):691–9.
61. Longo UG, Loppini M, Rizzello G, Ciuffreda M, Berton A, Maffulli N, et al. Remplissage, humeral osteochondral grafts, weber osteotomy, and shoulder arthroplasty for the management of humeral bone defects in shoulder instability: systematic review and quantitative synthesis of the literature. Arthroscopy. 2014;30:1650–66.

Arthroscopic Latarjet

5

Mirek Karel, Hean Wu Kang, Christopher Child, Kenneth Cutbush, Emilio Calvo, and Ashish Gupta

5.1 Introduction

The Latarjet procedure is common procedure for anterior shoulder instability in individuals participating in physically demanding activities or contact sports, especially those with glenoid bone loss or as revision surgery after a failed Bankart procedure. Traumatic glenohumeral dislocation is a prevalent shoulder injury, with incidence rates of 1.7–2% in the general population aged 18–70 years and 11.2–56.3/100,000 person-years [1] and even higher in the young athletic population [2]. The Latarjet procedure is indicated in patients with a high risk of postoperative recurrent instability [3]. The Latarjet procedure, initially described by M. Latarjet in 1954 [4], involves the transfer of the coracoid process with its conjoined tendon to the anterior glenoid rim for addressing recurrent anterior shoulder dislocation. Traditionally performed through an open deltopectoral approach, Lafosse introduced an arthroscopic Latarjet procedure in 2007 [5]. The primary indication for the Latarjet procedure is glenoid bone loss, while significant contraindications include glenoid bone loss exceeding the correctable range by a coracoid transfer [6, 7].

The Latarjet procedure achieves glenohumeral joint stability through three main mechanisms also called the triple-blocking effect: first, extending the glenoid arc with a bone block to replace lost or damaged anterior bone; second, using the conjoined tendon as a dynamic sling to resist anterior humeral translation during arm movement; and third, creating a tenodesis effect by transferring the conjoined tendon and coracoid process over the subscapularis tendon to reinforce the deficient anteroinferior capsule [5, 8]. Both open and arthroscopic Latarjet procedures have demonstrated excellent patient functional outcomes with low incidences of recurrent instability [8–10]. However, despite the favorable clinical outcomes, both approaches report similar overall complication rates between 6% [11] and 23.7% [3, 9]. Although more recent findings indicate a complication range more close to 4–7% when performed by high-volume practitioners [3, 12].

M. Karel · H. W. Kang · C. Child · K. Cutbush
Queensland Unit for Advanced Shoulder Research (QUASR), Queensland University of Technology, Brisbane, QLD, Australia

E. Calvo
Department of Orthopedic Surgery and Traumatology, Hospital Universitario Fundacion Jimenez, Universidad Autonoma, Madrid, Spain

A. Gupta (✉)
Queensland Unit for Advanced Shoulder Research QUASR, Queensland University of Technology, Brisbane, QLD, Australia

Greenslopes Private Hospital, Brisbane, QLD, Australia
e-mail: ashish@qoc.com.au

E. Calvo et al. (eds.), *Complex and Revision Problems in Shoulder Instability*, https://doi.org/10.1007/978-3-031-81389-4_5

Advantages of the arthroscopic Latarjet procedure include enhanced visualization for precise coracoid graft positioning, the capability to address intra-articular pathologies, reduced potential for postoperative scar tissue and stiffness, as well as benefits such as less pain, improved cosmesis, decreased stiffness, and faster functional recovery when compared to the open procedure [8, 13, 14]. Disadvantages of the arthroscopic Latarjet include increased surgical time and cost, with the procedure being more technically challenging compared to the traditional open approach, leading to reluctance in adopting this technique [6, 14]. Despite requiring advanced surgical skills the arthroscopic Latarjet demonstrates a manageable learning curve and shows fewer complications with increasing experience [14].

5.2 Preoperative Evaluation

Pathological changes after a first anterior dislocation predispose patients to recurrent instability. These changes include anteroinferior labrum avulsion (Bankart lesion), glenoid bony defects (bony Bankart), and posterosuperior humeral head or Hill-Sachs lesions. Bone graft stabilization procedures are recommended for glenoid bone loss over 15% to ensure successful postoperative outcomes [15]. Meta-analyses have indicated that risk factors for recurrence after arthroscopic Bankart repair include age $\leq$ 20 years, age $\leq$ 30 years, engagement in competitive sports, presence of Hill-Sachs lesion, off-track Hill-Sachs lesion, glenoid bone loss, anterior labroligamentous periosteal sleeve avulsion (ALPSA) lesion, more than one preoperative dislocation, surgical delay exceeding 6 months from the first-time dislocation to surgery, greater than 3, and ISIS greater than 6 [16]. Therefore, It is very important to identify the soft tissue lesions and the extent of glenoid and humeral bone loss preoperatively.

5.3 Indications and Contraindications

The decision to recommend a Latarjet procedure for a patient is multifactorial, primarily dependent upon the presence of glenoid bone loss. Young age, glenoid and/or humeral bone loss, a history of dislocation, and failed arthroscopic stabilization surgeries are relative indications for the procedure, with recent studies showing excellent clinical outcomes with careful patient selection and complication rates ranging from 4% to 7% in high-volume users [10, 12, 17]. Careful patient selection based on these indications is essential to enhance clinical outcomes and ensure patient satisfaction. An international consensus statement in 2022 supports the use of the Latarjet procedure in patients at high risk of postoperative recurrent instability, with a strong consensus (97%) indicating primary relative indications are (1) recurrent instability, (2) failed prior surgery, (3) collision athlete status, (4) significant glenoid bone loss (>15–20%), and (5) bipolar bone loss leading to an "off-track" lesion [3]. Bipolar bone loss refers to the presence of bone defects in both the glenoid rim and the head of the humerus (Hill-Sachs lesion) [18]. On the other hand, the primary relative contraindications include multidirectional instability, voluntary dislocators, uncontrolled epilepsy or seizure disorders, irreparable rotator cuff tears, and excessive glenoid bone loss beyond coracoid transfer capabilities, which warrant careful consideration before proceeding with the Latarjet procedure [3].

5.4 Diagnostic Imaging

Computed tomorgraphy (CT) imaging plays an important role in assessing patients for significant glenoid bone loss or other bony lesions. Specifically, the "en face" sagittal view with three-dimensional (3D) reconstruction allows for accurate assessment of glenoid dysplasia, bony Bankart lesions, and glenoid bone loss.

5.5 Glenoid Bone Loss

The extent of glenoid bone loss plays a crucial role in determining the choice between soft-tissue and bony reconstruction in the treatment of anterior shoulder instability. The estimated prevalence of glenoid bone loss varies; nonetheless, studies indicate that after an acute anterior instability event, 22% of patients display some degree of anterior glenoid bone loss, while up to 86% of patients with recurrent anterior instability also exhibit such bone loss [19].

Burkhart and De Beer [20] introduced the concept of "significant bone loss" as a crucial factor influencing the risk of failure in arthroscopic stabilization, emphasizing the anatomic relationship between bone loss on the humeral head and glenoid in critical positions. Critical bone loss was initially established 20–25% based on cadaveric studies [21, 22]. Today, the understanding of critical bone loss has evolved further to include what is now termed as "subcritical" glenoid bone loss, which has been shown to result in increased rates of failure in soft-tissue stabilization, particularly in cases with glenoid bone defects ranging from 13.5% to 17.3% [19, 23, 24]. This lower subcritical threshold prompts a shift in the treatment algorithm towards bony procedures like the coracoid graft (Latarjet procedure), iliac graft, or allograft [25].

5.6 Hill Sachs Lesions

Another important factor in determining the surgical treatment of anterior instability is the presence and the size of a Hill-Sachs lesion and whether it is an off-track Hill-Sachs lesion. The extent of glenoid bone loss correlates with a decrease in the glenoid track and an elevated risk of engagement. This suggests that both articular surfaces should be assessed collectively to ascertain a patient's susceptibility to dislocation [26]. The reported overall prevalence of Hill-Sachs defects is 50% with primary instability and 67% up to 90% in recurrent anterior shoulder instability [27, 28]. To determine if a Hill Sachs lesion is off track, the width of the glenoid track can be calculated according to the method of Di Giacomo et al. [25] glenoid track = 0.83 × A (glenoid diameter) − B (glenoid defect).

Recently, 3D reconstructions from magnetic resonance imaging (MRI) scans have become available and are comparable to 3D-CT in quantifying bone loss [29, 30]. Advantages of 3D MRI over CT are that MRI can evaluate soft tissue injury and is a radiation-free alternative for patients [29].

Calvo et al. [6] reported the results of arthroscopic Latarjet in a series of 51 shoulders with off-track Hill-Sachs lesions and found that Latarjet surgery was able to convert most off-track Hill-Sachs lesions into on-track Hill-Sachs. However, for 12% of patients with severe bony lesions the Latarjet was not able to restore glenoid track. The persistent postoperative off-track Hill-Sachs group showed a significant higher recurrence rate. Accordingly, the authors suggested adding a *remplissage* to the Latarjet procedure or using different bone techniques such as free bone graft for these shoulders with severe off-track Hill-Sachs lesions not amenable to be converted into on-track by the coracoid graft [6].

5.7 Three-Dimensional Quantification of Glenoid Bone Loss

Accurate quantification of bone loss is crucial for considering and planning surgical procedures and ensuring precise graft placement. Various methods exist to measure bone loss. The Sugaya method, or best-fit circle method, uses 3D reconstructed CT images but relies on two-dimensional (2D) measurements to calculate bone loss as a ratio of defect width to the best-fit circle's diameter based on the inferior glenoid rim [31]. The method by Giles et al. employs CT scans to measure glenoid height and predict native glenoid width, comparing this with actual width to assess bone loss [32]. However, both methods depend on 2D measurements from CT scans or 3D-reconstructed images and do not consider the glenoid's true anatomic surface area. In 2021, Launay et al. introduced the anatomic concave surface area (ACSA) method, which evaluates bone loss by quantifying the actual anatomic 3D surface area of the glenoid by mapping the concavity of the glenoid's 3D anatomic surface [33]. The ACSA method typically shows smaller bone loss percentages than the best-fit circle or height/width methods and minimizes measurement errors from 2D static images of 3D views.

5.8 Graft Fixation Methods

Optimal graft fixation in the Latarjet procedure is crucial for patient outcomes as graft complications such as graft osteolysis, nonunion, and fractures impact clinical results. The all-arthroscopic Latarjet procedure offers fixation methods including double-screw (SS), double-button (BB), and suture-button (SB) techniques. The overall preferred fixation method is the cannulated double-screw (SS) construct [34], but it is associated with a range of complications such as soft tissue irritation, intra- and postoperative fractures of the graft, proximal graft osteolysis, and subsequent screw breakage, due to factors like graft avascularity and stress shielding [35–37]. Moreover, imprecise screw placement and length have been correlated with higher complication rates, such as suprascapular nerve injury in the case of excessively long screws, and compromised stability leading to graft migration or nonunion with short screws [38, 39]. Therefore, BB fixation has been introduced as an alternative, aiming to enhance micromotion for improved bone union without the risk of hardware problems. On the other hand, the SB technique combines a single cannulated screw with a cortical suture button. Similarly, this fixation approach aims to promote graft micromotion and foster osteogenesis between the bone block and glenoid neck [40]. However, BB and SB fixations have been associated with fibrous nonunion. Previous biomechanical studies, involving both tensile and compressive testing, compared the mechanical strength of SS and BB fixation constructs [41]. Kazum et al. found no significant differences in failure load between SS and BB constructs in tensile testing on cadaveric specimens [41]. Saleky et al. observed no differences in failure load, elongation, or graft stiffness during compressive testing [42]. Williams et al. [43] reported significantly higher failure loads and lower graft displacement for SS compared to BB constructs, findings confirmed by Ziegenfuss et al. [40], which demonstrated that SS grafts withstood greater isolated loads, displaced less, and had longer survival times than BB constructs. The SB technique to balance structural strength and flexibility. flexibility, as it required significantly greater load and longer time to undergo graft displacement failure than the BB construct, but it was not as rigid as the SS construct, providing the potential to decrease the risk of graft osteolysis and other screw-related complications [40].

5.9 Surgical Technique

5.9.1 Anesthesia and Positioning

For anesthesia and positioning, general anesthesia combined with a regional nerve block is preferred. The patient is prepared similarly to a standard shoulder arthroscopic procedure, with particular attention to exposing a wider area medially for the most medial (M) portal. The patient is positioned in the beach chair position. Key technical considerations include securing the arm in an arm holder/positioner or is held by an assistant to avoid traction and have better positioning option. Important is to support the medial border of the scapula with a back support to facilitate posterior rotation of the scapula. This aids in laterally positioning the glenoid face and facilitates bone graft fixation to the glenoid. Additionally, it is crucial to check the joint line and assess the ideal location of the M portal.

5.9.2 Portals

Portal A: Standard posterior

Portal E: Standard anterior to access the rotator interval (RI)

Portal D: Anterolateral at the level of the anterolateral corner of the acromion

Portal I: Aligned with the coracoid process, just above the axillary fold

Portal J: Between I and D portal, parallel to the subscapularis fibers

Portal M: The most medial and anterior portal through the pectoralis major, aligned with the glenoid face. Check joint line and position M portal just after positioning

Portal H: Anterosuperior portal just above and slightly medial to the coracoid

5.9.3 Surgical Steps

The first all-arthroscopic Latarjet procedure was described by Lafosse et al. [5]. Today, current techniques are still the same or modifications regarding repair of the anterior capsule, the subscapularis split and graft fixation techniques. In brief, the authors' preference is positioning patients in beach chair with or without the use of a limb positioner. Portals are established as described by Lafosse et al. [5] using the A, D, J, I, H, and M portals. After arthroscopic intra-articular evaluation with 30° scope the anterior labrum and capsule are detached with or without preservation for later repair. First care has been taken to identify all anterior structures such as the subscapularis, coracoid, coracoacromial (CA) ligament, musculo cutaneous nerve, and axillary nerve. The J portal is created, enabling coracoid preparation while visualized from the I portal. The CA ligament is detached, and the pectoralis minor muscle is released medially from the coracoid. Both the axillary nerve and musculocutaneous nerve are identified. The coracoid graft is cleared from soft tissue. A small 5 mm burr is introduced through the M portal to carefully prepare the undersurface of the coracoid. The burr is used to create a flat coracoid undersurface matching the anterior glenoid to enhance healing. Subsequently, two 1.5 mm K wires are inserted through the superior H portal using a cannulated top hat drill system using the H portal (Fig. 5.1). The authors' preferred technique involves using a single button superiorly and a screw inferiorly. A single top hat is inserted inferiorly for the cannulated screw. Using the H portal a coracoid osteotomy is carefully performed to prevent intraoperative graft fracture. This is a very critical step and care must be taken so that the osteotomy does not breech the superior screw hole.

Once the osteotomy is performed, the Mitek Latarjet guide (DePuy Mitek, Raynham, MA) is introduced through the M portal, and the coracoid is prepared using a burr from the D portal. Visualization is achieved through the J portal (Fig. 5.2). The bursa in front of the subscapularis is cleared, and the axillary nerve, anterior cir-

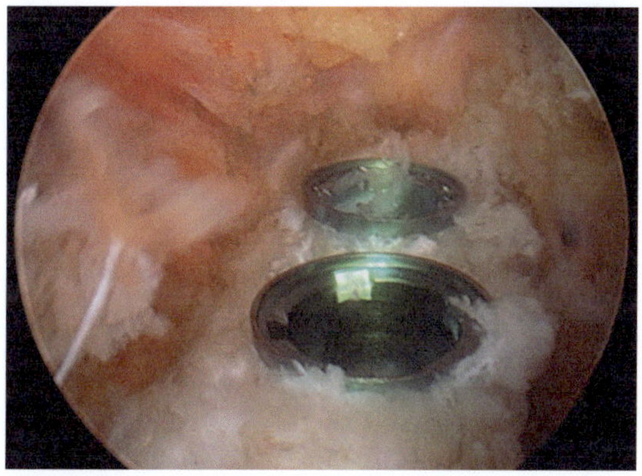

Fig. 5.1 Top hats inserted through coracoid process

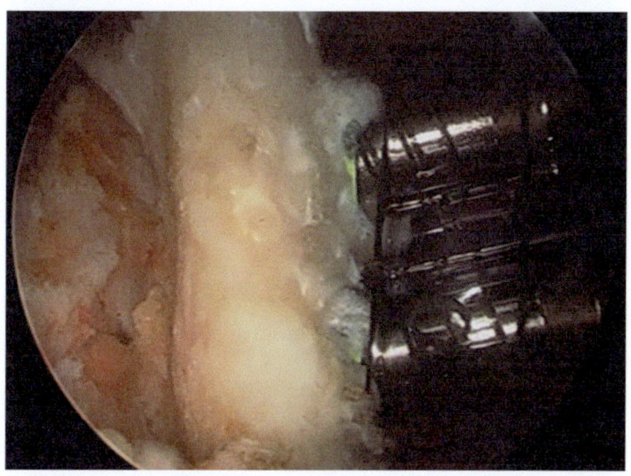

Fig. 5.2 Coracoid graft after the osteotomy attached to the double barrel transparent cannula (DePuy Mitek, Raynham, MA). The cannula permits coracoid handling and driving into the joint

cumflex vessels, and biceps groove are identified. The arm is internally rotated to avoid injury to the axillary nerve. A subscapularis split is performed from medial to lateral with constant visualization of the axillary nerve. Typically, a 2/3–1/3 subscapularis split is performed (Fig. 5.3). Once the subscapularis is split, two switching sticks are introduced—one from the transarticular portal and the second from an accessory I portal—to keep the subscapularis split retracted. Final glenoid neck preparation is then carried out (Fig. 5.4).

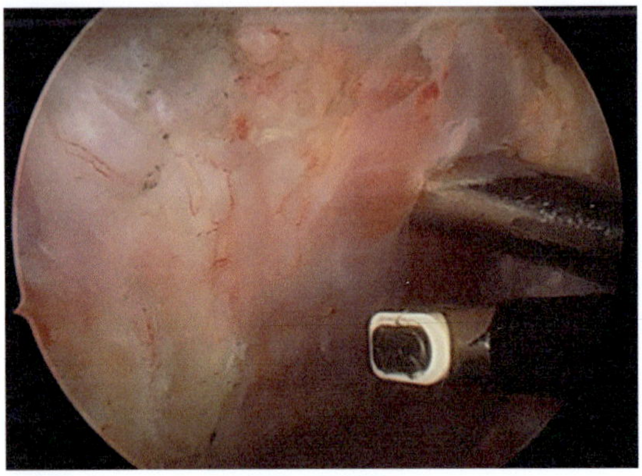

Fig. 5.3 Split level definition between the superior 2/3 and the inferior 1/3. Note the Wissinger rod is inserted from the posterior portal and piercing the subscapularis muscle at the level of the inferior glenoid equator

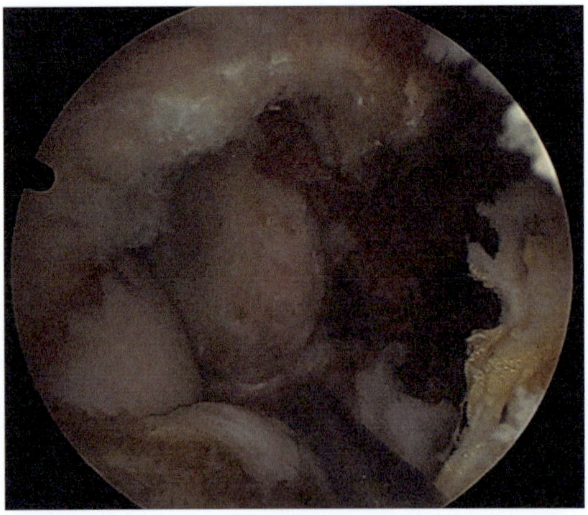

Fig. 5.4 Superior and inferior subscapularis are retracted after the split showing the access to the anterior glenoid rim which has been abraded

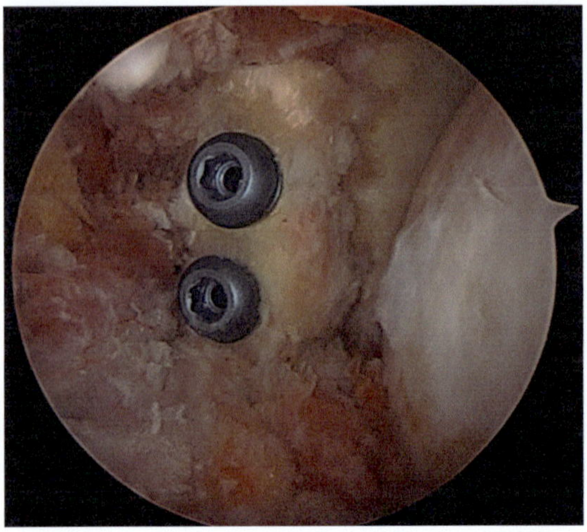

Fig. 5.5 Final appearance of the coracoid graft fixed with screws on the inferior equator of the glenoid. The graft should be positioned flush with the articular surface

The coracoid graft is then placed through the subscapularis split, viewed from the D portal. The graft is positioned with two K wires flush with the anterior glenoid surface, using the glenoid cartilage as the reference point during surgery to avoid any lateral overhang. Fixation of the graft onto the glenoid vault, between 3–5 o'clock (right shoulder) or 7–9 o'clock (left shoulder), is achieved using double-screw (SS), double-button (BB), or suture-button (SB) techniques (Fig. 5.5). Lastly, the anterior labral repair can be performed with two anchors, resulting in an extra-articular graft. The necessity of capsular and labral repair remains uncertain, and although not obligatory in every instance, it might offer benefits to certain patients [3].

5.10 Special Circumstances

5.10.1 Latarjet with Remplissage for Hill-Sachs Defects

When encountering a large engaging Hill-Sachs lesion, the authors prefer to pass the remplissage sutures at the beginning of the procedure. This approach has two benefits:

1. Once the remplissage sutures are passed through the rotator cuff, they serve as traction sutures, helping to distract the humeral head posteriorly. This creates space anteriorly, facilitating easier glenoid preparation.
2. At the end of the arthroscopic Latarjet, the subacromial space often swells due to fluid accumulation, making the remplissage procedure time-consuming and difficult if performed later.
3. Remplissage helps improve the symptoms of subluxation and associated instability which a Latarjet does not address in young patients who are often a bit ligamentous lax.

Visualization is carried out from the D portal, and a B portal is created to perform the remplissage. The anchor can be inserted through the A portal or an accessory posterior portal to ensure the correct trajectory. The arm should be maximally internally rotated to position the anchor perpendicular to the Hill-Sachs lesion. The authors prefer using PEEK anchors to avoid anchor pullout, as the cortical bone is deficient and weak in a Hill-Sachs lesion. They typically perform a single-anchor remplissage positioned at the junction of the supraspinatus and infraspinatus, allowing the humeral head to be tugged postero-superiorly. This approach helps avoid the subjective feeling of subluxation by the patient in conjunction with a Latarjet procedure.

5.10.2 Latarjet Post Bony Bankart Fracture

A malunited chronic bony Bankart lesion with significant bone loss is a common indication for a Latarjet procedure. Preparing the anterior glenoid neck can be challenging when there is a medialized united bone fragment. The authors recommend visualization from the anterolateral D portal. Using the E and I portals, the rotator interval is excised, an anterior glenoid capsulectomy is performed, and the pathological labrum is removed. The authors suggest using a coracoid osteotome to create an osteotomy at the anterior glenoid neck and separate the malunited fragment, making its removal quicker and easier. Bleeders encountered medial to the fragment usually require transiently raising the fluid pressure to coagulate the medial vessels. The bone fragment is then separated from the medial soft tissues and removed using graspers. A burr can be introduced via the C or I portal to finalize the glenoid preparation.

5.10.3 Latarjet Post Failed Bankart Repair

The Latarjet procedure is often performed as a revision surgery after failed soft tissue stabilization. This is a challenging yet common problem. The authors recommend anterior visualization through the D portal. The anterior glenoid neck and the subscapularis should be visualized both intra- and extra-articular. Using the I and C portals, the coracoid is identified. Exuberant scar tissue is usually present under the coracoid due to anterior recurrent instability. This scar tissue should be removed from the posterior surface of the coracoid, and the rotator interval should be completely excised. The gothic arch of the coracoid needs to be clearly visualized and freed of any scar tissue, which is critical to allow for subscapularis excursion postoperatively.

Following this, a meticulous anterior capsulectomy is performed using a mix of diathermy and a shaver. The labrum is completely excised, and the in situ sutures and anchors can make this step tedious. The authors prefer to introduce a 15-blade from the C portal to cut all the suture material intra-articularly, which makes excision of the scar and sutures much easier. The anchors are left in place unless the anchor heads are prominent, which necessitates removal.

The authors advise preparing the glenoid docking site before introducing the coracoid through the subscapularis. Guide wires are introduced, and screw tunnels are made. Preexisting anchors often cause difficulty in introducing the K wires and can lead to poor bone fixation. In this situation, the button construct is very useful for allowing suspensory fixation using bicortical compression. In the authors' experience, a one-screw, one-button construct is still preferred, but often the bone inferiorly is poor and deficient, necessitating a button inferiorly and a screw superiorly for stable, rotationally stable fixation.

5.11 Outcomes

5.11.1 Postoperative Clinical Outcomes

Arthroscopic Latarjet demonstrates promising results in stability, functional outcomes, and reliability, as reported by Cerciello et al. [8]. Return to sport is shown to be 91–100% of patients treated with arthroscopic Latarjet alongside excellent functional scores, with reliable constant values of the Rowe and Walch-Duplay (WD) scores >90 and a Western Ontario Shoulder Instability Index (WOSI) of 90.6 [27]. Cerciello showed in their study excellent mid-term functional outcomes too with the arthroscopic technique, exhibiting mean WD scores of 89.6 and Rowe scores of 90.2, even surpassing those of the open technique, which had mean WD scores of 90.1 and 84.5, respectively. The difference between arthroscopic and open Latarjet seems more pronounced within the first postoperative days, with reduced pain and analgesic consumption. The WOSI score, known for evaluating postoperative shoulder joint stabilization, has been shown to be more sensitive than the WD score in assessing patient satisfaction [44]. The systematic review and meta-analysis by Deng et al. [45] suggests similar overall outcomes in postoperative pain, function, and complications between arthroscopic Latarjet and open Latarjet procedures. Although arthroscopic Latarjet showed a lower WOSI score compared to open Latarjet, indicating slightly enhanced postoperative stabilization, the evidence is inconclusive due to limited data and potential biases. Theoretically, minimally invasive arthroscopic surgery is less painful for patients in the short term postoperatively, but few studies have reported immediate and short-term visual analogue scale (VAS) pain scores. Only the VAS score at the final follow-up was compared, showing no difference in postoperative pain in the long term [45].

Concerns have been raised regarding postoperative loss of external rotation. Kordasiewicz et al. [46] reported less loss of external rotation in open Latarjet procedures. However, Deng et al. [45] found no significant difference in external rotation between arthroscopic and open Latarjet at the last follow-up. Some authors suggest that restricted external rotation may result from subscapularis damage during the split necessary for precise bone block positioning [47]. On the other hand, Valencia et al. studied the function and structural integrity of subscapularis after arthroscopic Latarjet and reported a significant decrease of isokinetic performance of the muscle in internal rotation that was correlated with lower muscular attenuation. These findings did not result in decreased functional outcomes [48]. Nonetheless, arthroscopic procedures offer an advantage in limiting such damage. To minimize subscapularis damage, a (insulated) switching stick can be employed to identify the split location and perform a safe minimally invasive dissection window with protecting the axillary nerve.

For all of the functional scores Menendez et al. calculated the minimal clinically important difference (MCID) and patient acceptable symptomatic state (PASS) values for commonly used outcome measures to assess the smallest change in a treatment outcome that an individual patient would identify as important and which would indicate a meaningful change among patients undergoing the Latarjet procedure [49]. They found that the MCID and PASS values were, respectively, 9.6 and 86.0 for American Shoulder and Elbow Surgeons (ASES) shoulder score, 12.4 and 82.5 for single assessment numeric evaluation (SANE), 1.7 and 2.5 for VAS pain, and 254.9 and 571.0 for WOSI [49]. These findings are essential for incorporating patient perspectives into the clinical effectiveness of the Latarjet procedure and provide valuable parameters for the design and interpretation of clinical trials.

Lastly in patients with epilepsy, arthroscopic Latarjet stabilization can also lead to improved functional and subjective outcomes and should be considered for those with recurrent anterior glenohumeral instability. These results can be achieved regardless of the presence of bone defects and the postoperative control of seizures and are similar to those in patients without epilepsy [50].

5.11.2 Radiographic Graft Assessment

Graft position in the Latarjet procedure is crucial for its success. Arthroscopic techniques provide superior visualization, facilitating accurate graft placement compared to open procedures. The graft should ideally be flush with the glenoid articular surface to prevent recurrent instability and arthrosis. The extension of the glenoid arc and the sling effect of the conjoined tendon contribute to stability. This also promotes successful integration, indicated by bone bridge formation between the coracoid and glenoid, which is essential to prevent recurrence. Nonunions can be stable or unstable, with different signs of lysis or hardware complications.

To assess graft placement postoperatively, CT scans with 3D and multiplanar reformations offer detailed visualization for assessing bone-block position, with meticulous evaluation in the axial, coronal, and sagittal planes following Kraus et al.'s technique [44, 48, 51]. Especially during the learning curve, critical analysis of graft position can be valuable.

In the axial view, the bone block graft should ideally be flush with the glenoid rim, with an acceptable translation range of 4–5 mm medially [52]. Overhang, placing the graft too lateral, should be avoided at all costs. The lateralization of the bone graft during surgery can lead to increased peak contact pressure [53], potentially causing long-term osteoarthritis due to incongruent interaction between the humeral head cartilage and the graft. Peak contact pressure is particularly concerning between a lateralization of 1.5 and 3.0 mm [53]. The anterior glenoid cartilage thickness measures 2.3 mm (SD, 0.66 mm) [52], and it is noted to be underestimated by CT scan and it is thought that lateralization, measured on CT should not exceed 3 mm [20]. It is emphasized that maintaining the glenoid cartilage as a reference point during surgery is crucial. The advantage of an arthroscopic Latarjet is that graft placement can be accurately assessed intraoperatively in different angles by changing the camera view to different portals.

The precise positioning height in the anteroinferior quarter of the glenoid remains uncertain, with graft height being crucial as the recurrence rate could substantially increase when the coracoid is positioned too high [54]. Some authors caution against placing the bone-block directly over the equator (above 3 or 9 o'clock position) and recommend that the majority of the graft should be subequatorial to decrease the risk of recurrence [54]. Graft height is assessed using the "enface" clock system in the sagittal plane. To assess the graft's height the most superior aspect of the glenoid (tubercle superior = S) and the most inferior aspect of the glenoid (tubercle inferior = I) should be marked. The equator of the glenoid was defined as a line perpendicular to and bifurcating the line connecting points S and I. Several techniques can be addressed to measure the graft height however caution should be taken in interpreting results regarding the coracoid graft position on two-dimensional CT scans [55]. The ideal graft height is targeted subequatorial between 3–5 o'clock for the right shoulder or 7–9 o'clock for the left shoulder [56].

Lastly, screw orientation in relation to the glenoid is important and can be measured in the axial plane, following the methodology proposed by Ladermann et al. [57]. This involves determining the angle between the line connecting the posterior and anterior glenoid rim and the screw axis. When using a two-screw construct, screws should be positioned perpendicular to the glenoid rim without excessive penetration of the posterior cortex. Excess screw length can potentially lead to posterior impingement and suprascapular nerve lesions. Be mindful about the location of the M portal as this highly influences the screw orientation.

5.12 Complications

The literature highlights excellent clinical outcomes associated with the arthroscopic technique [8, 10], yet concerns persist regarding its complication rates, stemming from the procedure's technical complexity and steep learning curve, as highlighted by Bøe et al. [14]. While some initial studies reported a 30% complication rate, some studies indicate a range more close to 4–7% when performed by high-volume surgeons [7, 10]. Despite these challenges, the advantages of arthroscopic Latarjet procedures can serve as a compelling motivation for orthopedic surgeons. With increasing experience, there is potential for a reduction in complication rates and surgical time [14]. Experienced shoulder specialists generally require 30–50 cases to achieve operational efficiency with the arthroscopic Latarjet technique [12]. Surgeons in the early phase of the learning curve should prioritize joint exposure and mastering graft placement. To ensure proficiency, cadaveric training, collaborative surgeries, and surgical visitations are recommended [12]. Surgeons should also be familiar with an open Latarjet procedure in case they have to convert an arthroscopic Latarjet to an open procedure.

In 2022, a consensus statement outlined strategies for reducing complications, including meticulous dissection, precise nerve identification, preventing graft over-lateralization, and contour graft alignment with native cartilage [3]. Additionally, it recommended using tranexamic acid to minimize blood loss, ensuring accurate screw placement, and meticulous preparation of the glenoid neck and coracoid [3]. However, despite concerns over complications and the learning curve, mastering arthroscopic Latarjet techniques, particularly those involving the anterior shoulder and proximity to the plexus, offers valuable skills transferable to other arthroscopic procedures. Nonetheless, it is worth noting that arthroscopic Latarjet is a technically challenging procedure and is only advisable to perform in a high-volume setting. Hence, the decision to pursue arthroscopic Latarjet stabilization should not be solely based on concerns about potential complications and the learning curve.

5.12.1 Intraoperative Complications

The complication rate of arthroscopic Latarjet procedures ranges from 6% to 30%, with graft-related issues being common intraoperative complications. Accurate graft positioning is crucial to avoid complications such as fibrous nonunion, recurrent instability, and secondary osteoarthritis. Grafts placed too medially can increase recurrent instability, whereas those positioned too laterally may lead to early arthritic changes and should be avoided. Arthroscopic Latarjet offers the advantage of improved visualization of the glenoid from different portals, minimizing the risk of incorrect graft placement. Graft fractures, reported to occur at around 1.5%, can be prevented through circular decortication before the coracoid osteotomy. However, caution is necessary to avoid excessive decortication of the coracoid undersurface, which may compromise graft integrity. Among intraoperative complications, conversion to open surgery during arthroscopic Latarjet procedures is rare. Conversion to open is reported to be around 2% of cases, with a higher incidence observed in the initial learning curve [8]. Therefore, in the early stages of learning the procedure, surgeons should remain mindful of the potential to switch to the open technique during surgery. Other potential intraoperative complications may involve vascular and nerve injuries, although the risk of vascular injury, while possible, is relatively low [56].

5.12.2 Nerve Injuries

Reported nerve injury rates range from 0.7% to 1.8%, mostly resulting in transient neurapraxias that resolve without further treatment [27, 56, 58, 59]. During the transfer of the coracoid process in arthroscopic Latarjet procedures, close proximity to adjacent neurovascular structures poses risks to nerves such as the brachial plexus, axillary, musculocutaneous, and suprascapular nerves [14]. Compared to open Latarjet procedures, which carry a higher nerve injury risk of approximately 10% [60], arthroscopic techniques offer enhanced safety for neurovascular structures through direct visualization and magnification. Among the commonly affected nerves are the musculocutaneous and axillary nerves, with axillary nerve lesions frequently associated with coracoid graft transfer and fixation through the subscapularis split [56]. Delayed musculocutaneous nerve palsy remains a well-documented but rare complication of the arthroscopic Latarjet [56]. Prior to the subscapularis split in arthroscopic Latarjet, exploration of both the axillary and musculocutaneous nerves is deemed necessary, even though it may add to procedural time [14].

Transient suprascapular nerve palsy is a known risk, with screws directed towards the scapular spine potentially causing entrapment [57]. To prevent injury, attention should be given to the direction of the superior screw, ensuring it remains within a safe zone estimated by Shishido et al. [61] This safe zone involves an angle of <28° of medial tilt in the axial plane and <29° of inclination in the caudocranial direction (coronal plane). If suprascapular nerve injury is detected within the first 2 weeks postop, a CT scan should be performed to assess screw position. Urgent screw removal is warranted if mispositioned, while monitoring is warranted if placement of the screws are accurate and not protruding.

5.12.3 Early Postoperative Complications

Early postoperative complications of the arthroscopic Latarjet procedure involve hematoma and postoperative swelling, with delayed complications including infection and nerve issues. Hematoma, though infrequent, can be prevented through thorough hemostasis during the procedure. Additionally, a randomized controlled trial by Hurley et al. evaluated the use of tranexamic acid for the Latarjet procedure, where they found tranexamic acid to significantly reduce hematoma grade and subsequent pain levels, leading, in turn, to decreased opioid use [62]. While postoperative swelling is common and typically resolves within the first week, any extension beyond the shoulder or into the neck requires immediate attention and high-dependency monitoring. Implementing preventive measures such as low pump pressure, efficient operating time, and hypotensive anesthesia helps minimize soft tissue insufflation.

Infection risk after arthroscopic Latarjet procedures is very rare, generally ranging from 0.5% to 1.5%, often manifesting as superficial infections [9]. Infection poses a risk to coracoid graft integrity and may lead to instability recurrence, necessitating appropriate antibiotic therapy following thorough irrigation and debridement [56]. In severe cases, complete removal of metalwork may be necessary for complete infection eradication, often alongside an extended course of intravenous antibiotics.

5.12.4 Long-Term Complications

Long-term complications include recurrent instability, nonunion, osteolysis, graft resorption, persistent pain, and osteoarthritis. Recurrent instability postoperatively is reported to be between 0% and 8.3%, with most studies indicating recurrence rates below 4% [27, 63]. Intraoperative graft-related complications, such as placing the graft too medial, graft fractures, and resorption are associated with an increased risk of recurrence [46]. Other reasons for recurrent instability include postoperative trauma and patient factors such as voluntary dislocations, ligamentous laxity, or seizure disorders. Additional risk factors for recurrence include graft avulsion, subscapularis failure, and graft lysis [56]. The arthroscopic approach offers advantages compared to the open approach such as superior graft visualization, crucial for ensuring accurate placement. Notably, Hurley et al. observed no significant difference in recurrence instability rates between arthroscopic and open Latarjet procedures, while Metais et al. found similar rates of postoperative apprehension across various graft fixation methods [9, 59]. A systematic review and meta-analysis by Deng et al. [45], found that there was no statistically significant difference in persistent apprehension between the arthroscopic and open Latarjet at the last follow-up. Recurrences, if they occur, are often seen within the initial 12 months following surgery [58]. Promising outcomes have been reported by Zhu et al., who used a capsular repair as a modification to the Lafosse technique, resulting in zero recurrence among 52 patients during follow-ups exceeding 2 years [37].

5.12.5 Nonunion, Graft Osteolysis, and Resorption

Graft complications in the Latarjet procedure, including nonunion, osteolysis, and bone resorption, are critical considerations during follow-up and postoperative assessment. The systematic review by Griesser et al. found a 7.1% nonunion rate in arthroscopic Latarjet [58]. This underscores the importance of precise graft placement and postoperative management. This was also highlighted by Kordasiewicz et al. [46] that showed a higher nonunion rate in open Latarjet, coupled with a greater incidence of partial graft osteolysis in arthroscopic cases, emphasizes the need for careful surgical approach, especially around the proximal screw. Regardless of a nonunion, patients often achieve good to excellent functional outcomes despite incidental nonunion findings and highlights the potential resilience of the procedure [56]. Significant bone resorption after a Latarjet procedure is often seen on postoperative radiograph and CT. Especially concerning the proximal screw, which implies possible influences such as increased blood flow to the distal tip of the coracoid and enhanced mechanotransduction of the inferior part, emphasizing the complexity of graft integration [37]. Partial lysis of the coracoid, although frequent, rarely leads to persistent apprehension and unsatisfactory outcomes [63]. To mitigate the risk of nonunion and graft resorption in Latarjet procedures, meticulous graft preparation and parallel screw placement are crucial. Addressing factors such as smoking, unicortical or single screw fixation, and insufficient screw purchase can help prevent nonunion [63]. Standardized techniques, including preparing flat cancellous surfaces of the coracoid graft, correctly positioning the bone block, and using bicortical compression screws perpendicular to the graft, enhance stability and promote union.

5.12.6 Arthritis

The Latarjet procedure carries the potential long-term risk of glenohumeral arthritis. Studies by Domos et al. indicate a considerable incidence of glenohumeral arthritis, with rates reaching 20% at 20 years and varying degrees of severity observed in follow-up assessments [7, 63]. However, accurately quantifying arthropathy attributable to the surgical intervention remains challenging due to the overlapping natural evolution of posttraumatic arthropathy [49]. A more recent systematic review suggests a generally low incidence of osteoarthritis development post-Latarjet procedure, making it a safe option even for younger individuals and athletes [64]. Factors such as the positioning of the graft and screw obliquity can exacerbate arthritis onset [37, 65]. The major risk factor for joint degeneration is the lateral overhanging of the coracoid graft [64]. Notably, age, gender, time between dislocation and surgery, and number of dislocations do not significantly influence the onset of osteoarthritis following the procedure [64].

5.12.7 Reoperations

Reoperation rates for arthroscopic Latarjet procedures fall within the range of 6–8%, with symptomatic hardware failure accounting for 35% of cases, often necessitating arthroscopic screw removal [8, 13, 58]. Athwal et al. reported adverse event rates comparable to those of open Latarjet procedures, with hardware-related complications constituting 14% of adverse events [13]. Hardware complications occurring in 1.9% of patients after arthroscopic Latarjet, with similar proportions of screw breakage and loosening (1.0%) and symptomatic hardware (0.9%) [9]. To address these complications, nonrigid fixation methods such as cortical buttons have been proposed, offering success potentially due to their low profile, extra-articular placement, and positioning away from the commonly remodelled proximal pole of the graft, which exhibits more osteolysis.

5.13 Postoperative Rehabilitation and Follow-Up

Arthroscopic procedures are believed to result in less postoperative pain compared to open surgery. However, postoperative rehabilitation protocols vary among countries and hospitals. Typically, early mobilization is encouraged to prevent stiffness, with the use of a sling for the first 4–6 weeks. Strengthening exercises are usually prohibited for the initial 6 weeks, with the primary focus being on improving passive range of motion. Regular radiographs are taken to monitor graft position, with postoperative CT scans ordered at 6 weeks or 3 months for accurate assessment. Return to sport is advised after healing of the graft.

5.14 Summary

The arthroscopic Latarjet procedure, introduced by Lafosse in 2007, enhances glenohumeral joint stability through three mechanisms known as the triple-blocking effect: extending the glenoid arc with a bone block, using the conjoined tendon as a dynamic sling, and creating a tenodesis effect by transferring the conjoined tendon and coracoid process over the subscapularis tendon [5]. The primary indication for the Latarjet procedure is glenoid bone loss ranging from 15% to 20%. The arthroscopic approach offers advantages such as enhanced visualization for precise graft positioning, reduced postoperative scar tissue and stiffness, less pain, improved cosmesis, and faster recovery. The literature consistently highlights excellent clinical outcomes with low recurrence rates and with high return-to-sport rates. Despite concerns about complication rates due to technical complexity and surgical time, the arthroscopic Latarjet procedure offers significant benefits, especially improved visualization. These advantages can motivate orthopedic surgeons to master the technique, despite its learning curve. With increasing experience, complication rates and surgical time can potentially decrease, with shoulder specialists generally needing 30–50 cases to achieve operational efficiency.

References

1. Malmberg C, Andreasen KR, Bencke J, Hölmich P, Barfod KW. Anterior-posterior glenohumeral translation in shoulders with traumatic anterior instability: a systematic review of the literature. JSES Rev Rep Tech. 2023;3(4):477–93. https://doi.org/10.1016/j.xrrt.2023.07.002.
2. Galvin JW, Ernat JJ, Waterman BR, Stadecker MJ, Parada SA. The epidemiology and natural history of anterior shoulder instability. Curr Rev Musculoskelet Med. 2017;10(4):411–24. https://doi.org/10.1007/s12178-017-9432-5.
3. Hurley ET, Matache BA, Wong I, Itoi E, Strauss EJ, Delaney RA, et al. Anterior shoulder instability part II-Latarjet, remplissage, and glenoid bone-grafting—an international consensus statement. Arthroscopy. 2022;38(2):224–33.e6. https://doi.org/10.1016/j.arthro.2021.07.023.
4. Latarjet M. Treatment of recurrent dislocation of the shoulder. Lyon Chir. 1954;49(8):994–7.
5. Lafosse L, Lejeune E, Bouchard A, Kakuda C, Gobezie R, Kochhar T. The arthroscopic Latarjet procedure for the treatment of anterior shoulder instability. Arthroscopy. 2007;23(11):1242.e1–5. https://doi.org/10.1016/j.arthro.2007.06.008.
6. Calvo C, Calvo J, Rojas D, Valencia M, Calvo E. Clinical relevance of persistent off-track Hill-Sachs lesion after arthroscopic Latarjet procedure. Am J Sports Med. 2021;49(8):2006–12. https://doi.org/10.1177/03635465211019979.
7. Hovelius L, Sandström B, Olofsson A, Svensson O, Rahme H. The effect of capsular repair, bone block healing, and position on the results of the Bristow-Latarjet procedure (study III): long-term follow-up in 319 shoulders. J Shoulder Elbow Surg. 2012;21(5):647–60. https://doi.org/10.1016/j.jse.2011.03.020.
8. Cerciello S, Corona K, Morris BJ, Santagada DA, Maccauro G. Early outcomes and perioperative complications of the arthroscopic Latarjet procedure: systematic review and meta-analysis. Am J Sports Med. 2019;47(9):2232–41. https://doi.org/10.1177/0363546518783743.
9. Hurley ET, Schwartz LB, Mojica ES, Campbell KA, Matache BA, Meislin RJ, et al. Short-term complications of the Latarjet procedure: a systematic review. J Shoulder Elbow Surg. 2021;30(7):1693–9. https://doi.org/10.1016/j.jse.2021.01.024.

10. Valencia M, Calvo C, Novo U, Calvo C, Luengo-Alonso G, Martinez Catalan N, Foruria de Diego AM, Calvo E. Does preoperative bony defect size determines final graft position in Latarjet procedure? JSES Int. 2023;7:393–8. https://doi.org/10.1016/j.jseint.2023.02.006.
11. Calvo E, Granizo JJ, Fernández-Yruegas D. Criteria for arthroscopic treatment of anterior instability of the shoulder. J Bone Joint Surg. 2005;87-B:677–83. https://doi.org/10.1302/0301-620X.87B5.15794.
12. Valsamis EM, Kany J, Bonnevialle N, Castricini R, Lädermann A, Cunningham G, et al. The arthroscopic Latarjet: a multisurgeon learning curve analysis. J Shoulder Elbow Surg. 2020;29(4):681–8. https://doi.org/10.1016/j.jse.2019.10.022.
13. Athwal GS, Meislin R, Getz C, Weinstein D, Favorito P. Short-term complications of the arthroscopic Latarjet procedure: a North American experience. Arthroscopy. 2016;32(10):1965–70. https://doi.org/10.1016/j.arthro.2016.02.022.
14. Bøe B, Støen R, Blich I, Moatshe G, Ludvigsen TC. Learning curve for arthroscopic shoulder Latarjet procedure shows shorter operating time and fewer complications with experience. Arthroscopy. 2022;38(8):2391–8. https://doi.org/10.1016/j.arthro.2022.01.042.
15. Shin SJ, Koh YW, Bui C, Jeong WK, Akeda M, Cho NS, et al. What is the critical value of glenoid bone loss at which soft tissue bankart repair does not restore glenohumeral translation, restricts range of motion, and leads to abnormal humeral head position? Am J Sports Med. 2016;44(11):2784–91. https://doi.org/10.1177/0363546516656367.
16. Verweij LPE, van Spanning SH, Grillo A, Kerkhoffs G, Priester-Vink S, van Deurzen DFP, et al. Age, participation in competitive sports, bony lesions, ALPSA lesions, >1 preoperative dislocations, surgical delay and ISIS score>3 are risk factors for recurrence following arthroscopic Bankart repair: a systematic review and meta-analysis of 4584 shoulders. Knee Surg Sports Traumatol Arthrosc. 2021;29(12):4004–14. https://doi.org/10.1007/s00167-021-06704-7.
17. Haskel JD, Colasanti CA, Hurley ET, Matache BA, Jazrawi LM, Meislin RJ. Arthroscopic Latarjet procedure: indications, techniques, and outcomes. JBJS Rev. 2021;9(3) https://doi.org/10.2106/jbjs.Rvw.20.00071.
18. Nakagawa S, Iuchi R, Hanai H, Hirose T, Mae T. The development process of bipolar bone defects from primary to recurrent instability in shoulders with traumatic anterior instability. Am J Sports Med. 2019;47(3):695–703. https://doi.org/10.1177/0363546518819471.
19. Gouveia K, Rizvi SFH, Dagher D, Leroux T, Bedi A, Khan M. Assessing bone loss in the unstable shoulder: a scoping review. Curr Rev Musculoskelet Med. 2022;15(5):369–76. https://doi.org/10.1007/s12178-022-09773-4.
20. Burkhart SS, De Beer JF, Barth JR, Cresswell T, Roberts C, Richards DP. Results of modified Latarjet reconstruction in patients with anteroinferior instability and significant bone loss. Arthroscopy. 2007;23(10):1033–41. https://doi.org/10.1016/j.arthro.2007.08.009.
21. Itoi E, Lee SB, Berglund LJ, Berge LL, An KN. The effect of a glenoid defect on anteroinferior stability of the shoulder after Bankart repair: a cadaveric study. J Bone Joint Surg Am. 2000;82(1):35–46. https://doi.org/10.2106/00004623-200001000-00005.
22. Yamamoto N, Itoi E, Abe H, Kikuchi K, Seki N, Minagawa H, et al. Effect of an anterior glenoid defect on anterior shoulder stability: a cadaveric study. Am J Sports Med. 2009;37(5):949–54. https://doi.org/10.1177/0363546508330139.
23. Dickens JF, Owens BD, Cameron KL, DeBerardino TM, Masini BD, Peck KY, et al. The effect of subcritical bone loss and exposure on recurrent instability after arthroscopic bankart repair in intercollegiate American football. Am J Sports Med. 2017;45(8):1769–75. https://doi.org/10.1177/0363546517704184.
24. Shaha JS, Cook JB, Song DJ, Rowles DJ, Bottoni CR, Shaha SH, et al. Redefining "critical" bone loss in shoulder instability: functional outcomes worsen with "subcritical" bone loss. Am J Sports Med. 2015;43(7):1719–25. https://doi.org/10.1177/0363546515578250.
25. Di Giacomo G, Itoi E, Burkhart SS. Evolving concept of bipolar bone loss and the Hill-Sachs lesion: from "engaging/non-engaging" lesion to "on-track/off-track" lesion. Arthroscopy. 2014;30(1):90–8. https://doi.org/10.1016/j.arthro.2013.10.004.
26. Gowd AK, Liu JN, Cabarcas BC, Garcia GH, Cvetanovich GL, Provencher MT, et al. Management of recurrent anterior shoulder instability with bipolar bone loss: a systematic review to assess critical bone loss amounts. Am J Sports Med. 2019;47(10):2484–93. https://doi.org/10.1177/0363546518791555.
27. Saliken D, Boileau P. Arthroscopic Latarjet—learning curve, results, and complications. Ann Joint. 2017;2(11) https://doi.org/10.21037/aoj.2017.10.15.
28. Yiannakopoulos CK, Mataragas E, Antonogiannakis E. A comparison of the spectrum of intra-articular lesions in acute and chronic anterior shoulder instability. Arthroscopy. 2007;23(9):985–90. https://doi.org/10.1016/j.arthro.2007.05.009.
29. Cui DD, Long Y, Yan Y, Li C, Yang YT, Zhong JL, et al. 3D-MRI FRACTURE Sequence is equivalent to 3D-CT in quantifying bone loss and measuring shoulder morphology in patients with shoulder dislocation. Arthroscopy. 2024;40(6):1777–88. https://doi.org/10.1016/j.arthro.2023.12.016.
30. Ozaki R, Nakagawa S, Mizuno N, Mae T, Yoneda M. Hill-sachs lesions in shoulders with traumatic anterior instability: evaluation using computed tomography with 3-dimensional reconstruction. Am

J Sports Med. 2014;42(11):2597–605. https://doi.org/10.1177/0363546514549543.
31. Sugaya H. Techniques to evaluate glenoid bone loss. Curr Rev Musculoskelet Med. 2014;7(1):1–5. https://doi.org/10.1007/s12178-013-9198-3.
32. Giles JW, Owens BD, Athwal GS. Estimating glenoid width for instability-related bone loss: a CT evaluation of an MRI formula. Am J Sports Med. 2015;43(7):1726–30. https://doi.org/10.1177/0363546515581468.
33. Launay M, Choudhry MN, Green N, Maharaj J, Cutbush K, Pivonka P, et al. Three-dimensional quantification of glenoid bone loss in anterior shoulder instability: the anatomic concave surface area method. Orthop J Sports Med. 2021;9(6):23259671211011058. https://doi.org/10.1177/23259671211011058.
34. Sharareh B, Edwards TB, Shah A, Shybut T. Variation in technique and postoperative management of the Latarjet procedure among orthopedic surgeons. J Shoulder Elbow Surg. 2021;30(4):e157–64. https://doi.org/10.1016/j.jse.2020.07.027.
35. Di Giacomo G, Costantini A, de Gasperis N, De Vita A, Lin BK, Francone M, et al. Coracoid graft osteolysis after the Latarjet procedure for anteroinferior shoulder instability: a computed tomography scan study of twenty-six patients. J Shoulder Elbow Surg. 2011;20(6):989–95. https://doi.org/10.1016/j.jse.2010.11.016.
36. Sano H, Komatsuda T, Abe H, Ozawa H, Yokobori TA Jr. Proximal-medial part in the coracoid graft demonstrates the most evident stress shielding following the Latarjet procedure: a simulation study using the 3-dimensional finite element method. J Shoulder Elbow Surg. 2020;29(12):2632–9. https://doi.org/10.1016/j.jse.2020.03.037.
37. Zhu YM, Jiang CY, Lu Y, Li FL, Wu G. Coracoid bone graft resorption after Latarjet procedure is underestimated: a new classification system and a clinical review with computed tomography evaluation. J Shoulder Elbow Surg. 2015;24(11):1782–8. https://doi.org/10.1016/j.jse.2015.05.039.
38. Kany J, Flamand O, Grimberg J, Guinand R, Croutzet P, Amaravathi R, et al. Arthroscopic Latarjet procedure: is optimal positioning of the bone block and screws possible? A prospective computed tomography scan analysis. J Shoulder Elbow Surg. 2016;25(1):69–77. https://doi.org/10.1016/j.jse.2015.06.010.
39. Manfredi JN, Schick S, Paul KD, Elphingstone JW, Sowell J, Lameka M, et al. A systematic review of screw and suture button glenoid augmentation constructs. Orthop J Sports Med. 2023;11(10):23259671231186429. https://doi.org/10.1177/23259671231186429.
40. Ziegenfuss BL, Launay MM, Maharaj JC, Green NR, Stalin KA, Barlow G, et al. A biomechanical analysis of double-screw, double-button, and screw-button fixation constructs in patient-specific instrument-guided Latarjet procedure. J Shoulder Elbow Surg. 2023;32(7):1370–9. https://doi.org/10.1016/j.jse.2023.02.117.
41. Kazum E, Chechik O, Pritsch T, Mozes G, Morag G, Dolkart O, et al. Biomechanical evaluation of suture buttons versus cortical screws in the Latarjet-Bristow procedure: a fresh-frozen cadavers study. Arch Orthop Trauma Surg. 2019;139(12):1779–83. https://doi.org/10.1007/s00402-019-03269-6.
42. Saleky B, Hapa O, Isin Y, Güvençer M, Havıtçıoğlu H, Uzun B. Suture anchor fixation strength in the Latarjet procedure: a biomechanical study in cadavers. Eur J Orthop Surg Traumatol. 2019;29(8):1667–72. https://doi.org/10.1007/s00590-019-02476-6.
43. Williams RC, Morris RP, El Beaino M, Maassen NH. Cortical suture button fixation vs. bicortical screw fixation in the Latarjet procedure: a biomechanical comparison. J Shoulder Elbow Surg. 2020;29:1470–8. https://doi.org/10.1016/j.jse.2019.11.025.
44. Khiami F, Sariali E, Rosenheim M, Hardy P. Anterior shoulder instability arthroscopic treatment outcomes measures: the WOSI correlates with the Walch-Duplay score. Orthop Traumatol Surg Res. 2012;98(1):48–53. https://doi.org/10.1016/j.otsr.2011.09.013.
45. Deng Z, Zheng Y, Su J, Chen S, Deng Z, Zhu W, et al. Open versus arthroscopic latarjet for recurrent anterior shoulder instability: a systematic review and meta-analysis. Orthop J Sports Med. 2023;11(5):23259671231174476. https://doi.org/10.1177/23259671231174476.
46. Kordasiewicz B, Kiciński M, Małachowski K, Boszczyk A, Chaberek S, Pomianowski S. Arthroscopic Latarjet stabilization: analysis of the learning curve in the first 90 primary cases: early clinical results and computed tomography evaluation. Arthroscopy. 2019;35(12):3221–37. https://doi.org/10.1016/j.arthro.2019.07.007.
47. Lafosse L, Boyle S. Arthroscopic Latarjet procedure. J Shoulder Elbow Surg. 2010;19(2 Suppl):2–12. https://doi.org/10.1016/j.jse.2009.12.010.
48. Valencia M, Bermejo Fernández G, Martín Rios MD, Fernández Jara J, Morcillo D, Coifman I, Foruria A, Calvo E. Subscapularis structural integrity and function after arthroscopic Latarjet procedure at a minimum 2-year follow-up. J Shoulder Elbow Surg. 2020;29:104–12. https://doi.org/10.1016/j.jse.2019.05.027.
49. Menendez ME, Sudah SY, Cohn MR, Narbona P, Lädermann A, Barth J, et al. Defining minimal clinically important difference and patient acceptable symptom state after the Latarjet procedure. Am J Sports Med. 2022;50(10):2761–6. https://doi.org/10.1177/03635465221107939.
50. Dzidzishvili L, Calvo C, Valencia M, Calvo E. Outcomes of arthroscopic Latarjet procedure for anterior glenohumeral instability in patients with epilepsy: a case-control study. Am J Sports Med. 2022;50(3):708–16. https://doi.org/10.1177/03635465211067531.

51. Kraus TM, Graveleau N, Bohu Y, Pansard E, Klouche S, Hardy P. Coracoid graft positioning in the Latarjet procedure. Knee Surg Sports Traumatol Arthrosc. 2016;24(2):496–501. https://doi.org/10.1007/s00167-013-2651-4.
52. Zumstein V, Kraljević M, Conzen A, Hoechel S, Müller-Gerbl M. Thickness distribution of the glenohumeral joint cartilage: a quantitative study using computed tomography. Surg Radiol Anat. 2014;36(4):327–31. https://doi.org/10.1007/s00276-013-1221-2.
53. Martins R, Quental C, Folgado J, Ângelo AC, de Campos Azevedo C. Influence of graft positioning during the latarjet procedure on shoulder stability and articular contact pressure: computational analysis of the bone block effect. Biology (Basel). 2022;11(12):1783. https://doi.org/10.3390/biology11121783.
54. Nourissat G, Delaroche C, Bouillet B, Doursounian L, Aim F. Optimization of bone-block positioning in the Bristow-Latarjet procedure: a biomechanical study. Orthop Traumatol Surg Res. 2014;100(5):509–13. https://doi.org/10.1016/j.otsr.2014.03.023.
55. Barth J, Neyton L, Métais P, Panisset JC, Baverel L, Walch G, et al. Is the two-dimensional computed tomography scan analysis reliable for coracoid graft positioning in Latarjet procedures? J Shoulder Elbow Surg. 2017;26(8):e237–42. https://doi.org/10.1016/j.jse.2016.12.067.
56. Gupta A, Delaney R, Petkin K, Lafosse L. Complications of the Latarjet procedure. Curr Rev Musculoskelet Med. 2015;8(1):59–66. https://doi.org/10.1007/s12178-015-9258-y.
57. Lädermann A, Denard PJ, Burkhart SS. Injury of the suprascapular nerve during latarjet procedure: an anatomic study. Arthroscopy. 2012;28(3):316–21. https://doi.org/10.1016/j.arthro.2011.08.307.
58. Griesser MJ, Harris JD, McCoy BW, Hussain WM, Jones MH, Bishop JY, et al. Complications and re-operations after Bristow-Latarjet shoulder stabilization: a systematic review. J Shoulder Elbow Surg. 2013;22(2):286–92. https://doi.org/10.1016/j.jse.2012.09.009.
59. Metais P, Clavert P, Barth J, Boileau P, Brzoska R, Nourissat G, et al. Preliminary clinical outcomes of Latarjet-Patte coracoid transfer by arthroscopy vs. open surgery: prospective multicentre study of 390 cases. Orthop Traumatol Surg Res. 2016;102(8s):S271–6. https://doi.org/10.1016/j.otsr.2016.08.003.
60. Shah AA, Butler RB, Romanowski J, Goel D, Karadagli D, Warner JJ. Short-term complications of the Latarjet procedure. J Bone Joint Surg Am. 2012;94(6):495–501. https://doi.org/10.2106/jbjs.J.01830.
61. Shishido H, Kikuchi S. Injury of the suprascapular nerve in shoulder surgery: an anatomic study. J Shoulder Elbow Surg. 2001;10(4):372–6. https://doi.org/10.1067/mse.2001.115988.
62. Hurley ET, Lim Fat D, Pauzenberger L, Mullett H. Tranexamic acid for the Latarjet procedure: a randomized controlled trial. J Shoulder Elbow Surg. 2020;29(5):882–5. https://doi.org/10.1016/j.jse.2020.01.066.
63. Domos P, Lunini E, Walch G. Contraindications and complications of the Latarjet procedure. Shoulder Elbow. 2018;10(1):15–24. https://doi.org/10.1177/1758573217728716.
64. Menon A, Fossati C, Magnani M, Boveri S, Compagnoni R, Randelli PS. Low grade of osteoarthritis development after Latarjet procedure with a minimum 5 years of follow-up: a systematic review and pooled analysis. Knee Surg Sports Traumatol Arthrosc. 2022;30(6):2074–83. https://doi.org/10.1007/s00167-021-06771-w.
65. Mizuno N, Denard PJ, Raiss P, Melis B, Walch G. Long-term results of the Latarjet procedure for anterior instability of the shoulder. J Shoulder Elbow Surg. 2014;23(11):1691–9. https://doi.org/10.1016/j.jse.2014.02.015.

The Open Free Bone Graft Procedure

6

Pietro S. Randelli and Alfonso Liccardi

6.1 History and Indication of Free Bone Graft Procedure in Shoulder Instability

Shoulder instability is a relevant issue in the population, typically manifesting as anterior instability in about 95% of cases, with posterior and multidirectional presentations also occurring. Risk factors include contact sports, younger age, hyperlaxity, and previous glenohumeral dislocations [1]. Treatment options range from conservative measures to surgical interventions, including arthroscopic or open procedures.

Bone loss has long been recognized as a challenge in cases of shoulder instability. It is widely acknowledged that arthroscopic stabilization yields unsatisfactory outcomes when significant bone loss is present. Bone loss can be classified as monopolar or bipolar, with the former affecting either the glenoid or humerus alone, and the latter involving both. Glenoid bone loss occurs in up to 22% of cases after the initial traumatic dislocation event and may rise to 72% in cases of recurrent dislocations [2, 3].

The threshold for "critical" glenoid bone loss, deemed clinically significant, remains a topic of debate. Historically, 20% has been considered the threshold negatively impacting clinical outcomes following arthroscopic stabilization. However, recent studies suggest that even over 13.5% glenoid bone loss significantly reduces the Western Ontario Shoulder Instability (WOSI) score, resulting in an unacceptable outcome, labeling this threshold as "subcritical" [4, 5].

Glenoid bone loss can coincide with humeral Hill-Sachs lesions, leading to bipolar bone loss. This humeral lesion occurs due to the posterolateral impact of the humerus against the anteroinferior part of the glenoid and is present in 63–97% of initial dislocations and up to 100% in recurrent cases [6]. Recent focus has shifted towards evaluating the size, position, and dynamics of these injuries during movement rather than solely considering their magnitude. The introduction of the "on-track" and "off-track" injury concept [7] distinguishes between stable and unstable conditions during shoulder abduction and external rotation. Given these considerations, selecting the appropriate surgical approach is critical.

P. S. Randelli (✉)
Laboratory of Applied Biomechanics, Department of Biomedical Sciences for Health, Università degli Studi di Milano, Milan, Italy

U.O.C. 1° Clinica Ortopedica, ASST Gaetano Pini-CTO, Milan, Italy

Research Center for Adult and Pediatric Rheumatic Diseases (RECAP-RD), Department of Biomedical Sciences for Health, Università degli Studi di Milano, Milan, Italy
e-mail: pietro.randelli@unimi.it

A. Liccardi
Unità funzionale di chirurgia della spalla, Humanitas San Pio X, Milan, Italy

E. Calvo et al. (eds.), *Complex and Revision Problems in Shoulder Instability*,
https://doi.org/10.1007/978-3-031-81389-4_6

Before 1980, all cases of shoulder instability were managed through open procedures. Pioneering techniques include the Bankart repair in 1923 and subsequent advancements such as the Eden-Hybinette procedure in 1932, which utilized an iliac crest autograft to augment the anterior glenoid. The Magnuson-Stack procedure in 1934 involved subscapularis transfer, followed by the Putti-Platt technique in 1948, which combined subscapularis tendon transfer and anterior capsular imbrication. A significant development occurred in 1954 with Michel Latarjet's description of coracoid transfer to address glenoid defects. This procedure was later refined by Bristow-Helfet, exclusively transferring the coracoid tip. Various bone graft options, including autografts and allografts, have since been described [8].

Indications for bone graft usage include subcritical/critical bone loss, large engaging Hill-Sachs lesions, ISIS score > 6 [9], and recurrent instability [10].

6.2 Types of Bone Grafts in Shoulder Instability

Several types of bone grafts can be utilized, categorized into autografts and allografts.

6.2.1 Autografts

6.2.1.1 Coracoid Bone

Despite several decades having passed since its introduction, this type of graft is still considered the gold standard for treating glenoid bone loss in shoulder anteroinferior instability [11]. Initially described by Latarjet, the technique involves transferring the entire coracoid process and fixing it in the anteroinferior region of the glenoid surface using screws. Subsequently, Bristow modified the technique by suggesting the transfer of only the tip of the coracoid. This technique harnesses what is known as the "triple blocking effect": augmentation of bone due to the coracoid's profile, reinforcement of the lower subscularis and capsule through tension of the conjoint tendon during arm abduction and external rotation (sling effect), and stabilization of the glenohumeral joint through repair of the capsule and inferior glenohumeral ligament to the stump of the coracoacromial ligament [12]. Biomechanically, this technique yields remarkable effects, with excellent patient-reported outcomes, particularly among athletes, where it enables a return to play in up to 88% of cases, with 72% returning to their pre-injury level [13]. However, there are several disadvantages, notably its nonanatomical nature, making potential future revisions more challenging. Additionally, it is indicated only when bone loss does not exceed 31% of the native glenoid surface. A modification of this procedure is the "congruent arc technique," which involves augmenting the glenoid surface not with the lateral region of the coracoid but with its inferior surface, enabling reconstruction of defects up to 54% of the glenoid. However, the literature has shown a higher rate of complications and failures compared to the original technique, with osteolysis reported in 60% of cases [14]. Another drawback of the Latarjet procedure is the absence of cartilage on the coracoid surface, which could predispose to osteoarthritis. The primary concern with this technique is the rate of complications, ranging from 7% to 30% [15–17], including malpositioning of fixation devices, arthrosis, graft resorption, persistent instability, infections, graft mobilization, bone graft overhang, persistent pain, and nerve injuries.

6.2.1.2 Iliac Crest

Historically, this was the first described technique for glenoid bone loss in anterior and posterior shoulder instability. This involves tricortical bone removal from the iliac crest and transferring it to the site of glenoid bone loss, fixing it with screws or buttons. This technique can restore defects up to 35 mm in length, significantly more than the Latarjet procedure. Since it is an autograft, compatibility is maximal, and the bone graft source is almost always available. However, disadvantages include donor site morbidity and absence of a cartilaginous region, potentially predisposing to osteoarthritis. The reported complication rate is 19.9% [18], with main issues being persistent pain at the donor site, graft reabsorption, glenohumeral arthrosis, infection, iliac spine fracture, femorocutaneous nerve lesion-related hypoesthesia, and hardware-related complications. An interesting variant is the "J-bone graft technique," involving bicortical removal from the iliac bone shaped like a J and inserted using a press-fit technique at the glenoid defect level to avoid hardware complications [19].

6.2.1.3 Distal Clavicle

Among the latest techniques is the use of the lateral distal region of the clavicle as a bone graft for glenoid bone loss in anterior and posterior shoulder instability [20]. This technique offers the advantage of containing a cartilaginous region within the graft, utilizing an area usually available without reported donor site morbidity. Although it could be used for bone loss up to 44%, it's recommended for young patients with glenoid bone loss ranging between 15–30% [21]. Disadvantages include lack of soft tissue retention and that it's surgical demanding.

6.2.1.4 Scapular Spine

One of the most innovative techniques involves bone graft removal from the scapula spine in cases of anterior and posterior shoulder instability [22]. The scapula spine has shown compatibility with the glenoid profile, making it a potential graft source. A micromovement rate comparable to that utilized in the Latarjet procedure has also been demonstrated for this specific graft [23]. However, studies on this technique lack long-term follow-up data, so the rate of relative complications is yet to be defined.

6.2.2 Allografts

Over the years, various allograft sources have been used to bridge glenoid bone defects in anterior or posterior shoulder instability, including iliac crest, distal tibia, femoral head, and humeral head [24–26]. Fixation is usually intraarticular using screws, anchors, J-grafting, or buttons. Among these, the distal tibial allograft has shown a radius of curvature more compatible with the glenoid, especially the lateral part [8], making it an excellent source. Fresh distal tibial allograft contains dense, weightbearing corticocancellous bone, ideal for screw fixation, and a robust cartilaginous surface for anatomical, osteoarticular glenoid surface reconstruction. Clinical results are excellent, with high patient satisfaction, low recurrence rate, 89% allograft healing rate, and only 3% graft reabsorption rate [27]. Advantages of allografts include superior source compared to autografts, presence of cartilage, ability to fill larger defects, recreate bone surface, and absence of donor site morbidity. Disadvantages include cost, source availability, rare disease transmission possibility [28], and surgical technique complexity.

6.3 Surgical Approaches

6.3.1 Deltopectoral Approach

After the interscalene block and general anesthesia, the patient is positioned in the "beach chair" position. A support is positioned behind the scapula to stabilize it, enhance the angle of vision of the glenoid, and facilitate palpation of the coracoid. The arm can be left free or supported; in either case, sterile materials are used to prepare the arm, and be ready to mobilize it during surgery.

The incision, approximately 6–7 cm in length, starts at the level of the coracoid and follows the traditional deltopectoral approach (some surgeons prefer a more medial approach towards the axilla). The interval between the deltoid and the pectoralis major is identified, as this constitutes an internervous plane—the deltoid being innervated by the axillary nerve and the pectoralis major by the medial and lateral pectoral nerves. The cephalic vein is identified within the space between the two muscles, which can be ligated or gently retracted laterally; however, its medial branches are preferably ligated to prevent bleeding. The clavipectoral fascia is incised, and the conjoint tendon is identified, being carefully retracted medially to avoid injury to the underlying nerve structures (the musculocutaneous nerve enters the coracobrachialis muscle approximately 5–8 cm distal to the coracoid). The subscapularis muscle is exposed, and its upper and lower borders are delineated. An "L shape" cut is performed using Mayo scissors between the upper two-thirds and lower one-third of the tendon and muscle. The scissors are then vertically opened to expose the underlying capsule. To avoid unnecessary difficult steps of the procedure the capsule is removed till the level of the joint line and further, thus exposing the glenoid neck. A Bankart retractor medial on the scapula body, together with a Fukuda retractor for the humeral head, finally allows a perfect exposure of the glenoid and its neck. Some surgeons prefer to respect the subscapularis doing a split in line with the muscle fibers between the upper two-thirds and lower one-third [29]. This step reduces the invasiveness of the procedure but it is technically demanding and can make the glenoid visualization difficult with possible malpositioning of the graft.

6.3.2 Posterior Approach

The patient is positioned either prone or, more commonly, in the lateral decubitus position. Supports are placed on the slopes to prevent nerve compression and pressure sores. The initial incision is made just medially to the posterolateral corner of the acromion and extends for 6–7 cm towards the posterior axillary fold. Upon dissecting through the subcutaneous tissue, we reach the deltoid plane and proceed to retract it laterally. This exposes the internervous plane, consisting of the infraspinatus muscle and the teres minor muscle, with the former innervated by the suprascapular nerve and the latter by the axillary nerve. The infraspinatus are retracted medially meanwhile the teres minor are laterally retracted. This phase requires particular attention due to the proximity to the suprascapular nerve (located 0.5–2 cm medially to the glenoid neck) and the axillary nerve, as well as the axillary artery, which lie beneath the teres minor muscle in the quadrangular (or Velpeau) space. Finally the capsule is exposed, and a T-capsulotomy shape is performed, thereby exposing the posterior region of the glenoid.

6.4 Surgical Technique of Free Bone Graft Procedures

The main distinction between various bone grafts lies in their harvesting method.

6.4.1 Distal Tibial Allograft

Upon reaching the shoulder joint plane, bone loss is identified. A bone loss ranging from 25% to 30% generally indicates the need to augment approximately 8–9 mm of anterior glenoid bone. The glenoid is prepared with a burr to accommodate the graft. A fresh distal tibia is obtained from a donor cadaveric (Fig. 6.1) source, with the lateral third designated for grafting. The appropriate size of the graft is determined by comparing preoperative CT and in vivo intraoperative measurements. Once marked the needed size of the graft, a surgeon holds the graft in place while another surgeon cuts the outlined part with a sagittal saw. Throughout this process, the graft is continuously irrigated to prevent damage from the saw (Fig. 6.2a).

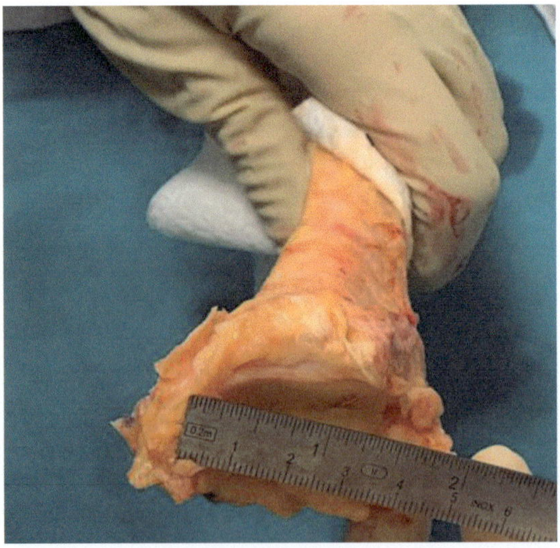

Fig. 6.1 Fresh distal tibial allograft

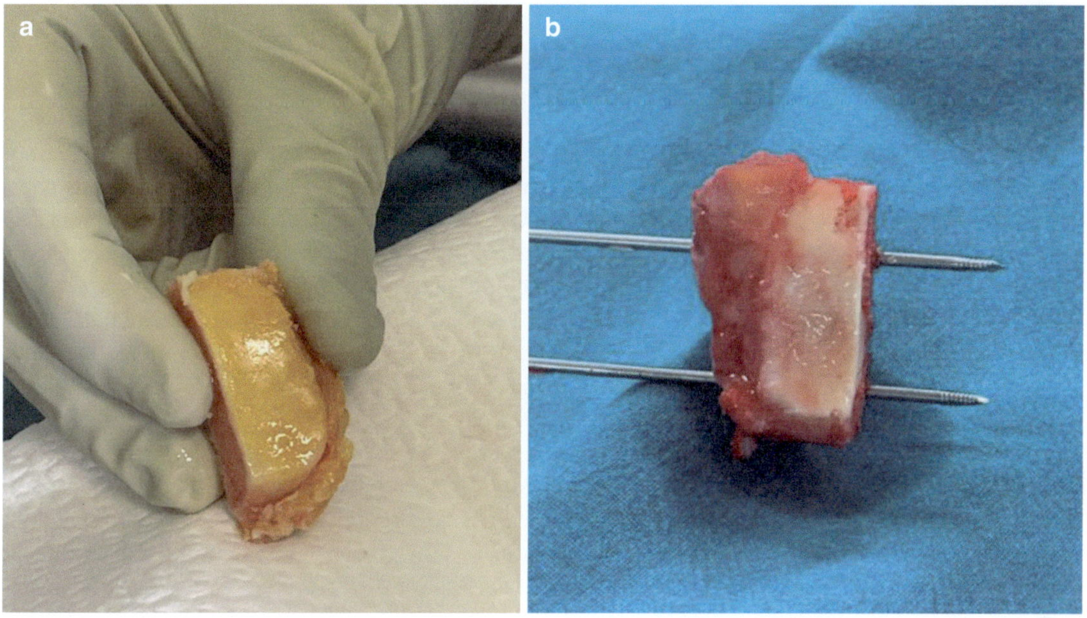

Fig. 6.2 (**a**, **b**) Preparation of the graft

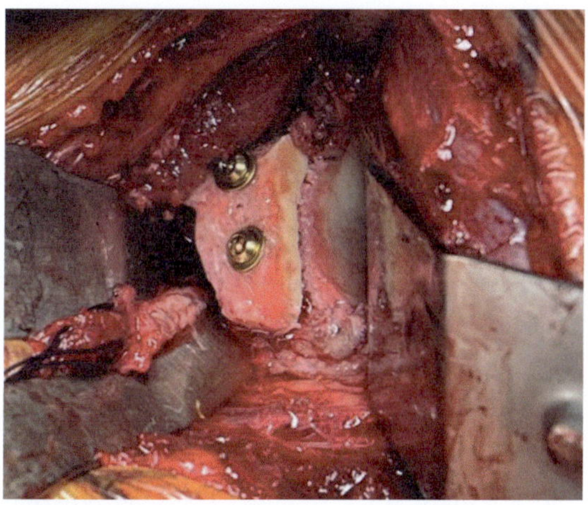

Fig. 6.3 Fixation of the graft

Subsequently, the graft is checked against the glenoid to ensure correct size and shape; if necessary, further adjustments are made. Once it fits perfectly, it is temporarily fixed with two 1.6 mm K-wires (Fig. 6.2b) before final fixation using two 3.5 mm diameter screws with washers (Fig. 6.3). Ideally, the capsule and the labrum are also repaired if desired by the surgeon, we never do it. Finally the subscapularis is well repaired with 2-0 reabsorbable sutures if a tendon "L shaped" incision has been done.

6.4.2 Iliac Crest Bone Graft

An incision approximately 4–5 cm long, parallel and just below the iliac crest, is made, starting 3 cm behind the anterior-inferior iliac spine to avoid damage to the lateral femorocutaneous nerve. Subperiosteal stripping of the iliacus muscle is performed, followed by its retraction to expose the ilium. The graft, obtained using a saw and an osteotome, varies in size depending on the glenoid bone defect. The wound is closed layer by layer upon completion.

6.4.3 Distal Clavicle Bone Graft

For grafts obtained from the lateral region of the clavicle, the incision is extended proximally. The bone plane is exposed, and care is taken to avoid damaging the coracoclavicular ligaments, located approximately 2–2.5 cm away from the lateral margin of the clavicle. The graft is harvested laterally to these ligaments using an oscillating saw. Soft tissue is removed from the graft, slight decortication is performed, and it is then shaped to fit the glenoid defect.

6.4.4 Scapular Spine Bone Graft

The midpoint of the scapula is identified, and a transverse incision of about 4 cm is made along the spine of the scapula. Dissection of the trapezius fascia, aponeurosis, and insertion of the posterior deltoid exposes the bone plane. A tricortical bone graft is harvested starting 49.6 mm laterally from the medial scapular edge, where the scapular spine is thickest [21]. The graft, measuring 20 mm × 10 mm × 8 mm [30], is obtained with an osteotome to bridge the glenoid defect. The graft can be fixed using screws, suture anchors [31], or cerclages with tape [32]. Closure is performed layer by layer, ensuring repair of the deltoid band while taking special care to avoid nerve damage, particularly to the axillary nerve during graft collection.

6.5 Results

A systematic review spanning 10 years of follow-up demonstrated excellent results in patient-reported outcome following Latarjet procedure in 86% of the patients, with over 90% expressing satisfaction with the treatment [33]. This is strongly linked to the procedure's high rate of return to sport [13]. Significant enhancements in scores for bone grafting in shoulder anterior instability procedures were observed. There was a notable increase in both the Constant Score, from 51 ± 5.5 to 90.2 ± 4.4 for the Latarjet procedure, and from 53.6 ± 6 to 89 ± 5 for other bone grafting procedures. Similarly, improvements were noted in the UCLA score, rising from 14.2 ± 3.1 to 31 ± 2.2 for the Latarjet procedure and from 15.4 ± 3 to 30.2 ± 2.2 for other bone grafting procedures [34]. The union rate of the graft was high, ranging from 78% to 100% [35].

Recurrence of dislocation exhibited a low occurrence rate in the literature, ranging between 2% and 5% [36, 37], often linked to new traumatic events, sports injuries, or seizure episodes. Osteoarthritis development remains a concern, affecting approximately 10% of patients undergoing these procedures.

Other reported complications include hardware issues such as breakdown or malpositioning, infections, undersized grafts, and nerve lesions.

Bone grafting for posterior instability yields slightly different results. While excellent outcomes are reported in the short and medium terms, long-term studies demonstrate a clinical deterioration with increased recurrence of instability and almost always progression of glenohumeral arthrosis [38]. Notably, graft reabsorption is frequent, with an incidence rate ranging from 18% to 62% [39], yet it appears not to be associated with instability recurrence.

Given the favorable outcomes, bone grafting procedures are deemed safe and recommended for cases of glenoid bone loss due to anterior and posterior shoulder instability.

6.6 Treatment Algorithm

Following a thorough objective examination and review of the X-rays in both the anteroposterior (AP) and Y-views of the scapula, we proceed with a request for a shoulder CT scan utilizing the PICO protocol and 3D reconstruction to evaluate glenoid bone deficiency, and humeral head as well. If the glenoid bone deficit measures less than 13.5%, our approach shifts towards arthroscopic stabilization. In cases where the glenoid bone deficit ranges between 13.5% and 20%, we conduct a comprehensive assessment with the patient. Depending on factors such as the type of sports activity engaged in, whether the injury is on- or off-track, and the numbers of dislocations, we determine whether to pursue an arthroscopic procedure involving Bankart repair with Remplissage or opt for stabilization according to the Latarjet technique. If the bone deficit exceeds 20%, our preference will lie on a procedure involving bone grafting. Typically, we favor performing a Latarjet procedure unless the deficit surpasses 30% or the patient presents issues related to the coracoid. In such instances, stabilization with a free bone graft is recommended. Distal Tibial Allograft is our preferred option.

References

1. Olds M, Ellis R, Donaldson K, et al. Risk factors which predispose first-time traumatic anterior shoulder dislocations to recurrent instability in adults: a systematic review and meta-analysis. Br J Sports Med. 2015;49:913–22.
2. Taylor DC, Arciero RA. Pathologic changes associated with shoulder dislocations: arthroscopic and physical examination findings in first-time, traumatic anterior dislocations. Am J Sports Med. 1997;25(3):306–11.
3. Hovelius LK, Sandström BC, Rösmark DL, Saebö M, Sundgren KH, Malmqvist BG. Long-term results with the Bankart and Bristow-Latarjet procedures: recurrent shoulder instability and arthropathy. J Shoulder Elb Surg. 2001;10(5):445–52.
4. Shaha JS, Cook JB, Song DJ, et al. Redefining "critical" bone loss in shoulder instability: functional outcomes worsen with "subcritical" bone loss. Am J Sports Med. 2015;43(7):1719–25.
5. Bois AJ, Mayer MJ, Fening SD, Jones MH, Miniaci A. Management of bone loss in recurrent traumatic anterior shoulder instability: a survey of North American surgeons. JSES Int. 2020;4(3):574–83.
6. Fox JA, Sanchez A, Zajac TJ, et al. Understanding the hill-Sachs lesion in its role in patients with recurrent anterior shoulder instability. Curr Rev Musculoskelet Med. 2017;10:469–79.
7. Di Giacomo G, Itoi E, Burkhart SS. Evolving concept of bipolar bone loss and the hill-Sachs lesion: from "engaging/non-engaging" lesion to "on-track/off-track" lesion, arthroscopy. J Arthrosc Relat Surg. 2014;30(1):90–8.
8. Fares MY, Boufadel P, Daher M, Koa J, Khanna A, Abboud JA. Anterior shoulder instability and open procedures: history, indications, and clinical outcomes. Clin Orthop Surg. 2023;15(4):521–33.
9. Balg F, Boileau P. The instability severity index score. J Bone Joint Surg Br. 2007;89-B(11):1470–7.
10. Skupinski J, Piechota MZ, Wawrzynek W, Maczuch J, Babinska A. The bony Bankart lesion: how to measure the glenoid bone loss. Pol J Radiol. 2017;82:58–63.
11. Griesser MJ, Harris JD, McCoy BW, Hussain WM, Jones MH, Bishop JY, Miniaci A. Complications and re-operations after Bristow-Latarjet shoulder stabilization: a systematic review. J Shoulder Elb Surg. 2013;22(2):286–92.
12. Bradley Edwards T, Walch G. The Latarjet procedure for recurrent anterior shoulder instability: rationale and technique. Oper Tech Sports Med. 2012;20(1):57–64.
13. Hurley ET, Montgomery C, Jamal MS, et al. Return to play after the Latarjet procedure for anterior shoulder instability: a systematic review. Am J Sports Med. 2019;47(12):3002–8.
14. Di Giacomo G, Costantini A, de Gasperis N, De Vita A, Lin BKH, Francone M, Rojas Beccaglia MA, Mastantuono M. Coracoid graft osteolysis after the Latarjet procedure for anteroinferior shoulder instability: a computed tomography scan study of twenty-six patients. J Shoulder Elb Surg. 2011;20(6):989–95.
15. Scanlon JP, Hurley ET, Davey MS, et al. 90-day complication rate after the Latarjet procedure in a high-volume center. Am J Sports Med. 2020;48(14):3467–71.
16. Menon A, Fossati C, Magnani M, Boveri S, Compagnoni R, Randelli PS. Low grade of osteoarthritis development after Latarjet procedure with a minimum 5 years of follow-up: a systematic review and pooled analysis. Knee Surg Sports Traumatol Arthrosc. 2022;30(6):2074–83.
17. Willemot L, De Boey S, Van Tongel A, et al. Analysis of failures after the Bristow-Latarjet procedure for recurrent shoulder instability. Int Orthop. 2019;43:1899–907.
18. Malahias MA, Chytas D, Raoulis V, et al. Iliac crest bone grafting for the management of anterior shoulder instability in patients with glenoid bone loss: a systematic review of contemporary literature. Sports Med Open. 2020;6:12.
19. Boesmueller S, Berchtold M, Lorenz G, et al. Implant-free iliac crest bone graft procedure shows anatomic remodelling without redislocation in recurrent anterior shoulder instability after short-term follow-up. Arch Orthop Trauma Surg. 2022;142:1047–54.
20. Tokish JM, Fitzpatrick K, Cook JB, Mallon WJ. Arthroscopic distal clavicular autograft for treating shoulder instability with glenoid bone loss. Arthrosc Tech. 2014;3(4):e475–81.
21. Petersen SA, Bernard JA, Langdale ER, Belkoff SM. Autologous distal clavicle versus autologous coracoid bone grafts for restoration of anterior-inferior glenoid bone loss: a biomechanical comparison. J Shoulder Elb Surg. 2016;25(6):960–6.
22. Rohman E, Gronbeck K, Tompkins M, Mittelsteadt M, Kirkham JA, Arciero RA. Scapular spine dimensions and suitability as a glenoid bone graft donor site. Am J Sports Med. 2019;47(10):2469–77.
23. Youssef Y, Heilemann M, Melcher P, et al. Assessment of micromotion at the bone-bone interface after coracoid and scapular-spine bone-block augmentation for the reconstruction of critical anterior glenoid bone loss—a biomechanical cadaver study. BMC Musculoskelet Disord. 2023;24:790. https://doi.org/10.1186/s12891-023-06914-9.
24. Provencher MT, Ghodadra N, LeClere L, Solomon DJ, Romeo AA. Anatomic osteochondral glenoid

reconstruction for recurrent glenohumeral instability with glenoid deficiency using a distal tibia allograft. Arthroscopy. 2009;25(4):446–52.

25. Zhao J, Huangfu X, Yang X, Xie G, Xu C. Arthroscopic glenoid bone grafting with nonrigid fixation for anterior shoulder instability: 52 patients with 2- to 5-year follow-up. Am J Sports Med. 2014;42(4):831–9.
26. Weng P-W, Shen H-C, Lee H-H, Wu S-S, Lee C-H. Open reconstruction of large bony glenoid erosion with allogeneic bone graft for recurrent anterior shoulder dislocation. Am J Sports Med. 2009;37(9):1792–7.
27. Provencher MT, Frank RM, Golijanin P, Gross D, Cole BJ, Verma NN, Romeo AA. Distal tibia allograft glenoid reconstruction in recurrent anterior shoulder instability: clinical and radiographic outcomes. Arthroscopy. 2017;33(5):891–7.
28. Buck BE, Malinin TI, Brown MD. Bone transplantation and human immunodeficiency virus. An estimate of risk of acquired immunodeficiency syndrome (AIDS). Clin Orthop Relat Res. 1989;240:129–36.
29. Bouju Y, Gadéa F, Stanovici J, Moubarak H, Favard L. Shoulder stabilization by modified Latarjet-Patte procedure: results at a minimum 10 years' follow-up, and role in the prevention of osteoarthritis. Orthop Traumatol Surg Res. 2014;100(4, Suppl):S213–8.
30. Taverna E, D'Ambrosi R, Perfetti C, Garavaglia G. Arthroscopic bone graft procedure for anterior inferior glenohumeral instability. Arthrosc Tech. 2014;3(6):e653–60.
31. Xiang M, Yang J, Chen H, Hu X, Zhang Q, Li Y, Jiang C. Arthroscopic autologous scapular spine bone graft combined with bankart repair for anterior shoulder instability with subcritical (10%–15%) glenoid bone loss. Arthroscopy. 2021;37(7):2065–74.
32. Moroder P, Kathi T, Lacheta L, Karpinski K, Paksoy A, Akgün D. Arthroscopic bone block cerclage technique using a tricortical scapular spine autograft for glenoid reconstruction in patients with anterior shoulder instability. Arthrosc Tech. 2022;11(3):e379–83.
33. Hurley ET, Jamal MS, Ali ZS, Montgomery C, Pauzenberger L, Mullett H. Long-term outcomes of the Latarjet procedure for anterior shoulder instability: a systematic review of studies at 10-year follow-up. J Shoulder Elbow Surg. 2018;28:e33–9.
34. Mahmoud HF, Farhan AH, Fahmy FS. Satisfactory functional results and complication rates after anterior glenoid bone block reconstruction in recurrent shoulder dislocation: a mean 4-year follow-up comparative study. J ISAKOS. 2022;7(4):47–53.
35. Gilat R, Wong SE, Lavoie-Gagne O, Haunschild ED, Knapik DM, Fu MC, Chahla J, Forsythe B, Cole BJ. Outcomes are comparable using free bone block autografts versus allografts for the management of anterior shoulder instability with glenoid bone loss: a systematic review and meta-analysis of "the non-Latarjet". Knee Surg Sports Traumatol Arthrosc. 2021;29(7):2159–74.
36. Allain J, Gutallier D, Glorion C, Creteil F. Long-term results of the Latarjet procedure for the treatment of anterior instability of the shoulder. J Bone Joint Surg. 1998;80(6):841–52.
37. Moroder P, Schulz E, Wierer G, Auffarth A, Habermeyer P, Resch H, et al. Neer award 2019: Latarjet procedure vs. iliac crest bone graft transfer for treatment of anterior shoulder instability with glenoid bone loss: a prospective randomized trial. J Shoulder Elb Surg. 2019;28(7):1298–307.
38. Meuffels DE, Schuit H, van Biezen FC, Reijman M, Verhaar JAN. The posterior bone block procedure in posterior shoulder instability. J Bone Joint Surg Br. 2010;92-B(5):651–5.
39. Villefort C, Stern C, Gerber C, Wyss S, Ernstbrunner L, Wieser K. Mid-term to long-term results of open posterior bone block grafting in recurrent posterior shoulder instability: a clinical and CT-based analysis. JSES Int. 2022;7(2):211–7.

7 The Arthroscopic Free Bone Graft Procedure

Taverna Ettore, Albizzini Ohin Caterina, Perfetti Carlo, and Guarrella Vincenzo

7.1 Introduction to Shoulder Instability

Shoulder instability is a common problem that can significantly impair the function and quality of life of affected individuals. It is characterized by the abnormal movement of the humeral head relative to the glenoid, often resulting in recurrent dislocations or subluxations. The primary cause of shoulder instability is damage to the structures that provide stability to the joint, including ligaments, labrum, and the glenoid bone. Traditionally, in case of bone defect, surgical options for the treatment of anterior shoulder instability involved open procedures, such as the Latarjet procedure, to address glenoid bone loss. However, these procedures were associated with significant morbidity and complications. In recent years, advancements in arthroscopic techniques have allowed for a less invasive and more effective surgical approach to shoulder instability. Arthroscopic Bankart repair, which involves repairing the torn labrum and stabilizing the joint using sutures, has become the gold standard for surgical treatment [1]. However, in cases where there is significant glenoid bone loss, arthroscopic soft tissue procedures may not be sufficient to restore stability. This is where the arthroscopic bone block procedure comes in. The arthroscopic bone block procedure is a relatively new advancement in the field of shoulder instability surgery. It is specifically designed for patients with recurrent anterior shoulder instability, young age, sportive activities, and glenoid defects that may result in a high risk of failure with traditional Bankart repair techniques.

The chapter content was already published in: A. Marinelli, E. Guerra, G. Bain. Classification of elbow stiffness, Journal of ISAKOS, Volume 9, Issue 2, 2024, 234-239, ISSN 2059-7754, https://doi.org/10.1016/j.jisako.2023.10.011. Reproduced with the permission of ISAKOS and Elsevier.

T. Ettore (✉)
Department of Shoulder Surgery, IRCCS OGSA—Ospedale Galeazzi Sant'Ambrogio, Milan, Italy
e-mail: Ettore.Taverna@eoc.ch; taverna@shoulder.it

A. O. Caterina
International Society of Arthroscopy, Knee Surgery and Orthopaedic Sports Medicine, Milan, Italy

P. Carlo · G. Vincenzo
IRCCS Istituto Ortopedico Galeazzi, Milan, Italy

E. Calvo et al. (eds.), *Complex and Revision Problems in Shoulder Instability*,
https://doi.org/10.1007/978-3-031-81389-4_7

7.2 Understanding Arthroscopic Bone Block

The arthroscopic bone block procedure aims to address glenoid bone loss and capsular deficiency, which are critical factors in recurrent shoulder instability [2]. Traditionally, open surgical procedures like the Latarjet procedure were used to address glenoid bone loss. However, these procedures are associated with a higher risk of complications. In recent years, the arthroscopic bone block procedure has gained popularity as a less invasive alternative. This procedure involves using arthroscopic techniques to perform a bone block transfer and stabilize the shoulder joint. During the arthroscopic bone block procedure, two glenoid tunnels are created from the posterior to the anterior side of the glenoid using a dedicated bone block guide [3]. Following the creation of the tunnels, a bone graft, autograft, allograft or xenograft, is harvested and prepared. The bone graft is then passed through the tunnels and fixed to the glenoid using buttons, while soft tissues are repaired using anchors. The arthroscopic bone block procedure offers several advantages over open surgical techniques. First and foremost, it is a minimally invasive procedure that allows for smaller incisions and less soft tissue dissection. This results in reduced postoperative pain, faster recovery, and improved cosmetic outcomes. Additionally, the arthroscopic bone block procedure allows for better visualization of the glenoid and surrounding structures, which enhances accuracy in graft placement [4]. Moreover, the arthroscopic bone block procedure preserves the native anatomy of the shoulder joint, minimizing the risk of complications. Furthermore, the arthroscopic bone block procedure offers the potential for better long-term outcomes in terms of stability and function.

7.2.1 Surgical Indications

The arthroscopic bone block procedure is specifically designed for patients with recurrent anterior shoulder instability, young age, sportive activities, and bone defects. Indications for the bone block procedure include an ISIS score greater than 3, up to 5 shoulder dislocation episodes, glenoid bone loss exceeding 15% or over 10% with a concurrent hill sachs lesion, and the first dislocation occurring within 3 years. Contraindications for the procedure include a history of failed previous surgery for shoulder instability, experiencing more than five episodes of shoulder dislocation, having above 20% glenoid bone loss, and chronic instability persisting for more than 3 years since the first episode. The surgical indications are shown in Table 7.1.

Table 7.1 Bone block procedure surgical indications

Arthroscopic bone block graft procedure indication
Anterior glenoid bone loss <20% with associated Bankart lesion
Anterior glenoid bone loss >10% but <20% with ISIS score of 3–6 points
First episode of dislocation ≤3 years earlier
≤5 episodes of dislocation

7.2.2 Detailed Procedure: The Free Arthroscopic Bone Block

The free arthroscopic bone block procedure is a specific technique for treating recurrent anterior shoulder instability with glenoid bone loss. This procedure involves the precise placement of a tricortical bone on the anterior glenoid neck. The procedure begins with the patient under general anesthesia and in the beach chair position or lateral decubitus. The surgeon starts by creating a standard arthroscopic portal for the camera and two additional portals for instrumentation. Through a posterior portal, the surgeon introduces an arthroscopic guide for the glenoid tunnels. The guide is positioned on the posterior glenoid neck, allowing for accurate placement of the tunnels on the anterior side of the glenoid (Fig. 7.1a, b). Next, the surgeon uses a motorized bur to decorticate the anterior glenoid rim and create a flat and bleeding bony surface [5]. Following decortication, the surgeon prepares the bone graft. Once the bone graft is prepared, it is passed inside the joint through a cannula and positioned on the anterior-inferior

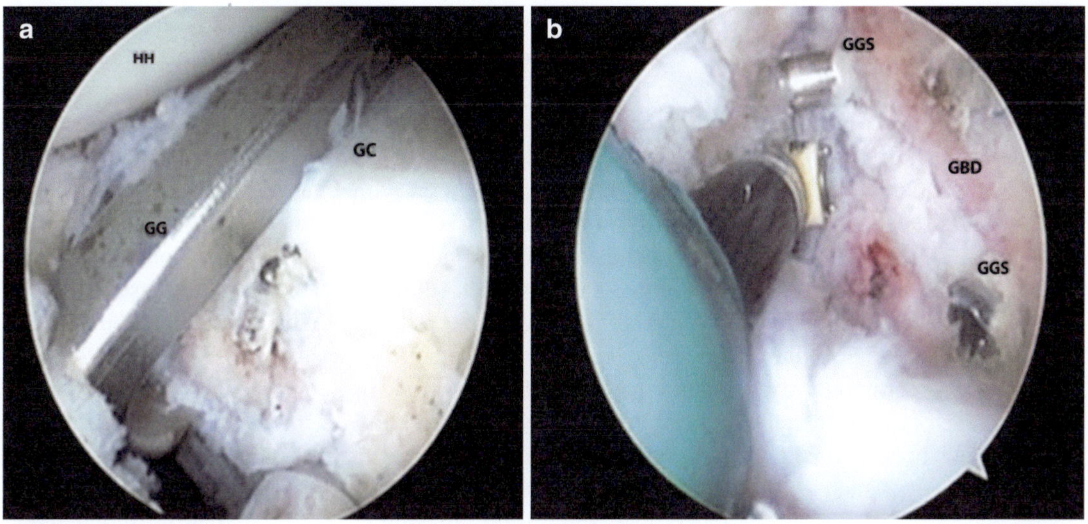

Fig. 7.1 (**a**) Arthroscopic view: glenoid guide positioning (*HH* humeral head, *GC* glenoid cartilage, *GG* glenoid guide). (**b**) Arthroscopic view: sleeve insertion (*GGS*, glenoid guide sleeve, *GBD* glenoid bone deficit)

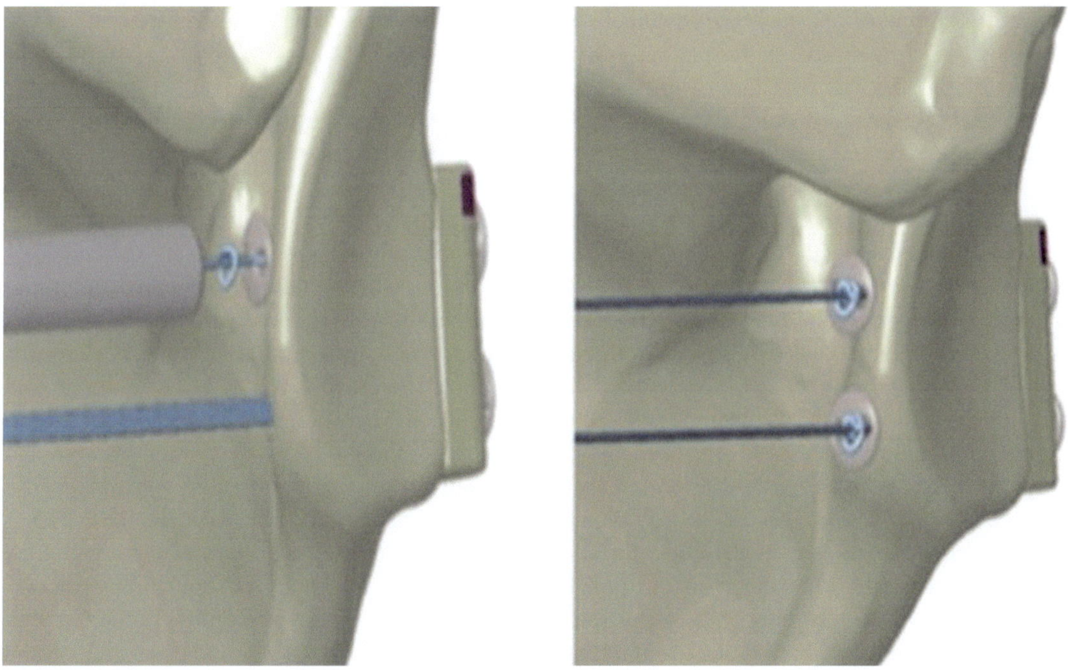

Fig. 7.2 Arthroscopic bone block procedure: endobuttons fixation

glenoid neck. Special buttons are used to secure the bone graft flush with the anterior glenoid rim under arthroscopic control (Fig. 7.2). The next step involves capsular, labral, and ligament reconstruction on the glenoid rim using suture anchors. These anchors stabilize as a standard Bankart repair. Advantages of this procedure include the possibility of adding surgical arthroscopic procedures such as remplissage and ASA technique (Arthroscopic Subscapularis Augmentation) [2, 6].

7.2.3 Bone Graft Options

There are several options for the bone graft used in the free arthroscopic bone block procedure. The bone graft can be harvested from the patient's own iliac crest (autograft), obtained from a tissue bank (allograft), or derived from an animal source (xenograft). The choice of bone graft depends on various factors such as patient preference, surgeon expertise, availability of graft material, and the specific needs of the individual case. Autografts are commonly used as they provide the advantage of osteoconductivity, meaning they promote new bone formation. Autografts offer general advantages such as availability (they are always accessible), without any added cost, and no risk of transmitting infectious diseases from the donor. In addition, autografts have a lower risk of graft rejection compared to allografts and xenografts. Autografts also have the advantage of providing a perfect match to the patient's own bone, reducing the risk of immune reactions. Iliac crest autograft and distal clavicle autograft are the most commonly used autografts in the free arthroscopic bone block procedure [7]. However, harvesting an autograft involves an additional surgical site and carries the risks associated with the donor site. Surgical time is also prolonged. Allografts, on the other hand, are readily available and do not require an additional surgical site for harvesting. They are obtained from tissue banks and undergo rigorous screening and sterilization processes to ensure safety. Allografts also have the advantage of providing a larger graft size compared to autografts, which can be beneficial in cases of larger bone defects. Other benefits include the option to customize size and shape, as well as reduced surgical time. The most commonly used allografts are the iliac crest allograft and distal tibia allograft [8]. Allografts have disadvantages such as a higher resorption rate compared to autografts, limited availability, increased cost, and the risk of transmitting infectious diseases. Xenografts, derived from an animal source, are another option for bone grafting in the free arthroscopic bone block procedure. Xenografts are typically sourced from animals such as horses, cows, or pigs and undergo a thorough sterilization process to minimize the risk of infection. Xenografts offer advantages such as no risk of transmitting infectious diseases due to sterilization, availability, absence of donor site morbidity and no need for additional surgical procedures, with reduced surgical time. However, they also come with disadvantages including added cost and inability to customize size and shape. Additionally, there is limited scientific literature on this topic. In recent years, biocompatible synthetic bone substitutes known as alloplasts have emerged as an alternative for autologous or allogeneic bone but more studies are needed to fully evaluate their efficacy and safety in the context of the free arthroscopic bone block procedure. In summary, the free arthroscopic bone block procedure for shoulder instability can utilize autografts, allografts, xenografts, or alloplasts as bone substitutes. Each type of graft has its own advantages and disadvantages [9].

7.2.4 Osteointegration and Bone Resorption

After the free arthroscopic bone block procedure, the bone graft undergoes a process called osteointegration, which allows it to become fully integrated with the scapular bone. During this process, the body's natural healing mechanisms stimulate the growth of new bone tissue around the graft, effectively fusing it to the glenoid rim. Over time, the bone graft becomes a stable and permanent part of the shoulder joint [10]. The process of osteointegration is crucial for the long-term success of the free arthroscopic bone block procedure. As the bone graft undergoes osteointegration, it becomes structurally integrated with the surrounding bone, providing stability and support to the shoulder joint (Fig. 7.3). This integration process is facilitated by the body's natural healing response, which promotes the formation of new bone tissue and the remodelling of the graft to conform seamlessly with the glenoid rim In addition to osteointegration, it is important to consider the possibility of bone resorption following the free arthroscopic bone block procedure. Bone resorption refers to the loss of bone

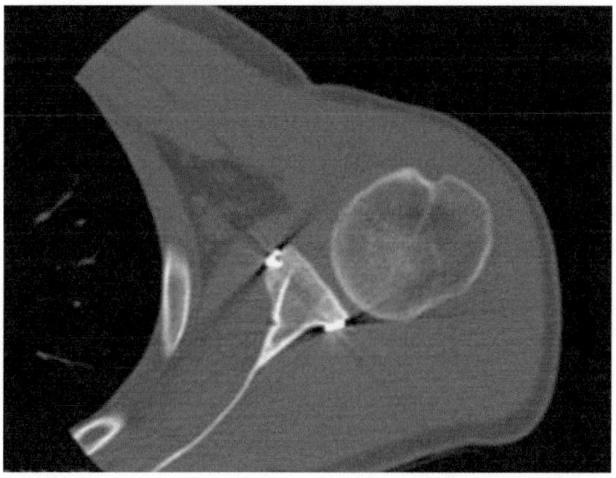

Fig. 7.3 Example of bone graft osteointegration

tissue over time and can potentially impact the stability of the graft. Understanding the factors that contribute to bone resorption and implementing strategies to minimize its occurrence are essential for ensuring the long-term success of the procedure. Factors that may contribute to bone resorption include inadequate initial fixation of the graft, poor blood supply to the graft site, and excessive mechanical stress on the graft. To address these potential issues, careful surgical technique and meticulous graft placement are crucial [11, 12].

7.2.5 Benefits and Risks of Arthroscopic Bone Block

The arthroscopic bone block procedure offers several benefits compared to traditional open procedures for treating glenoid bone loss in anterior shoulder instability [10]. One of the main benefits is that it preserves the native anatomy of the shoulder joint, allowing for better stability and function in the long term. Another benefit is the reduced morbidity associated with the arthroscopic approach. This includes smaller incisions, less soft-tissue dissection, and better visualization of the joint. Additionally, the use of special buttons to fix the bone graft eliminates the need for screws, reducing the risk of hardware complications such as loosening or irritation of surrounding structures. Furthermore, the arthroscopic technique allows for intraoperative modification of the surgical plan, providing the surgeon with greater flexibility and adaptability. However, it is important to note that the arthroscopic bone block procedure also carries certain risks and limitations. These include the potential for graft displacement or failure, infection, nerve or blood vessel injury, and the need for revision surgery in case of recurrent instability.

7.2.6 Recovery and Rehabilitation After the Procedure

After an arthroscopic bone block procedure for shoulder instability, the patient's recovery and rehabilitation play a crucial role in achieving successful outcomes. The goals of rehabilitation after an arthroscopic bone block procedure are to restore shoulder stability, improve range of motion, and regain strength in the affected shoulder muscles. The rehabilitation process typically begins with the patient wearing a sling to protect the shoulder and limit movement for 3 weeks. During this period, the patient can be allowed to start gentle passive physical therapy to prevent stiffness of shoulder and elbow. After 3 weeks, the patient has to start passive-assisted range of motion exercises. After 7 weeks from surgery the patient progresses to active range of motion exercises. Strengthening exercises for the rotator cuff muscles and scapular stabilizers are gradually introduced to improve shoulder stability and function at 12 weeks postop. Return to sports activities and overhead mobility is generally allowed around 4–6 months post-surgery, but this timeline may vary depending on the individual patient's progress and the surgeon's discretion. During the rehabilitation process, the patient will work closely with a physical therapist who will guide them through various exercises and activities to regain strength, range of motion, and stability in the shoulder joint.

7.3 Outcomes of Free Arthroscopic Bone Block for Anterior Shoulder Instability

In a retrospective study conducted, the authors evaluated the outcomes of arthroscopic bone block procedures in patients with anterior glenohumeral instability and glenoid bone loss. The study included 27 patients who underwent the arthroscopic bone block procedure, and they were followed up for an average of 29. months. The results showed that at the final follow-up, 25 patients had no signs of osteoarthritis, indicating a successful outcome [11]. The mean glenoid bony gain observed was 24.2%, indicating successful bone graft healing. Additionally, the study reported a recurrence rate of 0%, with a mean Walch-Duplay score of 93.2 and a mean Rowe score of 96. These findings suggest that the arthroscopic bone block procedure is an effective treatment option for anterior glenohumeral instability with glenoid bone loss, providing stability and improving functional outcomes. Another case study conducted evaluated the outcomes of arthroscopic bone block procedures in a group of athletes with recurrent shoulder instability. The study included 15 athletes who underwent the procedure and were followed up for an average of 24 months. The results showed that all 15 athletes had successful outcomes with no recurrence of instability. They were able to return to their pre-injury level of sports activities without experiencing any significant complications. These case studies provide further evidence for the effectiveness of the arthroscopic bone block procedure in treating glenohumeral instability.

7.4 Conclusion and Future Prospects of Arthroscopic Free Bone Block Techniques

The arthroscopic bone block procedure has emerged as a promising technique for the treatment of shoulder instability with glenoid bone loss [4]. With excellent clinical and radiological results, this procedure offers a viable option for restoring shoulder stability in patients with anterior glenohumeral instability [11]. Not only does it allow for bone graft healing and significant improvements in functional outcomes, but it also has a low recurrence rate and allows athletes to return to their pre-injury level of sports activities. However, further research is still needed to evaluate the long-term outcomes of this procedure and compare it to other surgical techniques. Additionally, advancements in arthroscopic techniques and instrumentation continue to improve the accuracy and success of the arthroscopic bone block procedure. These advancements include the use of computer-assisted navigation systems, which can aid in precise graft placement and reduce the risk of graft malpositioning. Furthermore, the development of new fixation methods, such as suture anchors and bioabsorbable materials, may provide additional options for securing the graft to the glenoid rim. Overall, the arthroscopic bone block procedure holds great promise for the treatment of anterior glenohumeral instability with glenoid bone loss. It offers a less invasive approach with excellent clinical outcomes and a low recurrence rate.

References

1. Beletsky A, Cancienne JM, Manderle BJ, Mehta N, Wilk KE. A comparison of physical therapy protocols between open Latarjet coracoid transfer and arthroscopic bankart repair. Sports Health. 2020;12:124. https://doi.org/10.1177/1941738119887396.
2. Russo R, Maiotti M, Taverna E, Rao C. Arthroscopic bone graft procedure combined with arthroscopic subscapularis augmentation for recurrent anterior instability with glenoid bone defect. Arthrosc Tech. 2018;7:e623. https://doi.org/10.1016/j.eats.2018.02.009.
3. Russo R, Maiotti M, Taverna E. Arthroscopic bone graft procedure combined with arthroscopic subscapularis augmentation (ASA) for recurrent anterior instability with glenoid bone defect: a cadaver study. J Exp Orthop. 2018;5:5. https://doi.org/10.1186/s40634-018-0121-0.
4. Owens BD. Been around the block before. Am J Sports Med. 2014;42(11):2557–9. https://doi.org/10.1177/0363546514556637.
5. Taverna E, Garavaglia G, Ufenast H, D'Ambrosi R. Arthroscopic treatment of glenoid bone loss. Knee

Surg Sports Traumatol Arthrosc. 2015;24:546. https://doi.org/10.1007/s00167-015-3893-0.
6. Armocida D, Rossi CM, Pietto FD, Romano M, Guastafierro A, Rotonda GD, Russo R. Arthroscopic subscapularis augmentation with xenograft glenoid bone block in patients with recurrent anterior shoulder instability. Arthrosc Sports Med Rehabil. 2023;5:e809. https://doi.org/10.1016/j.asmr.2023.04.008.
7. Levin JM, Whitlock K, Warren E, Klifto CS, Anakwenze O. Arthroscopic distal clavicle bone block technique for anteroinferior instability with critical bone loss. Arthrosc Tech. 2023;12(6):e787–94. https://doi.org/10.1016/j.eats.2023.02.055.
8. Liles J, Ganokroj P, Peebles AM, Mologne MS, Provencher MT. Primary distal tibia allograft for restoration of Glenohumeral stability with anterior glenoid bone loss. Arthrosc Tech. 2022;11(6):e1039–43. https://doi.org/10.1016/j.eats.2022.02.006.
9. Gilat R, Wong SE, Lavoie-Gagne O, Haunschild ED, Knapik DM, Fu MC, Chahla J, Forsythe B, Cole BJ. Outcomes are comparable using free bone block autografts versus allografts for the management of anterior shoulder instability with glenoid bone loss: a systematic review and meta-analysis of "the non-Latarjet". Knee Surg Sports Traumatol Arthrosc. 2020;29(7):2159–74. https://doi.org/10.1007/s00167-020-06194-z.
10. Taverna E, D'Ambrosi R, Perfetti C, Garavaglia G. Arthroscopic bone graft procedure for anterior inferior glenohumeral instability. Arthrosc Tech. 2014;3:e653. https://doi.org/10.1016/j.eats.2014.08.002.
11. Taverna E, Garavaglia G, Perfetti C, Ufenast H, Sconfienza LM, Guarrella V. An arthroscopic bone block procedure is effective in restoring stability, allowing return to sports in cases of glenohumeral instability with glenoid bone deficiency. Knee Surg Sports Traumatol Arthrosc. 2018;26(12):3780–7. https://doi.org/10.1007/s00167-018-4921-7.
12. Albizzini Ohin C, Guarrella V, Perfetti C, Larghi MM, Messina C, Sconfienza LM, Taverna E. CT-scan evaluation of osteointegration and osteolysis in different graft types and surgical techniques for the treatment of shoulder instability. Arch Bone Jt Surg. 2023;11(2):117–23.

8 Systems for Bone Graft Fixation: Screws, Buttons, Tapes

Nicholas F. Kwon, Yazdan Raji, Connor J. Sholtis, and Michael T. Freehill

8.1 Introduction

Anterior glenohumeral instability involving a bone defect remains a challenging orthopaedic condition, often necessitating complex surgical intervention to restore joint stability and function. Several techniques have been developed to address recurrent anterior instability, most commonly the Latarjet procedure [1, 2]. Regardless of the chosen technique, success is critically dependent on effective fixation of graft to glenoid, a task that demands meticulous attention to both biomechanics and patient-specific considerations [3–5]. Over the past decade, three primary methods of graft fixation have emerged: screw, suture button, and suture tape-based fixation, each with its own set of advantages, challenges, and indications [6–8].

Screw-based fixation, historically the more traditional approach, involves the use of one or two metallic screws to secure the coracoid graft to the glenoid. Several types of screws have been employed, including fully threaded solid cortical screws, partially threaded solid cancellous screws, and cannulated partially threaded cancellous screws [3, 6]. The choice among screw types is often based on surgeon preference, with considerations given to the biomechanical strength of the construct, the ease of achieving maximum compression for graft-to-bone healing, and the accuracy of screw placement to prevent migration of bone blocks during insertion. Despite the proven effectiveness of screw fixation in both healing rates and clinical outcomes, it is not without risk, including screw pullout or loosening, coracoid fracture, graft nonunion, neurovascular injury, and arthrosis secondary to screw prominence [4, 9, 10].

Suture button-based fixation offers an alternative approach that has gained popularity, especially in arthroscopic applications. Suture buttons provide several benefits, including ease of use in arthroscopy, reduced hardware complications, and potentially quicker rehabilitation times [3, 7, 11]. This technique leverages the mechanical stability and flexibility offered by these nonrigid devices to accommodate the dynamic forces within the shoulder joint. Clinical studies have reported satisfactory outcomes with suture button fixation, highlighting its viability as a method for graft fixation. Early biomechanical data has been promising, but debate persists surrounding the biomechanical properties of suture button compared to the more conventional screw fixation.

Other contemporary surgical approaches for anterior glenoid bone graft procedures propose use of arthroscopic techniques utilizing com-

N. F. Kwon · Y. Raji · C. J. Sholtis · M. T. Freehill (✉)
Department of Orthopaedic Surgery, Stanford University School of Medicine, Redwood City, CA, USA
e-mail: nickkwon@stanford.edu; Csholtis@stanford.edu

E. Calvo et al. (eds.), *Complex and Revision Problems in Shoulder Instability*,
https://doi.org/10.1007/978-3-031-81389-4_8

pletely metal-free constructs with ultra-high-strength sutures for graft stabilization and capsulolabral reconstruction. While there is a lack of comparative clinical studies assessing these novel approaches, these contributions collectively advance orthopaedic interventions for anterior shoulder instability, promising optimized patient outcomes and reduced iatrogenic risks.

The decision between screw, suture button, and tape fixation is influenced by multiple factors, including surgeon experience, anatomical and pathological specificity, and the potential for complications. The following section details these fixation strategies, with particular attention to technique and technical considerations, biomechanics, and clinical outcomes. The aim of this section is to provide an up-to-date summary of high-quality literature to guide surgeon decision-making in graft fixation for anterior shoulder instability with associated glenoid bone defect.

8.2 Screw Fixation

8.2.1 Solid Screws

Of the many design elements that can be modulated, screw length and diameter are among the key decision points. Larger screw diameter has been classically associated with greater implant strength; however, this must be carefully balanced with the consequent defect introduced by larger bore [12]. Similarly, increased screw length is also thought to impart greater stability; however, the risk of iatrogenic injury must also be carefully considered [10, 11, 13]. Screw diameter itself has not been shown to directly affect construct strength in biomechanical models thus far [13]. In a 2022 meta-regression by Huish et al. including eight biomechanical studies, screw diameter was not shown to affect the resistance to either tensile or shear forces [14]. Interestingly, however, increasing *drill* diameter was found to significantly decrease the ultimate failure load against shear force. Similarly, this same effect trended towards statistical significance against tensile force as well. The authors surmise that this is in part due to weakening of the graft by increased hole size, though this was not investigated directly.

Throughout the literature, screw length has mostly been studied in the context of number of cortices engaged by screws. The use of two screws with each achieving bicortical fixation has been thought to impart the greatest rigidity, and several studies have supported this notion [13, 15]. In simulated bone-block studies, both Schmiddem and Willemot found two screws placed in bicortical fashion to be biomechanically superior to alternative combinations utilizing unicortical configurations. However, achieving bicortical purchase with two screws can be technically challenging, especially given the significant risk of nerve injury associated with posterior screw prominence. Perhaps the most comprehensive study to examine this relationship was conducted by Shin et al. in 2017, in which five different combinations of screw types and cortical engagement were mechanically tested in both cyclic loading and load to failure [6]. Notably, neither screw type nor number of engaged cortices was found to significantly affect the measured biomechanical outcomes. This finding was replicated in Huish's meta-analysis, which showed no association between number of cortices engaged and mean ultimate failure load. To date, there is no evidence that bicortical fixation leads to higher union rates. A nonrandomized study from 2022 followed 184 patients that underwent Latarjet fixation with either unicortical or bicortical fixation and found no clinically significant difference in union rates, recurrent instability, or postoperative complication between either group at 8 weeks follow-up [16]. As such, the independent contribution of "double bicortical" engagement is not entirely clear, though the literature suggests that the ideal construct optimizes for both screw length and diameter while ensuring safe screw placement.

8.2.2 One- Versus Two-Screw Constructs

In addition to variation in screw implant design, there also exists variation in the number of screws used for graft fixation [6]. The choice between one and two screws is often a function of graft orientation, as is noted between the conventional Latarjet versus the Bristow procedures [17]. The decision between one and two screws may also be driven by the demand for earlier and more aggressive rehabilitation, during which more robust stability in the early postoperative period preceding bony union is clinically valuable. Biomechanically, the limited body of literature has shown two-screw constructs to confer greater overall stability. In a synthetic bone block model, two-screw constructs required a significantly higher load to failure compared to one-screw when load was applied directly to the synthetic coracoid bone block, mimicking the force experienced under maximum shoulder abduction and external rotation [18]. This was further supported in a 3D-printed polyurethane anatomic model by Azoulay et al. which showed two-screw constructs to have nearly 1.5 times the fixation rigidity of one-screw configurations [19]. Cadaveric and clinical correlates are unfortunately lacking. The only known cadaver study to examine this relationship was conducted by Weppe et al. [20], although two different techniques were compared, one utilizing a single bioabsorbable interference screw for coracoid bone plug fixation and the other utilizing two bicortical screws through a larger piece of the coracoid (Latarjet-Patte) [20]. Perhaps predictably, the ultimate failure load in the two-screw group was nearly double that of the single bioabsorbable screw, when force was applied directly in axis with the conjoint tendon. In all three of these studies, the two-screw configurations withstood physiologic loads without failure [3]. Taken together, these data suggest that two-screw constructs provide greater immediate stability compared to one-screw counterparts. However, the clinical significance of this difference remains unclear, including patient-reported outcomes, union rates, and complication rates.

8.2.3 Cannulated Screws

Cannulated screws offer a viable alternative to solid screws for anterior graft fixation, particularly in complex cases requiring precise graft placement (Fig. 8.1). Proponents of cannulated screws cite the ability to maintain graft positioning during screw insertion as a critical advantage, particularly in all-arthroscopic Latarjet procedures [21]. To date, cannulated screws have not been shown to be overwhelmingly different than solid screws from a biomechanical standpoint [22]. One of the first comparative biomechanical

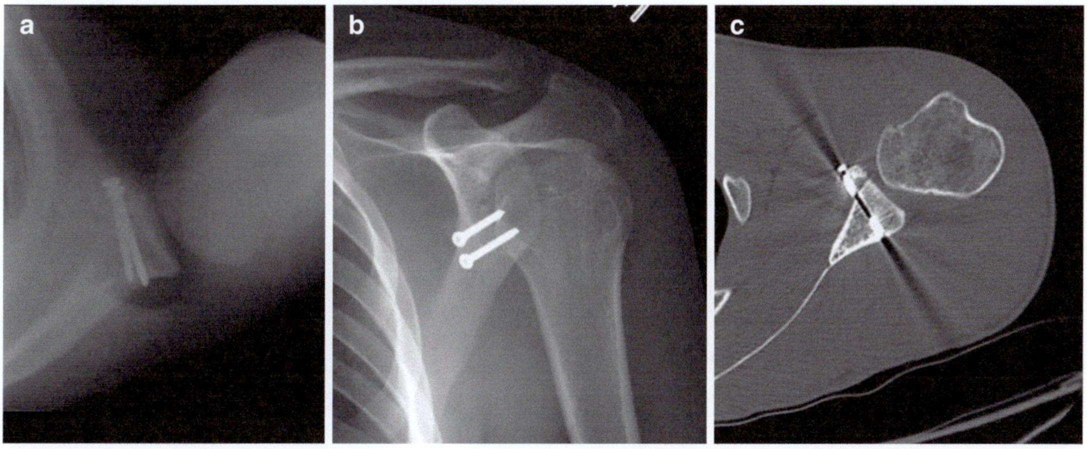

Fig. 8.1 (**a, b**) 3 month post-operative axillary lateral and anteroposterior radiographs of the left shoulder following Latarjet procedure with 4.0 mm cannulated titanium screw fixation. (**c**) Left shoulder axial sequence computed tomography scan 3 months post-operatively following Latarjet procedure with 4.0 mm cannulated titanium screw fixation. (Courtesy of Michael T. Freehill, MD)

studies by Alvi et al. evaluated solid versus cannulated screws in Latarjet fixation using the congruent-arc technique, finding no significant difference in mean cycles to failure between the two. This finding was supported by Shin et al., who demonstrated no significant difference in load to failure between cannulated and solid screws in Latarjet fixation using the classic technique. Furthermore, no differences were appreciated between unicortical and bicortical configurations involving cannulated screws. A study published the following year evaluating two different cannulated screw types demonstrated that a two-screw configuration could sufficiently resist physiologic cyclic loading if both screws had bicortical purchase [13]. Interestingly, this study did find that the Arthrex 3.75 mm cannulated screw was uniquely sensitive to number of cortices engaged under higher loads when compared with other proprietary instrumentation. This screw had smallest shaft diameter, the coarsest pitch, and the lowest shaft/thread length ratio of the three screws included for testing, implicating the screw design features as an important factor in graft stability, especially if bicortical engagement is not attainable. Most recently, a 2022 meta-regression by Huish et al., found no significant difference in mean ultimate failure load in both shear and tension between cannulated and solid screws.

However, some have argued that the biomechanical advantage plays a less important role in graft function than graft positioning. If such is the case, then the clinical advantage of cannulated screws may not be fully captured by biomechanical superiority alone. Indeed, graft malpositioning is known to contribute to a host of suboptimal outcomes including suprascapular nerve injury, serial instability, nonunion, and intraoperative fracture [23–25]. Unfortunately, the literature surrounding clinical outcomes following cannulated screw fixation remains sparse. This may be in part due to the results of a 48-patient series by Shah et al., which reported recurrent instability in four out of the five patients in this cohort treated with either 4.0-mm or 4.5-mm cannulated screw fixation [26]. Two of these failures occurred within 8 months, and screw loosening was noted in three of the four cases. A series of 124 primary Latarjet procedures performed by a single surgeon using only 4.5-mm cannulated screws demonstrated encouraging clinical results at 2-year follow-up, most notably a 100% graft fusion rate at 3 months, assessed on radiographs [21]. Other notable outcomes included 88% return to sport rate and high patient-reported outcome measures (Walch Dupay, SSV, VAS). To date, no other large studies have been performed using cannulated screws. As such, more robust data is needed to investigate the safety and efficacy of cannulated screws for graft fixation.

8.2.4 Screw Insertion Angle

While many studies have focused on screw quantity and material, others have suggested that screw trajectory may play an equally, if not more, influential role in stability [27–29]. Screw trajectory can be quantified using the alpha angle, which is measured between the screw and the glenoid surface (Fig. 8.2). Several key considerations are weighed when determining alpha

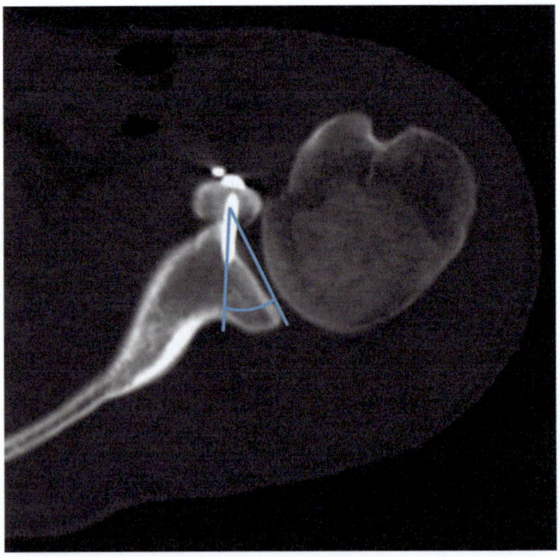

Fig. 8.2 Axillary lateral radiograph of the right shoulder of a patient presenting with post-operative pain and sensation of instability 3-month following Latarjet procedure at an outside facility with an elevated alpha angle. (Courtesy of Ettore Taverna, MD)

angle including risk of suprascapular nerve injury and graft stability. To date, no consensus has been established on optimal alpha angle, also referred to as divergence or insertion angle. Prior studies have been published on angles ranging from 0° to 50°, although the literature has trended towards smaller alpha angles in recent years [28]. Indeed, several studies have associated larger alpha angles with inferior biomechanical properties and clinical outcomes including nonunion, graft overhang, and suprascapular nerve injury [30, 31]. A recent study by Hsu et al., using a single screw construct, found no difference in graft displacement under cyclic loading between α angles of 0° and 15°, but significantly increased graft displacement at 30°. Similarly, in a bone-block simulated model, Frank et al. showed that both single- and double-screw constructs oriented at an alpha angle of 15 led to greater graft displacement and lower maximum load to failure compared to those placed at 0° [18]. Taken together, the limited literature seems to favor smaller alpha angles to maximize stability and decrease risk of complication, though more standardized biomechanical testing models are needed to draw direct comparisons.

8.2.5 Screw-Related Complications

Despite overall excellent outcomes following screw-based fixation, this method is not without challenge. The overall complication rate following screw fixation has been reported as high as 30%, with nonunion, graft resorption, graft fracture, nerve injury, and symptomatic hardware comprising the majority [3, 32–34]. In 2012, prior to the advent of suture button Latarjet procedures, Butt and Charalambous published a systematic review of complications following open coracoid transfer. In this analysis, hardware-related complications were reported at an overall rate of 6.5%, the most common being screw migration, loosening, breakage in addition to joint penetration, and soft tissue irritation/impingement [4] (Fig. 8.3). This was highlighted by a meta-analysis published the following year

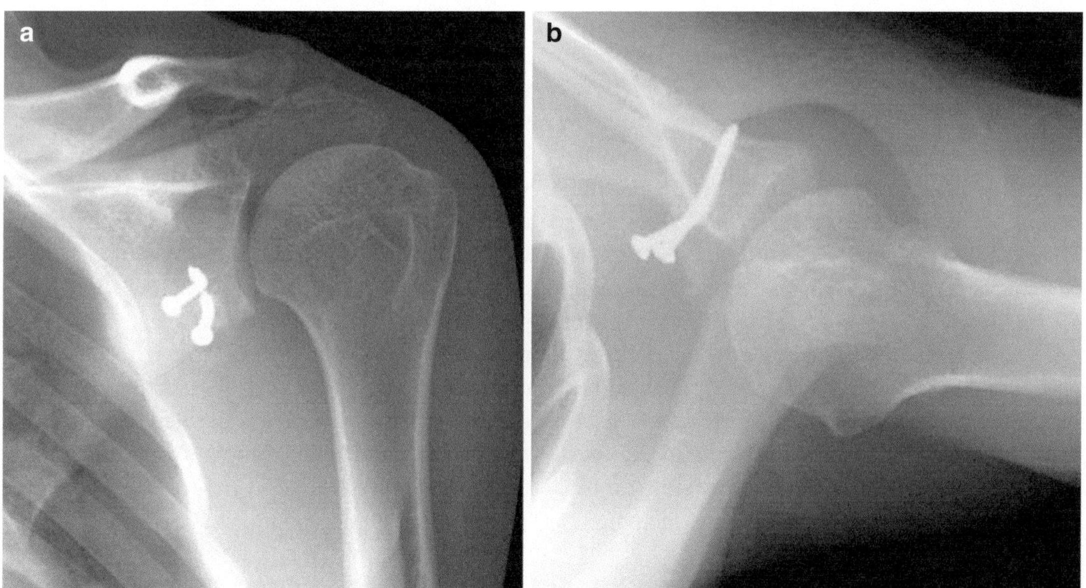

Fig. 8.3 (**a, b**) 6 month post-operative Grashey and axillary lateral radiographs of the left shoulder following Latarjet procedure with 3.5 mm solid stainless steel screw fixation with evidence of bending deformation. (Courtesy of Michael T. Freehill, MD)

which reported a 7% unplanned reoperation rate, of which 35% were due to symptomatic hardware [34]. Nerve injury, namely to the suprascapular and musculocutaneous nerves as well as the brachial plexus, can be a morbid complication following anterior instability procedures [10]. More contemporary literature has cited the rate of neurologic injury between 1.2% and 1.9% with screw fixation, while older studies have reported as high as 8.2% [4, 35, 36]. Some have pointed to excessive screw length as a contributor; however, excessively short screws run the risk of instability and possible nonunion [37]. Most agree that optimal screw placement and trajectory is critical to maximize biomechanical stability and minimize risk of iatrogenic nerve injury, but this has been shown to be quite challenging, particularly when performed arthroscopically [24, 38, 39]. Furthermore, the literature has not shown complication rates to decrease with more surgeon experience [9].

8.3 Alternative Screw-Materials

In attempts to avoid the deleterious effects that can be seen following metallic screw complications, alternative screw materials have been introduced. Bioabsorbable screws, which typically resorb during the initial months to years following surgery, offer the theoretical advantage of avoiding soft tissue and cartilage irritation, especially in the setting of osteolysis [40]. These screws, typically composed of polymers or mineralized compounds, have seen increasing use in other orthopaedic applications, such as ACL interference screws [41, 42]. However, their use has not yet been widely adopted in anterior stabilization shoulder surgery. A cadaver study by Bockmann et al. investigated the fixation strength of fully threaded stainless-steel screws compared to magnesium screws and poly L-lactic acid (PLLA) screws under several different loading conditions that a coracoid graft could experience [43]. They found that stainless-steel screws had the greatest primary fixation strength under direct graft loading, with a statistically significant difference between only stainless steel and PLLA screws. However, interestingly, all three constructs failed at greater than 200 N, suggesting reasonable fixation strength under physiologic conditions. Clinical studies investigating the use of bioabsorbable screws is also quite limited. A 2015 case series including 12 patients that underwent coracoid graft fixation with a polylactic acid and co-glycolic acid copolymer (PLGA) reported severe osteolysis in 67% of cases [44]. Mechanisms for failure were not clear, but the authors note that hydrolytic reaction surrounding the screws was not widely observed, which is a known effect seen in other bioabsorbable screw materials. It is worth noting that, like metallic implants, not all bioabsorbable screws are equal. There exists little biomechanical or clinical evidence directly comparing different metal screw materials, such as titanium and stainless-steel. Similarly, bioabsorbable screw materials vary widely in their composition and consequent interactions with surrounding tissue, and new technologies continue to emerge [42, 45]. Recently, a bioabsorbable screw composed of several different mineralized fibers was introduced [46]. The senior author favors the utilization of mineralized screws (Bio-Integrative OSSIOfiber® Compression Screws, Woburn, MA) due to their capacity for osseous bio-integration, high compression strength, pull-out and shear stability at time-zero as well as artifact-free imaging properties (Fig. 8.4). However, the current mechanical properties are primarily derived from priority testing, and additional comparative clinical studies are necessary to further validate their efficacy.

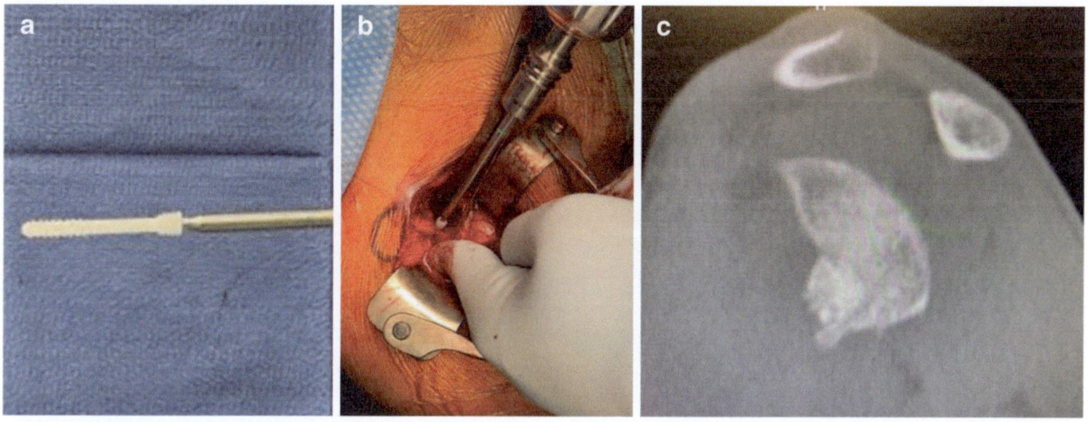

Fig. 8.4 (**a**) Mineralized 4.0 mm partially threaded cancellous screw (Bio-Integrative OSSIOfiber® Compression Screw). (**b**) Placement of mineralized screw during Latarjet procedure. (**c**) Left shoulder sagittal en face computed tomography scan sequence 6 months postoperatively following Latarjet procedure with mineralized partially threaded cancellous screws (Bio-Integrative OSSIOfiber® Compression Screws). (Courtesy of Michael T. Freehill, MD)

8.4 Suture Button Fixation

Suture button fixation, also referred to as nonrigid fixation, for anterior glenoid instability emerged in 2014, first described by Taverna, and later by Boileau as a novel fixation method that could overcome many of the challenges and drawbacks associated with screw fixation, including graft malpositioning, iatrogenic nerve injury, and hardware-associated complications [7, 47] (Fig. 8.5). Boileau's original study included 76 patients who all underwent suture button fixation with two cortical buttons (anterior and posterior) and reported a 91% union rate with no neurologic complications. Additionally, 96% of grafts were determined to be placed congruent to the glenoid articular surface, as determined by CT scan. Given the promising outlook of this technology, several biomechanical studies comparing screw and suture button fixation soon followed. With respect to ultimate load to failure, two cadaveric studies comparing double suture button constructs against double-screw constructs found no significant difference between the two groups [48, 49]. However, it is important to note that tensile force along the vector of the conjoint tendon—as studied by Provencher and Kazum—is not the only force that a newly fixed graft might experience. This important distinction was highlighted by Williams et al., who simulated direct loading onto the graft that could be imposed by the humeral head in the case of a fall onto the operative arm [50]. In doing so, they found significantly lower maximum cycle displacement and higher load to failure in the screw group compared to the suture button group. Notably, each of these studies found distinct differences in the modes of failure. Screw-based constructs typically fractured through the graft itself, often resulting in significant damage to both graft and surrounding structures. Conversely, suture button constructs tended to fail at either the glenoid or the interface of the cadaver and testing jig and did not usually induce significant surrounding destruction. These results may implicate the larger drill holes needed for screw fixation as a possible stress riser. Some have postulated that this tendency could afford suture-button constructs more options if the need for revision were to arise [50].

Following Taverna and Boileau's original technique descriptions, the body of literature focused on clinical outcomes after suture button fixation expanded meaningfully. This collection was nicely synthesized in a 2023 systematic

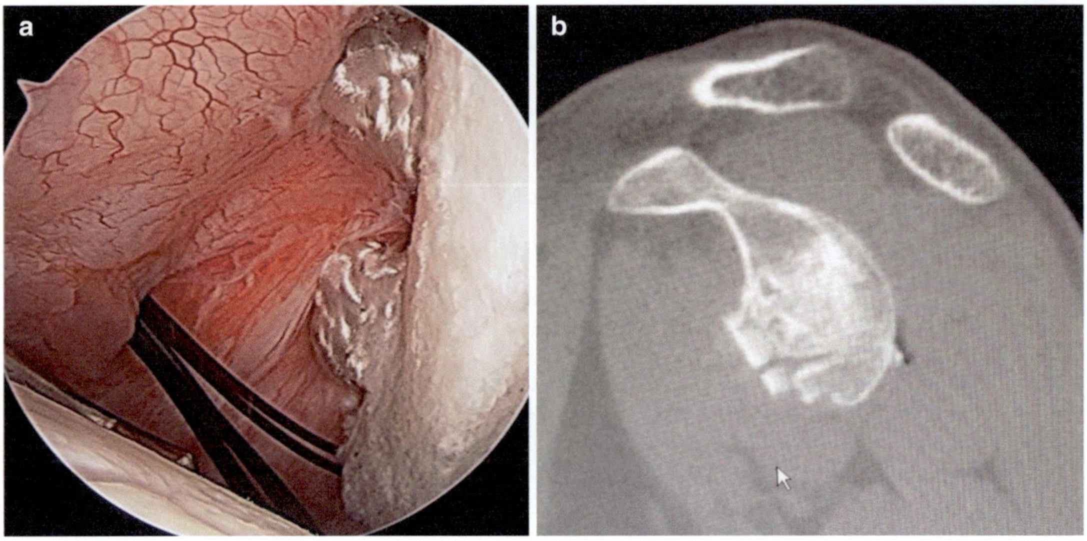

Fig. 8.5 (**a**) Intraoperative arthroscopic image of allograft bone block procedure using all-suture double-loaded anchor construct along with posterior suture button fixation of allograft on anterior glenoid. (**b**) 6 month post-operative sagittal en face computed tomography scan sequence demonstrating evidence of osseous healing. (Courtesy of Michael T. Freehill, MD)

review by Hali et al., which reported on seven different outcomes studies, including 1124 total patients. The results found no significant differences in patient-reported outcome metrics including Walch Duplay scores, Rowe Scores, and VAS between screw fixation and suture button fixation [51]. Similarly, no significant differences were seen in range of motion at final follow-up. This finding was further supported by another meta-analysis published the same year, which found no significant difference in the aforementioned PROMs, in addition to the ASES and the SSV [35]. The two groups differed, however, in rates of recurrent instability and complications. Recurrent instability, which was variably defined by each study, occurred at a higher rate in the suture button group (range 0–8.3%) compared to the screw fixation (range 0–2.5%) group, although this difference was only accounted for by a single study [52], with the remaining studies reporting no significant difference. Suture button fixation was originally proposed as an alternative solution to screws that could avoid screw-related complications such as screw bending/pullout, bone block fractures, and symptomatic hardware [11]. While not necessarily definitive, this proposition was supported by these studies, with no hardware-related complications reported in the suture button group. Even excluding hardware-associated complications, screw fixation had an overall higher range of complication rates (0–27%) compared to suture button fixation (0–12.5%).

Radiographic outcomes, including graft union, graft resorption, and graft positioning, were also included in the review. At final follow-up, there were no significant differences in graft union rate. However, at 6 months follow-up, overall graft union rates were higher in screw fixation group compared to suture button group. This was largely accounted for by a 2021 study by Bonnevialle, which used CT to compare union at 3 and 6 months in arthroscopic two-button Latarjet and two-screw open Latarjet [53]. At 3 months, 41% of the suture-button group achieved union compared to 100% for the screw group. At 6 months, this increased to 70%. However, the conclusions drawn from this study do not solely reflect differences in fixation method, given the additional variability contributed by the open versus arthroscopic approaches and a strict criterion used to determine union, which excluded fibrous unions. An alternative method to assess graft integration was introduced in a 2020 retrospective study by Weick et al., in which osseous integration was quantified on CT scan based on percentage of osseous bridging [54]. In this study, average osseous healing was found to be 74% and 68.9% at 26 weeks as determined by two independent musculoskeletal radiologists.

Graft osteolysis following anterior glenoid augmentation has been previously described, and some have suggested that osteolysis itself may lead to screw prominence [23, 33]. The exact mechanism leading to graft osteolysis is not entirely known, though the literature has implicated mechanical compression, stress shielding, and biologic preservation as key players in this process [17, 32, 33]. In the two studies included in Hali's analysis, screw fixation was found to have overall higher rates of graft resorption (range 25.2–47.6%) compared to suture button fixation (range 10.1–18.5%), as assessed on CT [55, 56]. The exact mechanism of this difference is not entirely clear, but authors have postulated that suture button fixation may decrease osteolytic reaction by decreasing focal stress experienced by the graft at the graft–fixation interface, thus better preserving its biology. Others have suggested that the nonrigid fixation afforded by suture buttons allows for more micromotion across the bone–bone interface, thus stimulating greater osteogenesis, although this has not been shown consistently across the literature [57].

Appropriate graft positioning has been increasingly recognized as a critical component in the Latarjet procedure to decrease the risk of adverse outcomes such as secondary osteoarthritis. Though the optimal graft position remains up for debate, suture button fixation has been suggested as a technology that may facilitate more precise graft positioning. Thus far, the majority of published studies have shown no significant differences in graft positioning between suture button and screw fixation, although Neyton et al. did report significantly lower graft positioning in the sagittal plane with suture button fixation compared to screw fixation [25]. However, the clinical significance of this finding is unclear given that most of the literature has focused on medial versus lateral graft positioning.

8.4.1 Suture Button System Modifications

Some have expressed concerns that a suture button system would not adequately resist rotational force or provide sufficient compression for bony integration, which could lead ultimately lead to graft nonunion [58, 59]. In response, several novel techniques have recently been described as a means of overcoming this issue. In 2022, Boileau et al. developed a device that applies measured tension to the suture button, intended to transform the nonrigid suture material into a more rigid "bolt." In the study, which included 34 shoulders treated with suture button fixation using hand tensioning and 35 using the novel device, they found a 74% union rate in the hand tensioned cohort compared to 94% in the mechanical tensioned cohort at 6 months [60]. Clinical scores did not differ significantly between the two groups at final follow-up (minimum of 24 months) and bone block position was not significantly affected by the tensioning method. The authors surmise that the nonunion in the hand tensioned group is likely a result of residual micromotion of the coracoid bone block after fixation, although they also point out that bony union is likely to continue beyond 6 months. Similarly, to address the claim that suture button fixation lacked rotational stability, the same group published a study that utilized a novel four-button construct (two sutures) for 23 patients with traumatic recurrent anterior shoulder instability. Compared to patients in their study that underwent the previously described two-button fixation (one suture), there were no differences in initial and final bone block positioning, rates of bone block healing, frequency of recurrent instability, return to sports, and patient satisfaction [61]. Taken together, these interesting results appropriately highlight the complex role that compression, rigidity, and biology contribute to graft stability and ultimately outcomes following anterior shoulder instability surgery.

8.5 All-Suture Fixation Construct

Similar to the use suspensory fixation for anterior glenoid bone graft procedures, all-suture fixation constructs offer the advantage of avoiding any metallic implants and inherently reducing the risk of iatrogenic arthritis while simultaneously providing substantial stability. Hachem et al. described an arthroscopic technique for anatomical reconstruction of the glenoid using a tricortical iliac crest with a metal-free construct using two ultra-high-strength sutures, allowing both graft stabilization, as well as capsulolabral reconstruction [62] (Fig. 8.6). The technique involves drilling two holes from posterior to anterior glenoid and subsequently shuttling loop sutures and the allograft bone block from anterior to posterior. Following appropriate insertion and positioning of the allograft, the sutures were interconnected and passed through a pretied racking hitch knot and subsequently tensioned and locked with a cerclage tensioner [62].

Iizawa et al. presented functional surgical technique and clinical outcomes for arthroscopic Bankart repair with bone graft augmentation employing either autologous iliac crest or artificial bone graft (dual hydroxyapatite composite of porous and solid parts; NEOBONE X2; MMT, Osaka, Japan), comparing this to arthroscopic Bankart repair alone. [63] In this technique, the bone graft is threaded down and secured to the anterior glenoid using soft anchors (JuggerKnot soft anchors; Zimmer Biomet, Warsaw, IN, USA) positioned in the defect bed approximately 5 mm medial to the articular surface [2]. The anchors were placed at the 2:00, 3:30, 4:30, and 5:00 positions, with the 3:30 and 4:30 suture limbs threaded through the graft and tied proximally and distally to it. The suture limbs from the other anchors were used for the capsulolabral repair and shift. Although both groups demonstrated comparable return-to-sport rates at the same pre-injury level, this study reports a higher mean Rowe score and a lower recurrence rate in the bone graft augmentation group [63].

Lastly, Zhao et al. report on the healing rate and clinical outcomes of glenoid bone grafting with nonrigid fixation for patients with recurrent anterior shoulder instability [64]. This technique involves preparing a 3-mm wide bone bed on the

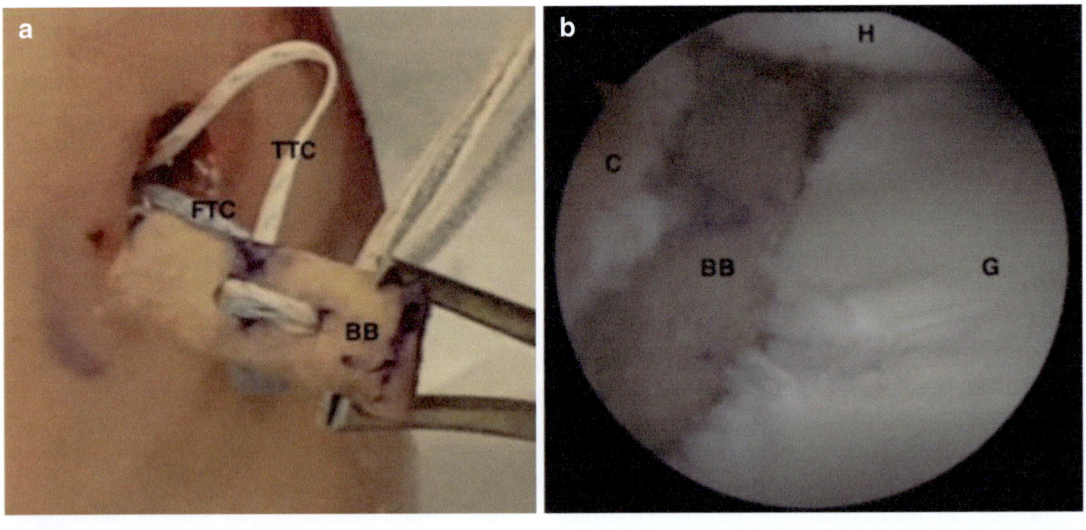

Fig. 8.6 Right shoulder. Patient is in the lateral decubitus position. (**a**) Shirt button allograft image before insertion through the interval portal. Right shoulder. (**b**) Intraoperative view of allograft positioning from the anterosuperior portal. *BB* bone block graft, *C* capsule, *FTC* FiberTape Cerclage, *G* glenoid, *H* humeral head, *TTC* TigerTape Cerclage. (Reproduced with permission from "Hachem et al., Arthroscopic Bone Block Cerclage: A Fixation Method for Glenoid Bone Loss Reconstruction Without Metal Implants, Arthroscopy Techniques, Volume 8, Issue 12, 2019, Pages e1591–e1597")

anterior glenoid and elevating the capsulolabral complex from the 1:00 to 5:00 positions. Two 3.5-mm double-loaded titanium suture anchors are then inserted on the anterior glenoid surface just posterior to the previously prepared bone bed at the 2:00–3:00 and 5:00 positions. A trapezoidal bicortical iliac crest graft (10 mm wide, 8–9 mm thick, and 30 mm long) is then contoured. The sutures are retrieved from the joint, passed through the graft and the graft is then shuttled to the anterior glenoid. Once appropriately positioned, the sutures are tied together to secure the graft to the anterior glenoid. In this study, the authors reported that all grafts healed at 3 or 6 months postoperatively and completed glenoid remodeling within 12 months postoperatively with a failure rate of 5.8% [64]. Functional outcomes, including the Oxford and Rowe score, improved significantly postoperatively [64]. Although the anchors had titanium metal, it was buried in the bone and not exposed.

8.6 Limitations and Other Considerations

Biomechanical studies provide valuable information to the surgeon, but they must be understood in the context of time-zero fixation strength. As much of the presented literature has pointed out, graft union and stability rely on many different factors, of which initial fixation strength is only one. Therefore, the critical reader must be cautious not to equate initial and final fixation quality. Despite the breadth of available literature on this subject, there remains poor consensus on optimal fixation methods. This issue perhaps stems from the wide variation in testing methods—both clinically and biomechanically [3, 6, 14, 51]. To date, the majority of the comparative data is retrospective and comes from single institutions [51, 56]. Biomechanical studies have utilized a wide range of tissues, synthetic materials and mechanical testing protocols. As such, it remains difficult to reliably assess the head-to-head efficacy and properties of the host of currently available technologies. Moving forward, this highlights the need for more robust and standardized biomechanical testing protocols and necessitates more rigorous clinical studies to guide clinical decision-making.

8.7 Conclusion

In conclusion, the selection of graft fixation methods in the treatment of anterior glenohumeral instability with bone defect presents a multifaceted decision-making process that must account for various biomechanical properties, surgical techniques, and individual patient factors. Screw fixation, with its robust historical data and proven effectiveness, remains a reliable choice. Different screw types are now available which may revolutionize this construct technique. However, complications such as screw migration and potential nerve damage necessitate careful consideration and precision during implantation. Meanwhile, suture button fixation offers an appealing alternative, especially in arthroscopic settings, due to its ease of use and reduced hardware-related complications. Its growing popularity is supported by early clinical studies that suggest viable efficacy and safety, though ongoing research and long-term data are needed to fully understand its comparative performance against traditional screw methods. All-suture constructs represent an innovative approach, particularly appealing for their metal-free nature and the reduced risk of iatrogenic complications associated with traditional implants. This technique, while still under clinical evaluation, promises significant benefits, particularly in terms of biocompatibility and the potential to minimize postsurgical complications. Ultimately, the choice of fixation method should be tailored to the individual patient's anatomy, surgeon experience, and patient-specific demands. Ongoing advancements in surgical techniques and fixation technologies continue to enhance our ability to address anterior shoulder instability effectively. As the field evolves, it remains vital for the shoulder surgeon to critically evaluate emerging research and developments, enabling them to make the best possible decisions for their patients.

References

1. Latarjet M. Treatment of recurrent dislocation of the shoulder. Lyon Chir. 1954;49(8):994–7.
2. Longo UG, Loppini M, Rizzello G, Ciuffreda M, Maffulli N, Denaro V. Latarjet, Bristow, and Eden-Hybinette procedures for anterior shoulder dislocation: systematic review and quantitative synthesis of the literature. Arthroscopy. 2014;30(9):1184–211.
3. Manfredi JN, Schick S, Paul KD, Elphingstone JW, Sowell J, Lameka M, et al. A systematic review of screw and suture button glenoid augmentation constructs. Orthop J Sports Med. 2023;11(10):23259671231186429.
4. Butt U, Charalambous CP. Complications associated with open coracoid transfer procedures for shoulder instability. J Shoulder Elb Surg. 2012;21(8):1110–9.
5. Bliven KCH, Parr GP. Outcomes of the Latarjet procedure compared with Bankart repair for recurrent traumatic anterior shoulder instability. J Athl Train. 2018;53(2):181–3.
6. Shin JJ, Hamamoto JT, Leroux TS, Saccomanno MF, Jain A, Khair MM, et al. Biomechanical analysis of Latarjet screw fixation: comparison of screw types and fixation methods. Arthroscopy. 2017;33(9):1646–53.
7. Boileau P, Gendre P, Baba M, Thélu CÉ, Baring T, Gonzalez JF, et al. A guided surgical approach and novel fixation method for arthroscopic Latarjet. J Shoulder Elb Surg. 2016;25(1):78–89.
8. Paul K, Elphingstone JW, Williams M, Manfredi JN, Jardaly A, Schick S, et al. Suspensory fixation for bone transfer procedures in shoulder instability is superior to screws in an angled construct: a biomechanical analysis. JSES Int. 2024;8(2):250–6.
9. Athwal GS, Meislin R, Getz C, Weinstein D, Favorito P. Short-term complications of the arthroscopic Latarjet procedure: a north American experience. Arthroscopy. 2016;32(10):1965–70.
10. Lädermann A, Denard PJ, Burkhart SS. Injury of the suprascapular nerve during Latarjet procedure: an anatomic study. Arthroscopy. 2012;28(3):316–21.
11. Boileau P, Saliken D, Gendre P, Seeto BL, d'Ollonne T, Gonzalez JF, et al. Arthroscopic Latarjet: suture-button fixation is a safe and reliable alternative to screw fixation. Arthroscopy. 2019;35(4):1050–61.
12. Viezens L, Sellenschloh K, Püschel K, Morlock MM, Lehmann W, Huber G, et al. Impact of screw diameter on pedicle screw fatigue strength-a biomechanical evaluation. World Neurosurg. 2021;152:e369–76.
13. Willemot LB, Wodicka R, Bosworth A, Castagna A, Burns J, Verborgt O. Influence of screw type and length on fixation of anterior glenoid bone grafts. Shoulder Elbow. 2018;10(1):32–9.
14. Huish EG Jr, Kelly SR, Cutter BM. Factors affecting biomechanical strength of Latarjet constructs: a systematic review and meta-regression. Shoulder Elbow. 2022;14(1):17–23.
15. Schmiddem U, Hawi N, Liodakis E, Dratzidis A, Kraemer M, Hurschler C, et al. Monocortical fixation of the coracoid in the Latarjet procedure is significantly weaker than bicortical fixation. Knee Surg Sports Traumatol Arthrosc. 2019;27(1):239–44.
16. Jassim SS, Amaranath J, Taylor DM, Warby SA, Hoy G. Unicortical fixation does not compromise bony union in the Latarjet procedure. JSES Int. 2022;6(4):555–62.
17. Sano H, Komatsuda T, Abe H, Ozawa H, Kumagai J, Yokobori TA. Intra-articular biomechanical environment following modified Bristow and Latarjet procedures in shoulders with large glenoid defects: relationship with postoperative complications. J Shoulder Elb Surg. 2021;30(10):2260–9.
18. Frank RM, Roth M, Wijdicks CA, Fischer N, Costantini A, Di Giacomo G, et al. Biomechanical analysis of plate fixation compared with various screw configurations for use in the Latarjet procedure. Orthop J Sports Med. 2020;8(7):232596712093139.
19. Azoulay V, Briot J, Mansat P, Swider P, Bonnevialle N. Mechanical behavior of screw versus endobutton for coracoid bone-block fixation. Orthop Traumatol Surg Res. 2020;106(6):1089–93.
20. Weppe F, Magnussen RA, Lustig S, Demey G, Neyret P, Servien E. A biomechanical evaluation of Bicortical metal screw fixation versus absorbable interference screw fixation after coracoid transfer for anterior shoulder instability. Arthroscopy. 2011;27(10):1358–63.
21. Rattier S, Druel T, Hirakawa Y, Gröger F, Van Rooij F, Neyton L. Use of cannulated screws for primary Latarjet procedures. Orthop J Sports Med. 2022;10(8):232596712211178.
22. Alvi HM, Monroe EJ, Muriuki M, Verma RN, Marra G, Saltzman MD. Latarjet fixation: a cadaveric biomechanical study evaluating cortical and cannulated screw fixation. Orthop J Sports Med. 2016;4(4):232596711664353.
23. Casabianca L, Gerometta A, Massein A, Khiami F, Rousseau R, Hardy A, et al. Graft position and fusion rate following arthroscopic Latarjet. Knee Surg Sports Traumatol Arthrosc. 2016;24(2):507–12.
24. Kany J, Flamand O, Grimberg J, Guinand R, Croutzet P, Amaravathi R, et al. Arthroscopic Latarjet procedure: is optimal positioning of the bone block and screws possible? A prospective computed tomography scan analysis. J Shoulder Elb Surg. 2016;25(1):69–77.
25. Neyton L, Barth J, Nourissat G, Métais P, Boileau P, Walch G, et al. Arthroscopic Latarjet techniques: graft and fixation positioning assessed with 2-dimensional computed tomography is not equivalent with standard open technique. Arthroscopy. 2018;34(7):2032–40.
26. Shah AA, Butler RB, Romanowski J, Goel D, Karadagli D, Warner JJP. Short-term complications of the Latarjet procedure. J Bone Joint Surg. 2012;94(6):495–501.
27. Hovelius L, Sandström B, Saebö M. One hundred eighteen Bristow-Latarjet repairs for recurrent anterior dislocation of the shoulder prospectively followed for fifteen years: study II—the evolution of dislocation arthropathy. J Shoulder Elb Surg. 2006;15(3):279–89.

28. Hsu KL, Yeh ML, Kuan FC, Hong CK, Chuang HC, Wang WM, et al. Biomechanical comparison between various screw fixation angles for Latarjet procedure: a cadaveric biomechanical study. J Shoulder Elb Surg. 2022;31(9):1947–56.
29. Meyer DC, Moor BK, Gerber C, Ek ETH. Accurate coracoid graft placement through use of a drill guide for the Latarjet procedure. J Shoulder Elb Surg. 2013;22(5):701–8.
30. Boileau P, Thélu CÉ, Mercier N, Ohl X, Houghton-Clemmey R, Carles M, et al. Arthroscopic Bristow-Latarjet combined with bankart repair restores shoulder stability in patients with glenoid bone loss. Clin Orthop. 2014;472(8):2413–24.
31. Hendy BA, Padegimas EM, Kane L, Harper T, Abboud JA, Lazarus MD, et al. Early postoperative complications after Latarjet procedure: a single-institution experience over 10 years. J Shoulder Elb Surg. 2021;30(6):e300–8.
32. Giacomo GD, Costantini A, de Gasperis N, De Vita A, Lin BKH, Francone M, et al. Coracoid bone graft osteolysis after Latarjet procedure: a comparison study between two screws standard technique vs mini-plate fixation. Int J Shoulder Surg. 2013;7(1):1–6.
33. Alp NB, Doğan O, Yılmaz TG, Kalay OC, Moussa AA, Karpat F, et al. Understanding the causes behind coracoid graft osteolysis in Latarjet procedure (finite element analysis and comparison of three fixation methods). Orthop Traumatol Surg Res. 2020;106(1):53–9.
34. Griesser MJ, Harris JD, McCoy BW, Hussain WM, Jones MH, Bishop JY, et al. Complications and re-operations after Bristow-Latarjet shoulder stabilization: a systematic review. J Shoulder Elb Surg. 2013;22(2):286–92.
35. Thamrongskulsiri N, Limskul D, Tanpowpong T, Kuptniratsaikul S, Itthipanichpong T. Clinical outcomes, union rates, and complications of screw versus button fixation in the Bristow-Latarjet procedure for anterior shoulder instability: a systematic review and meta-analysis. Clin Orthop Surg. 2023;15(6):1000.
36. Ho E, Cofield RH, Balm MR, Hattrup SJ, Rowland CM. Neurologic complications of surgery for anterior shoulder instability. J Shoulder Elb Surg. 1999;8(3):266–70.
37. Boileau P, Mercier N, Old J. Arthroscopic Bankart-Bristow-Latarjet (2B3) procedure: how to do it and tricks to make it easier and safe. Orthop Clin North Am. 2010;41(3):381–92.
38. Allain J, Goutallier D, Glorion C. Long-term results of the Latarjet procedure for the treatment of anterior instability of the shoulder. J Bone Joint Surg Am. 1998;80(6):841–52.
39. Gracitelli MEC, Ferreira AA, Benegas E, Malavolta EA, Sunada EE, Assunção JH. Arthroscopic Latarjet procedure: safety evaluation in cadavers. Acta Ortop Bras. 2013;21(3):139–43.
40. Barber FA, Dockery WD. Long-term absorption of poly-L-lactic acid interference screws. Arthroscopy. 2006;22(8):820–6.
41. Shiwaku K, Suzuki T, Matsumura T, Takashima H, Otsubo H, Yamashita T. Bioabsorbable interference screws can be used with less tunnel widening in anatomic rectangular tunnel anterior cruciate ligament reconstruction with a bone–patellar-tendon–bone graft. Knee. 2020;27(5):1293–9.
42. Mascarenhas R, Saltzman BM, Sayegh ET, Verma NN, Cole BJ, Bush-Joseph C, et al. Bioabsorbable versus metallic interference screws in anterior cruciate ligament reconstruction: a systematic review of overlapping meta-analyses. Arthroscopy. 2015;31(3):561–8.
43. Bockmann B, Jaeger E, Dankl L, Nebelung W, Frey S, Schmölz W, et al. A biomechanical comparison of steel screws versus PLLA and magnesium screws for the Latarjet procedure. Arch Orthop Trauma Surg. 2022;142(6):1091–8.
44. Balestro JC, Young A, Maccioni C, Walch G. Graft osteolysis and recurrent instability after the Latarjet procedure performed with bioabsorbable screw fixation. J Shoulder Elb Surg. 2015;24(5):711–8.
45. Fu X, Xin WG, Guang WC, Jun LZ. Comparison between bioabsorbable magnesium and titanium compression screws for hallux valgus treated with distal metatarsal osteotomies: a meta-analysis. Jt Dis Relat Surg. 2023;34(2):289–97.
46. Ebrahimi A, Sohn S, Lucaciu A, Ashkani-Esfahani S, Waryasz G. Short-term follow-up of patients receiving bio-integrative screws for Lisfranc injuries: a case series. J Orthop Case Rep. 2023;13(12):34–9.
47. Taverna E, D'Ambrosi R, Perfetti C, Garavaglia G. Arthroscopic bone graft procedure for anterior inferior glenohumeral instability. Arthrosc Tech. 2014;3(6):e653–60.
48. Provencher MT, Aman ZS, LaPrade CM, Bernhardson AS, Moatshe G, Storaci HW, et al. Biomechanical comparison of screw fixation versus a cortical button and self-tensioning suture for the Latarjet procedure. Orthop J Sports Med. 2018;6(6):2325967118777784.
49. Kazum E, Chechik O, Pritsch T, Mozes G, Morag G, Dolkart O, et al. Biomechanical evaluation of suture buttons versus cortical screws in the Latarjet–Bristow procedure: a fresh-frozen cadavers study. Arch Orthop Trauma Surg. 2019;139(12):1779–83.
50. Williams RC, Morris RP, El Beaino M, Maassen NH. Cortical suture button fixation vs. bicortical screw fixation in the Latarjet procedure: a biomechanical comparison. J Shoulder Elb Surg. 2020;29(7):1470–8.
51. Hali NZ, Tahir M, Jordan RW, Laprus H, Woodmass J, D'Alessandro P, et al. Suture button fixation in Latarjet has similar load to failure and clinical outcomes but lower bone resorption compared with screw fixation: a systematic review. Arthroscopy. 2023;40:S0749806323008654.
52. Hardy A, Sabatier V, Schoch B, Vigan M, Werthel JD, Study Investigators. Latarjet with cortical button fixation is associated with an increase of the risk of recurrent dislocation compared to screw fixation. Knee Surg Sports Traumatol Arthrosc. 2020;28(7):2354–60.
53. Bonnevialle N, Girard M, Dalmas Y, Martinel V, Faruch M, Mansat P. Short-term bone fusion with

arthroscopic double-button Latarjet versus open-screw Latarjet. Am J Sports Med. 2021;49(6):1596–603.
54. Weick JW, Kalia V, Pacheco E, Jacobson JA, Freehill MT. Osseous healing with nonrigid suture fixation in the arthroscopic Latarjet procedure. Orthop J Sports Med. 2020;8(11):232596712096448.
55. Wang Y, Zhou Z, Zhang Y, He C, Xue C, Xu W, et al. Early follow-up of arthroscopic Latarjet procedure with screw or suture-button fixation for recurrent anterior shoulder instability. Orthop Surg. 2020;12(5):1350–61.
56. Song Q, Zhang S, Cheng X, Xiao J, Lin L, Liu Q, et al. Clinical and radiographic outcomes after arthroscopic inlay Bristow surgery with screw versus suture button fixation: a comparative study of 117 patients with 3.3-year follow-up. Orthop J Sports Med. 2022;10(3):232596712210760.
57. Ziegenfuss BL, Launay MM, Maharaj JC, Green NR, Stalin KA, Barlow G, et al. A biomechanical analysis of double-screw, double-button, and screw-button fixation constructs in patient-specific instrument–guided Latarjet procedure. J Shoulder Elb Surg. 2023;32(7):1370–9.
58. Xu J, Liu H, Lu W, Deng Z, Zhu W, Peng L, et al. Modified arthroscopic Latarjet procedure: suture-button fixation achieves excellent remodeling at 3-year follow-up. Am J Sports Med. 2020;48(1):39–47.
59. Valenti P, Maroun C, Wagner E, Werthel JD. Arthroscopic Latarjet procedure combined with Bankart repair: a technique using 2 cortical buttons and specific glenoid and coracoid guides. Arthrosc Tech. 2018;7(4):e313–20.
60. Boileau P, Gendre P, Saliken DJ, Thélu CÉ, Trojani C. Tensioning device increases coracoid bone block healing rates in arthroscopic Latarjet procedure with suture-button fixation. J Shoulder Elb Surg. 2022;31(7):1451–62.
61. Barret H, Chelli M, Van Der Meijden O, Langlais T, Boileau P. Arthroscopic Latarjet: 2 or 4 cortical buttons for coracoid fixation? A case-control comparative study. Am J Sports Med. 2022;50(2):311–20.
62. Hachem AI, Del Carmen M, Verdalet I, Rius J. Arthroscopic bone block cerclage: a fixation method for glenoid bone loss reconstruction without metal implants. Arthrosc Tech. 2019;8(12):e1591–7.
63. Iizawa N, Yoneda M, Yamada S, Mizuno N, Goto K, Iwashita S, et al. Benefits of bone graft augmentation to arthroscopic Bankart repair for recurrent anterior shoulder instability with glenoid bone loss. Knee Surg Sports Traumatol Arthrosc. 2020;28(7):2325–33.
64. Zhao J, Huangfu X, Yang X, Xie G, Xu C. Arthroscopic glenoid bone grafting with nonrigid fixation for anterior shoulder instability: 52 patients with 2- to 5-year follow-up. Am J Sports Med. 2014;42(4):831–9.

9 The Dynamic Anterior Stabilization of the Shoulder

Clara de Campos Azevedo
and Ana Catarina Ângelo

9.1 Introduction

Several surgical treatment options for the management of anterior glenohumeral instability have been described to treat deficiencies of the anterior labrum, anterior glenoid, or humeral head, ranging from soft tissue to bony procedures, open or arthroscopic. The clinical studies of soft tissue procedures report increased recurrence rates in patients with subcritical (13.5–20%) to critical (>20%) anterior glenoid bone loss (GBL) [1, 2]. In this setting, a bony procedure is recommended. Nevertheless, bony procedures are associated with higher rates of more severe complications [3, 4]. Other theoretically safer soft tissue surgical techniques have emerged in recent years reporting promising outcomes in patients with minimal to subcritical anterior GBL [5, 6]. The arthroscopic dynamic anterior stabilization (DAS) is one of the alternative soft tissue procedures available, and it utilizes the transfer of the long head of the biceps (LHB) to the anterior glenoid [7–10]. The overall goal of the DAS is to increase anterior glenohumeral stability through a triple effect: the anterior labroplasty effect, restoring the concavity-compression provided by the missing or insufficient anterior labrum; the hammock effect [11], with the LHB exerting a downward force on the subscapularis tendon which is tensioned preventing the inferior glenohumeral dislocation during the first degrees of abduction and external rotation; and the sling effect [11], with the LHB in front of the humeral bead blocking humeral head anterior translation and glenohumeral dislocation during higher degrees of abduction and external rotation.

The current chapter presents the rationale of the DAS, the arthroscopic technique, and a literature review discussing the clinical outcomes.

9.2 Rationale

The arthroscopic DAS utilizing the LHB transfer from the superior labrum to the anterior glenoid through the subscapularis tendon split was first described in technical reports using the inlay type of fixation of the LHB, meaning that the LHB is fixed medial to the anterior glenoid articular cartilage [7, 9]. The inlay type of DAS relies on the hammock and the sling effect throughout the range of motion (ROM) to increase anterior glenohumeral stability, with the LHB exerting a downward force tensioning the subscapularis tendon preventing the inferior glenohumeral dislocation during the first degrees of abduction and external rotation, and with the LHB in front of the humeral bead preventing humeral head anterior translation and glenohumeral dislocation

C. de Campos Azevedo (✉) · A. C. Ângelo
Hospital dos SAMS de Lisboa, Lisbon, Portugal

Joaquim Chaves Saúde, Lisbon, Portugal
e-mail: claracamposazevedo@shoulder.pt

E. Calvo et al. (eds.), *Complex and Revision Problems in Shoulder Instability*,
https://doi.org/10.1007/978-3-031-81389-4_9

during higher degrees of abduction and external rotation [11]. Other authors described the arthroscopic DAS using the onlay type of fixation of the LHB [8, 10], meaning that the LHB is fixed on the anterior glenoid articular cartilage. The purpose of the onlay type of DAS is to restore the concavity-compression typically provided by the anterior labrum in patients who have capsulolabral insufficiency and do not have sufficient anterior labrum to perform a Bankart repair. Other authors described technical modifications to the DAS with the addition of the Hill-Sachs remplissage for treatment of anterior glenohumeral instability cases with off-track Hill-Sachs lesions in the setting of bipolar bony lesions [12–14]. Recent biomechanical studies have shown that the addition of the Hill-Sachs remplissage to the Bankart repair increases glenohumeral stability under high translational loads for off-track lesions in cadaveric specimens with 15% of anterior GBL, but restricts ROM, whereas the DAS restores the native glenohumeral stability in on-track lesions without restricting ROM, supporting the rationale of utilizing the DAS augmented by the Hill-Sachs remplissage in patients who have off-track Hill-Sachs lesions [15].

In the current chapter, the authors' preferred DAS technique is described in detail [16].

9.3 Surgical Technique

The patient is positioned in the beach chair position and a mechanical arm holder is used to place the shoulder in 70° of forward flexion with the elbow in full extension. Three arthroscopic portals are used for the DAS: the posterior, the anterior, and the anterolateral portals [17]. An additional posterolateral portal is used when a Hill-Sachs remplissage is performed as well (Fig. 9.1).

The posterior portal is established in the soft spot (Fig. 9.1). The 4-mm and 30° arthroscope is aimed at the coracoid process. Inspection of the humeral head, glenoid, rotator cuff tendon insertions, and LHB tendon are performed. The engagement of the Hill-Sachs lesion is tested by placing the shoulder at increased degrees of abduction and external rotation.

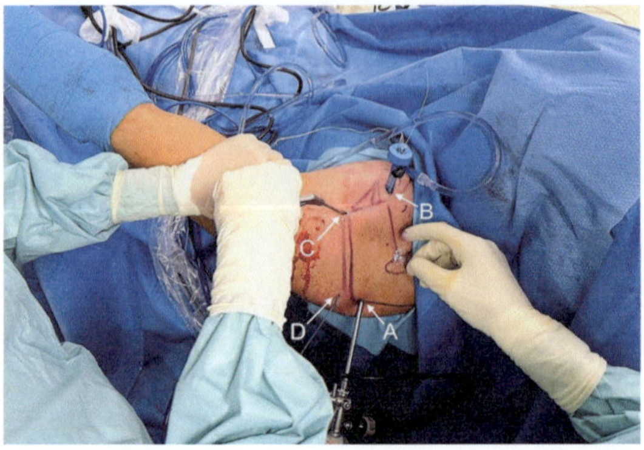

Fig. 9.1 Image showing the patient in the beach-chair position with the left shoulder placed in 70° of forward flexion with the elbow in full extension using a mechanical arm holder. The anatomical landmarks were drawn on the skin using a dermographic pen. Three arthroscopic portals were established for the DAS plus one portal for the Hill-Sachs remplissage augmentation: the posterior viewing portal (A) with the 4-mm 30° arthroscope placed through it; the anterior portal (B) with the 7-mm working canula placed through it and the four suture limbs of the first anchor of the DAS; the anterolateral portal (C) with a suture retriever going through it; and the fourth additional posterolateral portal (D) with the four suture limbs of the anchor that was placed in the Hill-Sachs defect for the Hill-Sachs remplissage augmentation of the DAS

The anterior portal is established from outside-in, under direct vision, using an 18-gauge spinal needle directed to the superior border of the subscapularis tendon, lateral to the conjoint tendon. A working cannula with an outflow connection, typically 7-mm × 85–mm, is placed through this portal. A gauged probe is used to dynamically identify and classify a SLAP tear, if present.

The anterolateral portal is established from outside-in, distal to the anterolateral aspect of the acromion, using the 18-gauge spinal needle directed laterally to the THL, parallel and slightly distal to the superior border of the subscapularis.

The placement of the suture anchors is marked on the anterior glenoid rim, at the 4 and 5 o'clock positions on a right shoulder, using the 3.5 × 130-mm bipolar radiofrequency ablator probe placed through the anterior portal. The middle glenohumeral ligament is excised until the muscle fibers of the subscapularis are visualized.

The bony bed of the Bankart lesion is debrided using the 4 × 125-mm automated shaver. The subscapularis tendon is longitudinally split using the radiofrequency ablator, which is introduced through the anterior portal, and is used to cut the tendon from medial to lateral at the middle to superior third of articular side of the subscapularis tendon, lateral to the conjoint tendon. The radiofrequency ablator is introduced from superficial to intra-articular, through the split, and is used to continue splitting the subscapularis tendon from medial to lateral, on the articular side of the subscapularis, under direct vision. The split is complete when the split is unobstructed by remnants of ligament or tendon.

First, one 1.8-mm all-suture anchor double-loaded with sutures is introduced through the anterior portal and the subscapularis tendon split and is implanted on the anteroinferior glenoid rim at the 5 o'clock position (right shoulder) (Fig. 9.2).

Each suture limb is passed through the LHB sequentially using an automatic suture passer which is introduced through the anterior portal. The first suture limb is passed through the LHB just proximal to the THL (Fig. 9.3), and is retrieved through the anterolateral portal, where it is parked.

The second suture limb chosen should be different colored and is passed posterior to the first and retrieved through the anterolateral portal, where it is parked as well; at this point, these two suture limbs are tied to make the first double-pulley knot and the suture limbs are cut; the third and fourth suture limbs are passed approximately 2-mm more proximal to the first double-pulley knot, following the same sequential steps as the first two suture limbs. These two suture limbs from the 5 o'clock anchor that have been passed through the LHB, are then referenced with a straight hemostat, and left parked in the anterolateral portal.

A second 1.8-mm all-suture double-loaded anchor is placed through the anterior portal and the subscapularis tendon split and is implanted on the anteroinferior glenoid rim at the 4 o'clock position (right shoulder) (Fig. 9.4).

Each of the four suture limbs is passed through the LHB sequentially, medially to the previous suture limbs and closer to the LHB anchor and

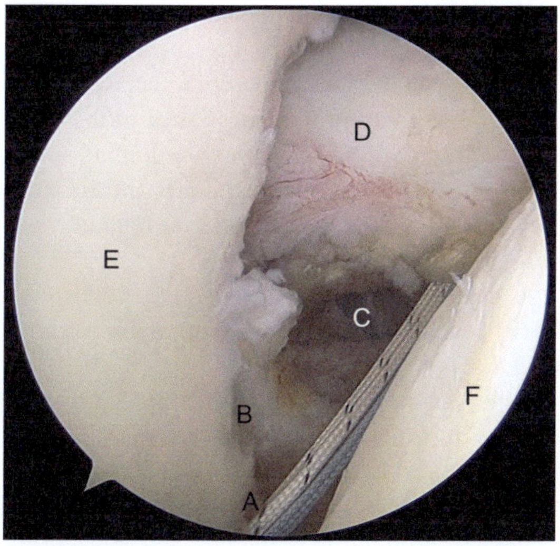

Fig. 9.2 Arthroscopic image of the posterior portal view of the right shoulder showing the 5 o'clock anchor implanted (A) and the marking of the 4 o'clock anchor (B) on the anterior glenoid with the four suture limbs of the 5 o'clock anchor going through the split (C) of the subscapularis tendon (D). (E) Glenoid articular cartilage; (F) humeral head articular cartilage

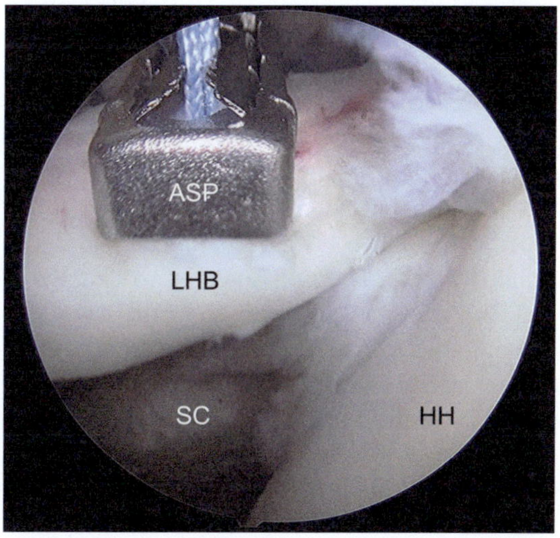

Fig. 9.3 Arthroscopic image of the posterior portal view of the right shoulder showing the first suture limb of the 5 o'clock anchor passing through the LHB just proximal to the THL with an automatic suture passer which is introduced through the anterior portal. *ASP* automatic suture passer, *HH* humeral head articular cartilage, *LHB* long head of biceps, *THL* transverse humeral ligament, *SC* subscapularis tendon

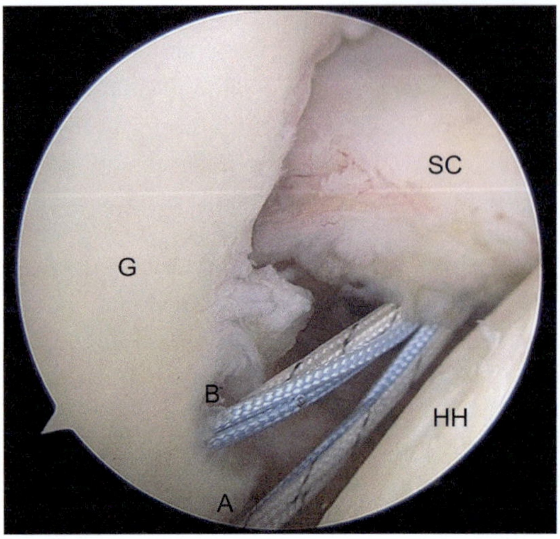

Fig. 9.4 Arthroscopic image of the posterior portal view of the right shoulder showing the 5 o'clock anchor (A) and the 4 o'clock anchor (B) implanted on the anterior glenoid with the eight suture limbs going through the split of the subscapularis tendon (SC). *G* glenoid articular cartilage, *HH* humeral head articular cartilage

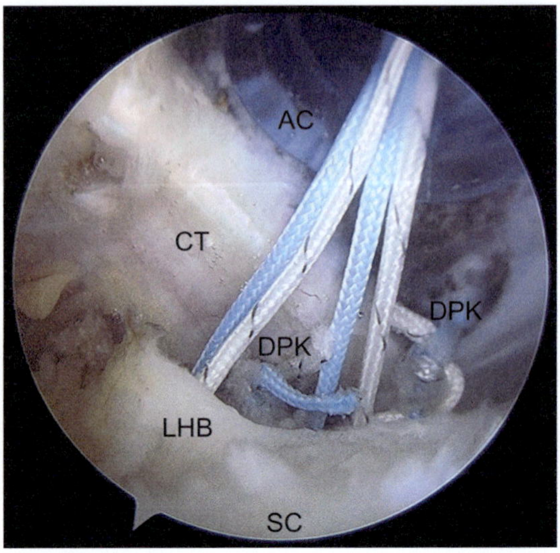

Fig. 9.5 Arthroscopic image of the posterior portal view of the right shoulder showing the LHB dislocated medially after the tenotomy the release of the THL with the two double pulley knots (DPK) and the four suture limbs going through anterior canula (AC). *CT* conjoint tendon, *LHB* long head of the biceps, *SC* subscapularis tendon

superior labrum, repeating the same steps used for the 5 o'clock anchor; after they have been passed through the LHB, two different colored suture limbs of the 4 o'clock anchor are tied to make the second double-pulley knot and the suture limbs are cut. The remaining two suture limbs of the 4 o'clock anchor that have been passed through the LHB are retrieved from the anterolateral portal to the anterior portal, referenced with a curved hemostat, and parked in the anterior portal. The two suture limbs of the 5 o'clock anchor are retrieved from the anterolateral portal to the anterior portal, referenced with a straight hemostat, and parked in the anterior portal as well. The remaining four opposing limbs of each of the two anchors are thus left parked in the anterior portal, and each pair of suture limbs is referenced with different types of hemostats to facilitate suture management.

The radiofrequency ablator probe is introduced through the anterolateral portal and is used to cut the THL laterally to the LHB tendon, until the LHB tendon is completely released from the bicipital groove and dislocates medially.

The LHB is tenotomized proximally to the most proximal limbs of the sutures and distally to the bicipital anchor on the superior labrum using the ablator or arthroscopic scissors. The four limbs of suture that are parked in the anterior portal are pulled and the two double-pulley knots push the tenotomized LHB intra-articularly through the subscapularis tendon split (Fig. 9.5).

The remaining suture limbs are tied when the LHB reaches the anteroinferior glenoid rim (Fig. 9.6).

One 1.3-mm all-suture single-loaded anchor may be implanted adjacent to the superior half of the transposed LHB tendon at the 3 o'clock position on the glenoid rim and after one suture limb is passed through the remaining anterior labrum and/or capsular tissue a simple knot is tied to plicate it onto the glenoid rim. Alternatively, two suture limbs from the 4 and 5 o'clock anchors

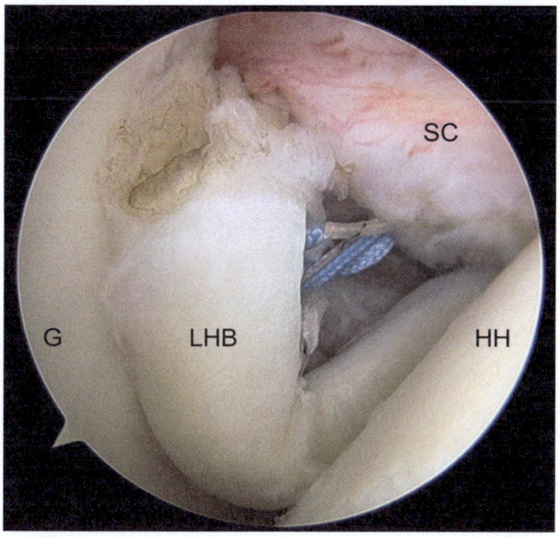

Fig. 9.6 Arthroscopic image of the posterior portal view of the right shoulder showing the LHB fixed to the anterior glenoid in an onlay position and for the labroplasty effect after all four knots were tied. *G* glenoid articular cartilage, *HH* humeral head articular cartilage, *LHB* long head of the biceps, *SC* subscapularis tendon

may be used to suture the remaining anterior labrum and/or capsular tissue instead.

9.4 Rehabilitation

For the first 3–6 weeks, patients are instructed to wear a sling and to remove it several times a day to perform active assisted, nonresistant, forward flexion shoulder and elbow exercises. Use of the sling is diminished from weeks 3 to 6. During this period, shoulder active assisted exercises are not limited in range and patients are instructed to perform forward flexion exercises, and external-internal rotation exercises, with the arm at the side, rotating from internal rotation to the full external rotation position as tolerated. Full range of flexion-extension active assisted nonresistant exercises of the elbow are allowed as well. However, until 6 weeks postoperatively, active resistant elbow exercises are not allowed. The purpose of the ROM exercises is to avoid postoperative adhesions to the subscapularis tendon while avoiding compromising the first stages of LHB tendon-to-bone healing to the anterior glenoid rim.

From week 6 onwards, patients undergo a supervised shoulder rehabilitation protocol that adds more active nonresistant ROM exercises until full ROM is achieved.

From weeks 6 to 8, active resistant exercises of the elbow progress from 1 to 2 kg. The purpose is to continue to protect the LHB tendon-to-bone healing to the anterior glenoid rim.

After week 8, active resistant elbow exercises progress according to patient tolerance. Active resistant abduction in external rotation exercises are avoided until 3 months postoperatively.

After 6 months, a full return to the previous level of sports activity is progressively allowed.

9.5 Clinical Results

Significantly improved postoperative outcomes after the DAS using the long head of the biceps are reported in clinical studies at short-term follow-up [17–19].

In the retrospective study by Collin et al. [18], of the DAS using the LHB fixed in an inlay position plus the Bankart repair [7], the authors reported significantly improved clinical outcomes, without restriction in postoperative ROM, at a minimum follow-up of 2 years postoperative. In 22 patients who had a mean GBL of 9.0% (range, 0–15.8%), with Hill-Sachs lesions in 68.2%, off-track lesions in 18%, and SLAP lesions in 9% of the patients, no postoperative Popeye deformity, LHB cramping, or other complications of the biceps were reported. Three (13.6%) patients had a recurrence of the instability early in the learning curve of the technique, of which two (9.1%) had to be revised with a Latarjet procedure. The authors concluded that the DAS can be an option for augmentation of a Bankart repair in patients with anterior shoulder instability and subcritical bone loss.

In the retrospective study by de Campos Azevedo and Ângelo [17], of the DAS using the LHB fixed in an onlay position [10, 16], the authors reported significant improvements in clinical outcomes, without restriction in postoperative ROM, at a minimum follow-up of 1 year. In 15 patients who had a mean GBL of 8.2%

(range, 0–20.24%) and SLAP lesions in 5 (33.3%) of the patients, each patient had a control magnetic resonance imaging confirming biceps healing to the anterior glenoid, no biceps, neurological, or other complications were reported. One severely hyperlax patient had an atraumatic recurrence of the instability (6.7% recurrence) which did not require revision surgery. The authors concluded that the all-arthroscopic all-suture anchor DAS using the LHB, and the double double-pulley technique was safe, and produced good clinical outcomes at 12, 24, and 48 months of follow-up in patients with GBL of 0–20% with no recurrences of anterior instability in the subgroup of patients without severe hyperlaxity.

In the retrospective comparative study by Wu et al. [19], a subgroup patients who underwent the DAS using the LHB fixed in an inlay position [9], was compared with a subgroup of patients who underwent the DAS using the conjoint tendon, and the authors reported significant improvements in clinical outcomes, without restriction in postoperative ROM, at a minimum follow-up of 3 years. In the subgroup of 33 patients who underwent the DAS using the LHB, the mean GBL was 10.5%, and off-track Hill-Sachs lesions were reported in ten patients (30.3%). No recurrent dislocations were reported. One patient (3.0%) had occasional recurrent subluxations, and one patient (3.0%) had a positive anterior apprehension test. The reported overall recurrent instability rate of the DAS using the LHB was 6.1% (two patients). No other complications such as hardware failures, neurological disorders, or infections were reported. The authors concluded that the DAS using the LHB achieved good shoulder function outcomes, high return-to-sports rates, and low recurrence and complication rates in patients with less than 15% of anterior GBL.

9.6 Discussion

Arthroscopic DAS utilizing the LHB tendon is a minimally invasive arthroscopic technique that utilizes an in situ autograft and avoids donor site morbidity because harvesting the iliac bone or harvesting other distant types of grafts is not necessary. The DAS can utilize soft suture anchors to fix the LHB to the glenoid, thereby avoids hardware-related complications and decreases the risk of implant-related postoperative complications in comparison with most bony and coracoid transfer procedures. The clinical studies of the DAS using the LHB have a limited minimum follow-up period (range, 1–3 years), and are of low level of evidence (range, level III to V). However, the clinical studies have shown that the DAS is a safe procedure, without any reports of neurological, vascular, or biceps complications, with instability recurrence rates ranging from 6.1% to 13.6%. Therefore, the DAS can be considered a burn-no-bridges technique in which the recurrence rate may be an acceptable trade-off for the reduced risk of severe hardware-related or bone-on-cartilage lesions in very young and active patients. The transfer of the LHB avoids the risks of bone-on-cartilage wear related to bony transfers and avoids the risk of neurological lesions caused by traction to the musculocutaneous nerve because the LHB is transposed instead of the conjoint tendon. Arthroscopic DAS utilizes standard arthroscopic instruments, and does not require specific arthroscopic guides, decreasing the need for bulky instrumentation sets, and adds an option to the surgeon's treatment armamentarium when faced intraoperatively with increased bony loss and engaging Hill-Sachs lesions in patients with preoperatively apparent on-track bipolar lesions. At postoperative time zero, DAS increases glenohumeral stability in subcritical GBL and in humeral head bone loss models in comparison with either an isolated Bankart repair [20], or conjoint tendon transfer procedures [21]. The LHB tendon combines the increased biologic healing potential and the decreased immunologic reaction potential of an autograft in comparison with either soft or bony allografts or xenografts. In patients with concomitant SLAP types I–III lesions, the DAS addresses the SLAP lesion and the anteroinferior glenohumeral instability with the tenodesis of the LHB to the anterior glenoid. In the Latarjet procedure the physiological scapular kinesis is permanently disturbed because the pectoralis minor is detached, and the vector and the working length of the coracobrachialis and the short head of the biceps are changed because the coracoid is transferred [22], whereas in the DAS the LHB alone is transferred and scapular kinesis changes are not expected.

9.7 Summary

The arthroscopic DAS utilizing the LHB is a safe option for the treatment of anterior glenohumeral instability with minimal to subcritical anterior GBL of less than 20% and is a useful addition to the armamentarium of the orthopedic surgeon that treats patients with anterior glenohumeral instability with concomitant SLAP tears and/or and bipolar bony lesions. In patients with Hill-Sachs lesions, the Hill-Sachs remplissage should be considered for augmentation of the DAS, especially when the Hill-Sachs lesion is off-track and/or the patient is severely hyperlax.

References

1. Imam MA, Shehata MSA, Martin A, Attia H, Sinokrot M, Bahbah EI, et al. Bankart repair versus Latarjet procedure for recurrent anterior shoulder instability: a systematic review and meta-analysis of 3275 shoulders. Am J Sports Med. 2021;49(7):1945–53.
2. Shaha JS, Cook JB, Song DJ, Rowles DJ, Bottoni CR, Shaha SH, et al. Redefining "critical" bone loss in shoulder instability: functional outcomes worsen with "subcritical" bone loss. Am J Sports Med. 2015;43(7):1719–25.
3. Cho CH, Na SS, Choi BC, Kim DH. Complications related to Latarjet shoulder stabilization: a systematic review. Am J Sports Med. 2021;51:3635465211042314.
4. Griesser MJ, Harris JD, McCoy BW, Hussain WM, Jones MH, Bishop JY, et al. Complications and reoperations after Bristow-Latarjet shoulder stabilization: a systematic review. J Shoulder Elb Surg. 2013;22(2):286–92.
5. Brzoska R, Laprus H, Michniowski P, Solecki W, Klon W, Blasiak A. Novel and effective arthroscopic extracapsular stabilization technique for anterior shoulder instability-BLS. Knee Surg Sports Traumatol Arthrosc. 2019;27(12):3897–904.
6. Maiotti M, Massoni C, Russo R, Schroter S, Zanini A, Bianchedi D. Arthroscopic subscapularis augmentation of Bankart repair in chronic anterior shoulder instability with bone loss less than 25% and capsular deficiency: clinical multicenter study. Arthroscopy. 2017;33(5):902–9.
7. Collin P, Ladermann A. Dynamic anterior stabilization using the long head of the biceps for anteroinferior glenohumeral instability. Arthrosc Tech. 2018;7(1):e39–44.
8. Milenin O, Toussaint B. Labral repair augmentation by labroplasty and simultaneous trans-subscapular transposition of the long head of the biceps. Arthrosc Tech. 2019;8(5):e507–12.
9. Tang J, Zhao J. Arthroscopic transfer of the long head of the biceps Brachii for anterior shoulder instability. Arthrosc Tech. 2017;6(5):e1911–7.
10. de Campos Azevedo C, Ângelo AC. All-suture anchor dynamic anterior stabilization produced successful healing of the biceps tendon: a report of 3 cases. JBJS Case Connect. 2021;11(1):e20.00149.
11. Goetti P, Denard PJ, Collin P, Ibrahim M, Hoffmeyer P, Lädermann A. Shoulder biomechanics in normal and selected pathological conditions. EFORT Open Rev. 2020;5(8):508–18.
12. Popescu IA, Neculau DC, Simion C, Popescu D. Modified dynamic anterior stabilization (DAS) and Hill-Sachs Remplissage for the treatment of recurrent anterior shoulder dislocation. Arthrosc Tech. 2022;11(2):e147–52.
13. Nair AV, Mohan PK, Jangale A, Kuntwad V, Kumar MP, Goud N, et al. Dynamic anterior stabilization using transosseous bone tunnel technique with the adjustable loop length cortical button incorporating high-strength suture augmentation for recurrent shoulder instability. Arthrosc Tech. 2022;11(11):e1929–35.
14. Purchase RJ, Wolf EM, Hobgood ER, Pollock ME, Smalley CC. Hill-Sachs "remplissage": an arthroscopic solution for the engaging Hill-Sachs lesion. Arthroscopy. 2008;24(6):723–6.
15. Wu C, Ye Z, Lu S, Fang Z, Xu J, Zhao J. Biomechanical analysis reveals shoulder instability with bipolar bone loss is best treated with dynamic anterior stabilization for on-track lesions and with remplissage for off-track lesions. Arthroscopy. 2024;40:1982.
16. de Campos Azevedo CI, Ângelo AC. Dynamic anterior stabilization of the shoulder: onlay biceps transfer to the anterior glenoid using the double double-pulley technique. Arthrosc Tech. 2023;12(7):e1097–106.
17. de Campos Azevedo CI, Ângelo AC. Onlay dynamic anterior stabilization with biceps transfer for the treatment of anterior glenohumeral instability produces good clinical outcomes and successful healing at a minimum 1 year of follow-up. Arthrosc Sports Med Rehabil. 2023;5(2):e445–57.
18. Collin P, Nabergoj M, Denard PJ, Wang S, Bothorel H, Ladermann A. Arthroscopic biceps transfer to the glenoid with Bankart repair grants satisfactory 2-year results for recurrent anteroinferior glenohumeral instability in subcritical bone loss. Arthroscopy. 2022;38(6):1766–71.

19. Wu C, Xu J, Fang Z, Chen J, Ye Z, Wang L, et al. Arthroscopic dynamic anterior stabilization using either long head of the biceps or conjoined tendon transfer for anterior shoulder instability results in a similarly low recurrence rate. Arthroscopy. 2023;39:1618.
20. Mehl J, Otto A, Imhoff FB, Murphy M, Dyrna F, Obopilwe E, et al. Dynamic anterior shoulder stabilization with the long head of the biceps tendon: a biomechanical study. Am J Sports Med. 2019;47(6):1441–50.
21. Bokshan SL, Gil JA, DeFroda SF, Badida R, Crisco JJ, Owens BD. Biomechanical comparison of the long head of the biceps tendon versus conjoint tendon transfer in a bone loss shoulder instability model. Orthop J Sports Med. 2019;7(11):2325967119883549.
22. Carbone S, Moroder P, Runer A, Resch H, Gumina S, Hertel R. Scapular dyskinesis after Latarjet procedure. J Shoulder Elb Surg. 2016;25(3):422–7.

Part II

Shoulder Instability and Difficult Conditions

10 The Unstable Painful Shoulder

Daichi Morikawa, Hirohisa Uehara, Yoshimasa Saigo, Kenta Shibuya, Yasutaka Yoshimura, Takayuki Kawasaki, and Muneaki Ishijima

10.1 Background

Unstable painful shoulder (UPS) is a recently introduced concept in the field of shoulder disorders. In 2011, UPS was defined as shoulder pain related to anteroinferior instability without any feeling of dislocation or subluxation [1]. However, similar shoulder disorders have been reported under different names since 1981. In 1981, a condition called "dead arm syndrome" in which the patient experiences sudden sharp or paralyzing shoulder pain during movement was reported [2]; this disorder is possibly caused by transient subluxation of the shoulder. Shoulder pain during abduction and external rotation (ER) in noncontact athletes may be attributed to anterior instability without any feeling of instability, also known as "occult subluxation" [3, 4]. Furthermore, shoulder pain secondary to shoulder laxity without any soft tissue injury or bony lesion may be caused by capsular laxity, also known as "minor shoulder instability" [5]. These types of shoulder disorders are commonly associated with minor instability of the glenohumeral joint without any feeling of instability.

10.2 Definitions of UPS

Currently, there are two definitions of UPS. In 2011, Boileau et al. [1] defined UPS as having two characteristics: (1) shoulder pain related to anteroinferior instability without any apparent history of dislocation or subluxation, and (2) anteroinferior instability confirmed by the discovery of "roll-over lesions" (Table 10.1). The term roll-over lesions is used to describe any posttraumatic soft tissue or bony lesion indicative of anteroinferior

Table 10.1 The definitions of unstable painful shoulder (UPS)

Boileau et al. [1]	Hoshika et al. [6]
1. Shoulder pain related to anteroinferior instability without any apparent history of dislocation or subluxation	1. Shoulder pain during daily or sports activity
2. Anteroinferior instability confirmed by the discovery of "roll over lesions"	2. Traumatic onset[a]
	3. No complaint of shoulder instability
	4. Soft-tissue or bony lesions, such as Bankart or HAGL lesions, can be confirmed by arthroscopy

[a] The biggest difference between the definitions of UPS in the studies by Boileau et al. and Hoshika et al.

D. Morikawa (✉) · H. Uehara · Y. Saigo · K. Shibuya
Y. Yoshimura · T. Kawasaki · M. Ishijima
Department of Orthopaedics, Juntendo University School of Medicine, Tokyo, Japan
e-mail: dmorikaw@juntendo.ac.jp; hi-uehara@juntendo.ac.jp; y.saigo.ux@juntendo.ac.jp; ke-shibuya@juntendo.ac.jp; y-yoshimura@juntendo.ac.jp; k-saki@luck.ocn.ne.jp; ishijima@juntendo.ac.jp

E. Calvo et al. (eds.), *Complex and Revision Problems in Shoulder Instability*,
https://doi.org/10.1007/978-3-031-81389-4_10

instability, including capsulolabral detachment (i.e., Bankart or humeral avulsion of the glenohumeral ligament [HAGL] lesions), capsular tears, glenohumeral fractures or erosions, or capsular distension allowing excessive glenohumeral translation on imaging or arthroscopy [1]. The presence of such findings confirms that the humeral head has subluxated at least once to the level of the anteroinferior edge of the glenoid [1]. In 2022, Hoshika et al. [6] defined the UPS differently to Boileau et al. [1]. Their definition of UPS is: (1) shoulder pain during daily or sports activity, (2) traumatic onset, (3) no complaint of shoulder instability, (4) soft tissue or bony lesions (such as Bankart or HAGL lesions) confirmed by arthroscopy (Table 10.1) [6]. The biggest difference between the definitions of UPS in the studies by Boileau et al. [1] and Hoshika et al. [6] was the traumatic onset (Table 10.1). Hoshika et al. [6] questioned whether atraumatic pathologies such as multidirectional shoulder instability should be included as causes of UPS [6]. Therefore, they added "traumatic onset" to their definition of UPS.

10.3 Epidemiology of UPS

The epidemiology of UPS has not been reported. We summarized the characteristics of patients with UPS in Table 10.2. Hoshika et al. [6] reported that approximately 4.7% (91/1952 shoulders) of shoulders undergoing arthroscopic stabilization surgery between 2007 to 2018 met the definition of UPS. In the studies by Boileau et al. [1] and Hoshika et al. [6], the mean ages at the time of surgery were 23 and 25 years, respectively, the percentages of male patients were 60% and 87%, respectively, and the percentages of cases affecting the dominant shoulder were 69% and 80%, respectively. The sports activity was contact, overhead, or resisted overhead activity in 80% (16/20) of patients with UPS in the study by Boileau et al. [1], and was collision and contact sports (60%), overhead sports (29%), others (7%), and none (4%) in the study by Hoshika et al. [6].

Table 10.2 Patients characteristics and clinical outcomes

Author, year	Number of shoulders and patients	Age years (range)	Sports	F/U years (range)	Technique variants	Outcome measures		
							Preop.	Postop.
							Mean ± SD (range)	Mean ± SD (range)
Boileau, JSES 2011	20 shoulders in 20 patients	25 (15–47)	–	>24	Standardized Bankart repair (18 shoulder, 90%)	UCLA score	24 ± 2	$32 \pm 2^{P<0.05}$
					Capsular plication (2 shoulders, 10%)	Rowe score	57 ± 16	$85 \pm 14^{P=0.001}$
						Walch-Duplay score	62 ± 22	$87 \pm 13^{P=0.002}$
						Satisfaction	–	95% very satisfied or satisfied
						aROM-AE	178 ± 6	$177 \pm 7^{N.S.}$
						aROM-ER	75 ± 19	$65 \pm 20^{P=0.029}$
						aROM-IR (level)	T9 ± 3	$T7 \pm 2^{P=0.065}$
						Return to sport [time]	–	75% at same level [7 months (2–18)]
Hoshika, JSES Int 2022	73 shoulders in 73 patients	23 (15–51)	Collision contact (60%)	44 (24–72)	Standardized Bankart repair (73 shoulders, 100%)	Rowe score	71 (20–100)	$95\ (45–100)^{P<0.001}$
			Overhead (29%)		Augmentation rotator interval closure (36 shoulders, 49.3%)	SSV score	42 (0–95)	$86\ (0–100)^{P<0.004}$
			Others (7%)		Hill-Sachs remplissage: (4 shoulders, 5.5%)	Pain VAS	34 (10–80)	$8\ (0–100)^{P<0.001}$
			None (4%)			aROM-AE	169 (140–180)	$168\ (135–180)^{N.S}$
						aROM-ER	65 (60–90)	$62\ (20–90)^{N.S}$
						aROM-IR (points)[a]	9 (4–10)	$9\ (4–10)^{N.S}$
						Return to sports [time]	–	60 % at same or nearly level [7 months (3–36)]
						Reinjury rate	–	9%

F/U follow-up, *SD* standard deviation, *UCLA* University of California, Los Angeles, *SSV* subjective shoulder value, *VAS* visual analog scale, *aROM* active range of mortion, *AE* anterior elavation, *ER* external rotation, *IR* internal roation

[a] Active internal rotation was scored as greater trochanter, 0; buttocks, 2; sacrum,4; L3, 6; Th12, 8; Th7-8, 10

10.4 Physical Examination Findings

It is important to note that the most significant sign of UPS is pain rather than instability or apprehension. There is no specific test for UPS. However, pain during the anterior apprehension test is reportedly useful in the diagnosis of UPS [1, 6].

Boileau et al. [1] reported recurrent pain with movement, described as deep anterior pain in 80% of patients, with radiation to the anterior arm in 40% of patients. Positions that are commonly painful for patients with UPS are the "siesta sign" in which the hand is placed behind the head and elbow backward, and the "suitcase sign" in which a heavy weight is carried with the arm extended along the body [1]. Anterior laxity of the glenohumeral joint is exhibited by 90% of patients with UPS, as indicated by more than 50% anterior translocation on the drawer test [1]. Glenohumeral laxity is exhibited by 85% of patients with UPS, as indicated by ER with the arm at the side of greater than 85° (anterior hyperlaxity) or greater than a 20° difference in hyperabduction (i.e., a positive Gagey test) compared with the contralateral side (inferior hyperlaxity) [1]. Asymmetrical inferior drawer (sulcus sign) is present in 25% of patients with UPS, while posterior drawer is present in 10% [1].

Hoshika et al. [6] also reported that 35% of patients with UPS exhibit glenohumeral hyperlaxity, as indicated by ER with the arm at the side of greater than 85°. Furthermore, they reported that the anterior apprehension test is positive in 20% of patients with UPS, and causes pain in 95% of patients with UPS [6].

10.5 Preoperative Imaging and Intraoperative Findings of UPS

Among the bony lesions in patients with UPS, Boileau et al. [1] reported that 20% are osseous glenoid lesions (erosion: 10%, glenoid fractures: 10%), while Hoshika et al. [6] reported that 50% are osseous glenoid lesions (erosion: 14%, fragment: 37%, normal: 49%). The reported prevalences of Hill-Sachs lesions are 30% [1] and 42% [6].

Among the capsulolabral lesions in patients with UPS, the reported prevalences of Bankart lesions are 74% [1] and 84% by magnetic resonance arthrogram and 100% by arthroscopy [6]. Superior labral anterior and posterior lesions were excluded from the study by Boileau et al. [1] and were reported as being present in 35% of patients with UPS by Hoshika et al. [6]. HAGL lesions were reported as being present in 5% of patients with UPS by Boileau et al. [1] and in 1% by Hoshika et al. [6]. Among patients with UPS, the prevalence of capsular tears is reportedly 2% [6], while the prevalence of capsular distension is reportedly 32% [1].

10.6 Nonoperative Treatment for UPS

Nonoperative treatment for UPS comprises immobilization in the internal rotation position for 3–4 weeks after injury, as for a traumatic dislocation. Initially, conservative treatment such as physical therapy is generally suggested. To return to athletic activities, it is necessary to improve the function of the shoulder joint complex and to improve the quality of the muscles (maximum muscle strength, instantaneous force, endurance, and coordination) and the range of motion (ROM). Most patients with UPS have a history of minor trauma; to prevent similar trauma, the patient must achieve proper form, improve any inappropriate positioning for contact, and strengthen their body balance before returning to competition [1, 6]. No study has investigated conservative treatment for UPS. Moreover, some patients with UPS show recurrence of pain or dislocation/subluxation when they return to sports after conservative treatment [6].

10.7 Surgical Treatment for UPS

10.7.1 Summary of Surgical Treatment for UPS

Surgical treatment is considered for patients with UPS who fail to respond to conservative treatment including rehabilitation for 6 months [1]. UPS is treated with arthroscopic soft tissue stabilization, which is the same procedure as for traumatic recurrent anterior shoulder instability and capsular plication [1, 6]. Furthermore, rotator interval closure is performed as an augmentation for patients with a high risk of recurrence, such as younger athletes or collision and contact athletes [6, 7]. Hill-Sachs remplissage is also performed for young collision and contact athletes with a Hill-Sachs lesion and glenoid bone loss [6, 8].

10.7.2 Rehabilitation After Surgical Treatment for UPS

After 3–4 weeks of immobilization using a sling, passive and assisted-active ROM exercises are initiated while avoiding pain. Strengthening is started between 8 and 12 weeks postoperatively. Full return to sport is allowed at 3–6 months postoperatively in accordance with the functional recovery of each patient [1, 6].

10.7.3 Clinical Results of Surgical Treatment for UPS

The results of arthroscopic soft tissue stabilization and capsular plication for UPS are shown in Table 10.2. However, these two studies of these specific techniques have relatively short-term follow-up periods [1, 6]. All clinical scores (University of California Los Angeles, Rowe, Walch-Duplay, and subjective shoulder value scores) were significantly improved postoperatively [1, 6]. Regarding the active ROM, Boileau et al. [1] reported that ER was significantly decreased (75 ± 19° to 65 ± 20°, $P = 0.029$) and internal rotation (IR) was significantly increased after surgery (T9 ± 3 to T7 ± 2, $P = 0.005$), with no change in anterior elevation (Table 10.2). Hoshika et al. [6] reported that there were no significant changes before versus after surgery for UPS in the active ROMs (anterior elevation, ER, and IR) (Table 10.2). Regarding return to sports after arthroscopic surgery for UPS, Boileau et al. [1] reported that 75% of patients were able to return to their preinjury level, while Hoshika et al. [6] reported that 46% and 14% of patients were able to return to their complete and nearly complete preinjury level at a mean time of 7 months, suggesting that 25–54% of patients were not able to return to their previous level of sports. Furthermore, Hoshika et al. [6] reported that six patients (9%), including five contact or collision athletes, experienced re-injury at around 1 year postoperatively.

10.8 Complications

The complications of surgical treatment for UPS have not been reported. Therefore, we have discussed the possible complications of standardized Bankart repair and capsular plication for other conditions that may also occur after the performance of the same procedures for UPS.

10.8.1 Nerve Injury

Iatrogenic nerve injury is a rare complication after arthroscopic stabilization, with an incidence of 0.3% [9]. Although the axillary nerve is not viewed during shoulder arthroscopy, it is in close proximity to the inferior glenoid, lying 10–15 mm from the 6 o'clock position on the glenoid [10]. Therefore, capsular plication stitches should be placed within 10 mm of the 6 o'clock position on the glenoid to avoid iatrogenic axillary nerve injury [10].

10.8.2 Stiffness

Biomechanical data suggest that arthroscopic remplissage commonly results in shoulder stiffness, and that reduced ER can affect shoulder function [11]. For overhead throwers, the decrease in ER of the shoulder that may be caused by remplissage should be considered. However, for collision athletes, decreased ER is less of a concern and is unlikely to affect their ability to return to sports.

10.8.3 Insufficient Anchors

Several studies have reported that an insufficient number of anchors results in an increased risk of anterior instability recurrence [12, 13]. Specifically, the use of fewer than four anchors, regardless of the size of the initial Bankart lesion, is associated with a higher incidence of arthroscopic Bankart repair failure. Therefore, a minimum of four anchors should be used for labral repair in Bankart repair.

10.9 Conclusions

To our knowledge, the UPS has only been investigated in two clinical studies [1, 6]. The definition of UPS differed between the two studies. However, most patient characteristics were consistent in the two studies, such as an age in the twenties, high prevalence of males, injury of the dominant arm, and high sports activity including collision and contact sports. Preoperative imaging and intraoperative findings showed that patients with UPS have a high incidence of capsular labrum lesions (including Bankart lesions), and 20–50% have bony lesions (including osseous glenoid lesions and Hill-Sachs lesions). There are no reports of nonoperative treatment for UPS. The two clinical studies reported surgical treatments for UPS [1, 6]. Almost all surgical treatments comprised standardized Bankart repair with or without augmentations including rotator interval closure and Hill-Sachs remplissage. The clinical results of surgical treatment for UPS showed that all clinical scores (University of California Los Angeles, Rowe, Walch-Duplay, and subjective shoulder value scores) were significantly improved postoperatively, with little or no reduction in active shoulder ROMs postoperatively [1, 6]. The two studies reported that 75% and 46% of patients, respectively, were able to return to their preinjury level at a mean time of 7 months postoperatively [1, 6]. Re-injury occurred in 9% of patients, including contact or collision athletes, at around 1 year postoperatively [6]. Therefore, UPS in collision and contact athletes should be treated not with standardized Bankart repair but with augmentation (Hill-Sachs remplissage or rotator interval closure) or coracoid transfer depending on the sports activity level, patient wishes, and presence of bony lesions.

Acknowledgments We thank Kelly Zammit, BVSc, from Edanz (https://jp.edanz.com/ac) for editing a draft of this manuscript.

References

1. Boileau P, et al. The unstable painful shoulder (UPS) as a cause of pain from unrecognized anteroinferior instability in the young athlete. J Shoulder Elb Surg. 2011;20(1):98–106.
2. Rowe CR, Zarins B. Recurrent transient subluxation of the shoulder. J Bone Joint Surg Am. 1981;63(6):863–72.
3. Jobe FW, Kvitne RS, Giangarra CE. Shoulder pain in the overhand or throwing athlete. The relationship of anterior instability and rotator cuff impingement. Orthop Rev. 1989;18:963–75.
4. Garth WP Jr, Allman FL Jr, Armstrong WS. Occult anterior subluxations of the shoulder in noncontact sports. Am J Sports Med. 1987;15:579–85.
5. Castagna A, Nordenson U, Garofalo R, Karlsson J. Minor shoulder instability. Arthroscopy. 2007;23:211–5.
6. Hoshika S, et al. Pathology and surgical outcomes of unstable painful shoulders. JSES Int. 2022;6(3):349–54.
7. Kvitne RS, Jobe FW. The diagnosis and treatment of anterior instability in the throwing athlete. Clin Orthop Relat Res. 1993;291:107–23.
8. Nakagawa S, et al. Glenoid rim morphology in young athletes with unstable painful shoulders: primarily painful vs. frankly unstable. JSES Int. 2023;7(5):720–9.
9. Owens BD, et al. Surgical trends in Bankart repair: an analysis of data from the American Board of

Orthopaedic Surgery certification examination. Am J Sports Med. 2011;39(9):1865–9.
10. Eakin CL, Dvirnak P, Miller CM, Hawkins RJ. The relationship of the axillary nerve to arthroscopically placed capsulolabral sutures. An anatomic study. Am J Sports Med. 1998;26(4):505–9.
11. Hartzler RU, et al. Remplissage of an off-track Hill-Sachs lesion is necessary to restore biomechanical Glenohumeral joint stability in a bipolar bone loss model. Arthroscopy. 2016;32(12):2466–76.
12. Randelli P, Ragone V, Carminati S, Cabitza P. Risk factors for recurrence after Bankart repair a systematic review. Knee Surg Sports Traumatol Arthrosc. 2012;20(11):2129–38.
13. Plausinis D, et al. Arthroscopic rotator interval closure: effect of sutures on glenohumeral motion and anterior-posterior translation. Am J Sports Med. 2006;34(10):1656–61.

Shoulder Instability in Hyperlaxity and Collagen Disorders

11

Filip Vuletić and Berte Bøe

11.1 Introduction

The shoulder joint provides an incredible range of motion, but mobility and stability are inversely proportional. Dynamic and static stabilizers balance the physiologic range of motion and shoulder stability [1, 2]. Static stabilizers include the glenohumeral articular congruity, glenoid labrum complex, glenohumeral ligaments, and the negative pressure created within the joint [1]. Dynamic structures responsible for joint stability include rotator cuff muscles, the tendon of the long head of the biceps, and periscapular musculature [2]. Disrupting the interplay between these stabilizers often causes multidirectional instability (MDI) [3]. There are two main ways in which a person may develop MDI [2]. The first is through microtrauma, where ligaments and capsules become loose over time, usually in sports that involve overhead movements like baseball, volleyball, or swimming [2]. It is important to note that this type of instability is not generally due to one specific traumatic event. The second way multidirectional instability can occur is through joint hypermobility caused by underlying conditions that affect connective tissues [2]. Conditions such as Ehler-Danlos syndrome (EDS), Marfan syndrome, osteogenesis imperfecta, and benign joint hypermobility syndrome increase the risk of shoulder joint instability due to the weakness of the connective tissues [4, 5].

Athletes frequently report symptoms of instability, which can lead to pain, emotional distress, and interrupted sports participation [6]. In addition, athletes can experience reduced work capacity and impaired shoulder-related quality of life [6]. The incidence of shoulder injuries in overhead sports can reach up to 3.3 per 1000 athlete exposure hours [6, 7]. Shoulder instability cases may be caused by hyperlaxity, which is found in roughly 5–15% of cases [8]. This condition can be an indicator of failure for soft tissue repair, whether it is the primary or revision surgery. Hyperlaxity is typically localized to the shoulder joint and can occur alone or, as mentioned earlier, as part of a hypermobility spectrum disorder (HSD) or a related disorder, such as hypermobile (Type III) EDS or hEDS [4, 5, 9]. Joint dislocations are a common problem for people with EDS. It is estimated that around 75% of patients with EDS experience this issue [10]. Instability is a common issue across subtypes of EDS, but it is particularly significant in people with hEDS [4]. In this group, over 95% of individuals report experiencing joint dislocations, often leading

F. Vuletić
Department for Orthopaedic and Trauma Surgery, University Hospital "Sveti Duh", Zagreb, Croatia

Faculty of Kinesiology, University of Zagreb, Zagreb, Croatia

B. Bøe (✉)
Division of Orthopaedic Surgery, Oslo University Hospital, Oslo, Norway
e-mail: uxbebm@ous-hf.no

E. Calvo et al. (eds.), *Complex and Revision Problems in Shoulder Instability*,
https://doi.org/10.1007/978-3-031-81389-4_11

them to undergo surgical interventions at some point in their lives [4]. While dislocations can occur in any joint, the shoulder joint is one of the most frequently affected joints [4, 6, 9].

11.2 Diagnosis and Etiology

There are different definitions for joint hypermobility in relation to its link with shoulder injuries. The Beighton scoring system for hypermobility is the most commonly used method in epidemiological research [11]. This system uses nine assessments to determine the presence of hypermobility in joints. A score of 1 is given for each hypermobile joint and 0 for non-hypermobile joints. The total score can range from 0 to 9, with a higher score indicating more joints exhibiting hypermobility [12]. Diagnostic maneuvers for assessing joint laxities are commonly positive, such as the load-and-shift, apprehension (in the abduction and external rotation), relocation, posterior load-and-shift tests, and Kim's test [13, 14]. Genuine instability is confirmed through the elicitation of apprehension or discomfort during examination. It is essential to consider other specific indicators of hypermobility in addition to the ones already identified. These include the Sulcus sign, which is evident during neutral rotation and remains unchanged upon external rotation, indicating rotator interval laxity [15]. Additionally, hyperlaxity can be indicated by a Gagey hyperabduction test result showing glenohumeral abduction exceeding 105°, along with increased movement observed during both anterior and posterior drawer tests and external rotation exceeding 90° when the patient is lying down [13]. The Jerk test may also produce a positive result, characterized by a noticeable clunk as the shoulder is horizontally abducted under posterior pressure [16]. In cases of hEDS, instability may manifest across multiple planes during mid-range shoulder movements and not just at the limits of movement [11]. Therefore, a comprehensive patient history is necessary to diagnose associated hyperlaxity, which includes details of previous subluxations, familial hyperlaxity history, and the nature of the initiating event. Symptoms such as pain, numbness, or tingling when lifting heavy objects, which may suggest inferior hyperlaxity, and the severity of instability symptoms, like dislocations during sleep or voluntary control over instability symptoms, should also be carefully considered [17]. Moreover, it is common for individuals diagnosed with hypermobile Ehlers-Danlos syndrome (hEDS) to experience scapular dyskinesia, which may be a compensatory response to recurring subluxations or dislocations and may also contribute to these issues [4].

Chronic and recurring subluxation episodes can cause uneven stress distribution across the joint. In individuals with Ehlers-Danlos Syndrome (EDS), joint hypermobility can cause significant pain even before any changes are observable through standard X-ray imaging [11, 18]. Besides, the traction or compression of peripheral nerves can lead to neuropathic pain in the distal upper extremities [11]. Those with hEDS, poor muscle tone, and reduced proprioception may further hinder the development of stable postural responses, leading to observable postural instability [4]. The precise causes and mechanisms of pain are not fully understood. Still, potential factors include nociceptive pain from structural alterations in joints, muscles, and connective tissues, neuropathic pain, decreased proprioception and muscle strength, and central sensitization [9, 19]. These factors may interact and contribute to the overall pathology. Biomechanical stress and chronic injury to soft tissues due to joint laxity and instability are the focus of current theories. Such repetitive microtrauma can alter joint kinematics, placing additional stress on neighboring joints and leading to widespread joint pain and musculoskeletal discomfort [20, 21]. As mentioned earlier, individuals often exhibit reduced proprioceptive sensitivity, increasing their risk of injury [9, 19]. In addition to biomechanical issues, neurological factors in HSD patients may also cause widespread musculoskeletal pain. A common symptom among these patients is generalized hyperalgesia, similar to fibromyalgia, which is thought to be caused by central sensitization [22]. The exact biochemical processes behind hyperalgesia in HSD remain unidentified, though it is speculated to potentially act as a protective mechanism against further joint instability [22–24].

Diagnostic imaging evaluates joint hyperlaxity and typically involves standard X-rays and MRI scans. However, these imaging techniques may only sometimes show the underlying cause of joint instability [11, 19]. In most cases, joint instability can be caused by capsular insufficiency rather than bony anatomy [19]. Patients with hypermobile Ehlers-Danlos syndrome (hEDS) may have glenoid dysplasia, which can be detected in Grashey and axillary views [25]. In such cases, a computed tomography scan of the shoulder can help measure the humeral head's inferior displacement and detect glenoid bone malformation [25]. Magnetic resonance imaging (MRI) can help detect soft-tissue findings consistent with connective tissue diseases, such as underdeveloped labral anatomy, extensive Hill-Sachs lesions, increased capsular volume, and a redundant capsule [26]. Magnetic resonance imaging, with or without contrast, is a more sensitive modality in detecting capsular laxity and redundancy [26]. An increase in the glenocapsular ratio on magnetic resonance arthrography is a finding that supports a diagnosis of hEDS [11].

Moreover, the absence of a labral tear on cross-sectional imaging of an unstable shoulder is often more suggestive of underlying hEDS rather than traumatic dislocations [4, 11]. However, recent research suggests that certain types of labral tears are not uncommon in individuals with multidirectional instability (MDI), contrary to traditional beliefs [27]. Patients with a longstanding history of subluxation and dislocation may eventually develop glenohumeral erosion later in life.

As mentioned, shoulder hyperlaxity can be innate or acquired over time due to repetitive stress, stretching, or minor injuries to the shoulder's static stabilizers, often observed in athletes performing overhead activities [2, 6]. Innate hyperlaxity includes various connective tissue disorders like HSDs, hEDS, and Marfan syndrome, which can lead to shoulder instability due to weakened static stabilizers [4, 5]. Hypermobile Spectrum Disorders (HSDs) are classified by increased joint flexibility, assessed through the Beighton scoring system, plus additional physical signs, including flat feet, kyphosis, scoliosis, or misaligned joints [28]. Symptomatic HSD/hEDS affects approximately 1 in 500 people [4, 9]. These conditions are usually hereditary, following an autosomal dominant pattern with varied expression and incomplete penetrance [4, 6, 9]. The hereditary factors contributing to hEDS remain unidentified, setting it apart from other EDS types that have been more clearly defined genetically [4]. HSD/hEDS can present with non-musculoskeletal symptoms, including autonomic nervous system dysfunction, gastrointestinal issues, and anxiety, making shoulder instability one of many challenges within this complex condition [29]. However, people with hEDS will have a particularly extensive and expanded capsule with very little static stability [4]. This capsular and ligamentous laxity can often lead to low-energy subluxations or dislocations [30]. Current perspectives highlight the role of biomechanical stress and ongoing damage to soft tissues caused by the looseness and instability of joints [11, 31]. Continuous minor injuries might result in changes to movement patterns, leading to additional stress on various joints and subsequent injuries to soft tissues, presenting as joint pain and widespread musculoskeletal discomfort [31]. People with HSD often exhibit a reduced ability to perceive joint movement, potentially increasing their risk of sustaining injuries [9].

11.3 Treatment

11.3.1 Nonsurgical Treatment

Nonsurgical treatment, including rehabilitation protocols and education of the patient, is usually preferred for initial shoulder dislocation incidents unless significant structural damage is present [32]. Information about their condition of joint hypermobility and/or collagen disorder and how this predisposes them to shoulder instability might enhance the probability to succeed in nonsurgical treatment. Activity modifications can be discussed to minimize the risk of exacerbating the shoulder instability. Early rehabilitation protocols aim to improve range of motion (ROM) and focus on the toning and proprioceptive abilities of the shoulder's active stabilizers [32]. Progressive resistance exercises and modern rehabilitation programs that include sensorimotor system training are essential to restore shoulder function [33]. Innovations in conservative treatment include using "shoulder pacemaker" devices, which involve electrical muscle stimulation (EMS) therapy to enhance muscle strength and stability [34]. This approach is particularly suitable for patients with a functional component of shoulder instability [33, 34]. Bracing and taping techniques might also be beneficial in providing external support to the shoulder. Management of shoulder instability in individuals with hEDS primarily involves rehabilitation and activity adjustments [4]. Most patients who undergo exercise therapy supervised by a physiotherapist have reported positive outcomes [4, 11]. However, the patients need ongoing support and guidance, the rehabilitation plan might need to be adjusted based on individual response and feedback. The rehabilitation objective for individuals with EDS is to achieve dynamic stability for daily and physical activities [4, 17]. Priority is given to developing an active range of motion (ROM) over passive ROM [17, 35]. Enhancing coordination between the scapula and humerus and addressing scapular dyskinesia is crucial [4]. Strengthening exercises targeting the rotator cuff, periscapular stabilizers, and deltoid muscles are emphasized to correct imbalances in the force couple system of the rotator cuff and deltoid, which could lead to issues such as subacromial compression [36, 37]. The protocol should involve core stability and postural training to address any underlying deficits in core stability and posture that may contribute to shoulder instability. Extensive physical therapy should be undertaken for at least 3 to 6 months before turning to more aggressive treatments [2]. Functional activities and sport-specific movement should be gradually incorporated. This therapy regimen has been proven successful due to the natural stiffening of the shoulder joint that occurs with age. As skeletal maturity nears, symptoms of instability reduce [2]. Observational studies have shown that specific isometric exercises can influence humeral head positioning, suggesting that physical therapy should include targeted exercises for managing impingement symptoms and addressing posterior-inferior instability [35–37]. Managing patient discomfort is a significant challenge in the effective conservative management of EDS. Surveys indicate that hEDS patients use pain relief medications frequently, with a focus on achieving a balance to avoid long-term dependency [38]. Multimodal pain management strategies that include a pain specialist are recommended to facilitate participation in physical therapy [38]. Psychological support may also be beneficial for some hEDS patients, especially considering the high prevalence of anxiety disorders within this group [22, 24]. Understanding and addressing psychological barriers is essential for the comprehensive care of patients with severe hEDS. Recent studies have explored the potential of crosslinking procedures using riboflavin and UV irradiation to enhance the elasticity and stiffness of collagen fibrils in diseased shoulder capsules [39]. These procedures offer a promising direction for future non-operative treatments in patients with recurrent shoulder instability due to damaged capsulolabral tissue [39].

11.3.2 Surgical Treatment

It is recommended to consider open or arthroscopic stabilization procedures only when all other long-term therapy options have been exhausted [32]. These procedures include capsular shift, rotator interval closure, and plication of redundant capsular tissue [40].

The extent of capsular reduction and stabilization should be customized to meet each patient's specific needs, especially for athletes who may require a broader range of motion than the general public. The open inferior capsular shift technique was introduced by Neer et al. in 1980 and targets the expanded inferior capsular pouch that is often observed in patients with hyperlaxity [41] (Fig. 11.1). Over time, this technique has

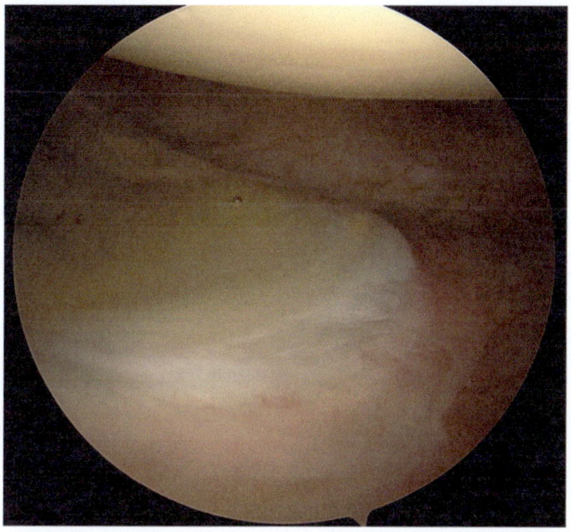

Fig. 11.1 Arthroscopic evaluation of a right shoulder in lateral decubitus with traction. Increased capsular laxity or redundancy, leading to excessive joint translation, may be observed

evolved and now includes posterior approaches and an arthroscopic variation [11]. To preserve a postoperative range of motion, it is recommended that the arm be positioned in reduced abduction and external rotation when tightening the capsule [42]. When chosen and executed correctly, the inferior capsular shift has consistently shown positive outcomes with minimal need for revision [42].

Arthroscopic capsular plication or capsulorrhaphy is becoming more popular due to its ability to precisely decrease capsular volume, enhance visibility, and reduce surgical morbidity [43]. Biomechanical research indicates that unilateral anteroinferior capsular shifts could increase posterior translation and the risk of joint degeneration [44]. Therefore, a more anatomical approach involving anterior and posterior capsular volume reduction is suggested for restoring natural joint biomechanics [43, 45]. This procedure can significantly decrease capsular volume and reestablish the normal tension of the posteroinferior glenohumeral ligament [43]. Various techniques for capsular plication or capsulorrhaphy have been proposed, including methods without glenoid fixation and those using suture anchors, which offer advantages such as a reduced risk of labral displacement and enhanced strength, particularly in the capsule's weaker posteroinferior quadrant [45, 46]. Arthroscopic pancapsular plication is considered the gold standard for addressing multidirectional hyperlaxity, with consistently positive outcomes reported [11]. For posterior instability, posteroinferior plication with a limited number of anchors has shown promise in achieving balanced capsular volume reduction, though further evidence is needed to confirm these findings [46].

Arthroscopic subscapularis augmentation (ASA) combined with classic Bankart repair presents a new solution for managing shoulder hyperlaxity, anterior instability, and glenoid bone loss, showing promising postoperative results and maintaining functional range of motion [47]. Rotator interval closure (RIC) techniques, which adjust the rotator interval directionally and can be performed via open or arthroscopic methods, aim to tighten the coracohumeral ligament to address inferior and posterior instability [48]. Despite varying techniques and indications, RIC has been shown to predominantly reduce glenohumeral translation inferiorly [49]. However, its effect on clinical stability varies, and some studies have linked it to a decreased range of motion [11].

Following surgical intervention, patients with hypermobility or collagen disorders may require longer rehabilitation periods due to delayed wound healing and potential complications associated with their underlying condition. Immobilization time might be prolonged, and close monitoring for recurrent instability and ongoing physical therapy are essential components of postoperative care.

The reoperation rates must be considered when deciding on the best surgical method. Recent reviews have shown that the reoperation rates for open and arthroscopic surgery were approximately 10% [50].

11.4 Conclusion

Shoulder instability in the context of hyperlaxity presents a complex challenge, requiring a comprehensive approach to diagnosis, treatment, and ongoing management. The balance between mobility and stability is crucial for the shoulder's function, with both static and dynamic stabilizers playing pivotal roles. Early and accurate diagnosis is essential, as well as employing clinical assessments and imaging techniques. Conservative treatment, focusing on physiotherapy, is the first line of management. Surgical interventions tailored to the individual's needs may be warranted when conservative measures are insufficient. Ultimately, the goal is to restore function, alleviate pain, and improve the overall quality of life for affected individuals.

Key Points

- **Prevalence and Diagnosis of Ehler-Danlos Syndrome (EDS):** EDS is a group of heritable connective tissue disorders with symptoms like hypermobile joints, hyperextensible skin, and fragile connective tissue. Joint instability is a common issue in classical and hypermobile types.
- **Hypermobility and Shoulder Instability:** Patients with hypermobility, such as hEDS, have severe shoulder instability due to connective tissue abnormalities, which require specialized treatment.
- **Multidisciplinary Approach:** Effective management of EDS involves a multidisciplinary team, including physiatrists, physiotherapists, occupational therapists, and orthopedic surgeons, to address the complex musculoskeletal features and recurrent joint instability.
- **Nonsurgical Treatment Options:** Specialized physiotherapy protocols focusing on strengthening periscapular muscles and improving sensorimotor control are promising nonsurgical treatments for shoulder instability in patients with hyperlaxity, potentially augmented by device-based interventions.
- **Surgical Interventions:** When necessary, arthroscopic techniques like pancapsular shift or plication are preferred and show favorable outcomes. However, the success of newer surgical innovations still needs to be fully established.
- **Patient-Specific Treatment:** Treatment success in connective tissue disorders is less predictable, necessitating a comprehensive evaluation of both nonoperative and operative interventions to tailor the treatment plan to the patient's specific needs.
- **Shoulder Hypermobility:** Shoulder hyperlaxity, ranging from isolated joint hyperlaxity to generalized ligamentous hyperlaxity, as seen in hEDS, increases joint translation and distractibility, leading to pathological instability when the balance of stabilizers is disrupted.
- **Etiology of Hyperlaxity:** Constitutional shoulder hyperlaxity affects up to 10% of the population, more commonly in females, and can be localized to the shoulder or generalized, affecting multiple joints.
- **Conservative Treatment Efficacy:** For patients without hEDS, conservative treatments after a first-time shoulder dislocation, focusing on proprioception and joint stability through specialized physiotherapy, show promise in managing hyperlaxity and instability.
- **Surgical Considerations:** In the absence of hEDS, surgical management, including capsular shift, rotator interval closure, and plication of redundant capsular tissue, is considered after exhausting long-term therapy options. The approach is customized to the patient's needs, especially for athletes requiring a broader range of motion.

References

1. DeFranco MJ, Bershadsky B. Shoulder instability: terminology and classification. Clin Sports Med. 2018;37(4):467–84. https://doi.org/10.1016/j.csm.2018.05.002.
2. Johnson DJ, Tadi P. Multidirectional shoulder instability. In: StatPearls. Treasure Island, FL: StatPearls Publishing; 2024. https://www.ncbi.nlm.nih.gov/books/NBK557726/.
3. Friedman LGM, Lafosse L, Garrigues GE. Global perspectives on management of shoulder instability: decision making and treatment. Orthop Clin North Am. 2020;51(2):241–58.
4. Broida SE, Sweeney AP, Gottschalk MB, Wagner ER. Management of shoulder instability in hypermobility-type Ehlers-Danlos syndrome. JSES Rev Rep Tech. 2021;1(3):155–64. https://doi.org/10.1016/j.xrrt.2021.03.002.
5. Malfait F, Hakim AJ, De Paepe A, Grahame R. The genetic basis of the joint hypermobility syndromes. Rheumatology. 2006;45(5):502–7.
6. Liaghat B, Pedersen JR, Young JJ, Thorlund JB, Juul-Kristensen B, Juhl CB. Joint hypermobility in athletes is associated with shoulder injuries: a systematic review and meta-analysis. BMC Musculoskelet Disord. 2021;22(1):389. https://doi.org/10.1186/s12891-021-04249-x.
7. Shanley E, Rauh MJ, Michener LA, Ellenbecker TS. Incidence of injuries in high school softball and baseball players. J Athl Train. 2011;46(6):648–54. https://doi.org/10.4085/1062-6050-46.6.648.
8. Kraeutler MJ, McCarty EC, Belk JW, Wolf BR, Hettrich CM, Ortiz SF, et al. Descriptive epidemiology of the MOON shoulder instability cohort. Am J Sports Med. 2018;46(5):1064–9.
9. Atwell K, Michael W, Dubey J, et al. Diagnosis and management of hypermobility spectrum disorders in primary care. J Am Board Fam Med. 2021;34(4):838–48. https://doi.org/10.3122/jabfm.2021.04.200374.
10. Stanitski DF, Nadjarian R, Stanitski CL, Bawle E, Tsipouras P. Orthopaedic manifestations of Ehlers-Danlos syndrome. Clin Orthopaedic Relat Res. 2000;376:213–21.
11. Rupp MC, Rutledge JC, Quinn PM, Millett PJ. Management of shoulder instability in patients with underlying hyperlaxity. Curr Rev Musculoskelet Med. 2023;16(4):123–44. https://doi.org/10.1007/s12178-023-09822-6.
12. Beighton P, Horan F. Orthopaedic aspects of the Ehlers-Danlos syndrome. J Bone Joint Surg Br. 1969;51(3):444–53.
13. Hippensteel KJ, Brophy R, Smith MV, Wright RW. Comprehensive review of provocative and instability physical examination tests of the shoulder. J Am Acad Orthop Surg. 2019;27(11):395–404.
14. Ropars M, Fournier A, Campillo B, Bonan I, Delamarche P, Crétual A, et al. Clinical assessment of external rotation for the diagnosis of anterior shoulder hyperlaxity. Orthop Traumatol Surg Res. 2010;96(8 Suppl):S84–7.
15. Harryman DT 2nd, Sidles JA, Harris SL, Matsen FA 3rd. The role of the rotator interval capsule in passive motion and stability of the shoulder. J Bone Joint Surg Am. 1992;74(1):53–66.
16. Goldenberg BT, Lacheta L, Rosenberg SI, Grantham WJ, Kennedy MI, Millett PJ. Comprehensive review of the physical exam for glenohumeral instability. Phys Sportsmed. 2020;48(2):142–50.
17. Johnson SM, Robinson CM. Shoulder instability in patients with joint hyperlaxity. J Bone Joint Surg Am. 2010;92(6):1545–57.
18. Schenk TJ, Brems JJ. Multidirectional instability of the shoulder: pathophysiology, diagnosis, and management. J Am Acad Orthop Surg. 1998;6(1):65–72.
19. Syx D, Wandele I, Rombaut L, Malfait F. Hypermobility, the Ehlers-Danlos syndromes and chronic pain. Clin Exp Rheumatol. 2017;35:S116–22.
20. Kumar B, Lenert P. Joint hypermobility syndrome: recognizing a commonly overlooked cause of chronic pain. Am J Med. 2017;130:640–7.
21. Castori M, Morlino S, Celletti C, et al. Re-writing the natural history of pain and related symptoms in the joint hypermobility syndrome/Ehlers-Danlos syndrome, hypermobility type. Am J Med Genet A. 2013;161A:2989–3004.
22. Rombaut L, Scheper M, De Wandele I, et al. Chronic pain in patients with the hypermobility type of Ehlers-Danlos syndrome: evidence for generalized hyperalgesia. Clin Rheumatol. 2015;34:1121–9.
23. Rombaut L, Malfait F, De Wandele I, et al. Muscle mass, muscle strength, functional performance, and physical impairment in women with the hypermobility type of Ehlers-Danlos syndrome. Arthritis Care Res (Hoboken). 2012;64:1584–92.
24. Scheper M, de Vries J, Verbunt J, et al. Chronic pain in hypermobility syndrome and Ehlers-Danlos syndrome (hypermobility type): it is a challenge. J Pain Res. 2015;8:591–601.
25. Longo UG, Rizzello G, Loppini M, Locher J, Buchmann S, Maffulli N, et al. Multidirectional instability of the shoulder: a systematic review. Arthroscopy. 2015;31(12):2431–43.
26. Lim JR, Lee HM, Yoon TH, Lee HM, Chun YM. Association between excessive joint laxity and a wider Hill-Sachs lesion in anterior shoulder instability. Am J Sports Med. 2021;49(14):3981–7.
27. Raynor MB, Horan MP, Greenspoon JA, Katthagen JC, Millett PJ. Outcomes after arthroscopic pancapsular capsulorrhaphy with suture anchors for the treatment of multidirectional glenohumeral instability in athletes. Am J Sports Med. 2016;44(12):3188–97.
28. What is HSD. 2021. https://www.ehlers-danlos.com/what-is-hsd/.
29. Tinkle B, Castori M, Berglund B, Cohen H, Grahame R, Kazkaz H, et al. Hypermobile Ehlers-Danlos syndrome (a.k.a. EhlersDanlos syndrome Type III and Ehlers-Danlos syndrome hypermobility type): clini-

cal description and natural history. Am J Med Genet C Semin Med Genet. 2017;175(1):48–69.
30. Rodeo SA, Suzuki K, Yamauchi M, Bhargava M, Warren RF. Analysis of collagen and elastic fibers in shoulder capsule in patients with shoulder instability. Am J Sports Med. 1998;26:634–43.
31. Sundemo D, Hamrin Senorski E, Karlsson L, Horvath A, Juul-Kristensen B, Karlsson J, et al. Generalised joint hypermobility increases ACL injury risk and is associated with inferior outcome after ACL reconstruction: a systematic review. BMJ Open Sport Exerc Med. 2019;5(1):e000620. https://doi.org/10.1136/bmjsem-2019-000620.
32. Abrams R, Akbarnia H. Shoulder dislocations overview. In: StatPearls. Treasure Island, FL: StatPearls Publishing; 2024. https://www.ncbi.nlm.nih.gov/books/NBK459125/.
33. Bateman M, Smith BE, Osborne SE, Wilkes SR. Physiotherapy treatment for atraumatic recurrent shoulder instability: early results of a specific exercise protocol using pathology-specific outcome measures. Should Elbow. 2015;7(4):282–8.
34. Moroder P, Plachel F, Van-Vliet H, Adamczewski C, Danzinger V. Shoulder-pacemaker treatment concept for posterior positional functional shoulder instability: a prospective clinical trial. Am J Sports Med. 2020;48(9):2097–104.
35. Spanhove V, De Wandele I, Kjaer BH, Malfait F, Vanderstukken F, Cools A. The effect of five isometric exercises on glenohumeral translations in healthy subjects and patients with the hypermobility type of the Ehlers-Danlos syndrome (HEDS) or hypermobility spectrum disorder (HSD) with multidirectional shoulder instability: an observational study. Physiotherapy. 2020;107:11–8. https://doi.org/10.1016/j.physio.2019.06.010.
36. Ericson WB Jr, Wolman R. Orthopaedic management of the Ehlers-Danlos syndromes. Am J Med Genet C Semin Med Genet. 2017;175:188–94. https://doi.org/10.1002/ajmg.c.31551.
37. Page P. Shoulder muscle imbalance and subacromial impingement syndrome in overhead athletes. Int J Sports Phys Ther. 2011;6:51–8.
38. Chopra P, Tinkle B, Hamonet C, Brock I, Gompel A, Bulbena A, et al. Pain management in the Ehlers-Danlos syndromes. Am J Med Genet C Semin Med Genet. 2017;175(1):212–9.
39. Cornette P, Jaabar IL, Dupres V, et al. Impact of collagen crosslinking on dislocated human shoulder capsules-effect on structural and mechanical properties. Int J Mol Sci. 2022;23(4):2297. https://doi.org/10.3390/ijms23042297.
40. Gervasi E, Sebastiani E, Spicuzza A. Multidirectional shoulder instability: arthroscopic labral augmentation. Arthrosc Tech. 2017;6(1):e219–25.
41. Neer CS 2nd, Foster CR. Inferior capsular shift for involuntary inferior and multidirectional instability of the shoulder. A preliminary report. J Bone Joint Surg Am. 1980;62(6):897–908.
42. Lewicky YM, Lewicky RT. Simplified arthroscopic rotator interval capsule closure: an alternative technique. Arthroscopy. 2005;21(10):1276.
43. Mayer SW, Kraszewski AP, Skelton A, Kontaxis A, Warren R. What are the effects of capsular plication on translational laxity of the glenohumeral joint: a study in cadaveric shoulders. Clin Orthop Relat Res. 2018;476(7):1526–36.
44. Ahmad CS, Wang VM, Sugalski MT, Levine WN, Bigliani LU. Biomechanics of shoulder capsulorrhaphy procedures. J Shoulder Elbow Surg. 2005;14(1 Suppl S):12s–8s.
45. Provencher MT, Verma N, Obopilwe E, Rincon LM, Tracy J, Romeo AA, et al. A biomechanical analysis of capsular plication versus anchor repair of the shoulder: can the labrum be used as a suture anchor? Arthroscopy. 2008;24(2):210–6.
46. Chiang ER, Wang JP, Wang ST, Ma HL, Liu CL, Chen TH. Arthroscopic posteroinferior capsular plication and rotator interval closure after Bankart repair in patients with traumatic anterior glenohumeral instability—a minimum follow-up of 5 years. Injury. 2010;41(10):1075–8.
47. Maiotti M, Russo R, Zanini A, Castricini R, Castellarin G, Schröter S, et al. Bankart repair with subscapularis augmentation in athletes with shoulder hyperlaxity. Arthroscopy. 2021;37(7):2055–62.
48. Provencher MT, Peebles LA. Editorial commentary: rotator interval closure of the shoulder continues to be a challenge in consensus on treatment. Arthroscopy. 2018;34(11):3109–11.
49. Coughlin RP, Bullock GS, Shanmugaraj A, Sell TC, Garrigues GE, Ledbetter L, et al. Outcomes after arthroscopic rotator interval closure for shoulder instability: a systematic review. Arthroscopy. 2018;34(11):3098–108.e1.
50. Prasetia R, Purwana SZB, Rasyid HN. Multidirectional instability of shoulder joint: a review. Orthop J Sports Med. 2023;11(2 Suppl):2325967121S00838. https://doi.org/10.1177/2325967121S00838.

12 Concomitant Rotator Cuff Tear After Shoulder Dislocation

Weihan Yu and Jiwu Chen

Stevens et al. [1] first reported rotator cuff tears (RCTs) following anterior shoulder dislocation in 1926. In 1934, Codman et al. [2] also reported that the possibility of RCT should be a concern in elderly patients with shoulder dislocation. Since then, a lot have been reported about the concomitant RCTs after shoulder dislocation in literature [3–6], and the condition was indicated to have higher incidence in older patients. It has been recognized that the natural history of anterior shoulder dislocations in patients older than 40 years is markedly different from the younger population. In the older patients, after shoulder dislocation the primary issue is not the recurrence of the dislocation but the concomitant RCTs, which might result in the persistent shoulder pain, dysfunction, and instability.

12.1 The Epidemiology of Concomitant RCT in Shoulder Dislocation

The concomitant RCTs after anterior shoulder dislocation were mainly reported in older patients, but with various incidences with different evaluation methods. Hawkins et al. [3] reported 90% RCTs after shoulder dislocations over the age of 40 through clinical examination. Reeves et al. [4] and Itoi et al. [5] found that RCT occurred in more than 30% of patients over the age of 40 and 57% of patients over the age of 50. Loew et al. [6] and Simank et al. [7] showed that the incidence of concomitant RCT was 100% in patients with a mean age > 70 years. In the ultrasonographic studies, the incidences of concomitant RCTs were reported as 38% in patients older than 40 years by Toolanen et al. [8] and 56% in the patients older than 60 years by Berbig et al. [9]. With clinical or MRI study, 17 cuff lesions in 52 patients (32%) with the mean age of 56 years were found by Pevny et al. [10], 58 RCTs (61%) of 108 patients (20%) aged more than 60 years were diagnosed by Gumina and Postacchini [11]. In conclusion, the concomitant RCTs after shoulder dislocation have correlation with age. The older patients with shoulder dislocation would have higher rates of the concomitant RCTs.

The concomitant RCTs secondary to shoulder dislocation were believed to be infrequent in young patients by some authors. Shin et al. [12] reported that only 1 of 33 patients with primary dislocation under the age of 30 had a partial rotator cuff injury, while Kim et al. [13] found one partial rotator cuff injury in 33 patients. Contrarily, some studies indicated that the concomitant RCTs were not rare in young patients. Rahu et al. [14] reported 16 male patients (mean age, 21 years [range, 16–25 years]) with a first-time traumatic anterior shoulder dislocation

W. Yu · J. Chen (✉)
Department of Sports Medicine, Shanghai General Hospital, Shanghai Jiao Tong University School of Medicine, Shanghai, China

E. Calvo et al. (eds.), *Complex and Revision Problems in Shoulder Instability*,
https://doi.org/10.1007/978-3-031-81389-4_12

without bony Bankart lesions. The articular-sided partial-thickness RCTs were found in 9 of the 16 patients. Zhou et al. [15] found 5.56% of 324 cadets with a mean age of 20.53 ± 1.80 years had RCTs in MRI before the shoulder stabilization surgery. Therefore, the concomitant RCTs in young patients were less than those in patients older than 40, but still need to be considered, especially in the athletes with cuff degeneration probably.

12.2 The Stabilzing Mechanism of Rotator Cuff

The mechanisms contributed to the shoulder stability include the static mechanisms from bone, capsule, and labrum, and the dynamic mechanism from rotator cuff and other muscles around shoulder. The rotator cuff plays active and passive roles through its muscles and tendons to prevent the glenohumeral instability.

12.2.1 The Direct Roles of Rotator Cuff in Stabilizing Shoulder

1. The rotator cuff muscles help to maintain the shoulder stability through their volume and tension.
2. The active contraction of rotator cuff muscles contributes to the stability of the shoulder joint through the compression mechanism to increase pressure between the articular surfaces and allow the concentric rotation. The rotator cuff muscle forces are ideally aligned for effective compression of the glenohumeral joint at all shoulder positions. This concavity-compression mechanism is the primary factor for shoulder stability during the middle ranges of motion when the capsular ligaments are lax, and also important at terminal ROM to limit motion and decrease strain on the glenohumeral ligaments. Although the four rotator cuff muscles played the similar role for anterior joint stability, the subscapularis was less effective than the other rotator cuff muscles for stabilizing the glenohumeral joint in end-range positions [16].
3. The movement of the joints directed by the rotator cuff could indirectly tighten the surrounding structures for static stability.
4. The contracted rotator cuff muscles would act as anterior or posterior barriers to enhance the shoulder stability, such as the subscapularis in anterior, and the supraspinatus, infraspinatus, and teres minor in posterior.

12.2.2 The Scapulohumeral Balance Mechanism: The Indirect Role of Rotator Cuff

The scapulohumeral balance mechanism involves synchronous contractions of the muscles around the shoulder joint. The lines of force acting on the humeral head pass through the arc formed by the glenoid and labrum, ensuring that the humeral head remains in the glenoid fossa during relative motion with the glenoid. This stabilization mechanism would be disrupted if muscle contractions were not synchronized, such as rotator cuff tear or muscle fatigue. Warner et al. [17] found the abnormal Moiré pattern in 64% of instability cases and 18% of asymptomatic individuals in the dynamic Moiré test. Paletta et al. [18] observed the significant differences in scapulohumeral rhythm between anterior glenohumeral joint instability and controls. When a rotator cuff injury was present, an increase in upward rotation of the scapula would be observed in many studies, and might be a positive compensation to maximize arm height without full rotator cuff function. Subsequently, it could lead to other problems with the shoulder muscles, resulting in scapular-thoracic abnormal motion (STAM), which further aggravates shoulder instability.

Edouard et al. [19] found the strength values of rotator cuff muscle in the shoulder with anterior instability were lower than those of normal. Gagey et al. [20] carefully detached the rotator cuff tendons from their insertion without damage to the underlying capsule in 80 cadaver shoulders, and proved that the humeral head dislocated easily with less extensive capsuloligamentous lesions when RCTs were present. Rodosky et al. [21] found a 50% decrease in the rotator cuff muscle forces resulted in nearly a 50% increase in anterior displacement of the humeral head in response to external loading at all glenohumeral joint positions.

12.3 The Pathophysiology of Concomitant RCT

12.3.1 Concomitant RCTs

After shoulder dislocation, the anterior capsular ligamentous structures most commonly injured in the younger patients, while the posterior structures fail frequently in the older patients with the degenerated rotator cuff. The subscapularis tendon tear was always thought to be the primary factor leading to the recurrent anterior shoulder dislocation in older patients. In 1993, Neviaser et al. [22] reported 37 patients over the age of 40 with primary anterior shoulder dislocations. Eleven of these patients experienced recurrent anterior instability due to subscapularis and anterior capsule rupture from the lesser tuberosity. The tear of the subscapularis tendon appears to be associated with shoulder instability due to its stabilizing role in the glenohumeral joint; however, the involvement of the subscapularis tendon after shoulder dislocation is controversial. Kim et al. [13] and Porcellini et al. [23] did not observe the associations between subscapularis tendon tear and glenohumeral instability in their studies.

McLaughlin [24] postulated that either the anterior or the posterior supporting structures of the shoulder can be disrupted after an anterior dislocation. The supraspinatus tendon tear was always found, and most often as an isolated tear in the study by Itoi et al. [5]. Berbig et al. [9] reported 75% of associated RCTs were isolated supraspinatus tendon tears, 25% of shoulder joints had combined subscapularis or infraspinatus tendon injuries, and no cases of subscapularis tendon involvement. Craig [25] popularized the "posterior mechanism" and suggested that injuries of the supraspinatus and infraspinatus tendons caused shoulder dislocation. Conversely, some other authors [11, 23] believed that these posterosuperior RCTs were secondary to the recurrent dislocations rather than the primary cause of instability, especially in the cases with seven or more episodes of anterior dislocations [26].

12.3.2 Concomitant RCTs and Nerve Injury

Shoulder dislocation could be associated with nerve injury in addition to rotator cuff tears. Gonzalez and Lopez [27] reported two patients in 1991, Guven et al. [28] reported one patient in 1994 and called this combination of injuries the "unhappy triad," and Groh and Rockwood [29] reported two patients in 1995 and called this combined injury the "terrible triad of the shoulder." Electromyography is recommended, as nerve injury can be easily missed in patients with massive RCTs [10]. Vise versa, the concomitant RCTs should be always suspected when axillary nerve or brachial plexus injury is found. Some authors recommended prompt rotator cuff repair to prevent further retraction and atrophy during nerve recovery, which can take 12–18 months; but the outcomes of rotator cuff repair in the patients with nerve injury were inferior to those with isolated rotator cuff injury [10, 30, 31].

12.4 Diagnosis

It was not rare that the concomitant RCTs were not diagnosed in patients with shoulder anterior instability. In 1993, Neviaser et al. [22] reported that the RCTs in all 37 patients older than 40 years with shoulder anterior dislocation were missed, and the mean time from dislocation to diagnosis of RCTs was 7.2 months. Additionally, the persistent dysfunction was often mistakenly attributed to presumed nerve palsy, resulting in delayed diagnosis of the cuff tear.

For patients experiencing persistent pain and dysfunction following shoulder dislocation, particularly those over 40 years of age, contact or overhead athletes, or individuals with nerve injuries, a thorough evaluation of the rotator cuff should be conducted [32]. Mancini et al. [33] reported that shoulder ultrasound was a reliable tool for diagnosing shoulder dislocation with rotator cuff tears. MRI can more accurately show shoulder joint injuries following dislocation, while arthroscopy can both diagnose and treat the injury simultaneously.

12.5 Management

In patients with persistent pain, dysfunction, and/or recurrent dislocations, repair of the concomitant RCTs should be recommended for function improvement and pain relief.

It was reported that surgical repair of concomitant RCTs after acute shoulder dislocation could have better prognosis than nonoperative treatment and delayed repair [34, 35].

At the time of surgery, the surgeon must decide whether capsulolabral repair, rotator cuff repair, or both should be performed in patients with concomitant RCTs after dislocation. Before selecting an operative option, the surgeon must assess the patient's age, functional status, time since first dislocation, capsular status, and degree of bone loss [32].

12.5.1 For Patients Below 40 Years

Although instability and cuff tear vary greatly, it is rare for young patients to require surgery for both conditions. In high-demand athletes, the challenge lies in achieving secure surgical fixation while also fully restoring motion. Brislin et al. [36] suggest performing a mini open cuff repair with combined suture anchors and sutures, or an arthroscopic repair in case of a small lesion, followed by an open Bankart repair using nonabsorbable anchors.

For the concomitant RCTs with partial thickness, Rahu et al. [14] reported a study of 16 male patients, mean age of 21 years, with first-time traumatic anterior shoulder dislocation. All patients underwent an arthroscopic Bankart procedure. For patients with articular-sided partial-thickness rotator cuff tears (APTRCT), intra-articular rotator cuff injuries were debrided with a shaver. At 2 years after surgical treatment, there were no significant differences between the patients with and without APTRCTs in terms of the Rowe score and ASES score. Hawkins et al. [37] recommended repair surgery for capsular ligament complexes and rotator cuffs in patients younger than 40 years of age. If the Bankart lesion is related to a partial rotator cuff tear on the side of the bursa and involves only 50% or less of the tendon, Bankart repair alone can be done.

12.5.2 For Patients Above 40 Years

12.5.2.1 Isolated Cuff Repair

In 1988, Neviaser et al. [38] reported eight patients, with the subscapularis tendon and anterior part of the capsule ruptured from the lesser tuberosity. Recurrent instability developed in all eight patients, and repair of these structures alone was successful in restoring stability. Five years later, Neviaser et al. [22] conducted a clinical investigation involving 11 patients aged over 40 years who presented with recurrent anterior shoulder instability secondary to avulsion of the subscapularis tendon and anterior capsule from the lesser tuberosity. The tear of the subscapularis tendon appears to be associated with shoulder instability due to its stabilizing role in the glenohumeral joint. No patient had a Bankart lesion. Repairing the capsule and subscapularis restored stability in all patients. Itoi et al. [5] diagnosed 16 rotator cuff tears in 109 shoulders in 104 patients with a traumatic anterior dislocation. A surgical repair of the cuff was carried out in 11 and the results were satisfactory in 8 (73%) regardless of a Bankart lesion. The repair of a torn cuff seems to be sufficient to stabilize the shoulder in elderly patients, even when a Bankart lesion is present and is not repaired. Gumina and Postacchini [11] repaired only the torn rotator cuff in eight older patients with a primary dislocation and concomitant RCTs. The results showed no recurrence of dislocation after surgery, and the patients achieved good functional scores. Recently, Marsalli et al. [39] reported the results of rotator cuff repair alone in patients over

40 years of age with first traumatic dislocation. The study included 84 patients with a mean age of 57 years (range: 40–75 years). Regardless of the factors including the incidence of significant Hill–Sachs defects, anterior glenoid defects, bipolar bone defects, size of the RC injury, and tendon re-tears, the isolated rotator cuff repair after traumatic shoulder dislocation was useful to prevent the recurrent glenohumeral dislocation in active patients over 40 years.

In addition, rotator cuff repair alone is a suitable option to restore function and stability for patients older than 60 or with low functional demands.

12.5.2.2 Shoulder Stability Reconstruction and Rotator Cuff Repair

Theoretically, the repair of rotator cuff involved in the posterior mechanism of instability could restore the concavity-compression mechanism to stabilize the glenohumeral joint. However, anterior capsulolabral detachment has been identified as a clinically significant finding in patients over 40 years of age following shoulder dislocation, necessitating appropriate diagnostic recognition and therapeutic intervention [40]. Several authors recommended to repair both torn cuff and capsulolabral lesion [23, 41, 42].

Walch et al. [43] treated 28 shoulders between 1988 and 2002 with mean age of 47 years at first dislocation, and claimed that isolated repair of the cuff should not be performed because of the fear of higher rate of postoperative instability leading to RC re-tear。.

Gumina and Postacchini [11] studied 16 older patients who required surgery for shoulder dislocations. Among the eight patients who had a single dislocation with rotator cuff tears, only the torn rotator cuff was repaired. The remaining eight patients had recurrent dislocations and rotator cuff tears, five of them required stabilization surgery with rotator cuff repair or rotator cuff repair only. All patients who underwent surgery achieved satisfactory results, except for of those with multiple re-dislocations and rotator cuff tears who had repair of the cuff only. Studies have shown that surgery is necessary to repair the torn rotator cuff or stabilize the shoulder joint in older patients with shoulder dislocations. Patients with recurrent dislocations may require two types of surgery.

Voigt and Lill [44] proposed an algorithm for the surgical treatment of associated instability and tendon lesions in patients younger than 60 years. The algorithm recommends performing both capsulo-ligament reconstruction and cuff repair.

In patients over the age of 70, where a cuff lesion is likely to have preceded the dislocation, and repair is not possible, tendon transfer, inverse prosthesis, or conservative management should be considered.

References

1. Stevens JH. Dislocation of the shoulder. Ann Surg. 1926;83:84–103.
2. Codman EA. The shoulder: rupture of the supraspinatus tendon and other lesions in or about the subacromial Bursa. Boston: Thomas Todd; 1934.
3. Hawkins RJ, Bell RH, Hawkins RH, et al. Anterior dislocation of the shoulder in the older patient. Clin Orthop Relat Res. 1986;206:192–5.
4. Reeves B. Acute anterior dislocation of the shoul der: clinical and experimental studies. Ann R Coll Surg Engl. 1969;44:255–73.
5. Itoi E, Tabata S, Prim J. Rotator cuff tears in anterior dislocation of the shoulder. Int Orthop. 1992;19:240–4.
6. Loew M, Thomsen M, Rickert M, et al. Injury pattern in elderly people shoulder. Unfallchirurg. 2001;104:115–8.
7. Simank HG, Dauer G, Schneider S, et al. Incidence of rotator cuff tears in shoulder dislocations and results of therapy in older patients. Arch Orthop Trauma Surg. 2006;126:235–40.
8. Toolanen G, Hildingsson C, Hedlund T, et al. Early complications after anterior dislocation of the shoulder in patients over 40 years. Acta Orthop Scand. 1993;64:549–52.
9. Berbig R, Weishaupt D, Prim J, Shahin O. Primary anterior shoulder dislocation and rotator cuff tears. J Shoulder Elb Surg. 1999;8:220–5.
10. Pevny T, Hunter RE, Freeman JR. Primary traumatic anterior shoulder dislocation in patients 40 years of age and older. Arthroscopy. 1998;14:289–94.
11. Gumina S, Postacchini R. Anterior dislocation of the shoulder in elderly patients. J Bone Joint Surg Br. 1979;79:540–3.
12. Shin SJ, Ko YW, Lee J. Intra-articular lesions and their relation to arthroscopic stabilization failure in young patients with first-time and recurrent shoulder dislocations. J Shoulder Elb Surg. 2016;25(11):1756–63.

13. Kim TK, Rauh PB, McFarland EG. Partial tears of the subscapularis tendon found during arthroscopic procedures on the shoulder: a statistical analysis of sixty cases. Am J Sports Med. 2003;31:744–50.
14. Rahu M, Kartus JT, Põldoja E, Pedak K, Kolts I, Kask K. Do articular-sided partial-thickness rotator cuff tears after a first-time traumatic anterior shoulder dislocation in young athletes influence the outcome of surgical stabilization? Orthop J Sports Med. 2018;6(6):2325967118781311.
15. Zhou L, Gee SM, Posner MA, Cameron KL. Concomitant glenohumeral instability and rotator cuff injury: an epidemiologic and case-control analysis in military cadets. J Am Acad Orthop Surg Glob Res Rev. 2022;6(4):e22.00049.
16. Blasier RB, Guldberg MS, Rothman ED. Anterior shoulder stability: contributions of rotator cuff forces and the capsular ligaments in a cadaver model. J Shoulder Elb Surg. 1992;1:140–50.
17. Warner JJ, Micheli LJ, Arslanian LE, Kennedy J, Kennedy R. Scapulothoracic motion in normal shoulders and shoulders with glenohumeral instability and impingement syndrome. A study using Moire topographic analysis. Clin Orthop Relat Res. 1992;285:191–9.
18. Paletta GA Jr, Warner JJ, Warren RF, Deutsch A, Altchek DW. Shoulder kinematics with two-plane x-ray evaluation in patients with anterior instability or rotator cuff tearing. J Shoulder Elb Surg. 1997;6:516–27.
19. Edouard P, Degache F, Beguin L, Samozino P, Gresta G, Fayolle-Minon I, Farizon F, Calmels P. Rotator cuff strength in recurrent anterior shoulder instability. J Bone Joint Surg Am. 2011;93(8):759–65.
20. Pouliart N, Gagey O. Concomitant rotator cuff and capsular ligamentous lesions of the shoulder: a cadaver study. Arthroscopy. 2006;22:728–35.
21. Rodosky MW, Harner CD, Fu FH. The role of the long head of the biceps muscle and superior glenoid labrum in anterior stability of the shoulder. Am J Sports Med. 1994;22:121–30.
22. Neviaser RJ, Neviaser TJ, Neviaser JS. Anterior dislocation of the shoulder and rotator cuff rupture. Clin Orthop Relat Res. 1993;291:103–6.
23. Porcellini G, Paladini P, Campi F, et al. Shoulder instability and related rotator cuff tears: arthroscopic finding and treatment in patients aged 40 to 60 years. Arthroscopy. 2006;22:270–6.
24. McLaughlin H. Injuries of the shoulder and arm. In: McLaughlin H, Harrison L, editors. Trauma. Philadelphia: Saunders; 1959. p. 233–96.
25. Craig EV. The posterior mechanism of acute anterior shoulder dislocations. Clin Orthop Relat Res. 1984;190:212–6.
26. Porcellini G, Caranzano F, Campi F, et al. Glenohumeral instability and rotator cuff tear. Sports Med Arthrosc Rev. 2011;19(4):395–400.
27. Gonzalez D, Lopez R. Concurrent rotator cuff tear and brachial plexus palsy associated with anterior dislocation of the shoulder: a report of two cases. J Bone Joint Surg Am. 1991;73:620–1.
28. Guven O, Akbar Z, Yalcin S, et al. Concomitant rotator cuff tear and brachial plexus injury in association with anterior shoulder dislocation: unhappy triad of the shoulder. J Orthop Trauma. 1994;8(429):430.
29. Groh G, Rockwood C. The terrible triad: anterior dislocation of the shoulder associated with rupture of the rotator cuff and injury to the brachial plexus. J Shoulder Elb Surg. 1995;4:51–4.
30. Brown T, Newton P, Steinmann S, et al. Rotator cuff tears and associated nerve injuries. Orthopedics. 2000;23:329–32.
31. Simonich SD, Wright TW. Terrible triad of the shoulder. J Shoulder Elb Surg. 2003;12:566–8.
32. Sekiya JK, Gomberawalla MM. Rotator cuff tear and glenohum feral instability a systematic review. Clin Orthop Relat Res. 2014;472:2448–56.
33. Mancini GB, Malaspina C, Scalercio AM, Ferranti R. Anterior shoulder dislocation and injuries of the rotator cuff in patients aged over 40 years. Clinical and sonographic study. Chir Organi Mov. 2001;86(1):37–44.
34. Bassett RW, Cofield RH. Acute tears of the rotator cuff: the timing of surgical repair. Clin Orthop Relat Res. 1983;175:18–24.
35. Lahteenmaki HE, Virolainen P, Hiltunen A, Heikkila J, Nelimarkka OI. Results of early operative treatment of rotator cuff tears with acute symptoms. J Shoulder Elb Surg. 2006;15:148–53.
36. Brislin K, Rubenstein D, Wetzler M, et al. Operative repair of anterior instability and rotator cuff tears in athlete. Oper Tech Sports Med. 2002;10(2):64–8.
37. Hawkins RJ, Mohtadi NG. Controversy in anterior shoulder instability. Clin Orthop Relat Res. 1991;272:152–61.
38. Neviaser RJ, Neviaser TJ, Neviaser JS. Concurrent rupture of the rotator cuff and anterior dislocation of the shoulder in the older patient. J Bone Joint Surg Am. 1988;70:1308–11.
39. Marsalli M, Errázuriz JD, Morán NI, Cartaya MA. Recurrence of glenohumeral instability in patients with isolated rotator cuff repair after a traumatic shoulder dislocation. Arch Orthop Trauma Surg. 2023;143(7):3857–62.
40. Araghi A, Prasarn M, St Clair S, Zuckerman JD. Recurrent anterior glenohumeral instability with onset after forty years of age: the role of the anterior mechanism. Bull Hosp Jt Dis. 2005;62:99–101.
41. Hawkins RJ, Morin WD, Bonutti PM. Surgical treatment of full- thickness rotator cuff tears in patients 40 years of age or younger. J Shoulder Elb Surg. 1999;8:259–65.
42. Voos JE, Pearle AD, Mattern CJ, Cordasco FA, Allen AA, Warren RF. Outcomes of combined arthroscopic rotator cuff and labral repair. Am J Sports Med. 2007;35:1174–9.
43. Jouve F, Graveleau N, Nové-Josserand L, Walch G. Recurrent anterior instability of the shoulder associated with full thickness rotator cuff tear: results of surgical treatment. Rev Chir Orthop Reparatrice Appar Mot. 2008;94:659–69.
44. Voigt C, Lill H. Shoulder instability and rotator cuff tear (in German). Orthopade. 2009;38:70–4.

Shoulder Instablity in Patients with Seizure Disorders

13

Davide Cucchi, Tobias Baumgartner, Amadeo Touet, Sofia Fragedakis, and Pietro S. Randelli

13.1 Introduction

Shoulder injuries, including dislocations, fractures, and rotator cuff lesions, are frequent among patients with epilepsy (PWE). These patients experience a higher incidence of rare injuries, such as proximal humerus fracture-dislocations and bilateral shoulder lesions. The literature on the types, frequency, and outcomes of these injuries in PWE is limited. This chapter explores the dynamics and pathomechanics of shoulder injuries in PWE, emphasizing the mechanisms and unique challenges they present and summarize the treatment options of seizure-related shoulder instability.

D. Cucchi · A. Touet · S. Fragedakis
Department of Orthopaedics and Trauma Surgery, University Hospital Bonn, Bonn, Germany

T. Baumgartner
Department of Epileptology, University Hospital Bonn, Bonn, Germany

P. S. Randelli (✉)
Laboratory of Applied Biomechanics, Department of Biomedical Sciences for Health, Università degli Studi di Milano, Milan, Italy

Clinica Ortopedica, ASST Centro Specialistico Ortopedico Traumatologico Gaetano Pini-CTO, Milan, Italy
e-mail: pietro.randelli@unimi.it

13.2 Characteristics of Patients and Lesions

13.2.1 Dynamics of Injury and Pathomechanics

Among musculoskeletal injuries in PWE, shoulder injuries, including dislocations, fractures, and rotator cuff lesions, are significant. This subgroup experiences a higher incidence of rare injuries, such as proximal humerus fracture-dislocations and bilateral shoulder lesions [1, 2]. Limited literature exists on the types, frequency, and outcomes of these injuries in PWE. Three mechanisms of shoulder injury in PWE are described: uncontrolled muscular contraction during tonic-clonic seizures, unprotected falls (tonic, atonic, tonic-clonic, myoclonic, or facio-brachial dystonic seizures), and loss of consciousness during other activities leading to high-energy accidents (any type of seizures) [3–6]. Injuries from muscular contractions during tonic-clonic seizures are a distinctive characteristic of PWE, particularly in younger patients, but their pathomechanics remain unclear [7].

During a tonic-clonic seizure, muscle activation imbalance can dislocate the humerus or cause a proximal humerus or glenoid fracture, depending on the force exerted and bone quality. The exact muscular activation pattern is unknown, but clinical observations suggest that during the tonic extensor phase of generalized tonic-clonic sei-

E. Calvo et al. (eds.), *Complex and Revision Problems in Shoulder Instability*, https://doi.org/10.1007/978-3-031-81389-4_13

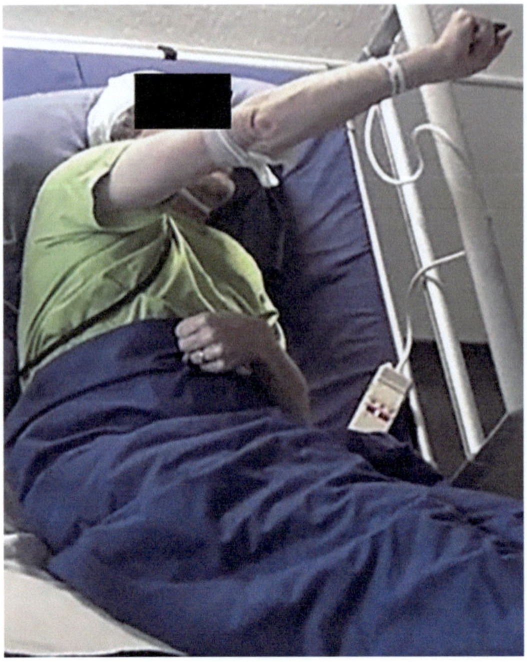

Fig. 13.1 Clinical example of a patient assuming the so-called figure of four position during a tonic-clonic seizure: the right arm is adducted, internally rotated, and flexed

zures, the shoulder is often adducted, internally rotated, and flexed (Fig. 13.1). In this position, muscle contractions can force the humeral head posteriorly, leading to a posterior dislocation or fracture. In focal to bilateral tonic-clonic seizures, the "fencing position" (arm abducted and externally rotated) may cause an anteroinferior pull, potentially resulting in an anterior dislocation [8–10]. However, both anterior and posterior shoulder dislocations have been reported, challenging the idea of a single pathological mechanism [7]. Muscular imbalance during seizures may also cause plastic deformations, especially in developing children. PWE with frequent tonic-clonic seizures can exhibit slightly increased glenoid retroversion compared to those with rare seizures, which may result from repeated posteriorly directed muscular contractions. This could be the effect of a plastic deformation of the glenoid during growth, but its clinical impact on posterior instability remains to be clarified [11]. A further hypothesis for shoulder injuries in PWE involves differing activation timing and frequency of periscapular and shoulder muscles. This is being tested with electromyography, but no conclusive results on muscle roles in dislocations are available yet [12–15].

Table 13.1 General risk factors for sustaining fractures in patients with epilepsy and seizures

First tonic-clonic seizure
Seizure frequency
Type of seizure (tonic-clonic >> atonic, tonic, myoclonic)
Generalized onset
Inappropriate patient positioning during seizure
Psychiatric comorbidities
Less independent living situation
Number & type of ASMs
Response to therapy
Patients' compliance with ASMs

13.2.2 Musculoskeletal Injuries in Patients with Epilepsy and Seizures

Compared to the general population, PWE face a higher risk of accidental injuries and fractures, significantly impacting their quality of life [16–20]. Incidence rates of injuries range up to 45% over a 12-month or lifetime period, with studies based on outpatient settings reporting higher rates than those focusing on emergency care or hospital admissions [6, 16, 21–26]. A recent systematic review highlighted bilateral posterior shoulder fracture-dislocations as the most common injury from tonic-clonic seizures, though the quality of evidence was low due to the predominance of case reports [1]. Risk factors for seizure-related injuries include seizure frequency, type, generalized onset, number of anti-seizure medications (ASMs), living situation, and psychiatric comorbidities [24]. While specific studies on dislocation risk are lacking, fracture risk is well-studied, showing higher rates in the first 2 years post-diagnosis, possibly decreasing as patients develop injury prevention strategies and seizure frequency declines over time [5, 19, 27–29]. Therapy response and ASM compliance also influence injury risk, with poorly controlled epilepsy associated with higher risk [30–32]. Table 13.1 summarizes key risk factors for fractures in PWE [5, 6, 19, 20, 22, 33–41].

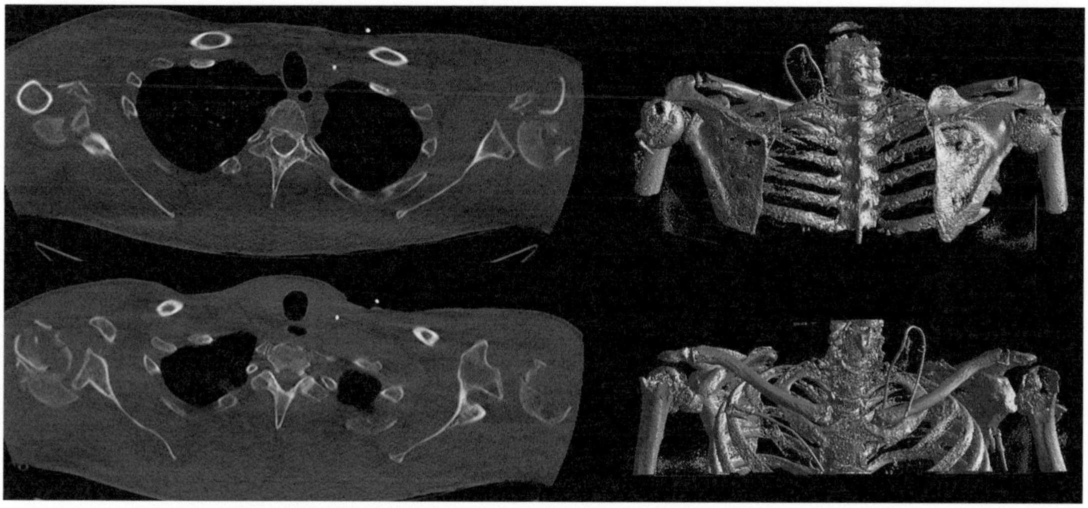

Fig. 13.2 Axial and 3D CT scan reconstructions of a 39-year-old male patient with bilateral posterior fracture dislocations sustained during the first episode of a tonic-clonic seizure

13.2.3 Epidemiology and Risk Factors of Shoulder Instability in PWE

Literature on shoulder dislocations in PWE is scarce, with few studies dedicated to their epidemiology and risk factors. While large cohorts and cross-sectional studies often categorize shoulder injuries broadly, smaller orthopaedic-focused studies provide detailed but limited data, often lacking neurological history [19, 40, 42–45]. Shoulder injuries predominantly affect young (20–40 years old) males, with varying mean ages reported across studies [7, 42–44, 46, 47]. Direction of instability varies in reports, with posterior dislocations often linked to seizures and surpassing general population incidence, while anterior instability remains predominant [7, 42–44, 46, 48, 49]. Bilateral shoulder injuries, typically rare and mostly seen in case reports, are more common in PWE, especially younger ones. They can occur simultaneously or as a consequence of separate seizure episodes and have anterior as well as posterior direction (Fig. 13.2) [7, 43, 46, 48–52].

Few specific shoulder-injury risk factors are known for PWE: epilepsy has been confirmed as an independent risk factor for associated fractures in patients with shoulder dislocations [53] and compliance with ASMs appears crucial, with over 10% of PWE experiencing seizure-related shoulder injuries after ASM discontinuation [7]. Therefore, caution is warranted when considering ASMs discontinuation, especially in older (>35 years) male PWE who experience particularly negative results after shoulder-related injuries. Older age, male sex, and ASM discontinuation are characteristic features of patients with posterior dislocation episodes [2].

13.3 Approach and Treatment: The Neurologist's Point of View

13.3.1 General Considerations

Seizure and epilepsy types are classified by the International League Against Epilepsy (ILAE) 2017 definition. Seizures are categorized into focal onset, generalized onset, or unknown onset, while epilepsy types include focal, generalized, or unknown epilepsy [54–56]. Tonic-clonic seizures fall under focal or generalized onset, depending on diagnostic findings and semiology.

Shoulder injuries can occur in patients with a first seizure or chronic epilepsy, mostly from tonic-clonic seizures. Specific shoulder injuries (proximal humerus fracture-dislocations, posterior instability and bilateral shoulder lesions as well as shoulder lesions with unknown onset or after loss of consciousness of unknown aetiology) suggest tonic-clonic seizures, aiding diagnosis when seizures are unobserved [1, 7]. Neurological assessment is crucial in managing shoulder injuries in PWE in four specific situations: emergency care, diagnostic workup, preoperative evaluation, and postoperative management.

13.3.2 Emergency Management of Patients with Tonic-Clonic Seizures

Recognizing shoulder injuries in the emergency department after a tonic-clonic seizure can be challenging due to neurological treatment prioritization (e.g., in acute-symptomatic seizures due to stroke, cerebral venous sinus thrombosis, or alcohol withdrawal) and post-seizure symptoms. Muscle pain, soreness, and haematomas are common, leading to initially missed injuries [57]. After a postictal observation, patients may be discharged for outpatient follow-up or admitted, with diagnostic and therapeutic approaches varying based on whether it is their first seizure or they have a diagnosis of epilepsy [54–56].

13.3.3 Diagnostic Workup After Seizures: Patients with a First Seizure

In patients who injure their shoulder during a first seizure, assessing relapse risk is crucial for identifying those who may benefit from ASM. Risk depends on anamnestic and diagnostic findings; for provoked seizures (e.g., alcohol withdrawal, hypoglycemia, stroke), medication is usually not necessary, as relapse risk is low [58, 59]. Unprovoked seizures carry a 40–50% risk of recurrence within 2 years, increasing to more than 60% within 10 years if EEG or MRI reveal epileptiform discharges or lesions [60–62]. ASM may also be considered in specific situations, such as perioperatively, to mitigate seizure-related risks, even if supporting data is missing in most situations and only the administration of benzodiazepines after a seizure due to alcohol withdrawal is sufficiently well confirmed [63]. Moreover, efforts should be made to minimize potential provoking factors for seizures in this delicate phase, whenever feasible.

13.3.4 Diagnostic Workup After Seizures: PWE

PWE reporting seizure-related shoulder injuries require thorough treatment evaluation. This includes assessing potential triggers (e.g., sleep deprivation), ASM selection, and ASM adherence. Approximately 30–40% of epilepsy cases are pharmacoresistant, but therapy optimization can reduce tonic-clonic seizure frequency. Avoidance of ASMs that are associated with an increased risk of osteoporosis should be considered in patients who sustained a fracture or are at risk of sustaining fractures. New medications offer hope of achieving seizure freedom in pharmacoresistant patients, and epilepsy surgery or vagus nerve stimulation may be considered in complex cases, warranting referral to an epilepsy centre [64–68].

13.3.5 Preoperative Evaluation of Patients Undergoing Shoulder Surgery

In acute settings or when strict immobilization is needed, adjusting ASM may be necessary, with transient benzodiazepine use considered appropriate. For elective surgeries, preoperative neurological consultation is vital to assess and minimize postoperative seizure risks [69, 70]. Predicting seizure remission in drug-resistant epilepsy is challenging, with developmental delay, structural epilepsy, and ASM failures identified as negative predictors [71, 72]. The risk of seizure relapse decreases with the time passed since the last seizure, although risk factors for a relapse after achieving seizure freedom are unknown [73, 74]. Therefore, a 6-month seizure-free interval is usually recommended before elective surgery, which may be shortened to three for very debilitating clinical situations [8]. Perioperative ASM administration is crucial for PWE to prevent increased seizure incidence, with consideration given to potential drug interactions and proconvulsive effects of anaesthetics [69]. When using analgesics, it should be considered that tramadol is suspected of being able to trigger seizures, recommending use of alternative analgesics if available [75–80]. Collaboration between orthopaedic surgeons and neurologists is essential for optimal surgical planning and also to avoid inappropriate conservative treatment due to fear of perioperative seizures, which can lead to poor outcomes. In patients who suffer from uncontrolled seizures, the indication for surgery should first be critically evaluated against the risk of failure due to recurrent seizure and specific surgical technical considerations should be made for these patients [2].

13.3.6 Postoperative Management of Operated Patients

Postoperative management of patients with epilepsy who have undergone surgery is a critical aspect of ensuring a successful recovery and minimizing potential complications. Proper ASM administration is vital, with adjustments as needed based on patient response and interactions with other medications. Follow-up with neurologists is essential to assess ASM efficacy and perform comprehensive epilepsy diagnostics if not done pre-surgery.

13.4 Approach and Treatment: The Surgeon's Point of View

13.4.1 History, Clinical Assessment, and Radiological Investigations

Alongside the neurological evaluation outlined in the previous section, prompt orthopaedic and radiological examination is crucial following a seizure-related shoulder injury to avoid delayed diagnosis and treatment. Diagnosing shoulder injuries in postictal patients or those under sedation can be challenging, leading to missed diagnoses, especially of posterior dislocations [81–83]. A comprehensive medical history, including details on the accident, seizure frequency, and physical activity, is important. Physical examination should assess range of movement, neurovascular status, strength, and shoulder function including laxity assessment and appropriate provocative tests. Radiological exams are essential, starting with basic radiography (true-AP, scapular-Y, axillary, or Velpeau views) and potentially advancing to CT scans if needed. Especially in the emergency setting, where the support of a dedicated musculoskeletal radiologist may lack, it is worth reminding that posterior dislocations may be overseen if only ap-view radiographs are performed (Fig. 13.3).

Radiological assessment for seizure-related shoulder injuries follows similar principles as in non-epileptic patients but with a focus on glenohumeral bone defects, more common in PWE [43, 84]. CT scans with multiplanar and 3D reconstructions provide precise detection and measurement of these defects [85–88]. Among the numerous methods proposed to quantify glenoid bone defects, the PICO method has established itself as a reliable and reproducible technique [85–88]. PWE are prone to Hill-Sachs and reverse Hill-Sachs lesions (RHSL or McLaughlin fractures), possibly following atypical patterns or associated with concomitant prox-

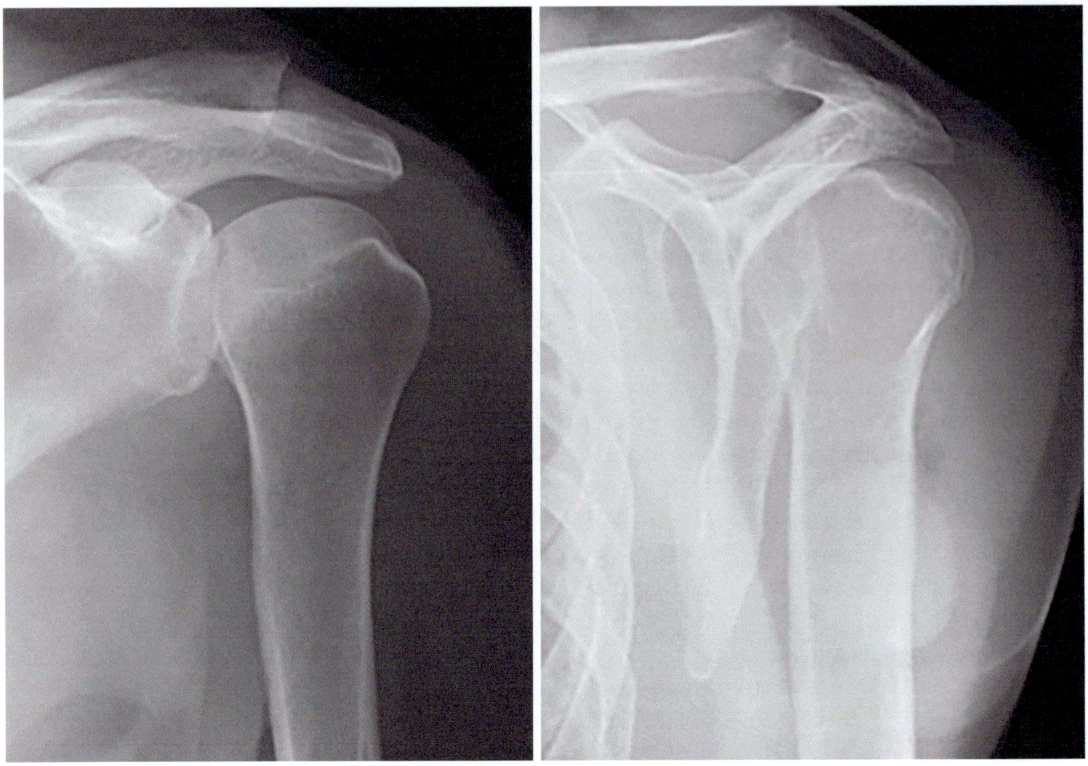

Fig. 13.3 AP view and scapular-Y view of a posterior shoulder dislocation. Various radiological signs may indicate a posterior dislocation, but they are not always present. The "light-bulb" sign, showing the loss of the greater tuberosity contour due to fixed internal rotation, is pathognomonic. The "trough line" sign results from impaction of the humeral head. The "rim sign" indicates an enlarged glenohumeral space, while the "vacant glenoid sign" may also suggest a posterior dislocation

imal humerus fractures [2]. Over the past 25 years, treatment concepts based on bone loss quantification have advanced. For anteroinferior dislocations, the critical bone loss benchmark at the glenoid has been reduced and bipolar bone loss evaluation through 3D evaluation has gained importance [89–99]. For RHSL, the γ-angle is a reliable measurement method, adapted to consider bipolar loss by adding 2°/mm of glenoid defect and with a suggested cutoff set at 90°, with higher thresholds acceptable in older patients with limited range of motion [100–103]. Ultrasound and MRI are less relevant for bone defects but useful for rotator cuff and capsule-ligament complex injuries.

13.4.2 General Considerations and Conservative Treatment

Seizure-related shoulder injuries in PWE pose significant treatment challenges and no standardized guidelines exist, so treatments typically follow protocols for non-epileptic patients [7, 42, 43]. Treatment decisions must consider patient-specific factors like age, functional expectations, individual anatomy, epilepsy severity, compliance, and possible psychiatric comorbidities. PWE have higher rates of perioperative complications both of surgical and of medical nature (in hospital adverse events such as mechanical ventilation and deep vein thrombosis) and of injury recurrence due to persistent seizures and larger bone defects leading to higher recurrence rate [43, 84, 104, 105]. Proper management of these patients with such unfavourable profile requires orthopaedic and neurologic expertise; in case of lack of sufficient experience or of essential structural requirements, transfer to an appropriate facility should be considered [43].

Time is critical in treating seizure-related shoulder injuries, both in terms of time between injury and diagnosis and of time between last seizure and treatment start. Delays or missed diagnoses can severely impair treatment success, which occurs frequently in epilepsy patients [81, 83]. A study showed an average of 66 days elapsed between injury and diagnosis for posterior shoulder fracture dislocations, with 55% initially overlooked [83]. During this time, the joint incongruity and the locked position can lead to rapid bone loss, which is associated with a significantly poorer prognosis [42, 96]. Prompt diagnosis and effective seizure control improve surgical outcomes, but in cases with a prolonged missed interval and concomitant risk factors such as advanced age or poorly controlled epilepsy, surgical neglect and conservative treatment may be the most appropriate options [81, 105].

Considering all seizure-related shoulder injuries, only a minority is treated conservatively; although conservative therapy is a respectable treatment option if performed with correct indications and frequent follow-up appointments, inappropriate conservative treatment guided either by lack of expertise in treating shoulder pathology or by fear of complications due to the underlying neurological disease will lead to extremely unsatisfying clinical results [2]. Conservative treatment of instability episodes in PWE does not differ from that in non-epileptic subjects, including reduction, initial movement restriction, analgesia, physiotherapeutic exercises, and patient education [106]. A detailed description of reduction techniques is beyond the scopes of this chapter; it shall only briefly be reminded on the importance of adequate pain control and muscular relaxation during reduction and on the importance to avoid forced external rotation in the case of locked dislocations, as this is associated with an increased risk of fracture.

13.4.3 Operative Treatment

Treatment approaches for instability can be divided into soft tissue and bony stabilization, which can be further subdivided into anatomical and nonanatomical techniques. Thangarajah et al. observed that bony stabilization resulted in significantly fewer recurrent dislocations compared to soft tissue stabilization methods (28% vs. 71%), yet to date, there are no reliable studies comparing the results and long-term data [42].

13.4.3.1 Soft Tissue Stabilization Procedures

Arthroscopic Bankart repair is a well-established soft tissue stabilization technique for traumatic anterior dislocations, showing a recurrence rate of about 15% in the general population [96, 107–109]. However, Thangarajah et al. reported a 92% failure rate in PWE after primary Bankart repair [42]. Other soft tissue stabilization techniques, such as capsular shift, Bankart repair augmentation, and remplissage, are also used, but research on their effectiveness in PWE is limited. Agha et al. suggested that the remplissage is more frequently used in PWE and Guity et al. reported good midterm results and a 17.2% recurrence rate for PWE with glenoid defects <20% using Bankart repair combined with remplissage, though recurrence rose to 71.4% in patients with persistent seizures [84, 110]. Soft tissue stabilization is therefore advised only for patients with well-controlled epilepsy (Fig. 13.4) [110]. The reversed remplissage technique is used for RHSLs [111, 112], with promising results in isolated epileptic cases [113].

13.4.3.2 Bony Procedures

Given the limitations of soft tissue procedures for glenohumeral stabilization, bony stabilization should be strongly considered for PWE, especially if seizure control cannot be guaranteed [9, 114]. The MOON Shoulder Group reported that PWE with shoulder stabilization often had more previous dislocations and extensive preoperative bone loss, associated with a higher likelihood of requiring open stabilization procedures [84].

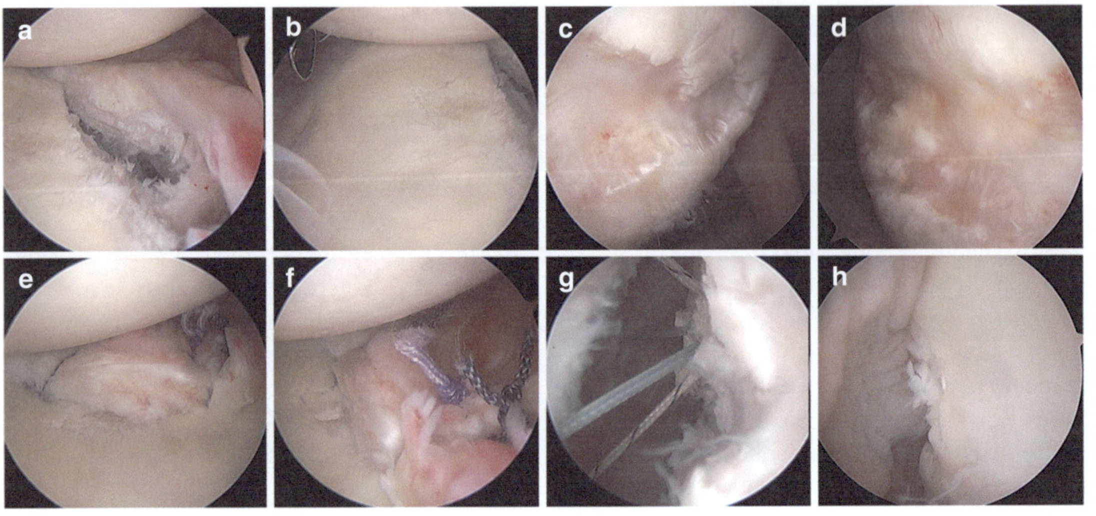

Fig. 13.4 Arthroscopic images of surgical intervention for anteroinferior instability with a bipolar component: capsulolabral detachment and chondral lesions are evident on the glenoid side (**a, b**), while a Hill-Sachs lesion is visible on the humeral side (**c, d**). Following capsulolabral repair (**e, f**), the remplissage technique is employed to convert the intra-articular Hill-Sachs lesion into an extra-articular one (**g, h**)

Glenoid Procedures

The literature on the Latarjet procedure in epilepsy patients shows varied recurrence rates (9–80%) [105, 115–117]. Raiss et al. observed a 43% re-dislocation rate and a mean postoperative Rowe-score of 76, which they concluded as unacceptable for patients at risk of seizures [115]. Similary, Thon et al. reported an 80% recurrence rate in patients with postoperative seizures, which increased the risk of recurrent instability by almost 40 times and Makaram et al. identified epilepsy as a risk factor for poorer outcomes [116, 118]. These conclude therefore that the Latarjet procedure should only be used in well-controlled patients with minimal risk of a recurrent seizure (Fig. 13.5). In contrast, Erşen et al. found a lower recurrence rate of 9%, but with a small sample size and low postoperative seizure rate (33% vs. 76% in Raiss et al.) and Dzidzishvili et al. documented comparable results for epileptic and non-epileptic patients after arthroscopic Latarjet procedures [105, 117].

Postoperative seizures are the main predictors of re-dislocation after the Latarjet procedure, significantly impacting its success, as demonstrated by Khater et al. in 73 patients treated for tramadol-induced seizures, who reported a low seizure relapse rate (9%) post-tramadol discontinuation, contrasting with results in PWE [119]. The role of seizure control is also highlighted in a 2022 consensus, which indicated the Latarjet procedure as a relative contraindication in patients with uncontrolled and poorly managed epilepsy [120]. The procedure's failure is attributed to the extreme stress exerted on the conjoint tendon during seizures compounded by the limited size of the bone block; therefore, free bone blocks (autograft or allograft) and osteochondral transplants (distal tibia allograft, DTA) offer valid alternatives for severe bone loss cases.

The Eden-Hybinette procedure was initially criticized due to the high revision rates (71% in the cohort studied by Bühler and Gerber [43]), yet a more recent low-level evidence exist also reporting satisfying results [121]; an anterior bone buttress with tricortical iliac crest or an allogenic femoral head proved to be successful in 14 PWE despite persistent seizures in 62% of cases [122]. In all these studies, the follow-up period is too short to assess secondary risks such as glenohumeral osteoarthritis. DTA has recently proved to be a good choice for the anatomical recon-

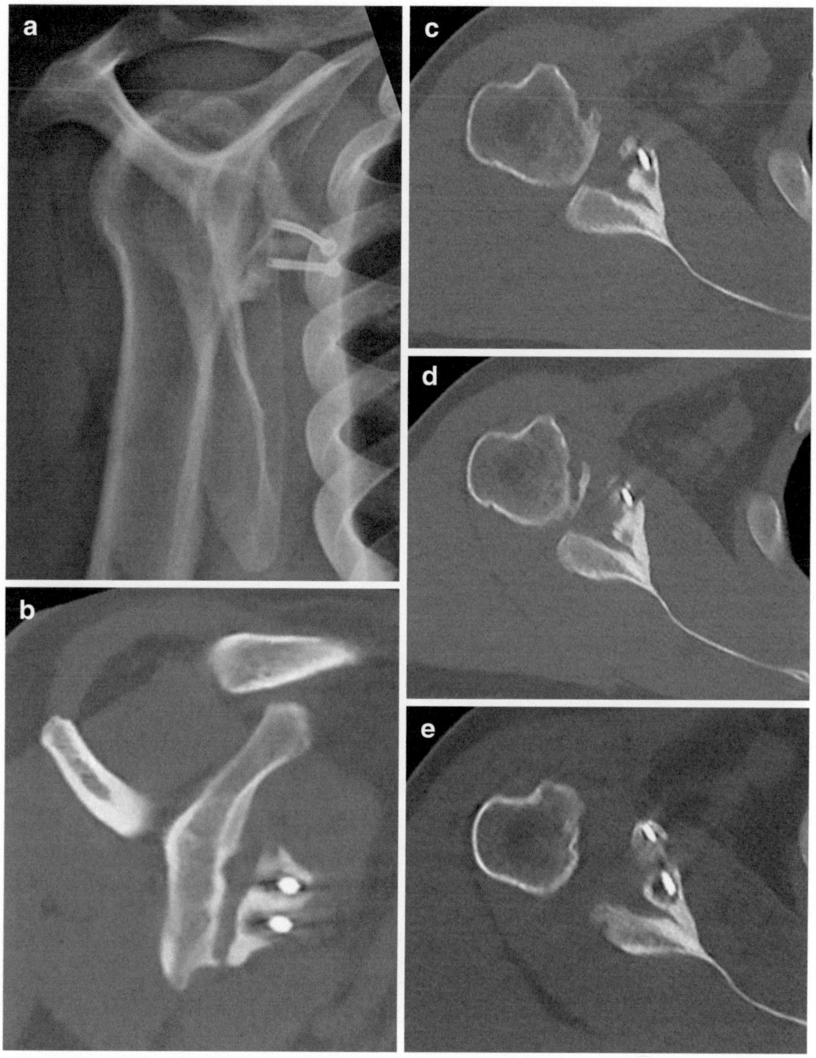

Fig. 13.5 Catastrophic failure of a Latarjet procedure in a 28-year-old patient suffering from tonic-clonic seizures since the age of 25, without ever achieving seizure freedom. Scapular-Y view radiograph (**a**) and sagittal and axial CT scans (**b**–**e**) obtained 4 years after the procedure show the coracoid graft dislocated, screw bent, lack of bony fusion, persistent instability, and humeral arthritis

struction of glenoid defects due to its shape and configuration, but there are no real data for PWE yet [123, 124].

Glenoid bone block surgery for posterior stabilization essentially follows the same principles as anterior procedures, with allograft or bone blocks restoring stability in a reproducible way [43]. Neuromuscular paralysis with botulinum toxin was experimentally used to protect grafts during the early postoperative phase [125]. Glenoid osteotomies can address abnormal glenoid version in shoulder instability, possibly combined with a bone block (Fig. 13.6), though dedicated reports on their outcomes in PWE are lacking [126, 127].

Humeral Procedures

Humeral defects may occur in the posterosuperior or anterior part of the humeral head, based on dislocation direction. Treatment of humeral defects (HSL and RHSL) depends on defect size and pathologies, with techniques like remplissage, reversed remplissage, subscapularis tendon transposition, and transfer of the lesser tuberosity (McLaughlin procedure and its modifications) being successful options for limited defects (Fig. 13.7) [128]. A "humeroplasty", using balloon osteoplasty and bone grafts, substitutes, or cement, is a further possibility for acute HSL and RHSL [129, 130]. Roach et al. described humeral head allografts with screws for HSL in patients

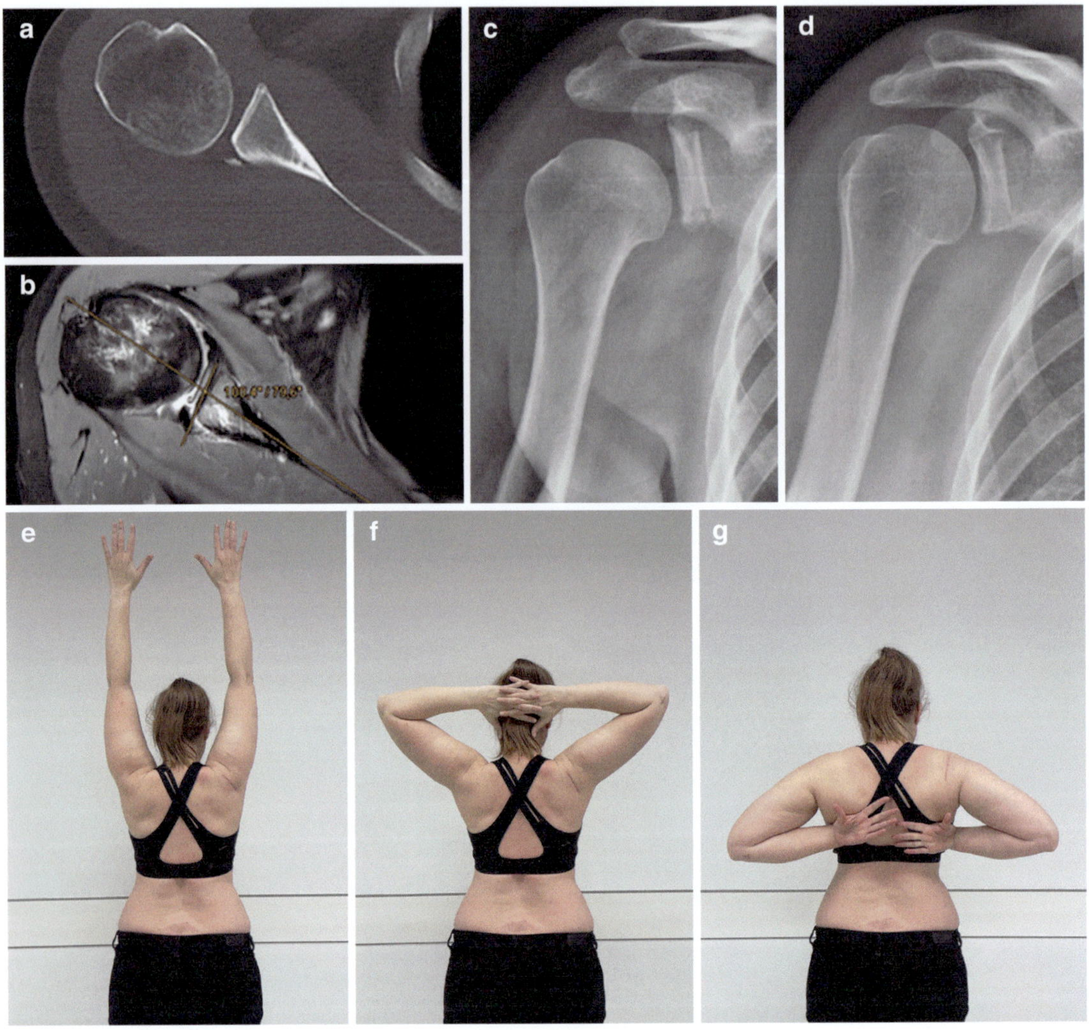

Fig. 13.6 Axial CT and MRI reconstructions of a 37-year-old female patient suffering from generalized tonic-clonic seizures since the age of 6 and experiencing seizure-related recurrent posterior shoulder dislocations. At presentation, the posterior glenoid was rounded and the reverse bony Bankart lesion almost completely resorbed (**a, b**). The patient had increased glenoid retroversion and posterior subluxation of the humeral head and was treated with a posterior J-graft from the iliac crest (**c**). Three months postoperative (**d–g**): osteotomy healing, almost full range of motion, no instability, and complete return to work as a fitness studio trainer

with uncontrolled seizure disorders; the glenoid was treated with capsulolabral repair and only one re-dislocation occurred over 4.8 years, despite recurrent seizures postoperatively in all patients [131]. RHSL in posterior dislocation, locked posterior dislocation, and chronic locked posterior dislocation do not differ in terms of localization but show significant differences in size [103]. Accordingly, locked posterior shoulder dislocation may require a treatment strategy focused on fracture management rather than conventional dislocation protocols [132]. For patients with large RHSL (30–50%) following locked posterior dislocations, Gerber et al. reported excellent long-term results using segmental reconstruction, primarily with fresh-frozen femoral or humeral heads (Fig. 13.8) [130]. Posterior fracture dislocations can achieve good postoperative outcomes by open reduction, allo–/autograft augmentation, and screw fixation for the RHSL

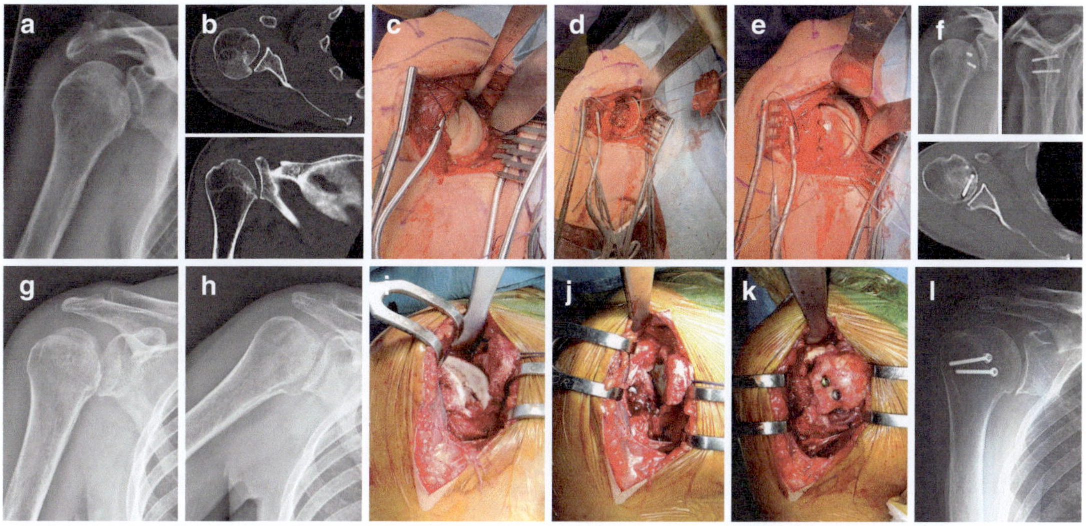

Fig. 13.7 Treatment of acute and chronic RHSL: In the acute setting (**a, b**), the still vital impacted articular fragment of the humeral head (**c**) can be elevated, reduced, grafted, and fixed with cannulated headless compression screws and additional sutures for subscapularis refixation allowing for joint surface restoration (**d–f**). In chronic cases (**g, h**), a modified McLaughlin procedure can be performed with debridement of the avital bone and cartilage (**i, j**) and advancement of the lesser tuberosity, which is then fixed with cannulated screws and washers (**k, l**)

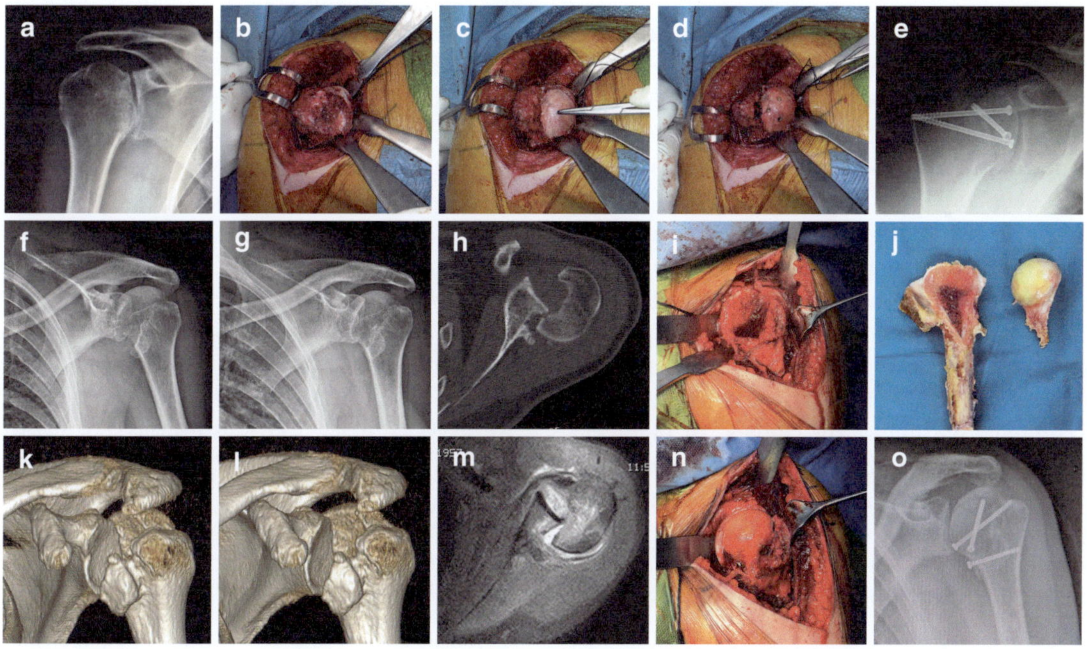

Fig. 13.8 Two cases of chronic locked posterior dislocations treated with allografts. Case 1: Preoperative radiographs (**a**) of a 31-year-old male anticipate the irreparably damaged anterior part of the humeral head (**b**). Grafting was performed with a femoral head segment and fixed with three cannulated screws (**c–e**). Case 2: Plain radiographs, axial and 3D CT reconstructions, and MRI scan (**f–h, k–m**) of a 60-year-old male with neglected posterior dislocation after an initial reduction of a posterior dislocation. A humeral head allograft was cut to fill and reconstruct the joint surface defect (**i, j**) and fixed with cannulated screws (**n, o**)

graft ([133], 42% seizure related, yet no subgroup analyses on seizure patients) and possibly considering double plating for complex and unstable proximal humeral fractures [134]. Augmentation may also be performed to increase construct stability, possibly reducing secondary dislocation [135]. Anatomical reconstruction is preferred in young patients, with fracture prostheses being alternatives associated burdened by poorer functionality and higher revision rates [134].

Seizure-induced bilateral injuries (dislocations, fractures, or fracture-dislocations) demand careful consideration [7, 136]. Current literature mostly includes case reports, highlighting the high complication rates due to persistent seizures [52, 137–141]. Treatment varies widely, from one-stage to two-stage procedures, sometimes combining arthroplasty and osteochondral autograft from the most to the least damaged side [139, 141].

13.4.3.3 Arthroplasty and Arthrodesis

For large, non-reconstructable bone defects or failed stabilizations with progressive osteoarthritis, arthroplasty or arthrodesis may be considered. Arthroplasty is effective for glenohumeral osteoarthritis and fracture sequelae but shows higher loosening and revision rates in younger patients [142, 143]. Given the often very young patient population with high functional demands and the persisting seizure activity, the application of these techniques is controversially discussed, and there are no representative long-term studies. In eight epileptic patients, Thangarajah et al. reported no further instability after anatomic arthroplasty despite continued seizures; however, 40% of hemiarthroplasties required revision due to glenoid erosion within 4.7 years follow-up, suggesting very restrictive indications [144]. Arthrodesis, a last resort for recurrent instability and failed surgeries with significant functional limitations, achieved bony fusion without postoperative instability in six patients, though one required revision for material loosening [145].

13.5 Conclusions

PWE face distinct challenges in managing shoulder injuries due to the unique dynamics and pathomechanics involved. Muscular contractions during seizures can lead to various shoulder injuries, complicating treatment. Conservative treatments are similar to those for non-epileptic patients but require careful consideration of seizure frequency and control, whereby inappropriate indications due to a lack of expertise can lead to unsatisfying results. For elective operations, a 6-month seizure-free interval is recommended before surgery, which may be shortened to three for very debilitating clinical situations. Surgical interventions, including soft tissue and bony stabilization, have varied success rates, with higher recurrence in uncontrolled epilepsy. Given the limitations of soft tissue procedures in PWE, humeral and/or glenoid bony stabilization should be strongly considered, especially if seizure control cannot be guaranteed. Arthroplasty and arthrodesis are options for severe cases but come with significant limitations and higher revision rates. The need for multidisciplinary collaboration between neurologists and orthopaedic surgeons is essential for optimizing outcomes, emphasizing the importance of tailored treatment strategies for this population.

References

1. Grzonka P, Rybitschka A, De Marchis GM, Marsch S, Sutter R. Bone fractures from generalized convulsive seizures and status epilepticus—a systematic review. Epilepsia. 2019;60:996.
2. Cucchi D, Walter SG, Baumgartner T, Menon A, Egger L, Randelli PS, Surges R, Wirtz DC, Friedrich MJ. Poor midterm clinical outcomes and a high percentage of unsatisfying results are reported after seizure-related shoulder injuries, especially after posterior proximal humerus fracture-dislocations. J Shoulder Elb Surg. 2023;33:1340. https://doi.org/10.1016/j.jse.2023.09.023.
3. Kristiansen B, Christensen S. Fractures of the proximal end of the humerus caused by convulsive seizures. Injury. 1984;16:108–9.

4. Aboukasm AG. Nocturnal vertebral compression fracture. A presenting feature of unrecognized epileptic seizures. Arch Fam Med. 1997;6:185–7.
5. Vestergaard P, Tigaran S, Rejnmark L, Tigaran C, Dam M, Mosekilde L. Fracture risk is increased in epilepsy. Acta Neurol Scand. 1999;99:269–75.
6. Tan M, D'Souza W. Seizure-related injuries, drowning and vehicular crashes—a critical review of the literature. Curr Neurol Neurosci Rep. 2013;13:361.
7. Cucchi D, Baumgartner T, Walter SG, Menon A, Ossendorff R, Surges R, Burger C, Wirtz DC, Friedrich MJ. Epidemiology and specific features of shoulder injuries in patients affected by epileptic seizures. Arch Orthop Trauma Surg. 2023;143:1999–2009.
8. Atwan Y, Wang A, Labrum JT, Sanchez-Sotelo J, Barlow JD, Dines JS, Camp CL. Management of shoulder instability in patients with seizure disorders. Curr Rev Musculoskelet Med. 2023;16:201–10.
9. Goudie EB, Murray IR, Robinson CM. Instability of the shoulder following seizures. J Bone Joint Surg Br. 2012;94-B:721–8.
10. DeToledo JC, Lowe MR, Ramsay REE. Restraining patients and shoulder dislocations during seizures. J Shoulder Elb Surg. 1999;8:300–2.
11. Cucchi D, et al. Kann die Belastung durch wiederholte tonisch-klonische Anfälle die Glenoidversion bei Epilepsiepatienten beeinflussen? German Medical Science GMS Publishing House; 2023.
12. Beniczky S, Conradsen I, Henning O, Fabricius M, Wolf P. Automated real-time detection of tonic-clonic seizures using a wearable EMG device. Neurology. 2018;90:e428. https://doi.org/10.1212/WNL.0000000000004893.
13. Conradsen I, Wolf P, Sams T, Sorensen HBD, Beniczky S. Patterns of muscle activation during generalized tonic and tonic-clonic epileptic seizures. Epilepsia. 2011;52:2125–32.
14. Conradsen I, Moldovan M, Jennum P, Wolf P, Farina D, Beniczky S. Dynamics of muscle activation during tonic–clonic seizures. Epilepsy Res. 2013;104:84–93.
15. Baumgartner C, Whitmire LE, Voyles SR, Cardenas DP. Using sEMG to identify seizure semiology of motor seizures. Seizure. 2021;86:52–9.
16. Beghi E, Cornaggia C, RESt-1 Group. Morbidity and accidents in patients with epilepsy: results of a European cohort study. Epilepsia. 2002;43:1076–83.
17. Téllez-Zenteno JF, Hunter G, Wiebe S. Injuries in people with self-reported epilepsy: a population-based study. Epilepsia. 2008;49:954–61.
18. Kwon C-S, Liu M, Quan H, Wiebe S, McChesney J, Wirrell E, Hamiwka L, Jetté N. The incidence of injuries in persons with and without epilepsy—a population-based study. Epilepsia. 2010;51:2247–53.
19. Persson HBI, Alberts KA, Farahmand BY, Tomson T. Risk of extremity fractures in adult outpatients with epilepsy. Epilepsia. 2002;43:768–72.
20. Friedman DE, Chiang S, Tobias RS. Do recurrent seizure-related head injuries affect seizures in people with epilepsy? Epilepsy Behav. 2012;23:159–61.
21. Mahler B, Carlsson S, Andersson T, Tomson T. Risk for injuries and accidents in epilepsy. Neurology. 2018;90:e779–89.
22. Tomson T, Beghi E, Sundqvist A, Johannessen SI. Medical risks in epilepsy: a review with focus on physical injuries, mortality, traffic accidents and their prevention. Epilepsy Res. 2004;60:1–16.
23. Buffo TH, Guerreiro MM, Tai P, Montenegro MA. Seizure related accidents and injuries in childhood. Arq Neuropsiquiatr. 2008;66:458–61.
24. Salas-Puig X, Iniesta M, Abraira L, Puig J. Accidental injuries in patients with generalized tonic–clonic seizures. A multicenter, observational, cross-sectional study (QUIN-GTC study). Epilepsy Behav. 2019;92:135–9.
25. Neufeld M, Vishne T, Chistik V, Korczyn A. Life-long history of injuries related to seizures. Epilepsy Res. 1999;34:123–7.
26. Finelli PF, Cardi JK. Seizure as a cause of fracture. Neurology. 1989;39:858.
27. Annegers JF, Melton LJ, Sun CA, Hauser WA. Risk of age-related fractures in patients with unprovoked seizures. Epilepsia. 1989;30:348–55.
28. Tellez-Zenteno J, Nguyen R. Injuries in epilepsy: a review of its prevalence, risk factors, type of injuries and prevention. Neurol Int. 2009;1:20.
29. Cockerell OC, Johnson AL, Sander JW, Hart YM, Shorvon SD. Remission of epilepsy: results from the National General Practice Study of Epilepsy. Lancet. 1995;346:140–4.
30. Beghi E. Injuries in patients with epilepsy. Lancet Neurol. 2005;4:71–2.
31. Orozco-Hernandez JP, Quintero-Moreno JF, Duque-Salazar C, Gil-Restrepo A, William-Martinez J, Lizcano-Meneses A, Carmona-Villada H. Predictors of seizure related injuries in adult patients with epilepsy in Colombia: a case-control study. Rev Neurol. 2017;65:546–52.
32. Willems LM, Watermann N, Richter S, Kay L, Hermsen AM, Knake S, Rosenow F, Strzelczyk A. Incidence, risk factors and consequences of epilepsy-related injuries and accidents: a retrospective, single center study. Front Neurol. 2018;9:1–9.
33. Lawn ND, Bamlet WR, Radhakrishnan K, O'Brien PC, So EL. Injuries due to seizures in persons with epilepsy: a population-based study. Neurology. 2004;63:1565–70.
34. Vestergaard P. Epilepsy, osteoporosis and fracture risk—a meta-analysis. Acta Neurol Scand. 2005;112:277–86.
35. Souverein PC, Webb DJ, Petri H, Weil J, Van Staa TP, Egberts T. Incidence of fractures among epilepsy patients: a population-based retrospective cohort study in the general practice research database. Epilepsia. 2005;46:304–10.
36. Petty SJ, Hill KD, Haber NE, Paton LM, Lawrence KM, Berkovic SF, Seibel MJ, O'Brien TJ, Wark

JD. Balance impairment in chronic antiepileptic drug users: a twin and sibling study. Epilepsia. 2010;51:280–8.
37. Carbone LD, Johnson KC, Robbins J, Larson JC, Curb JD, Watson K, Gass M, LaCroix AZ. Antiepileptic drug use, falls, fractures and BMD in postmenopausal women: findings from the Women's Health Initiative (WHI). J Bone Miner Res. 2010;25:873–81.
38. Asadi-Pooya AA, Nikseresht A, Yaghoubi E, Nei M. Physical injuries in patients with epilepsy and their associated risk factors. Seizure. 2012;21:165–8.
39. Henning O, Nakken KO, Lossius MI. People with epilepsy and their relatives want more information about risks of injuries and premature death. Epilepsy Behav. 2018;82:6–10.
40. DeToledo JC, Lowe MR. Seizures, lateral decubitus, aspiration, and shoulder dislocation: time to change the guidelines? Neurology. 2001;56:290–1.
41. Langenbruch L, Rickert C, Gosheger G, Schorn D, Schliemann B, Brix T, Elger CE, Meuth SG, Kovac S. Seizure-induced shoulder dislocations—case series and review of the literature. Seizure. 2019;70:38–42.
42. Thangarajah T, Lambert S. The management of recurrent shoulder instability in patients with epilepsy: a 15-year experience. J Shoulder Elb Surg. 2015;24:1723–7.
43. Bühler M, Gerber C. Shoulder instability related to epileptic seizures. J Shoulder Elb Surg. 2002;11:339–44.
44. Robinson CM, Akhtar A, Mitchell M, Beavis C. Complex posterior fracture-dislocation of the shoulder. J Bone Joint Surg. 2007;89:1454–66.
45. Kelly MJ, Holton AE, Cassar-Gheiti AJ, Hanna SA, Quinlan JF, Molony DC. The aetiology of posterior glenohumeral dislocations and occurrence of associated injuries. Bone Joint J. 2019;101-B(1):15–21.
46. Huizing JW, Monteban PE. Bilateral posterior fracture dislocation of the shoulders: review of case reports and treatment. Acta Orthop Belg. 2020;86:193–9.
47. Cucchi D, Baumgartner T, Walter SG, Ossendorff R, Wimmer M, Menon A, Friedrich MJ. Epidemiology and characteristics of shoulder injuries in patients affected by epileptic seizures. J Shoulder Elb Surg. 2022;31:e158.
48. Shaw JL. Bilateral posterior fracture-dislocation of the shoulder and other trauma caused by convulsive seizures. J Bone Joint Surg Am. 1971;53:1437–40.
49. Pushpakumara J, Sivathiran S, Roshan L, Gunatilake S. Bilateral posterior fracture-dislocation of the shoulders following epileptic seizures: a case report and review of the literature. BMC Res Notes. 2015;8:704.
50. Rudy BS, Hennrikus WL. Bilateral anterior shoulder dislocation. JAAPA. 2017;30:25–7.
51. Kasha S, Bandari G. Bilateral posterior fracture-dislocation of shoulder following seizures secondary to cavernous sinus venous thrombosis—a rare association. J Orthop Case Rep. 2018;8:49–52.
52. Ploeger MM, Pennekamp PH, Müller MC, Kabir K, Burger C, Wirtz DC, Schmolders J. Bilateral dislocation fracture of the humeral head (right AO 11C3.3; left AO 11A1.3) without direct trauma due to first clinical manifestation of seizure—a case report and review of the literature. Z Orthop Unfall. 2015;153:643–7.
53. Delattre Sousa S, Houze-Cerfon CH, Le Gourrierec T, Charpentier S, Dubucs X, Balen F. Risk factors for the presence of important fractures in ED patients with shoulder dislocation: a retrospective cohort study. Emerg Med J. 2022;39:662–5.
54. Fisher RS, Acevedo C, Arzimanoglou A, et al. ILAE official report: a practical clinical definition of epilepsy. Epilepsia. 2014;55:475–82.
55. Fisher RS, Cross JH, French JA, et al. Operational classification of seizure types by the international league against epilepsy: position paper of the ILAE Commission for Classification and Terminology. Epilepsia. 2017;58:522–30.
56. Scheffer IE, Berkovic S, Capovilla G, et al. ILAE classification of the epilepsies: position paper of the ILAE commission for classification and terminology. Epilepsia. 2017;58:512–21.
57. Kokkalis ZT, Iliopoulos ID, Antoniou G, Antoniadou T, Mavrogenis AF, Panagiotopoulos E. Posterior shoulder fracture–dislocation: an update with treatment algorithm. Eur J Orthop Surg Traumatol. 2017;27:285–94.
58. De Herdt V, Dumont F, Hénon H, Derambure P, Vonck K, Leys D, Cordonnier C. Early seizures in intracerebral hemorrhage: incidence, associated factors, and outcome. Neurology. 2011;77:1794–800.
59. Leung T, Leung H, Soo YOY, Mok VCT, Wong KS. The prognosis of acute symptomatic seizures after ischaemic stroke. J Neurol Neurosurg Psychiatry. 2017;88:86–94.
60. Randomized clinical trial on the efficacy of antiepileptic drugs in reducing the risk of relapse after a first unprovoked tonic-clonic seizure. First Seizure Trial Group (FIR.S.T. Group). Neurology. 1993;43:478–83.
61. Marson A, Jacoby A, Johnson A, Kim L, Gamble C, Chadwick D. Medical Research Council MESS study group immediate versus deferred antiepileptic drug treatment for early epilepsy and single seizures: a randomised controlled trial. Lancet. 2005;365:2007–13.
62. Fisher RS, Scharfman HE, DeCurtis M. How can we identify ictal and interictal abnormal activity? Adv Exp Med Biol. 2014;813:3–23.
63. D'Onofrio G, Rathlev NK, Ulrich AS, Fish SS, Freedland ES. Lorazepam for the prevention of recurrent seizures related to alcohol. N Engl J Med. 1999;340:915–9.
64. Chen Z, Brodie MJ, Liew D, Kwan P. Treatment outcomes in patients with newly diagnosed epilepsy

treated with established and new antiepileptic drugs. JAMA Neurol. 2018;75:279.
65. Brodie MJ, Barry SJE, Bamagous GA, Norrie JD, Kwan P. Patterns of treatment response in newly diagnosed epilepsy. Neurology. 2012;78:1548–54.
66. Chung SS, French JA, Kowalski J, Krauss GL, Lee SK, Maciejowski M, Rosenfeld WE, Sperling MR, Mizne S, Kamin M. Randomized phase 2 study of adjunctive cenobamate in patients with uncontrolled focal seizures. Neurology. 2020;94:e2311. https://doi.org/10.1212/WNL.0000000000009530.
67. Sperling MR, Abou-Khalil B, Aboumatar S, et al. Efficacy of cenobamate for uncontrolled focal seizures: post hoc analysis of a phase 3, multicenter, open-label study. Epilepsia. 2021;62:3005–15.
68. Engel J. What can we do for people with drug-resistant epilepsy? Neurology. 2016;87:2483–9.
69. Perks A, Cheema S, Mohanraj R. Anaesthesia and epilepsy. Br J Anaesth. 2012;108:562–71.
70. Voss LJ, Sleigh JW, Barnard JPM, Kirsch HE. The howling cortex: seizures and general anesthetic drugs. Anesth Analg. 2008;107:1689–703.
71. Callaghan B, Schlesinger M, Rodemer W, Pollard J, Hesdorffer D, Allen Hauser W, French J. Remission and relapse in a drug-resistant epilepsy population followed prospectively. Epilepsia. 2011;52:619–26.
72. Callaghan BC, Anand K, Hesdorffer D, Hauser WA, French JA. Likelihood of seizure remission in an adult population with refractory epilepsy. Ann Neurol. 2007;62:382–9.
73. Sillanpää M, Saarinen M, Schmidt D. Long-term risks following first remission in childhood-onset epilepsy. A population-based study. Epilepsy Behav. 2012;25(2):145–9.
74. Choi H, Heiman G, Pandis D, Cantero J, Resor SR, Gilliam FG, Hauser WA. Seizure remission and relapse in adults with intractable epilepsy: a cohort study. Epilepsia. 2008;49:1440–5.
75. Sneyd JR. Propofol and epilepsy. Br J Anaesth. 1999;82:168–9.
76. Kofke WA. Anesthetic management of the patient with epilepsy or prior seizures. Curr Opin Anaesthesiol. 2010;23:391–9.
77. Morrow RL, Dormuth CR, Paterson M, Mamdani MM, Gomes T, Juurlink DN. Tramadol and the risk of seizure: nested case-control study of US patients with employer-sponsored health benefits. BMJ Open. 2019;9:e026705.
78. Beyaz S, Sonbahar T, Bayar F, Erdem A. Seizures associated with low-dose tramadol for chronic pain treatment. Anesth Essays Res. 2016;10:376.
79. Gardner JS, Blough D, Drinkard CR, Shatin D, Anderson G, Graham D, Alderfer R. Tramadol and seizures: a surveillance study in a managed care population. Pharmacotherapy. 2000;20:1423–31.
80. Gasse MC, Derby L, Vasilakis-Scaramozza C, Jick H. Incidence of first-time idiopathic seizures in users of tramadol. Pharmacotherapy. 2000;20:629–34.
81. Robinson CM, Aderinto J. Posterior shoulder dislocations and fracture-dislocations. J Bone Joint Surg Am. 2005;87:639–50.
82. Haritinian EG, Stoica IC, Popescu R, Gheorghievici GL, Nové-Josserand L. Treatment and outcomes of chronic locked posterior shoulder dislocations: a retrospective case series. BMC Musculoskelet Disord. 2023;24:82.
83. Magnussen AP, Watura C, Torr N, Walker M, Amiras D, Griffiths D. Missed posterior shoulder fracture dislocations: a new protocol from a London major trauma Centre. BMJ Open Qual. 2020;9:e000550.
84. Agha O, Rugg CM, Lansdown DA, Ortiz S, Hettrich CM, Wolf BR, Feeley BT. Surgical stabilization of shoulder instability in patients with or without a history of seizure: a comparative analysis. Arthroscopy. 2020;36:2664–73.e3.
85. Verweij LPE, Schuit AA, Kerkhoffs GMMJ, Blankevoort L, van den Bekerom MPJ, van Deurzen DFP. Accuracy of currently available methods in quantifying anterior glenoid bone loss: controversy regarding gold standard—a systematic review. Arthroscopy. 2020;36:2295–313.e1.
86. Chuang T-Y, Adams CR, Burkhart SS. Use of preoperative three-dimensional computed tomography to quantify glenoid bone loss in shoulder instability. Arthroscopy. 2008;24:376–82.
87. Baudi P, Righi P, Bolognesi D, Rivetta S, Rossi Urtoler E, Guicciardi N, Carrara M. How to identify and calculate glenoid bone deficit. Chir Organi Mov. 2005;90:145–52.
88. Bois AJ, Fening SD, Polster J, Jones MH, Miniaci A. Quantifying glenoid bone loss in anterior shoulder instability. Am J Sports Med. 2012;40:2569–77.
89. Yamamoto N, Shinagawa K, Hatta T, Itoi E. Peripheral-track and central-track Hill-Sachs lesions: a new concept of assessing an on-track lesion. Am J Sports Med. 2020;48:33–8.
90. Li RT, Kane G, Drummond M, Golan E, Wilson K, Lesniak BP, Rodosky M, Lin A. On-track lesions with a small distance to dislocation are associated with failure after arthroscopic anterior shoulder stabilization. J Bone Joint Surg. 2021;103:961–7.
91. Di Giacomo G, Itoi E, Burkhart SS. Evolving concept of bipolar bone loss and the hill-sachs lesion: from "engaging/non-engaging" lesion to "on-track/off-track" lesion. Arthroscopy. 2014;30:90–8.
92. Arciero RA, Parrino A, Bernhardson AS, Diaz-Doran V, Obopilwe E, Cote MP, Golijanin P, Mazzocca AD, Provencher MT. The effect of a combined glenoid and Hill-Sachs defect on glenohumeral stability. Am J Sports Med. 2015;43:1422–9.
93. Yamamoto N, Kawakami J, Hatta T, Itoi E. Effect of subcritical glenoid bone loss on activities of daily living in patients with anterior shoulder instability. Orthop Traumatol Surg Res. 2019;105:1467–70.
94. Shin S-J, Kim RG, Jeon YS, Kwon TH. Critical value of anterior glenoid bone loss that leads to

recurrent glenohumeral instability after arthroscopic Bankart repair. Am J Sports Med. 2017;45:1975–81.
95. Shaha JS, Cook JB, Song DJ, Rowles DJ, Bottoni CR, Shaha SH, Tokish JM. Redefining "critical" bone loss in shoulder instability. Am J Sports Med. 2015;43:1719–25.
96. Burkhart SS, De Beer JF. Traumatic glenohumeral bone defects and their relationship to failure of arthroscopic Bankart repairs. Arthroscopy. 2000;16:677–94.
97. Yamamoto N, Itoi E, Abe H, Minagawa H, Seki N, Shimada Y, Okada K. Contact between the glenoid and the humeral head in abduction, external rotation, and horizontal extension: a new concept of glenoid track. J Shoulder Elb Surg. 2007;16:649–56.
98. Moroder P, Damm P, Wierer G, Böhm E, Minkus M, Plachel F, Märdian S, Scheibel M, Khatamirad M. Challenging the current concept of critical glenoid bone loss in shoulder instability: does the size measurement really tell it all? Am J Sports Med. 2019;47:688–94.
99. Nakagawa S, Uchida R, Yokoi H, Sahara W, Mae T. Changes of bipolar bone defect size after arthroscopic Bankart repair for traumatic anterior shoulder instability: evaluation using a scoring system and influence on postoperative recurrence. Orthop J Sports Med. 2019;7(11):2325967119885345.
100. Festbaum C, Minkus M, Akgün D, et al. Conservative treatment of acute traumatic posterior shoulder dislocations (type a) is a viable option especially in patients with centred joint, low gamma angle, and middle or old age. Knee Surg Sports Traumatol Arthrosc. 2022;30:2500–9.
101. Moroder P, Plachel F, Tauber M, Habermeyer P, Imhoff A, Liem D, Lill H, Resch H, Gerhardt C, Scheibel M. Risk of engagement of bipolar bone defects in posterior shoulder instability. Am J Sports Med. 2017;45:2835–9.
102. Moroder P, Runer A, Kraemer M, et al. Influence of defect size and localization on the engagement of reverse Hill-Sachs lesions. Am J Sports Med. 2015;43:542–8.
103. Moroder P, Tauber M, Scheibel M, et al. Defect characteristics of reverse Hill-Sachs lesions. Am J Sports Med. 2016;44:708–14.
104. Churchill J, Menendez ME, Ponce BA. Early postoperative complications after shoulder arthroplasty in patients with epilepsy. Orthopedics. 2016;39:e1075. https://doi.org/10.3928/01477447-20160714-02.
105. Dzidzishvili L, Calvo C, Valencia M, Calvo E. Outcomes of arthroscopic Latarjet procedure for anterior glenohumeral instability in patients with epilepsy: a case-control study. Am J Sports Med. 2022;50:708–16.
106. Alkaduhimi H, van der Linde JA, Willigenburg NW, van Deurzen DFP, van den Bekerom MPJ. A systematic comparison of the closed shoulder reduction techniques. Arch Orthop Trauma Surg. 2017;137:589–99.
107. Randelli P, Ragone V, Carminati S, Cabitza P. Risk factors for recurrence after Bankart repair a systematic review. Knee Surg Sports Traumatol Arthrosc. 2012;20:2129–38.
108. Zhang M, Liu J, Jia Y, Zhang G, Zhou J, Wu D, Jiang J, Yun X. Risk factors for recurrence after Bankart repair: a systematic review and meta-analysis. J Orthop Surg Res. 2022;17:113.
109. Chen AZ, Greaves KM, DeMeireles AJ, Fortney TA, Saltzman BM, Trofa DP. Clinical outcomes of arthroscopic bony Bankart repair for anterior instability of the shoulder: a systematic review. Am J Sports Med. 2023;51:2758–65.
110. Guity MR, Sobhani Eraghi A. Mid-term results of arthroscopic Bankart repair and remplissage for recurrent anterior shoulder instability in patients with a history of seizures. BMC Musculoskelet Disord. 2022;23:12.
111. Krackhardt T, Schewe B, Albrecht D, Weise K. Arthroscopic fixation of the subscapularis tendon in the reverse Hill-Sachs lesion for traumatic unidirectional posterior dislocation of the shoulder. Arthroscopy. 2006;22:227.e1–6.
112. Lavender CD, Hanzlik SR, Pearson SE, Caldwell PE. Arthroscopic reverse Remplissage for posterior instability. Arthrosc Tech. 2016;5:e43–7.
113. Bitar AC, Medina G, Ribas L, Smid J, Adoni T. Arthroscopic reverse Remplissage in a bilateral seizure-related posterior shoulder dislocation: technique description and 3-year follow-up case report. Arch Bone Jt Surg. 2021;9:350–4.
114. Thangarajah T, Lambert SM. Management of recurrent shoulder instability in patients with epilepsy. J Shoulder Elb Surg. 2016;25:1376–84.
115. Raiss P, Lin A, Mizuno N, Melis B, Walch G. Results of the Latarjet procedure for recurrent anterior dislocation of the shoulder in patients with epilepsy. J Bone Joint Surg Br. 2012;94-B:1260–4.
116. Thon SG, Branche K, Houck DA, Didinger T, Vidal AF, Frank RM, Bravman JT. Effectiveness of Latarjet for anterior shoulder instability in patients with seizure disorder. JSES Int. 2021;5:171–4.
117. Erşen A, Bayram S, Birişik F, Atalar AC, Demirhan M. The effectiveness of the Latarjet procedure for shoulder instability in patients with epilepsy. Orthop Traumatol Surg Res. 2017;103:1277–82.
118. Makaram NS, Nicholson JA, Yapp LZ, Gillespie M, Shah CP, Robinson CM. Factors affecting a patient's experience following the open Latarjet procedure to treat recurrent anterior shoulder instability. Bone Joint J. 2023;105-B:389–99.
119. Khater AH, Sobhy MH, Said HG, Kandil A, Reda W, Seifeldin AF, Moustafa R, Elassal MA, Kamel EM. Latarjet procedure for anterior shoulder instability due to tramadol-induced seizures. Am J Sports Med. 2016;44:957–62.
120. Hurley ET, Matache BA, Wong I, et al. Anterior shoulder instability part II—Latarjet, remplissage, and glenoid bone-grafting—an international consensus statement. Arthroscopy. 2022;38:224–33.e6.

121. Mittal R, Jain S. Eden-Hybinette procedure for revision surgery in recurrent anterior shoulder instability in epilepsy. Indian J Orthop. 2021;55:728–33.
122. Hutchinson JW, Neumann L, Wallace WA. Bone buttress operation for recurrent anterior shoulder dislocation in epilepsy. J Bone Joint Surg Br. 1995;77:928–32.
123. Liles JL, Ganokroj P, Peebles AM, Mologne MS, Provencher CMT. Fresh distal tibial allograft: an updated graft preparation technique for anterior shoulder instability. Arthrosc Tech. 2022;11:e1027–31.
124. Grossi J, Danahy P, Rosenthal OD, Ackerman GP. Management of a failed distal tibial allograft procedure for anterior shoulder instability in a patient with epilepsy: a case report. Cureus. 2024;16:e51477. https://doi.org/10.7759/cureus.51477.
125. Edwards MD, Koontz EH, Revuelta GJ, Edwards JC, Slone HS, Woolf SK. Perioperative botulinum toxin a in the surgical management of seizure-related shoulder instability. JBJS Case Connect. 2021;11 https://doi.org/10.2106/JBJS.CC.20.00688.
126. Waltenspül M, Häller T, Ernstbrunner L, Wyss S, Wieser K, Gerber C. Long-term results after posterior open glenoid wedge osteotomy for posterior shoulder instability associated with excessive glenoid retroversion. J Shoulder Elb Surg. 2022;31:81–9.
127. Malik SS, Jordan RW, Tahir M, MacDonald PB. Does the posterior glenoid osteotomy reduce the rate of recurrence in patients with posterior shoulder instability—a systematic review. Orthop Traumatol Surg Res. 2021;107:102760.
128. Banerjee M, Balke M, Bouillon B, Wafaisade A, Helm P, Akoto R, Shafizadeh S. Excellent results of lesser tuberosity transfer in acute locked posterior shoulder dislocation. Knee Surg Sports Traumatol Arthrosc. 2013;21:2884–8.
129. Ratner D, Backes J, Tokish JM. Arthroscopic reduction and balloon humeroplasty in the treatment of acute Hill-Sachs lesions. Arthrosc Tech. 2016;5:e1327–32.
130. Gerber C, Catanzaro S, Jundt-Ecker M, Farshad M. Long-term outcome of segmental reconstruction of the humeral head for the treatment of locked posterior dislocation of the shoulder. J Shoulder Elb Surg. 2014;23:1682–90.
131. Roach RP, Crozier MW, Moser MW, Struk AM, Wright TW. Management of bipolar shoulder injuries with humeral head allograft in patients with active, uncontrolled seizure disorder: case series and review of literature. JSES Int. 2022;6:132–6.
132. Schliemann B, Muder D, Geßmann J, Schildhauer TA, Seybold D. Locked posterior shoulder dislocation: treatment options and clinical outcomes. Arch Orthop Trauma Surg. 2011;131:1127–34.
133. Heilmann LF, Katthagen JC, Raschke MJ, Schliemann B, Lill H, El Bajjati H, Jensen G, Dey Hazra R-O. Promising mid-term outcomes after humeral head preserving surgery of posterior fracture dislocations of the proximal Humerus. J Clin Med. 2021;10:3841.
134. Warnhoff M, Jensen G, Dey Hazra R-O, Theruvath P, Lill H, Ellwein A. Double plating—surgical technique and good clinical results in complex and highly unstable proximal humeral fractures. Injury. 2021;52:2285–91.
135. Biermann N, Prall WC, Böcker W, Mayr HO, Haasters F. Augmentation of plate osteosynthesis for proximal humeral fractures: a systematic review of current biomechanical and clinical studies. Arch Orthop Trauma Surg. 2019;139:1075–99.
136. Königshausen M, Rausch V, Mempel E, von Glinski A, Ull C, Bernstorff M, Schildhauer T, Seybold D, Gessmann J. Bilateral proximal Humerus fracture—a rare combination with a high complication rate after surgery. Z Orthop Unfall. 2018;156:646–52.
137. Murphy JD, Braunlich PR, Bansal M, Edge L, Harker JN. Bilateral posterior four-part fracture-dislocation of the proximal Humerus after first-time seizure. Cureus. 2021;13:e17688. https://doi.org/10.7759/cureus.17688.
138. Pangopoulos A, Papagiannis S, Koutas K, Kokkalis ZT. Bilateral locked posterior fracture-dislocation of the shoulder after epileptic seizures secondary to cavernous hemangioma: a case report and literature review. Am J Case Rep. 2023;24:e940141. https://doi.org/10.12659/AJCR.940141.
139. Torrens C, Santana F, Melendo E, Marlet V, Caceres E. Osteochondral autograft and hemiarthroplasty for bilateral locked posterior dislocation of the shoulder. Am J Orthop (Belle Mead NJ). 2012;41:362–4.
140. Uppal HS, Robinson PW, Packham I, Crowther M. The management of bilateral posterior fracture dislocations of the shoulder: a case series illustrating management options. Shoulder Elbow. 2016;8:111–7.
141. Ivkovic A, Boric I, Cicak N. One-stage operation for locked bilateral posterior dislocation of the shoulder. J Bone Joint Surg Br. 2007;89-B:825–8.
142. Crowley M, Ghattas Y, Collins AP, Levin S, Service BC. Systematic review and meta-analysis of locked posterior dislocation of the shoulder treated with shoulder arthroplasty: improved outcomes for total shoulder arthroplasty are associated with increased age. Orthop Surg. 2023;15:1730–41.
143. Davies A, Lloyd T, Sabharwal S, Liddle A, Reilly P. Anatomical shoulder replacements in young patients: a systematic review and meta-analysis. Shoulder Elbow. 2023;15:4–14.
144. Thangarajah T, Falworth M, Lambert SM. Anatomical shoulder arthroplasty in epileptic patients with instability arthropathy and persistent seizures. J Orthop Surg. 2017;25:230949901771719.
145. Thangarajah T, Alexander S, Bayley I, Lambert SM. Glenohumeral arthrodesis for the treatment of recurrent shoulder instability in epileptic patients. Bone Joint J. 2014;96-B:1525–9.

The Humeral Avulsion of the Glenohumeral Ligament (HAGL) Lesion

14

Richard D. J. Smith, Alec Reihl, Evan Stieler, Blake M. Bacevich, Ian Hutchinson, and Augustus D. Mazzocca

14.1 Introduction to History and Anatomy

14.1.1 Introduction

The shoulder, the most mobile joint in the human body, is commonly associated with instability. Shoulder instability is a common musculoskeletal problem with an incidence of 1.84 per 1000 person-years [1]. Recurrent anterior glenohumeral instability can cause significant disability, affecting approximately 1–2% of the population [2]. Posterior shoulder instability is less common, accounting for just 2–12% of all cases of shoulder instability [1]. Shoulder instability has a negative impact on a patient's quality of life by causing pain and dysfunction.

14.1.2 History

Nicola and Bach et al. were among the first people to publish articles relating to humeral avulsion of glenohumeral ligaments (HAGL) lesions in 1942 and 1988, respectively [3, 4]. In 1988, Wolf et al. published a seminal article implicating HAGL lesions as contributing factors to shoulder instability. Their study of 64 shoulders with anterior instability revealed HAGL lesions in 9.3% of cases, and repair of this complex could restore anterior stability [5]. The incidence of HAGL lesions has been reported between 7.5% and 9.3% in patients with shoulder instability [6]. HAGL lesions often occur concurrently with other causes of instability, which can potentially lead to the underdiagnosis and undertreatment of these lesions [7].

14.1.3 Anatomy

Shoulder stability relies upon a combination of dynamic and static stabilizers. Dynamic stabilizers include the muscular structures that exert force on the glenohumeral joint, such as the deltoid, biceps, and rotator cuff muscles. Static stabilizers include the labrum, bony structures, capsule, and glenohumeral ligaments. The labrum is particularly important because it deepens the glenoid cavity and serves as the attachment site for the glenohumeral ligaments [8]. Within the capsuloligamentous complex, the coracohumeral ligament, superior glenohumeral ligament (SGHL), middle glenohumeral ligament (MGHL), and inferior glenohumeral ligament (IGHL) all play vital roles [7].

R. D. J. Smith · A. Reihl · E. Stieler · B. M. Bacevich
I. Hutchinson
Department of Orthopaedic Surgery, Massachusetts General Hospital, Harvard Medical School, Boston, MA, USA

A. D. Mazzocca (✉)
Harvard Medical School, Sports Medicine, Massachusetts General Brigham, Boston, MA, USA
e-mail: amazzocca@mgh.harvard.edu

E. Calvo et al. (eds.), *Complex and Revision Problems in Shoulder Instability*,
https://doi.org/10.1007/978-3-031-81389-4_14

Conceptualizing the glenoid as a clock face provides a helpful framework for understanding the trajectories of the glenohumeral ligaments. The SGHL runs from the superior aspect of the glenoid and coracoid process, around 12 o'clock, extending to the superior aspect of the lesser tuberosity. Initially the SGHL is anterior before becoming inferior to the long head of the biceps tendon [9]. The MGHL arises from the glenoid just inferior to the SGHL and runs in a similar trajectory. It typically attaches at the inferior aspect of the lesser tuberosity, just below the SGHL attachment [10]. Bächler et al. demonstrated considerable anatomic variation of the MGHL, with instances of a combined insertion with the SGHL, IGHL, long head of the biceps, or a combination thereof [11]. The IGHL originates from the inferior two-thirds of the labrum and is comprised of an anterior band, posterior band, and axillary pouch. The anterior band originates from 2 to 4 o'clock position, while the posterior band originates from 7 to 9 o'clock on the glenoid [12, 13]. The axillary pouch is located between these two bands. Functionally, the IGHL is the most important glenohumeral ligament as it is the primary static stabilizer during shoulder abduction [14]. During external rotation and abduction, the anterior band of the IGHL restrains anterior and inferior humeral translation. During flexion and internal rotation, the posterior band of the IGHL provides posterior stability [13, 15]. Avulsions of the glenohumeral ligaments can occur at the labral attachment, the mid-substance, or the humeral attachment [15]. Cadaveric studies have shown that the least common site of failure is the humeral attachment of the IGHL [16].

The glenohumeral capsule receives its blood supply from the anterior humeral circumflex artery (AHCA), posterior humeral circumflex artery (PHCA), suprascapular artery, and circumflex scapular artery [17]. The glenohumeral ligaments are predominantly supplied by the AHCA and PHCA. These arteries course horizontally and form vertical branches that anastomose, creating an intracapsular network. The capsule also receives arterial contributions from vessels that supply the overlying rotator cuff tendons [12, 17].

HAGL lesions are typically caused by trauma, often occurring during glenohumeral dislocations or subluxation events. These events can lead to the separation of the capsular complex from the anterior glenoid, affecting structures like the labrum, SGHL, and/or MGHL, or result in avulsion of the IGHL from the humerus. HAGL lesions are most commonly seen when the arm is externally rotated and hyper-abducted [7]. These lesions lead to glenohumeral instability, especially when the arm is abducted and externally rotated because of an incompetent IGHL complex. In terms of prevalence, anterior HAGL lesions constitute 93% of cases, with posterior HAGL lesions accounting for the remaining 7% [18].

When assessing patients for possible HAGL lesions, certain aspects of their medical history are crucial to understand. Details such as the arm position during the injury, the direction of instability, and any history of recurrent instability provide valuable insights into the underlying pathology. Patients often report nonspecific symptoms such as pain and limited function, making it essential for physicians to be vigilant for HAGL lesions. Notably, these lesions are frequently discovered after a patient has undergone unsuccessful surgery for glenohumeral instability.

14.2 Physical Exam and Imaging

14.2.1 Physical Exam

When examining the shoulder, it is important to follow a systematic approach to avoid missing subtle issues. The examination should begin with inspection, ensuring both shoulders are exposed for comparison to check for signs of trauma, scarring, muscle atrophy, and asymmetry. Next, range of motion should be evaluated. A typical shoulder should demonstrate flexion of 150–180°, extension of 40–60°, abduction of 150–180°, external rotation of 60–90°, and internal rotation of 50–70° [19]. It is important to test the subscapularis strength and competency, as a tear in the subscapularis tendon is often associated with an

HAGL lesion [20]. The subscapularis is primarily tested with the Gerber test, but if the patient does not have the prerequisite flexibility, the belly press-down test is an alternative. Following this, specific provocative physical exam maneuvers are employed to assess for instability.

An important distinction is made between shoulder laxity and shoulder instability; shoulder laxity refers to the degree of looseness of the passive stabilizers of the shoulder [21]. In contrast, shoulder instability refers to symptoms experienced due to increased laxity [22]. Several physical exam maneuvers can be used to assess anterior shoulder instability. The Apprehension Test involves placing the patient supine, abducting their shoulder to 90°, and externally rotating their shoulder. Eliciting pain indicates a positive Apprehension Test. This is often performed in tandem with the Relocation Test, where a posteriorly directed force is placed over the humeral head. If this force reduces the pain associated with the Apprehension Test, the Relocation Test is considered positive. The Load and Shift Test involves quantifies anteroposterior translation in the glenohumeral joint and can be performed sitting or supine [23]. The Jerk test assesses for posterior shoulder instability and involves flexing, adducting, and internally rotating the shoulder, while flexing at the elbow. An axial force is applied along the humerus to induce a posterior subluxation and the test is considered positive if pain is elicited [24]. The sulcus sign test can be used to assess for inferior glenohumeral laxity. The test is positive if a dimple appears below the acromion when the arm is pulled inferiorly [25]. Of note, HAGL lesions may mimic bony avulsions, causing midrange motion apprehension or instability, despite negative x-rays and CT scans.

14.2.2 Imaging

To radiographically assess the glenohumeral joint, the most important views to obtain are the anteroposterior (AP), Grashey, and axillary x-ray views. Axillary view is crucial for evaluating glenohumeral joint congruency. In cases of instability, the axillary view may reveal abnormal glenoid anatomy resulting from traumatic dislocations or demonstrate abnormal glenoid version or hypoplasia, which can predispose individuals to instability. These x-ray views can reveal glenohumeral alignment, humeral head impaction fractures, glenoid fractures, and glenoid dysplasia. Parameswaran et al. demonstrated that scalloping along the medial aspect of the humeral neck is indicative of HAGL lesions [26]. Bony HAGL manifests as an avulsion fracture from the medial cortex of the humeral neck, appearing radiographically as a fleck of bone inferior to the humeral neck [27].

MRI imaging helps to detect HAGL lesions, with damage to the IGHL complex best visualized on coronal or sagittal T2-weighted images. MR arthrography of the shoulder enhances diagnostic accuracy by distending the joint, facilitating improved visualization of the glenohumeral ligaments [28]. If an HAGL lesion is suspected, MR arthrogram is key. Typically, the IGHL complex appears U-shaped on imaging due to fluid distension of the axillary pouch, but in cases of HAGL lesions, it may appear J-shaped on MRI due to extravasation of joint fluid across the torn capsule [15]. MRI findings suggestive of HAGL lesions include increased signal intensity, thickening of the inferior capsule, contrast extravasation, and/or joint effusion along the medial humeral neck (Figs. 14.1 and 14.2). Occasionally, bony avulsions from the medial humeral cortex may accompany these lesions, raising suspicion on plain films [29]. Chronic HAGL lesions can be difficult to see, even on MRI, since the torn edges often scar into the capsule [26].

Several studies have highlighted the challenge of detecting HAGL lesions on MRI through retrospective MRI analysis of patients who were diagnosed with HAGL lesions via arthroscopy. [30]. Currently, the sensitivity and specificity of MRI in detecting HAGL lesions remain unknown, and definitive diagnosis still requires arthroscopic evaluation.

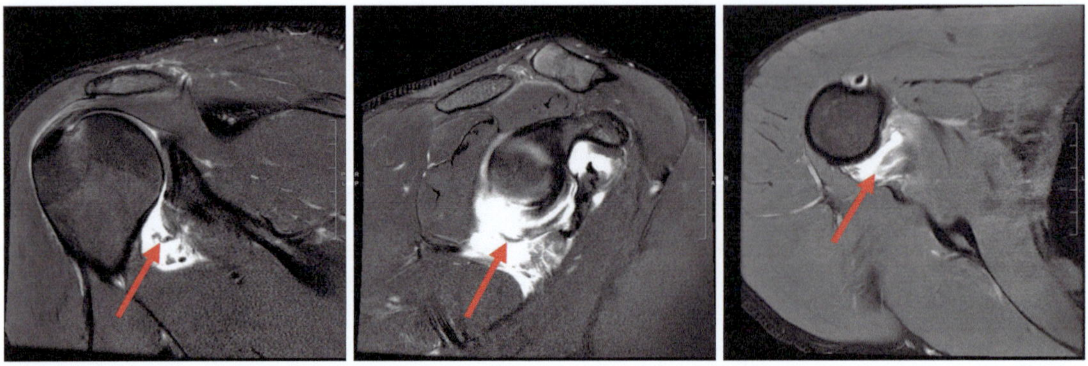

Fig. 14.1 Coronal, sagittal, and axial T2-weighted MRI of an HAGL lesion highlighted by red arrows

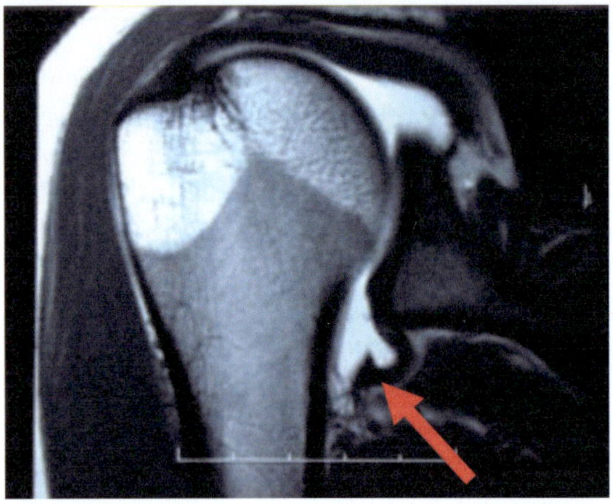

Fig. 14.2 Coronal T1 MRI with gadolinium with red arrow demonstrating the characteristic J-Sign of the IGHL

14.3 Classification

14.3.1 An Evolutionary Perspective

The endeavor to identify and classify HAGL lesions has undergone significant evolution since its inception. The journey began in 1988 when Bach et al. made a pivotal contribution to the understanding of shoulder instability by reporting on two patients with recurrent shoulder dislocation due to avulsion of the capsule from its lateral humeral attachment [3]. This work highlighted the significance of considering lateral humeral avulsion in the diagnostic and therapeutic algorithms for shoulder dislocation but did not yet introduce a classification system for HAGL lesions. Similarly, Wolf et al. further advanced the understanding of anterior shoulder instability by focusing on the HAGL lesion's role and incidence [5]. Their study identified HAGL lesions in a subset of patients with anterior instability, underscoring the importance of this pathology, especially in the absence of a primary Bankart lesion. However, they did not propose a formal classification system. Thus, the culmination of these efforts set the stage for the development of the West Point nomenclature [15]. This sophisticated system synthesizes the insights garnered from its predecessors, presenting a holistic approach to the classification of HAGL lesions.

14.3.2 West Point Nomenclature

Cadaveric studies examining the tensile properties of the IGHL have highlighted three possible locations for injury to occur: the IGHL labral complex at the glenoid origin (40%), intrasubstance tears (35%), and the humeral insertion point (25%) [16]. Informed by these foundational studies, the West Point nomenclature identifies six distinct types of HAGL lesions, classified according to the involvement of the IGHL's anterior or posterior band, the occurrence of bony avulsion, and the presence of associated labral tears (Table 14.1) [15]. This detailed classification not only clarifies the discourse surrounding humeral-sided lesions but also significantly informs therapeutic decision-making, facilitating a customized approach to surgery when deemed necessary.

Table 14.1 West point classification for HAGL lesions

Anterior lesions	
AHAGL	Anterior HAGL without a bony avulsion
ABHAGL	Anterior HAGL with a bony avulsion from the medial cortex of the humeral neck
FAIGHL	Anterior HAGL with a concurrent detachment of the anterior ligamentous–labral complex from the glenoid rim (i.e., a Bankart lesion)
Posterior lesions	
PHAGL	Posterior HAGL without a bony avulsion
PBHAGL	Posterior HAGL with a bony avulsion from the medial cortex of the humeral neck
FPIGHL	Posterior HAGL with a concurrent detachment of the posterior ligamentous–labral complex from the glenoid

Most HAGL lesions involve the anterior band of the IGHL, observed in up to 93% of cases. Anterior band tears manifest in two distinct forms: as an Anterior HAGL (AHAGL) without bony avulsion, or as an Anterior bony HAGL (ABHAGL) when accompanied by a bony avulsion from the medial cortex of the humeral neck. While less common, injuries to the posterior band also mirror this classification pattern. Posterior band tears are categorized as either a Posterior HAGL (PHAGL) without a bony avulsion, or as a Posterior bony HAGL (PBHAGL) when a bony avulsion is present [15].

Additionally, this classification system accounts for scenarios in which concurrent detachment of the ligamentous–labral complex from the glenoid rim leads to a "floating" IGHL condition. Such phenomena are categorized as a Floating Anterior IGHL (FAIGHL) when associated with a Bankart lesion, and as a Floating Posterior IGHL (FPIGHL) in the presence of a posterior ligamentous–labral tear [15].

The evolution from Bach's initial report to the nuanced West Point system underscores the orthopedic community's dedication to improving diagnostic and treatment strategies for patients with shoulder instability. Understanding the classification of HAGL lesions, particularly through the comprehensive lens of the West Point nomenclature, is important for orthopedic surgeons. This framework not only enables accurate diagnosis of HAGL lesions but also assists in management strategies, whether conservative or surgical interventions.

14.4 Treatment

14.4.1 Arthroscopic Technique

The arthroscopic technique allows for smaller and more cosmetic incisions but is more technically challenging due to the location of the HAGL lesion [31]. This arthroscopic technique has previously been published by both Fritz et al. and Cross et al. [32, 33].

14.4.1.1 Preoperative Evaluation

Both the mini-open and the arthroscopic repair require the same preoperative evaluation. This begins with a comprehensive clinical history and physical examination conducted in the office setting. If signs and symptoms of shoulder instability are present, the next step is obtaining imaging of the affected shoulder. Standard radiographs of the shoulder should be completed including anteroposterior, Grashey, and axillary views. Magnetic resonance imaging should also be completed with HAGL lesion best identified on T2-weighted sequences. Images highlighting notable pathology should be available in the operating room for review during the case. As HAGL lesions are often associated with concomitant pathology, it is vital to do a thorough evaluation of the shoulder MRI before entering the operating room.

14.4.1.2 Positioning

Arthroscopic repair of HAGL lesions may be completed in either the beach-chair or the lateral decubitus positions. After endotracheal intubation, the patient is positioned in the attending surgeon's preferred position. This author prefers the beach-chair position. While upright in the beach-chair, care must be taken to ensure that the patient's head is in a neutral position, the surgical shoulder is appropriately exposed, and a pillow should be placed under the patient's legs to prevent slipping down the bed. Prior to prepping and draping the patient, the surgeon should examine the shoulder while under anesthesia, comparing the exam to the contralateral side. A pneumatic arm holder should be used to allow for stabilization and manipulation throughout the case.

14.4.1.3 Diagnostic Arthroscopy

The first step of the procedure involves and external assessment with palpation and marking of the bony landmarks of the shoulder. Using an 11-blade, a portal incision is made about two finger breaths both inferior and medial to the acromion's posterior lateral border. A 30° arthroscopic camera is inserted, and a diagnostic arthroscopy can now be performed. Once the camera is inserted, an anterior working portal should be created through the rotator interval. As previously discussed, HAGL lesions are often associated with additional pathology in the shoulder. For this reason, the surgeon must conduct a thorough diagnostic arthroscopy, ensuring meticulous examination and probing of the relevant anatomy. This includes assessing the anterior and posterior labrum, long head of the biceps tendon, rotator cuff, and articular cartilage of both the humerus and glenoid, along with the HAGL lesion. When an HAGL lesion is present (Fig. 14.3), the fibers of the subscapularis can be seen between the humeral neck and the inferior capsule.

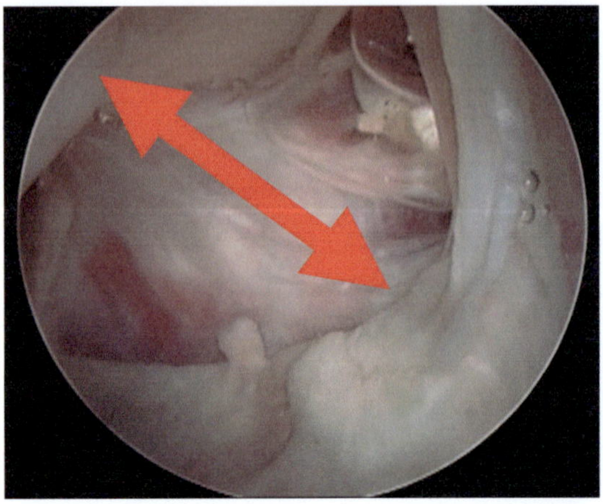

Fig. 14.3 Arthroscopic view of HAGL lesion from the standard posterior portal, with defect spanning from capsule to bony surface, as indicated by double-headed red arrow

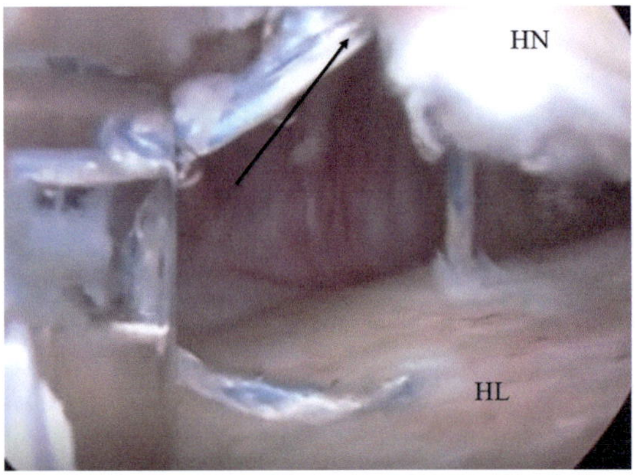

Fig. 14.4 Arthroscopic view from the posterior portal. The suture anchor (black arrow) has been placed into the humeral neck. One of the limbs of the suture has been passed through the detached portion of the HAGL lesion and is being tied down to the humeral neck. *HL* HAGL lesion, *HN* humeral neck. (Image taken from Fritz et al. [32])

14.4.1.4 Surgical Technique

A posterior inferior working portal is created under direct visualization from the standard posterior portal. The anterior humeral neck and avulsed inferior glenohumeral ligament should be identified. Using an arthroscopic grasper, the HAGL lesion's excursion should be tested to ensure that it can reach its native humeral neck insertion. With the use of an arthroscopic shaver through the posterior inferior working portal, the anterior humeral neck should be debrided down to bleeding bone, creating a surface for the HAGL lesion to heal. A 2.4-mm drill and guide are used to create a pilot hole on the humeral neck ensuring that the pilot hole is inferior to the articular surface. Without removing the guide, a 3.0-mm suture anchor is inserted into the pilot hole. A suture lasso loaded with a wire loop is passed through the avulsed anterior band of the inferior glenohumeral ligament. Once passed through the HAGL lesion (Fig. 14.4), the surgeon may use an arthroscopic suture grasper to retrieve the wire loop. The suture attached to the anchor (repair suture) may then be shuttled through the lesion using the wire loop. If using a knotless anchor, a knot pusher can be used to tighten the HAGL lesion to the humeral neck and the free end of the suture is cut once the desired tension is achieved. If using a standard suture anchor, an arthroscopic knot should be tied such that the HAGL lesion is brought back to its insertion on the humeral neck and both sutures should be cut once the desired tension is achieved. A second anchor is then placed laterally and inferiorly in a similar fashion. Once both anchors are placed, the repair is complete and the shoulder should be examined to ensure subluxation is no longer present. The portals are closed with nylon suture and the patient is placed in a sling before leaving the operating room.

14.4.1.5 Arthroscopic Complications

Grundshtein et al. reported the 2-year outcomes and associated complications of 23 patients who underwent arthroscopic HAGL repair [34]. They reported intraoperative anchor failure in four patients (17.4%) that required anchor replacement. One patient (4.3%) developed a musculocutaneous sensory deficit postoperatively, which recovered spontaneously. One patient (4.3%) developed significant venous bleeding around the lower anterior portal, which required admission to the pediatric intensive care unit and transfusion of 1 unit of packed red blood cells. Revision surgeries were performed in three patients (13%).

14.4.2 Mini-Open Technique

The mini-open technique allows for direct visualization of the HAGL defect and an anatomic repair. Both Arciero et al. and Grimm et al. have previously published the mini-open technique, which is outlined below [35, 36].

14.4.2.1 Preoperative Imaging

Standard radiographs of the affected shoulder should be obtained including anteroposterior, Grashey, axillary, and scapular-Y views. HAGL lesions are best characterized by magnetic resonance imaging. A coronal T2-weighted image demonstrating the HAGL lesion should be available for review in the operative room during the procedure. As concomitant injuries are common in patients with HAGL lesions, it is important to complete a full assessment of the MRI before entering the operative room.

14.4.2.2 Positioning

The patient is positioned supine with the operative shoulder hanging over the lateral side of the bed to allow for a free range of motion. When applying the sterile drapes, the arm should be placed on a sterile padded Mayo stand. The bed should be flexed, raising the patient's back to place the patient in a reclined beach-chair position.

14.4.2.3 Surgical Approach

The anterior skin incision is made with the most inferior portion starting at the axillary fold extending approximately 4 cm in the direction of the coracoid process. Dissection is then completed down to the deltopectoral interval. The cephalic vein is identified and protected while the deltopectoral interval is opened. Using a dissecting scissor, the clavipectoral fascia is divided extending superiorly to the coracoid process. Using a self-retaining retractor, the conjoint tendon is retracted medially and the deltoid is retracted laterally (Fig. 14.5). Care should be taken to identify ascending branches of the anterior humeral circumflex vessels. An L-shaped incision should be planned and marked with the vertical portion of the incision through the inferior subscapularis insertion and the horizontal incision extending medially toward the lesser tuberosity just proximal to the ascending branch of the anterior circumflex vessels.

It is vital to ensure that the axillary nerve is identified both medial and inferior to the horizontal portion of the incision before the incision is made. Tagging sutures are placed through the cut edge of the subscapularis tendon. While gently retracting the tagging sutures, blunt dissection is performed at the corner of the L-shaped incision lifting the subscapularis in the superior and medial direction. The HAGL lesion will be identified deep to the subscapularis tendon. Tagging sutures are then placed in the free humeral edge

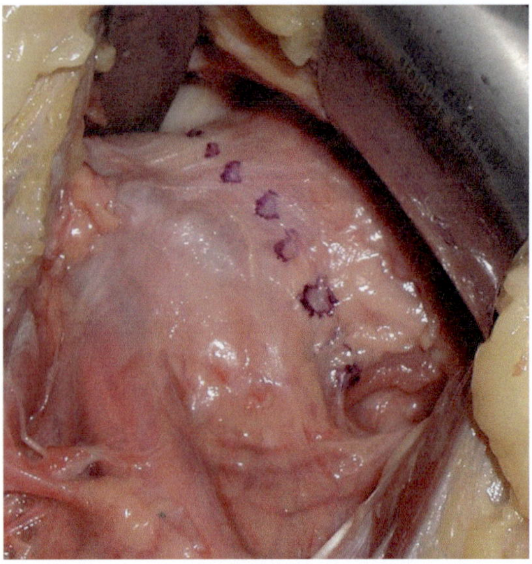

Fig. 14.5 The vertical portion of the incision through the inferior subscapularis is marked. A large enough stump is left attached to the bone so that a repair can be completed

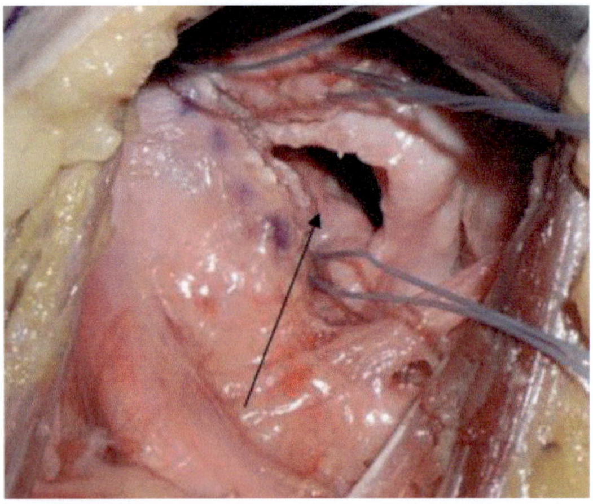

Fig. 14.6 Suture anchors are placed into the humerus and the suture is passed through the HAGL lesion (identified by the black arrow) to reattach the lesion to the humeral neck

of the inferior glenohumeral ligament. The glenohumeral joint may be inspected with superior and medial retraction of both the subscapularis and the inferior glenohumeral ligament. Using suture anchors, the avulsed inferior glenohumeral ligament is reattached to the anatomic attachment on the humeral neck (Fig. 14.6).

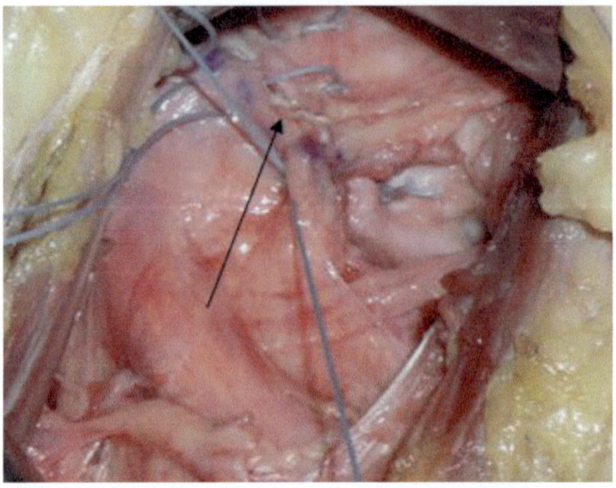

Fig. 14.7 Side-to-side repair of the subscapularis tendon, identified by the black arrow

Using a heavy suture, the subscapularis tendon is repaired in a side-to-side fashion as shown (Fig. 14.7).

The wound is then irrigated with sterile saline. Closure of the deltopectoral interval is completed with simple sutures. The subcuticular layer is also closed with interrupted sutures and finally, a running monofilament suture is used for the skin. Steri-strips are placed over the wound and a sterile dressing is applied.

14.4.3 Post-op Rehab

After surgery, the patient should be discharged with instructions to be non-weight-bearing in a sling for the first 3–5 weeks [27, 32, 36–38]. During this time, the patient should come out of the sling for pendulum exercises [37]. Some protocols discuss the use of Codman exercises and supine well-arm-assisted forward elevation in the first 3–5 weeks [36]. External rotation should be prohibited past 0° during the first 3–5 weeks to protect the repair. After 3–5 weeks the patients should work with a physical therapist first on passive motion including external rotation, then active motion, and finally strengthening exercises with a focus on the rotator cuff and scapular muscles [32, 37]. There is some variance in the literature in regards to when activity restrictions are lifted with a range of 4–9-months postoperatively [36, 37].

14.5 Outcomes

14.5.1 Introduction

Patients with HAGL lesions are initially recommended to undergo a trial of nonoperative management. However, if patients continue to experience persistent symptoms, operative intervention should be considered [39]. A systematic review by Longo et al. examined the outcomes of nonoperative and operative management of HAGL lesions at a median follow-up of 25.5 months [40]. The review revealed recurrent instability in 90% (9 of 10) of patients managed nonoperatively, whereas none of the patients (0 of 25) managed operatively experienced recurrent instability [40].

14.5.2 Open Repair

Numerous studies have demonstrated favorable clinical outcomes associated with open repair of HAGL lesions. Bhatia et al. observed significant improvements in the postoperative Oxford Shoulder Instability Score (OSIS) and Western Ontario Shoulder Instability Index (WOSI) scores among seven patients who underwent a modified Laterjet procedure concurrently with HAGL repair [41]. Rhee et al. investigated five patients with HAGL lesions who underwent diagnostic arthroscopy followed by open surgical repair [42]. While they noted increases in postoperative Rowe score and Constant score, a slight reduction in range of motion (ROM) was observed, including a 1° loss of forward flexion and a 15° loss of external rotation at follow-up [42]. Despite this limitation, two patients, including professional athletes, were able to return to sports, while the others resumed their daily activities without any issues. Warner et al. documented a case of a 15-year-old football player with combined Bankart and HAGL lesions who underwent open surgical repair for both injuries [43]. After 26 months, the patient regained full ROM comparable to the uninjured shoulder and returned to his pre-injury level of sports participation [43]. Schippinger et al. reported a successful open HAGL repair in a 17-year-old competitive skier who had previously undergone arthroscopic Bankart repair [44]. At the 1-year follow-up, the patient had returned to his pre-injury level of competitive skiing [44]. Similarly, Shah et al. described a case of a professional basketball player who underwent arthroscopic Bankart repair combined with open HAGL repair [45]. After 3 years, the patient successfully returned to his pre-injury level of basketball performance and even led the league in scoring post-return [45].

14.5.3 Arthroscopic Repair

Several studies have also reported positive outcomes after arthroscopic repair of HAGL lesions.

Castagna et al. performed an arthroscopic repair on nine patients with posterior HAGL lesions, all of whom experienced significant improvements in their UCLA shoulder score, Constant score, and Simple Shoulder Test (SST) score at a mean 34.2 month follow-up [38]. Additionally, all patients returned to their desired sporting activities without limitations or recurring symptoms [38]. Huberty et al. arthroscopically treated six patients with anterior HAGL lesions, resulting in improved UCLA shoulder scores for all patients at an average 31.8 month follow-up [46]. Taljanovic et al. reported successful arthroscopic repair of HAGL lesions in three Division I collegiate volleyball players, all of whom resumed full volleyball competition within 8 months postsurgery [47]. Flury et al. achieved successful arthroscopic repair of anterior HAGL lesions in six patients, with improved Rowe scores at a median follow-up of 29 months compared to preoperative assessments [48]. Schmiddem et al. described outcomes of arthroscopic HAGL repair in 16 patients, showing significant improvements in Rowe Score and Q-DASH score at a median follow-up of 59 months [49]. However, median external rotation was reduced compared to the contralateral shoulder, and there was one reported case of recurrent dislocation, with five patients unable to return to their pre-injury sports level [49].

14.5.4 Arthroscopic Versus Open Repair

Two studies have compared outcomes of open versus arthroscopic repair for HAGL lesions. Provencher et al. studied 27 military patients with various types of HAGL lesions, with 17 undergoing open repair for anterior or combined lesions, and ten undergoing arthroscopic repair for reverse lesions [39]. Both groups showed significant improvements in postoperative WOSI and SANE scores, with no complications reported and all patients returning to full active duty [39]. Lee et al. compared 11 patients undergoing open HAGL repair to 7 patients undergoing arthroscopic repair [50]. Both groups experienced significant improvements in SANE and WOSI scores postoperatively [50]. However, the arthroscopic group had higher WOSI scores [50]. There were no differences in range of motion between the two groups, and no instances of recurrent symptoms [50].

14.6 Conclusion

Both open and arthroscopic HAGL repair offer better clinical outcomes than nonoperative management. In the future, a multi-center randomized controlled trial could compare the effectiveness of open and arthroscopic approaches for treating HAGL lesions.

References

1. Galvin JW, Ernat JJ, Waterman BR, Stadecker MJ, Parada SA. The epidemiology and natural history of anterior shoulder instability. Curr Rev Musculoskelet Med. 2017;10:411–24.
2. Varacallo M, Musto MA, Mair SD. Anterior shoulder instability. StatPearls Publishing; 2019.
3. Bach BR, Warren RF, Fronek J. Disruption of the lateral capsule of the shoulder. A cause of recurrent dislocation. J Bone Jointt Surg Br Vol. 1988;70(2):274–6.
4. Nicola T. Acute anterior dislocation of the shoulder. J Bone Joint Surg Am. 1949;31A(1):153–9.
5. Wolf EM, Cheng JC, Dickson K. Humeral avulsion of glenohumeral ligaments as a cause of anterior shoulder instability. Arthroscopy. 1995;11(5):600–7.
6. Nelson C, Reiter C, Cyrus J, Satalich J, O'Connell R, Vap A. Indications, management, and outcomes of humeral avulsions of the glenohumeral ligament: a systematic review. Orthop Rev (Pavia). 2022;14(3):37830.
7. George MS, Khazzam M, Kuhn JE. Humeral avulsion of glenohumeral ligaments. J Am Acad Orthop Surg. 2011;19(3):127–33.
8. Lugo R, Kung P, Ma CB. Shoulder biomechanics. Eur J Radiol. 2008;68(1):16–24.
9. Robinson PJ. Essential radiology for sports medicine. Springer; 2010.
10. Bencardino JT, Beltran J. MR imaging of the glenohumeral ligaments. Radiol Clin. 2006;44(4):489–502.
11. Bächler J, Bergman S, Lancigu R, Hubert L, Ropars M, Rony L. Arthroscopic anatomy of the middle glenohumeral ligament. A series of 300 cases. Morphologie. 2020;104(346):187–95.
12. O'Brien SJ, Neves MC, Arnoczky SP, Rozbruck SR, Dicarlo EF, Warren RF, et al. The anatomy and histology of the inferior glenohumeral ligament complex of the shoulder. Am J Sports Med. 1990;18(5):449–56.
13. Burkart AC, Debski RE. Anatomy and function of the glenohumeral ligaments in anterior shoulder instability. Clin Orthop Relat Res. 2002;400:32–9.
14. Rockwood CA. The shoulder, vol. 1. Elsevier Health Sciences; 2009.
15. Bui-Mansfield LT, Banks KP, Taylor DC. Humeral avulsion of the glenohumeral ligaments: the HAGL lesion. Am J Sports Med. 2007;35(11):1960–6.
16. Bigliani LU, Pollock RG, Soslowsky LJ, Flatow EL, Pawluk RJ, Mow VC. Tensile properties of the inferior glenohumeral ligament. J Orthop Res. 1992;10(2):187–97.
17. Andary JL, Petersen SA. The vascular anatomy of the glenohumeral capsule and ligaments: an anatomic study. JBJS. 2002;84(12):2258–65.
18. Freshman RD, Zhang AL, Benjamin Ma C, Feeley BT, Ortiz S, Patel J, et al. Factors associated with humeral avulsion of Glenohumeral ligament lesions in patients with anterior shoulder instability: an analysis of the MOON shoulder instability cohort. Orthop J Sports Med. 2023;11(10):23259671231206756.
19. Bakhsh W, Nicandri G. Anatomy and physical examination of the shoulder. Sports Med Arthrosc Rev. 2018;26(3):e10–22.
20. Martetschläger F, Ames JB, Millett PJ. HAGL and reverse HAGL lesions. In: Shoulder arthroscopy: principles and practice. Springer; 2013. p. 411–8.
21. Tzannes A, Murrell GAC. Clinical examination of the unstable shoulder. Sports Med. 2002;32:447–57.
22. Bigliani LU. The unstable shoulder. American Academy of Orthopaedic Surgeons; 1996.
23. Silliman JF, Hawkins RJ. Current concepts and recent advances in the athlete's shoulder. Clin Sports Med. 1991;10(4):693–705.
24. Matesen FI. Glenohumeral instability. In: The shoulder. Saunders; 1998.

25. Provencher MT, Midtgaard KS, Owens BD, Tokish JM. Diagnosis and management of traumatic anterior shoulder instability. J Am Acad Orthop Surg. 2021;29(2):e51–61.
26. Parameswaran AD, Provencher MT, Bach BR Jr, Verma N, Romeo AA. Humeral avulsion of the glenohumeral ligament: injury pattern and arthroscopic repair techniques. Orthopedics. 2008;31(8):773.
27. Oberlander MA, Morgan BE, Visotsky JL. The BHAGL lesion: a new variant of anterior shoulder instability. Arthroscopy. 1996;12(5):627–33.
28. Melvin JS, MacKenzie JD, Nacke E, Sennett BJ, Wells L. MRI of HAGL lesions: four arthroscopically confirmed cases of false-positive diagnosis. Am J Roentgenol. 2008;191(3):730–4.
29. Stoller DW. MR arthrography of the glenohumeral joint. Radiol Clin North Am. 1997;35(1):97–116.
30. Magee T. Prevalence of HAGL lesions and associated abnormalities on shoulder MR examination. Skeletal Radiol. 2014;43:307–13.
31. Markus DH, Morgan AM, Campbell KA, Alaia MJ, Jazrawi LM, Strauss EJ. Outcomes following arthroscopic repair of humeral avulsion of the glenohumeral ligament (HAGL) lesion: a systematic review. J Clin Orthop Trauma. 2023;102166:102166.
32. Fritz EM, Pogorzelski J, Hussain ZB, Godin JA, Millett PJ. Arthroscopic repair of humeral avulsion of the glenohumeral ligament lesion. Arthrosc Tech. 2017;6(4):e1195–200.
33. Cross AG, Tramer JS, Guo EW, Muh SJ, Makhni EC. Arthroscopic repair of humeral avulsion of the glenohumeral ligament lesion with capsular plication in the lateral decubitus position. Arthrosc Tech. 2021;10(2):e569–74.
34. Grundshtein A, Kazum E, Chechik O, Dolkart O, Rath E, Bivas A, et al. Arthroscopic repair of humeral avulsion of glenohumeral ligament lesions: outcomes at 2-year follow-up. Orthop J Sports Med. 2021;9(8):23259671211004970.
35. Grimm NL, Jimenez AE, Levy BJ, Bell R, Arciero RA. The original mini-open technique for repair of humeral avulsion of the glenohumeral ligament. Arthrosc Tech. 2020;9(12):e1865–70.
36. Arciero RA, Mazzocca AD. Mini-open repair technique of HAGL (humeral avulsion of the glenohumeral ligament) lesion. Arthroscopy. 2005;21(9):1152–e1.
37. Field LD, Bokor DJ, Savoie FH III. Humeral and glenoid detachment of the anterior inferior glenohumeral ligament: a cause of anterior shoulder instability. J Shoulder Elb Surg. 1997;6(1):6–10.
38. Castagna A, Snyder SJ, Conti M, Borroni M, Massazza G, Garofalo R. Posterior humeral avulsion of the glenohumeral ligament: a clinical review of 9 cases. Arthroscopy. 2007;23(8):809–15.
39. Provencher MT, McCormick F, Leclere L, Sanchez G, Golijanin P, Anthony S, et al. Prospective evaluation of surgical treatment of humeral avulsions of the glenohumeral ligament. Am J Sports Med. 2017;45(5):1134–40.
40. Longo UG, Rizzello G, Ciuffreda M, Locher J, Berton A, Salvatore G, et al. Humeral avulsion of the glenohumeral ligaments: a systematic review. Arthroscopy. 2016;32(9):1868–76.
41. Bhatia DN, DasGupta B. Surgical treatment of significant glenoid bone defects and associated humeral avulsions of glenohumeral ligament (HAGL) lesions in anterior shoulder instability. Knee Surg Sports Traumatol Arthrosc. 2013;21:1603–9.
42. Rhee YG, Cho NS. Anterior shoulder instability with humeral avulsion of the glenohumeral ligament lesion. J Shoulder Elb Surg. 2007;16(2):188–92.
43. Warner JJP, Beim GM. Combined Bankart and HAGL lesion associated with anterior shoulder instability. Arthroscopy. 1997;13(6):749–52.
44. Schippinger G, Vasiu PS, Fankhauser F, Clement HG. HAGL lesion occurring after successful arthroscopic Bankart repair. Arthroscopy. 2001;17(2):206–8.
45. Shah AA, Selesnick FH. Traumatic shoulder dislocation with combined bankart lesion and humeral avulsion of the glenohumeral ligament in a professional basketball player: three-year follow-up of surgical stabilization. Arthroscopy. 2010;26(10):1404–8.
46. Huberty DP, Burkhart SS. Arthroscopic repair of anterior humeral avulsion of the glenohumeral ligaments. Tech Shoulder Elbow Surg. 2006;7(4):186–90.
47. Taljanovic MS, Nisbet JK, Hunter TB, Cohen RP, Rogers LF. Humeral avulsion of the inferior glenohumeral ligament in college female volleyball players caused by repetitive microtrauma. Am J Sports Med. 2011;39(5):1067–76.
48. Flury M, Rickenbacher D, Audigé L. Arthroscopic treatment of anterior shoulder instability associated with a HAGL lesion—a case series. J Shoulder Elb Surg. 2016;25(12):1989–96.
49. Schmiddem U, Watson A, Perriman D, Liodakis E, Page R. Arthroscopic repair of HAGL lesions yields good clinical results, but may not allow return to former level of sport. Knee Surg Sports Traumatol Arthrosc. 2019;27:3246–53.
50. Lee S, Krych AJ, Peebles AM, Rider D, Dekker TJ, Arner JW, et al. Outcomes of open versus arthroscopic treatment of HAGL tears. Am J Sports Med. 2023;51(6):1581–7.

15 Evolving Concepts: Pathoanatomy and Pathomechanics of Labral Injuries in the Disabled Throwing Shoulder (DTS)—Moving Beyond the Slap

W. Ben Kibler, Austin V. Stone, W. Jeffrey Grantham, Aaron Sciascia, and Giovanni Di Giacomo

15.1 Introduction

Clinical disorders involving the superior labrum and biceps anchor are common and well-known pathologic entities but the most effective methods for their diagnosis and management are far from clear. The conclusion that the SLAP lesion was responsible for the large majority of the clinical symptoms and dysfunction in the throwing athlete became the basis for evaluation and treatment for both athletes and workers. This organizational framework led to the concepts that (1) the labral injury most commonly exists from 11:00–1:00 on the glenoid rim; (2) the pathoanatomy is detachment of the labrum from the rim; (3) history and physical exam are not always sufficiently reliable or specific to make the diagnosis; (4) the pathoanatomy of the detachment can be delineated by MRI, with or without contrast; (5) arthroscopy may be the best method to confirm the pathoanatomy [1]; and (6) arthroscopic repair should reattach the superior labrum at 11:00 and 1:00 by high strength anchors and sutures, similar to repair of inferior labral injuries [2, 3]. Peer-reviewed studies regarding treatments utilizing these concepts reported outcomes collected from patient-reported questionnaires, clinical exam, performance parameters, or the incidence of failed or revision surgeries. The studies and their results varied widely, but generally suggested dissatisfying results and less than optimal outcomes, with varying relief of pain and return to activity [4–8]. This inconsistency in proposed treatments suggests that a review and possible reconsideration of the evolving scholarship may produce a more accurate understanding of the problem and may point to different methods of evaluation and treatment.

This chapter reviews the anatomy, pathoanatomy, pathomechanics, and clinical evaluation process that create the diagnosis of a labral injury and suggests directions for treatment. It will dis-

W. B. Kibler · W. J. Grantham
Department of Orthopedics-Sports Medicine, Shoulder Center of Kentucky, Lexington Clinic, Lexington, KY, USA
e-mail: wgran@lexclin.com

A. V. Stone
Division of Sports Medicine, Department of Orthopedic Surgery and Sports Medicine, University of Kentucky Lexington, Lexington, KY, USA
e-mail: Austin.stone@uky.edu

A. Sciascia (✉)
Institute for Clinical Outcomes and Research, Lexington Clinic, Lexington, KY, USA
e-mail: ascia@lexclin.com

G. Di Giacomo
Orthopedics and Traumatology Unit, Concordia Hospital, Rome, Italy
e-mail: concordia@iol.it

E. Calvo et al. (eds.), *Complex and Revision Problems in Shoulder Instability*,
https://doi.org/10.1007/978-3-031-81389-4_15

cuss: (1) Anatomy, mechanics, and functional roles of the labrum in the overhead throwing motion; (2) The role of the biceps in throwing athletes and its relationship to the glenoid labrum; (3) Pathoanatomy and pathomechanics of clinically significant labral injuries and their role in the clinical dysfunction of the disabled throwing shoulder (DTS); (4) Evaluation techniques in the athlete with DTS; and (5) Treatment guidelines and concepts of functional rehabilitation.

15.2 Anatomy and Mechanics of the Labrum

The glenohumeral (GH) joint is mechanically considered to be a "continuous controlled skid bed," a term applied to joint surfaces where rotation and translation takes place between the bony components of the joint [9]. Humeral motion on the glenoid exhibits the "skid bed" characteristics throughout arm motion, with small amounts of anterior and superior translations at low levels of arm elevation, before becoming centered on the glenoid and rotating at higher levels of arm elevation. In passive arm elevations from 30–90° the instant center of rotation (ICR) of the humerus moves anteriorly 1.5 mm, then from 90–150° moves posteriorly toward the center of the glenoid. In active elevation from 60–90° it moves anteriorly 1 mm then at 120° it moves 0.5 mm posteriorly towards the center of the glenoid. In passive arm elevations it moves superiorly 0.5 mm from 60–90° and then inferiorly 1 mm from 90–150°. In active arm elevations it is 1 mm superior at 60°, then moves inferiorly to be centered on glenoid between 90–150° [10]. GH joint reactive forces (JRF) demonstrate this same pattern. As the arm abducts up to 120°, the JRF moves medially to increase compression as well as anteriorly and inferiorly to center in the socket [11]. The ICR and JRF do not move posteriorly in any part of arm elevation, minimizing shear or compression loads on the posterior labrum. This controlled system allows continuous and smooth motion of the arm while creating and maintaining GH concavity-compression and ball and socket kinematics, especially at higher levels of arm elevation [12].

The labrum is considered to have specific roles as a part of this integrated system of dynamic and static restraints that contribute to GH stability [13–15]. Specific properties of the labrum contribute to its ability to fulfill its roles (Fig. 15.1) [12, 15–20]. Labral anatomy varies according to its position on the glenoid. It has two distinct parts and an area of transition between the two parts [21]. The superior portion of the labrum, from approximately 10:30 to 1:30 on the right glenoid face, has a limited bony attachment on the glenoid rim and not on the glenoid face, has more mobility, has a concave articular surface, and is designed to be loaded in tension created by joint motion and biceps muscle activation, similar to a tension band. It has been characterized as a "mobile organ of tension." Its tension band function is coupled with the long head of the biceps and with the superior and middle glenohumeral ligaments to provide dynamic restraint to the humeral head translations [15, 22]. The inferior portion of the labrum, from approximately 10:30 around to 2:00 on the right glenoid face, has a rigid attachment on the glenoid rim and glenoid face, has a convex articular surface, is designed to be loaded in compression, and is in direct continuity with the inferior glenohumeral ligaments (IGHL) all of which create the bumper for edge stability [23]. It has been characterized as a "static organ of compression." Its function is coupled with rotator cuff activation as a compressor cuff and with developed tension in the IGHL to confer dynamic concavity/compression and precise ball and socket kinematics to optimize GH stability. The area of transition between the two parts, approximately at the 10:00 to 10:30 position on the right glenoid face, is the posterior attachment and anchor point for the mobile superior part, which allows the tension band function, and the superior attachment and anchor point for the immobile inferior part, which allows the bumper/edge stability function. It can be considered as a "rip stop," keeping tears that may arise from tensile or shear loads from propagating along the posterior glenoid rim.

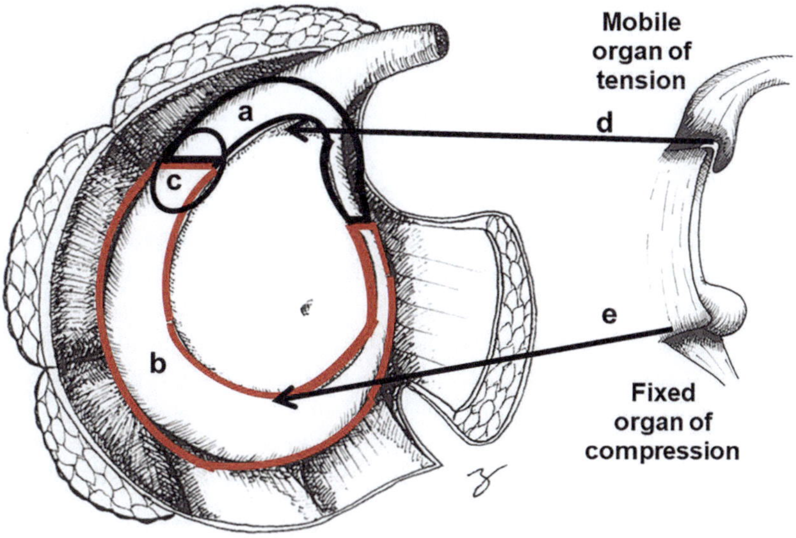

Fig. 15.1 Normal labral anatomy with call out illustrating the two anatomical areas, the mobile organ of tension (**a**) in the superior area, and the fixed organ of compression (**b**) in the inferior area, with the point of transition between the two areas, the rip stop (**c**). Arrows (**d, e**) illustrate the differences in the type of attachment to the glenoid of the organ of tension and organ of compression. (Figure used with permission from Andrew J. Sheean, MD, FAAOS)

Based on these anatomical and biomechanical findings, it appears that the labrum can play both dynamic and static roles in contributing to glenohumeral stability. The relatively mobile superior labrum, being anchored at the rip stop point, allows a large range of excursion in IR and ER through which the biceps can travel and still optimize tension to control humeral head translation. The inferior labrum, anchored superiorly at the rip stop point, can act as a static mechanical bumper to provide edge stability against shear forces, and as an attachment site for the ligaments [15, 23]. The entire labrum also can act as a dynamic deformable washer, spreading loads evenly across joint surfaces and increasing joint congruity when compression is applied through muscle activations [19, 24]. This property would facilitate the best mating of the two surfaces for joint lubrication, mobility, and stability [18, 25]. In addition, the deformable peripheral edges, by conforming to the surfaces and creating a stable circumferential boundary, maintain the intraarticular pressure that affects joint stability [24]. All of these roles allow the labrum to be the most precise of the restraints for control of GH stability, especially at high speeds of rotation, large changes in bone positions, and high compression, tension, and shear loads. Treatment of clinically significant anatomic labral injury should be directed at restoring these capabilities.

Integral to and facilitating the labral roles is the position and motion of the scapula. Scapular motions place the glenoid in mechanical positions that maximize GH concavity-compression and minimize humeral head translation within the glenoid [16, 26]. In the important ranges of 30–100° of arm elevation, the scapula is mechanically coupled through the tensed acromioclavicular and coracoclavicular ligaments and the acromioclavicular joint articulation with the clavicle to create the claviscapula segment. This integrated segment can produce smooth and consistent motion that places the glenoid in mechanically stable alignment with the humerus [9, 27]. Scapular motion in throwing athletes has two functions. First, the claviscapula develops specific three-dimensional constrained motions around the sternoclavicular, acromioclavicular, and scapulothoracic joints, guided by coupled activation of muscles attached to the ribs, spine, and core, to place the scapula, glenoid, and arm in position to perform the task. Second the claviscapula develops three-dimensional motions in horizontal ab/adduction, flexion/extension, ab/adduction, and internal/external rotation to maintain GH joint ball and socket kinematics throughout the entire range of arm motion in overhead activity and the throwing motion. Alterations in this composite motion are termed scapular dyskinesis [27, 28]. The dyskinesis is considered an impairment of the efficient mobility of the claviscapula segment of the shoulder complex [29, 30], creating possible shear and compression loads on the labrum [31].

15.3 The Role of the Biceps

The long head of the biceps is intimately associated with the labrum in shoulder anatomy, function, and dysfunction, and plays significant roles in shoulder biomechanics in the throwing athlete. It is an important stabilizing structure to the shoulder by facilitating GH joint concavity compression as well as by serving as a mechanical barrier to translation [32–36]. Due to its anatomic attachment at the supraglenoid tubercle and the posterior superior labrum, there is a degree of mobility of the biceps/labrum complex away from the glenoid with arm motion [13, 14]. The large majority of the biceps tendon fibers course into and are in continuity with the posterior superior labrum creating the biceps labrum complex, which constitutes a key element in the mechanical system around the glenohumeral joint serving to produce GH concavity/compression and optimal mechanics [14, 16, 25].

There is consistent evidence that the biceps plays an active role in producing optimal dynamic glenohumeral GH stability. Electromyographic data indicate that peak biceps muscle activation occurs in cocking (the maximum GH abduction/external rotation position) and in follow through (the maximum joint distraction position) [20, 22, 37, 38] pointing to a role of dynamically tensing the posterior labrum in these two high load positions that have been characterized as the critical positions in the throwing motion. This would be most important in throwing athletes who require the most efficient kinematics and kinetics. Biceps activation dynamizes the relatively loose attachment of the superior labrum and approximates it to the glenoid, creating the tension band effect on the superior labrum to increase joint stability throughout the entire range of shoulder motion [15, 21, 39]. It also produces a shoulder proximal force to resist and control the high distraction forces generated in throwing [38]. Biceps activation diminished strain on the anterior inferior GH ligaments in the abducted externally rotated position [41] and diminished GH translations in all directions and significantly centered the humeral axis of rotation in both external and internal rotation and posterior humeral head translation in external rotation was greatly lessened [40]. Biceps activation diminished strain on the anterior inferior glenohumeral GH ligaments in the abducted externally rotated position [41] and diminished glenohumeral GH translations in all directions [42–44]. These studies, in addition to electromyographic data are all in concordance with the role of the biceps as providing a significant restraint to excessive humeral head translation, especially in extremes of rotational motion [42].

Motion of the biceps, either by muscle activation or resulting from arm motion from maximum GH internal to external rotation, is very large. This motion places mainly shear and tensile strains on the biceps/labrum complex, which appear to be adequately dissipated in the radial and circumferential directions by normal biceps flexibility and an intact labrum with good attachments to the glenoid, especially posteriorly at the rip stop point. Biceps flexibility appears to be an important element in maintaining optimal biceps roles. Excessive biceps tension can result in increased labral strain and will increase the possibility of tear propagation of a labral injury that extends beyond the posterior superior attachment rip stop point (10:30 on the right shoulder, 1:30 on the left) [45]. The inflexibility can also create altered GH external rotation in abduction/external rotation and contribute to altered GH kinematics [46]. The biceps has been demonstrated to become adaptively tight following exposure to repetitive tensile strain [47, 48]. Conversely, excessive biceps flexibility has been demonstrated to result in increased humeral head translation on the glenoid in the mechanically undesired posterior and superior directions [34], which can place increased compression/shear loads on the posterior labrum.

15.4 Pathoanatomy and Pathomechanics of Clinically Significant Labral Injuries

Labral pathoanatomy has been traditionally described in relation to the injury to the superior labral and biceps attachment to the glenoid. This injury was believed to be the underlying pathology, and all the other tears seen were thought to be varieties of or extensions on the basic SLAP lesion. The original classification by Snyder included types I-IV [49]. Subsequent modifications described labral tears around the glenoid face, increasing the types from V-X [25, 50–54]. This classification system is based on arthroscopic findings, and is not related to specific injury mechanisms, physical exam findings, or clinical symptoms.

Recent literature has suggested that not all labral injuries or clinical symptoms in throwing athletes are associated with superior labral injuries [55–61]. Many asymptomatic players may show labral separation from the superior glenoid. This anatomy was described as "adaptive pathology," enabling throwers to achieve optimum the abduction/external rotation position to facilitate arm velocity [55, 62]. These studies demonstrate that injuries in multiple areas of the glenoid labrum may be clinically relevant and suggest that study of the incidence and location of labral injuries for these injuries may help increase understanding of the pathoanatomy involved in the DTS. Injuries located at the posterior labrum were the most common, comprising 78–86% of all labral injuries. Combined superior/posterior (SLAP VIII) injuries occurred in 48–49%, isolated posterior injuries occurred in 16–26%. Isolated superior labral injuries were uncommon—occurring in 7–8% of all labral injuries. Also, labral injuries involving more than one anatomic area of the glenoid (superior, anterior, posterior) were twice as common as those isolated into one area [58, 59].

These anatomic findings, in conjunction with the previously recorded relatively poor outcomes of treatment protocols based on the concept of the SLAP injury being the main pathoanatomy, move the emphasis regarding the pathoanatomy to a more holistic view of the labral injury. The term "SLAP" may not be the most inclusive or effective term through which investigation of pathoanatomy, pathophysiology, pathomechanics, and treatment of injuries in the DTS should proceed. The term clinically significant labral injury (CSLI) has been suggested as a concept to describe more specifically which labral tears represent the actual pathoanatomy and warrant surgical fixation [25, 63]. The CSLI concept, by focusing on injuries that may occur at several places on the entire glenoid, can be used as a framework for evaluating all possible anatomic alterations and as a basis for more specific surgical techniques. A CSLI lesion is defined as an anatomic injury occurring in any area of the glenoid labrum that results in clinical dysfunction that can be related to loss of specific roles of the labrum and can be identified by history, exam, and imaging with appropriate clinical symptoms. The main treatment implication of the CSLI concept is that arthroscopic evaluation of labral injuries should include inspection of all the areas of the glenoid, careful palpation and probing of the labral anatomy and contour to evaluate the different possible tear injury characteristics, and awareness of the possibility of sites of injury that may not involve the superior labrum [57–59, 61].

The pathomechanics associated with labral injuries in throwing athletes appear to be related to loss of control of normal humeral head translation so that there is either absolute or relative posterior humeral head motion in relation to the glenoid. Andrews et al. [20], Snyder et al. [49], Kuhn et al. [22], and Hwang et al. [45] suggested that the labral injury was mainly due to a traction injury from biceps tension in the extremes of shoulder cocking and follow through, described as the

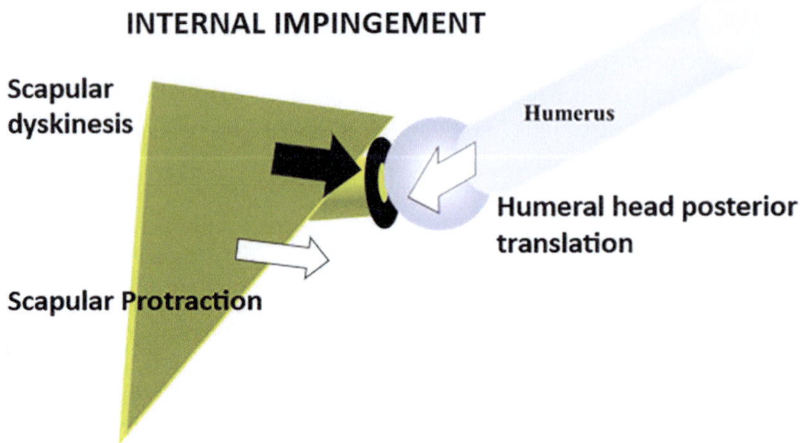

Fig. 15.2 Internal impingement results from a combination of scapular protraction and humeral head posterior translation (white arrows) which creates compression and shear forces (black arrow) across the posterior labrum (black ring)

"weed pulling" mechanism. Other authors suggested a mechanism more based on internal impingement involving the superior and posterior areas of the glenoid and labrum [55, 64–68]. Internal impingement represents a mechanical malalignment of the normal scapulohumeral axis and consists of excessive dynamic scapular protraction and posterior humeral head translation as the arm is placed in abduction and external rotation (Fig. 15.2) [26, 49, 65]. Causative factors for creating scapular protraction include excessive scapular internal rotation, anterior tilt, and loss of upward rotation, resulting from a combination of weakness/inhibition of the serratus anterior and lower trapezius muscles and tightness of the pectoralis minor and latissimus dorsi muscles. Causative factors for humeral head translation include alterations in GH joint IR and ER, biceps tightness, and increased humerus external rotation. The effect is to increase the amount of humeral head compression and shear on the posterior labrum [66].

The data demonstrate that both mechanisms can be present, probably dependent on other biomechanical and exposure factors. The studies demonstrating that a high percentage of CSLI injuries involve the superior/posterior labrum (SLAP II-IV, SLAP VIII, SLAP IX) or the posterior labrum (isolated posterior) agree with the two proposed mechanisms of causation.

In the overhead throwing motion, the superior and posterior labrum act statically and dynamically to facilitate glenohumeral concavity/compression in the two key high loading phases of cocking and follow through. In cocking, the labrum provides a bumper and an edge stability to mitigate posterior translation. In follow through, the biceps labral complex helps to control superior, anterior, and posterior translation because of its tension band and labral dynamization function. Labral injury can compromise these roles. The mechanical symptoms and "dead arm" most reported by injured athletes result from loss of the concavity/compression and edge stability from injury to the organ of compression, and the anterior symptoms may be related to the alteration of biceps tension in the organ of tension by loss of its rip stop anchor.

The biceps, as part of the biceps labral complex, plays roles in creating and maintaining dynamic glenohumeral concavity/compression and glenohumeral stability. The exact need for optimal biceps function may vary according to the mechanical needs of the individual athlete for arm position, force generation, and accuracy during the shoulder task. It appears to be most crucial for the baseball throwing motion, compared to other overhead athletic motions [69]. When the biceps anchor sites on the labrum are not intact, especially with posterior anchor injury at the rip stop, the loss of stability can be experienced as anterior shoulder pain. Treatment may be misdirected to focus on the biceps, when the actual pathoanatomy is the posterior labral injury.

15.5 Evaluation Techniques

Throwing athletes with CSLI pathoanatomy may have a variable presentation and history because of the pathomechanics. Pain is the most common presenting symptom [3, 70]. The pain may be experienced during all phases of the throwing motion, and may be associated with popping or catching during throwing, limited motion, and anterior/posterior instability. The pain reported is sometimes nonspecific and vague, but commonly it can be localized to the posterosuperior joint line, deep within the shoulder joint, most commonly in cocking to ball release, or it can radiate to the anterior aspect of the shoulder correlating with biceps-related symptoms in ball release to follow through. Pain can develop insidiously in the setting of chronic overuse or present acutely in the setting of an acute traumatic or acute on chronic event mechanism. Additionally, patients may present with mechanical symptoms such as clicking, locking, snapping, grinding, or instability depending on the extent of the injury. They may describe a feeling of a "dead arm," meaning decreased force production and difficulty in movement [71]. Alterations in performance parameters may include a decrease in velocity and control [72]. Decreased velocity and accuracy with associated shoulder discomfort are such common symptoms in throwing athletes with a CSLI injury that their presence should point towards that diagnosis. A poll of experienced shoulder surgeons reported that mechanical problems (clicking, catching, popping), difficulty in abduction/external rotation position, acute onset of symptoms, and stiffness were the most important findings in the history [70]. Overall, while the diagnostic accuracy of a patient's history is useful in identifying glenoid labral tears, it is most helpful when used in combination with the physical examination findings [73].

The physical exam is organized around range of motion, biceps evaluation, labral provocative tests, and scapular evaluation. Many patients will demonstrate altered GH range of motion, both in internal and external rotation. Alterations in external rotation have been demonstrated to be important as injury risk factors [74, 75] and external rotation can be affected by forearm position, indicating a role for biceps tightness [48]. Side to side differences in internal rotation greater than 18–20°, and total range of motion greater than 5° have been reported as increasing injury risk [74, 76–78].

To determine pathoanatomical sources of pain and/or dysfunction, an assessment of the long head of the biceps, the glenoid labrum, and other possible structures should be performed. The long head of the biceps can be examined by a combination of clinical tests. Tenderness to palpation over the biceps groove indicates some inflammation in the groove, although this should be compared to the contralateral non-throwing shoulder as biceps sensitivity is very common. Most clinical provocative tests evaluate increased tension in the biceps muscle/tendon. The Speed's test [79], the active compression test [80], and the upper cut test [81] are considered positive when the testing position and loading maneuvers produce pain on the anterior joint line and reproduce the clinical symptoms. Biceps tightness can be also estimated by the biceps eccentric test. The arm is placed at 90° abduction in the plane of the body, the elbow is flexed to maximum, then extended as the forearm is rotated into maximum pronation. Pain along the tightened biceps may be felt from the shoulder down to the elbow, indicating tightness as the biceps is lengthened [48].

Mechanical symptoms can sometimes be reproduced when the shoulder is placed in an abducted and externally rotated position. Multiple special tests have been described to assist in the diagnosis of a labral tear; however, these tests are highly variable in their reported clinical utility [51, 80–100]. These special tests do have diagnostic utility in the context of the complete history and shoulder examination, which is suggestive of labral pathology. Precision appears to be increased by selecting a combination of tests that can be consistently well performed in the examiner's hands to fortify their clinical suspicion for labral injuries. Although further assessments are required to determine its inclusion in a testing battery, the clinical test with the highest reported clinical utility is the Modified Dynamic

Labral Shear test [81]. A positive test is pain in the posterior joint line and is highly correlated with arthroscopic evidence of labral injury.

To determine if shoulder pain and/or dysfunction is being driven by scapular dysfunction or shoulder pathoanatomy, clinicians can establish the presence or absence of scapular dyskinesis with the scapular dyskinesis test and the scapular evaluation pathway to determine the causative factors for the dyskinesis [25, 30, 101–103].

While the great majority of symptomatic throwing athletes will have advanced imaging as part of the diagnostic evaluation, the exact role of imaging is still not clear. Many asymptomatic Major League Baseball pitchers and other throwers have SLAP, labral, and other shoulder pathologies [104, 105] and recent studies have shown that there is no correlation between MRI findings and location or clinical significance of the labral tear [59]. In addition, ascertainment of what are important thrower adaptations versus pathologic findings based solely on imaging is challenging. In summary, imaging should be best considered as confirmative, rather than solely diagnostic, especially as an individual modality.

15.6 Treatment Guidelines and Concepts of Functional Rehabilitation

Multiple surgical techniques are advocated to achieve the surgical goals of restoring optimal anatomy while minimizing morbidity. Several technical principles appear to optimize surgical success: First, avoid over-constraint of the biceps superior labrum complex. The entire complex is inherently mobile [15], and overly rigid suture constructs with high strength suture and anchors placed too close to the biceps origin will result in over-constraint and prevent the thrower from attaining full external rotation. An anchor placed anterior to or within 1 cm on either side of the biceps base (i.e.more superior than 10:30 positioning) will produce too much restriction of biceps mobility and prevent the increase in humeral external rotation needed for velocity plus reduce the biceps function as a tension band [106]. Many of the failures of labral repairs to return athletes to overhead sports activities can be shown to be due to the acquired biceps tightness and consequent loss of GH external rotation. Second, restore the bumper function of the inferior labrum. Restoration of labral height has been correlated with improved outcomes [107]. Anchors for repair of the inferior labrum should be placed 4 mm onto the glenoid surface in order to reproduce native anatomy [15]. Knotless anchors may allow a more anatomic repair to restore the bumper function [108]. Third, evaluate for and address the posterior and combined injuries. These are the most common types of labral injuries, and the failure to restore the posterior bumper function will compromise edge stability [58, 59]. The "Kim Lesion," an injury to the posterior labrum and the attachment of the PIGHL [60], must be sought, since the important PIGHL attaches to the glenoid and posterior inferior labrum at around 6:30–7:00 [23]. One way to discern if native anatomy is restored is to inspect tension of the PIGHL. Repair of the tear at this level will reconstitute normal tension in this critical structure. Fourth, conduct a careful evaluation before considering employing a biceps tenodesis as part of or the only treatment of labral injuries. Biceps tenodesis can result in early pain relief but it may be at the expense of introducing instability, excessive posterior translation, and increased shear forces on the glenoid surface due to increased translation at motion extremes accompanied by inability to return to throwing activities [34, 43, 69, 109]. One study demonstrated that biceps tenodesis could be recommended in certain types of athletes who perform overhead motions, but not in baseball throwing athletes [69], who require the extra dynamic humeral head control and ball and socket kinematics throughout the large ranges of motion and high compression and distraction loads that result in the most effective "launch window" that optimizes velocity and ball location [72]. In some cases of overhead athletes with anterior shoulder pain around the biceps, the actual pathoanatomy will be a posterior labral tear with loss of the rip stop so that there is excessive biceps tensile load. Treatment for these cases is posterior labral repair and rehabilitation of biceps tightness. These athletes will demonstrate biceps tightness and positive tests for labral injury.

15.7 Rehabilitation

Rehabilitation has not been evaluated or demonstrated to provide an enhancement of blood supply or scarring to or around the injured labrum suggesting "healing" has occurred. Although the impact on the labral injury is minimal, rehabilitation can reduce or eliminate impairments often seen with known labral injury. For example, Fedoriw et al. [110] reported a 40% return-to-play rate for 21 professional-level baseball pitchers with verified SLAP lesions who were treated with nonoperative methods that focused on mobility improvement and improving scapular-based impairments. These rates were relatively similar for the 27 pitchers who underwent operative treatments (48% return-to-play). Conversely, although a 39% return-to-play rate was noted for 10 position players treated nonoperatively, the return-to-play rate for 13 position players who underwent surgery was 85%. This suggests that nonoperative measures may have similar expected outcomes between positions, but surgical interventions likely favor non-pitching positions in baseball. Hashiguchi et al. [111] retrospectively examined the outcomes of baseball players participating at various levels (high school through professional teams). The group identified that patients with improvement in total range of motion and internal rotation after 2 months of treatment had increased chances of having successful nonoperative treatment (13.8 times and 5.8 times respectively). Finally, Yoon et al. [112], administered a comprehensive 12-week program to 13 baseball players with shoulder instability (cause of instability was not specified) and 12 control subjects without instability. The program was reported to be effective at reducing pain and increasing proprioception in the subjects with instability.

Nonoperative management of labral injury in a combination of athletes and nonathletes has also been examined. Edwards et al. [113] reported improvements in pain and self-reported function following nonoperative use of nonsteroidal anti-inflammatory drugs and multimodal rehabilitation in patients who are identified as recreational or competitive athletes. Shin et al. [114] reported improvements in similar metrics in a cohort that was between 30–45 years old and who underwent corticoteroid injection with combined rotator cuff and scapular muscle strengthening. Jang et al. [115] described predictors of failing nonoperative treatment of type II SLAP injuries, with the significant risk factors of a negative outcome being overhead activity (19 times likely), presence of trauma (9.8 times likely), and a positive compression-rotation test (8.8 times likely). The sample included 63 patients, with a 71% success rate; however, the sample included a heterogenous portion of 17 overhead athletes representing multiple sports. Across the studies, the treatment programs were multifaceted containing interventions such as electrical modalities, stretching, scapular exercises, rotator cuff exercises, proprioception training, and/or plyometrics. However, frequency of performance, intensity/loading, and/or sets/repetitions were not reported, so the results must be interpreted with caution. Although these reports show nonoperative treatments may have value, further comparative studies with and between groups should be conducted along with empirical studies investigating the effectiveness of specific interventions.

In a recent clinical commentary, Sciascia noted that scapular dysfunction (dyskinesis) most often occurs due to an imbalance between the scapular kinematics where the scapula is predominantly positioned or moving into internal rotation and anterior tilt which places the glenoid face in an anterior-inferior orientation [116]. As a result, scapular dyskinesis could negatively impact the glenoid labrum because the humeral head will not be centered within the joint during arm movement. Thus, the humeral head will contact the glenoid earlier than anticipated in arm elevation or abduction which in turn creates atypical contact/compressive forces on the anterior glenoid face/rim and labrum resulting in unexpected pain. This phenomenon provides an explanation as to why altered scapular positioning or posture correlates with a variety of conditions [117–124]. It also explains why there can be difficulty in identifying clinically significant labral injury in overhead athletes [39, 57, 125]. The repetitious nature of overhead activity combined with an anterior-inferior oriented glenoid creates a potential scenario where the early contact of the humeral head on the glenoid can irritate or injure the labrum. Accounting for scapular position as a possible contributor to shoulder pain and/or labral involvement is important because clinicians need to discern if the patient has labral "symptoms" versus labral injury. Labral symptoms would align with the presentation of labral injury (pain, positive labral specific special tests, and possible subjective complaints of "dead arm") except that the symptoms reduce or eliminate when the scapula is properly repositioned on clinical examination via the scapular assistance test and/or scapular retraction test [29, 30, 126]. This suggests that pathoanatomic sources of pain attributed to labral injury should be comprehensively evaluated before surgical treatment is rendered. If symptoms can be positively modified on examination (i.e., reduced or eliminated), then labral injury may not necessarily be present which allows clinicians to employ conservative treatment as an initial intervention [110, 113].

One of the common impairments present in patients with labral injury is altered mobility. Alterations in mobility (glenohumeral internal rotation, external rotation, and total arc of motion) have been linked with increased injury risk in the shoulder and elbow in overhead athletes [74, 77, 78, 127–134]. Considering that not all deficits in motion are pathologic, it is not recommended that every patient participate in a preemptive mobility program. It is recommended that these objective thresholds be utilized to employ interventions to enhance mobility for the examination to guide the treatment. Common interventions such as stretching, massage, and/or joint mobilization can be employed for addressing mobility deficits. However, a comprehensive review of commonly seen rotational range of motion deficits noted that there is no clear "best" method for addressing soft tissue inflexibilities in overhead athletes [76]. Using the literature and clinical experience as a guide, the authors of that review suggested the following: (1) clinicians should employ low load, long duration stretching but not as a part of pre-throwing warm-up regimens; (2) static stretching, self-stretching, and plyometric-based stretching are encouraged to be performed as part of the pre-activity (warm-up) regimens; (3) joint mobilizations are permissible but the clinician needs to account for joint position, load applied, technique (oscillations, tractions, or both), and number of bouts; and (4) objective range of motion and subjective end-feels should be assessed prior to employing joint mobilizations to determine if this type of manual therapy technique is applicable to the individual patient [76]. Using these principles as a guide, clinicians have the autonomy to develop mobility programs that are specific to each patient's needs, but in most cases, the latissimus dorsi, pectoralis major and minor, posterior rotator cuff muscles, and biceps brachii muscles in addition to the shoulder capsule will be the points of focus.

Another impairment that will likely exist is a deficit in strength of one or more muscle groups around the scapula and shoulder. It should be noted that strength deficits are typically noted to exist based on manual muscle testing findings. Manual muscle testing is flawed due to the frequent use of subjective grading of strength (force output as measured by dynamometers can be utilized but this is not standard practice), lack of standardized hand placement for resistance between clinicians, and assuming a manual test provides information specific to a single muscle [135–138]. Objective measurements of the ability to generate force are best captured with devices that provide quantifiable output such as spring balance gauges, digital handheld dynamometers, or isokinetic units should be utilized [136, 139–151]. As strength relates to the integrity of the labrum, a recent study that comprised of non-overhead athletes (American football and wrestling athletes) reported decreased peak force 3–4 months after labral repair within the injured arm but no differences in a physical performance test that assesses dynamic balance [152].

If strength is to be addressed during rehabilitation, the intent is to reestablish scapulohumeral rhythm through increasing scapular muscle activation and control along with optimizing rotator cuff concavity-compression. To best achieve these goals, it is recommended patients perform exercises in upright positions rather than supine or prone positions to simulate functional demands and reduce joint position sense errors [153]. Arm motions should be initiated using the legs and trunk to facilitate activation of the scapula and shoulder muscles. This is known as kinetic chain sequencing that drives upper extremity function [154–166]. The lever arm on the shoulder and trunk is recommended to be shortened in earlier phases of rehabilitation to reduce the load and torque on the injured arm. The exercises shown to elicit high amounts of muscle activity require the arm to be maintained in a set position throughout a range of motion and involve the arm to be further away from the body (also known as long lever exercises) thus increasing the demands on the muscles i.e., increased force output and torque generation [167]. Conversely, exercises that are performed with the elbow in 90° of flexion and/or with the arm close to the body (i.e., short lever exercises) elicit lower levels of muscle activity and have decreased demands on the muscles [168–170]. Either long lever or short lever exercises are acceptable to use in rehabilitation; however, the timing of implementation may cause different outcomes. Due to the physical demands of long lever exercises, patients may experience irritation or soreness during or after the performance of the maneuvers when they are employed early in the rehabilitation process. Additionally, it is also assumed that the greater demands require more effort be exerted to perform the exercises, which may conflict with a patient attempting to establish scapular control early in the rehabilitation program. This could potentially create a situation where the patient becomes fatigued early in treatment sessions which in turn could cause the patient to utilize compensatory movement patterns during exercise performance. Short lever exercises allow patients to focus on the stability function of the scapula in order to establish the foundation for rotator cuff and global muscle activation.

Sciascia and Kibler have opined that due to the known flaws with clinical strength testing, it is possible that motor control may be more effective compared to focusing on strengthening during rehabilitation [103]. They noted that patients are inherently disadvantaged when attempting to learn proper scapular motion because the scapula cannot be visualized due to its posterior location on the thorax. The lack of visual feedback leads to the alterations in motion known as scapular dyskinesis. This concept has merit based on the previous reports which have shown that intentional attempts at repositioning the scapula prior to elevating and/or rotating the humerus and various uses of feedback (visual, auditory, and kinesthetic) have been shown to positively influence scapular muscle activity and positioning [171–178]. Considering the scapula as a "link" within the kinetic chain and the labrum is positioned on the scapula, the feedback approach may be better suited for reestablishing scapular control and scapulohumeral rhythm as it relates to the sequential activation within the kinetic chain. Although previous works have verified increased shoulder and scapular muscle activation when trunk and/or leg movements are integrated into the exercise maneuvers, there are no empirical reports or randomized trials that have compared a motor control/kinetic chain focused program against a program that does not utilize this approach [168, 169, 179–182]. Instead, clinical recommendations supporting motor control/kinetic chain-based rehabilitation approaches have been made via expert opinion/consensus papers [29, 30, 55, 183–185], with the key guidelines being:

1. Short lever progression.
2. Sitting and standing preferred over prone or supine exercises.
3. Target impairments in the order of mobility, motor control, strength (if necessary), and endurance.
4. Utilize longer lever maneuvers later in the rehabilitation program.
5. Advance to plyometric-based maneuvers just prior to discharge.

When clinical examinations reveal obvious physical impairments (weakness, inflexibility, early fatigue with motion, compensatory movements, etc.) or pathology, activity restriction and the development of a formal rehabilitation program are recommended. Removing the insulting or exacerbating activity can minimize loading and allow rehabilitation to reintroduce the proper activations that create scapulohumeral rhythm [110]. However, in many instances, a patient will report symptoms yet the clinician does not identify any impairments or causes for concern from the clinical physical examination. In these instances, it is recommended that clinicians consider biomechnical causes of pain and dysfunction. It is possible that arm mechanics are faulty and are creating loads and stresses that result in irritation, pain, and/or injury. Although there is no standardized method to throw, serve, swing, or otherwise use the arm overhead, there are mechanics that should be avoided as they have been shown to alter the loads and stresses seen at various joints during activity [38, 186–193]. Biomechanical consultations may be needed to identify if flaws exist that could be contributing to the patients complaints.

Finally, nonoperative rehabilitation and postoperative rehabilitation for the labrum do not differ substantially. The interventions employed for improving symptoms, mobility, strength, motor control, and other physiological components are similar, but will differ in the timing of implementation [55, 194, 195]. The timing differs primarily due to the range of motion and loading restrictions implemented following surgical repair [195]. However, the decision to manage a labral injury nonoperatively or surgically requires communication between the rehabilitation clinician and surgeon. In nonoperative scenarios, communication should include whether labral injury is suspected based on clinical examination versus imaging (or both), whether any concomitant injury is present, and the timeframe for removal from activity. These items are important as the rehabilitation clinician will need to manage third-party payer implemented caps on rehabilitation visits and plan accordingly in terms of rest and progression. In postoperative scenarios, it is vitally important to share the surgical technique and anatomical tissue details between providers. The number of and location of anchors is crucial to discuss. Anchors placed superiorly between 11:00 and 1:00, especially anchors placed at 12:00, can create stiffness in the biceps tendon which in turn can create a ceiling effect in glenohumeral range of motion restoration. Clinicians who are aware of persistent tissue stiffness but not aware of anchor placement are at risk of applying higher than tolerated loads during rehabilitation which can result in biceps tendonitis or other load-based consequences. Similarly, sharing the integrity of the long head of the biceps tendon, capsule thickness, and presence of arthritic changes will assist the rehabilitation clinician with selecting interventions and timeframes for implementation.

References

1. Lubowitz JH. Lesions of the superior labrum from anterior to posterior (SLAP) are a slap in the face to the traditional trinity of history, examination, and imaging. Arthroscopy. 2015;31:2470–1.
2. Knesek M, Skendzel JG, Dines JS, Altchek DW, Allen AA, Bedi A. Diagnosis and management of superior labral anterior posterior tears in throwing athletes. Am J Sports Med. 2013;41:444–60.
3. Keener JD, Brophy RH. Superior labral tears of the shoulder: pathogenesis, evaluation, and treatment. J Am Acad Orthop Surg. 2009;17:627–37.
4. Gorantla K, Gill C, Wright RW. The outcome of type II SLAP repair: a systematic review. Arthroscopy. 2010;26(4):537–45.
5. Sciascia AD, Myers N, Kibler WB, Uhl TL. Return to pre-injury levels of play following superior labral repair in overhead athletes: a systematic review. J Athl Train. 2015;50(7):767–77.
6. Werner BC, Brockmeier SF, Miller MD. Etiology, diagnosis, and management of failed slap repair. J Am Acad Orthop Surg. 2014;22:554–65.
7. Taylor SA, Newman AM, Nguyen J, et al. Magnetic resonance imaging currently fails to fully evaluate the biceps-labrum complex and bicipital tunnel. Arthroscopy. 2016;32:238–44.
8. Calcei JG, Boddapati V, Altchek DW, Camp CL, Dines JS. Diagnosis and treatment of injuries to the biceps and superior labral complex in overhead athletes. Curr Rev Musculoskelet Med. 2018;11:63–71.
9. Dvir Z, Berme N. The shoulder complex in elevation of the arm: a mechanism approach. J Biomech. 1978;11:219–25.

10. Graichen H, Stammberger T, Bonel H, Karl-Hans E, Reiser M, Eckstein F. Glenohumeral translation during active and passive elevation of the shoulder—a 3D open-MRI study. J Biomech. 2000;33(5):609–13.
11. Gupta S, van der Helm FCT. Load transfer across the scapula during humeral abduction. J Biomech. 2004;37:1001–9.
12. Howell SM, Galinat BJ. The glenoid-labral socket, a constrained articular surface. Clin Orthop Relat Res. 1989;243:122–5.
13. Cooper DE, Arnoczky SP, O'Brien SJ, Warren RF, DiCarlo E, Allen AA. Anatomy, histology, and vascularity of the glenoid labrum. J Bone Joint Surg Am. 1992;74A(1):46–52.
14. Vangsness CT, Jorgenson SS, Watson T, Johnson DL. The origin of the long head of the biceps from the scapula and glenoid labrum. An anatomical study of 100 shoulders. J Bone Joint Surg Br. 1994;76(6):951–4.
15. Bain GI, Galley IJ, Singh C, Carter C, Eng K. Anatomic study of the superior glenoid labrum. Clin Anat. 2013;26:367–76.
16. Lippitt S, Vanderhooft JE, Harris SL, Sidles JA, Harryman Ii DT, Matsen Iii FA. Glenohumeral stability from concavity-compression: a quantitative analysis. J Shoulder Elb Surg. 1993;2(1):27–35.
17. Soslowsky LJ, Flatow EL, Bigliani LU, Mow VC. Articular geometry of the glenohumeral joint. Clin Orthop Relat Res. 1992;285:181–90.
18. Soslowsky LJ, Flatow EL, Bigliani LU, Pawluk RJ, Ateshian GA, Mow VC. Quantitation of in situ contact areas at the glenohumeral joint: a biomechanical study. J Orthop Res. 1992;10:524–34.
19. Carey J, Small CF, Pichora DR. In situ compressive properties of the glenoid labrum. J Biomed Mater Res. 2000;51(4):711–6.
20. Andrews JR. Glenoid labrum tears related to the long head of the biceps. Am J Sports Med. 1985;13(5):337–41.
21. Bain GI, Phadnis J, Itoi E, et al. Shoulder crane: a concept of suspension, stability, control, and motion. Joint Dis Orthop Sports Med 2019;4 2:63–70.
22. Kuhn JE, Lindholm SR, Huston LJ, Soslowsky LJ, Blasier RB. Failure of the biceps-superior labral complex: a cadaveric biomechanical investigation comparing the positions of late cocking and early deceleration. Arthroscopy. 2003;19(4):373–9.
23. Koga A, Itoigawa Y, Wada T, et al. Anatomic analysis of the attachment of the posteroinferior labrum and capsule to the glenoid: a cadaveric study. Arthroscopy. 2020;36:2814–9.
24. Veeger HEJ, van der Helm FCT. Shoulder function: the perfect compromise between mobility and stability. J Biomech. 2007;40:2119–29.
25. Eichinger JK, Li X, Cohen SB, et al. American shoulder and elbow surgeons slap/biceps anchor study group evidence review: pathoanatomy and diagnosis in clinically significant labral injuries. J Shoulder Elb Surg. 2023;32:e179–90.
26. Jobe FW, Kvitne RS, Giangarra CE. Shoulder pain in the overhand or throwing athlete the relationship of anterior instability and rotator cuff impingement. Orthop Rev. 1989;18(9):963–75.
27. Kibler WB, Sciascia A, Grantham WJ. The shoulder joint complex in the throwing motion. J Shoulder Elb Surg. 2024;33:443–9.
28. Kibler WB, McMullen J. Scapular dyskinesis and its relation to shoulder pain. J Am Acad Orthop Surg. 2003;11:142–51.
29. Kibler WB, Ludewig PM, McClure PW, Uhl TL, Sciascia AD. Scapula Summit 2009. J Orthop Sports Phys Ther. 2009;39(11):A1–A13.
30. Kibler WB, Ludewig PM, McClure PW, Michener LA, Bak K, Sciascia AD. Clinical implications of scapular dyskinesis in shoulder injury: the 2013 consensus statement from the "scapula summit". Br J Sports Med. 2013;47:877–85.
31. Yeh ML, Linter D, Luo ZP. Stress distribution in the superior labrum during the throwing motion. Am J Sports Med. 2005;33:395–401.
32. Itoi E, Kuechle DK, Newman SR, Morrey B, An KN. Stabilising function of the biceps in stable and unstable shoulders. J Bone Joint Surg Br. 1993;75(4):546–50.
33. Pagnani MJ, Deng X, Warren RF, Torzilli PA, O'Brien SJ. Role of the long head of the biceps brachii in glenohumeral stability: a biomechanical study in cadavera. J Shoulder Elb Surg. 1996;5:255–62.
34. Rauck RC, Jahandar A, Kontaxis A, et al. The role of the long head of the biceps tendon in posterior shoulder stabilization during forward flexion. J Shoulder Elb Surg. 2022;31:1254–60.
35. Burns JP, Bahk MS, Snyder SJ. Superior labral tears: repair versus biceps tenodesis. J Shoulder Elb Surg. 2011;20:S2–8.
36. Patzer T, Habermeyer P, Hurschler C, et al. The influence of superior labrum anterior to posterior (SLAP) repair on restoring baseline glenohumeral translation and increased biceps loading after simulated SLAP tear and the effectiveness of SLAP repair after long head of biceps tenotomy. J Shoulder Elb Surg. 2012;21:1580–7.
37. DiGiovine NM, Jobe FW, Pink M, Perry J. An electromyographic analysis of the upper extremity in pitching. J Shoulder Elb Surg. 1992;1(1):15–25.
38. Fleisig GS, Barrentine SW, Escamilla RF, Andrews JR. Biomechanics of overhand throwing with implications for injuries. Sports Med. 1996;21:421–37.
39. Kibler WB, Sciascia A, Tokish JT, et al. Disabled throwing shoulder: 2021 update: part 2—pathomechanics and treatment. Arthroscopy. 2022;38:1727–48.
40. Rodosky MW, Harner CD, Fu FH. The role of the long head of the biceps muscle and superior glenoid labrum in anterior stability of the shoulder. Am J Sports Med. 1994;22(1):121–30.
41. Youm T, ElAttrache NS, Tibone JE, McGarry MH, Lee TQ. The effect of the long head of the biceps

on glenohumeral kinematics. J Shoulder Elb Surg. 2009;18(1):122–9.
42. Alexander S, Southgate DFL, Bull AMJ, Wallace AL. The role of negative intraarticular pressure and the long head of biceps tendon on passive stability of the glenohumeral joint. J Shoulder Elb Surg. 2013;22:94–101.
43. Garg R, Boydtsun SM, Shafer BI, McGarry MH, Adamson GJ, Lee TQ. Role of the biceps tendon as a humeral head depressor. In: Romeo AA, Erickson BJ, Griffin JW, editors. The management of biceps pathology. Champaign: Springer; 2021. p. 77–85.
44. Kumar VP, Satku K, Balasubramianium P. The role of the long head of biceps brachii in the stabilization of the head of the humerus. Clin Orthop Relat Res. 1989;244:172–5.
45. Hwang E, Hughes RE, Palmer ML, Carpenter JE. Effects of biceps tension on the torn superior glenoid labrum. J Orthop Res. 2015;33(10):1545–51.
46. Mihata T, McGarry MH, Kinoshita M, Lee TQ. Excessive glenohumeral horizontal abduction as occurs during the late cocking phase of the throwing motion can be criticial for internal impingement. Am J Sports Med. 2010;38(2):369–82.
47. Jones DA, Newham DJ, Clarkson PM. Skeletal muscle stiffness and pain following eccentric exercise of the elbow flexors. Pain. 1987;30:233–42.
48. Kibler WB, Sciascia A, Pike JSM, Howell M, Wilk KE. Effect of forearm position on glenohumeral external rotation measurements in baseball players. Sports Health. 2022;14:577–84.
49. Snyder SJ, Karzel RP, Del Pizzo W, Ferkel RD, Friedman MJ. SLAP lesions of the shoulder. Arthroscopy. 1990;6(4):274–9.
50. Maffet MW, Gartsman GM, Moseley B. Superior labrum-biceps tendon complex lesions of the shoulder. Am J Sports Med. 1995;23(1):93–8.
51. Morgan CD, Burkhart SS, Palmeri M, Gillespie M. Type II SLAP lesions: three subtypes and their relationships to superior instability and rotator cuff tears. Arthroscopy. 1998;14(6):553–65.
52. Clavert P. Glenoid labrum pathology. Orthop Traumatol Surg Res. 2015;101:S19–24.
53. Elser F, Braun S, Dewing CB, Giphart JE, Millett PJ. Anatomy, function, injuries, and treatment of the long head of the biceps brachii tendon. Arthroscopy. 2011;27:581–92.
54. Ilahi OA, Labbe MR, P. C. Variants of the anterosuperior glenoid labrum and associated pathology. Arthroscopy. 2002;18:882–6.
55. Kibler WB, Kuhn JE, Wilk KE, et al. The disabled throwing shoulder—Spectrum of pathology: 10 year update. Arthroscopy. 2013;29(1):141–61.
56. Kibler WB, Sciascia A. New paradigms for the throwing shoulder: labral injury, surgery, and rehabilitation. In: Huddleston JI, Lieberman JR, editors. Instructional course lectures, vol. 68. Rosemont: American Academy of Orthopaedic Surgeons/Wolters Kluwer; 2019. p. 500–12.
57. Sheean AJ, Kibler WB, Conway J, Bradley JP. Posterior labral injury and glenohumeral instability in overhead athletes: current concepts for diagnosis and management. J Am Acad Orthop Surg. 2020;28:628–37.
58. Kibler WB, Grantham WJ, Pike JSM, Sciascia AD. Glenoid labral injuries are more common posteriorly than superiorly and are combined across multiple areas of the glenoid. Arthrosc Sports Med Rehabil. 2022;4:e535–44.
59. Alexeev M, Kercher JS, Levina Y, Duralde XA. Variability of glenoid labral tear patterns: a study of 280 sequential surgical cases. J Shoulder Elb Surg. 2021;30:2762–6.
60. Kim SH, Ha KI, Yoo JC, Noh KC. Kim's lesions: an incomplete and concealed avulsion oof the postero inferior labrum. Arthroscopy. 2004;20:712–20.
61. Kim JH, Ahn J, Shin SJ. Occult, incomplete, and complete posterior labral tears without glenohumeral instability on imaging underestimate labral detachment. Arthroscopy. 2024;40:58–67.
62. Kuhn JE. Adaptive pathology: new insights into the physical examination and imaging of the thrower's shoulder and elbow. J Shoulder Elb Surg. 2024;33:474–93.
63. Kibler WB. What is a clinically important superior labrum anterior to posterior tear? In: Pagano MW, Hart RA, editors. Instructional course lectures, vol. 62. Rosemont: American Academy of Orthopaedic Surgeons; 2013. p. 483–9.
64. Burkhart SS, Morgan CD, Kibler WB. The disabled throwing shoulder: spectrum of pathology part I: pathoanatomy and biomechanics. Arthroscopy. 2003;19(4):404–20.
65. Mihata T, Jun BJ, Bui CN, et al. Effect of scapular orientation on shoulder internal impingement in a cadaveric model of the cocking phase of throwing. J Bone Joint Surg Am. 2012;94(17):1576–83.
66. Itami Y, Mihata T, McGarry MH, et al. Effect of increased scapular internal rotation on glenohumeral external rotation and elbow valgus load in the late cocking phase of throwing motion. Am J Sports Med. 2018;46:3182–8.
67. Gelber JD, Soloff L, Schickendantz MS. The thrower's shoulder. J Am Acad Orthop Surg. 2018;26:204–13.
68. Kibler WB, Sciascia A, Tokish JT, et al. Disabled throwing shoulder 2021 update: part 1—anatomy and mechanics. Arthroscopy. 2022;38:1714–26.
69. Klemt C, Toderita D, Reilly P, Bull AMJ. Biceps tenodesis cannot be used as primary treatment option in baseball pitchers with intact rotator cuff muscles. Clin Biomech. 2022;100:105819.
70. Kibler WB, Sciascia A. Current practice for the diagnosis of a superior labral anterior to posterior (slap) lesion: systematic review and physician survey. Arthroscopy. 2015;31(12):2456–69.
71. Burkhart SS, Morgan CD, Kibler WB. Shoulder injuries in overhead athletes, the "dead arm" revisited. Clin Sports Med. 2000;19(1):125–58.

72. Stone AV, Platt BN, Collofello BS, Sciascia AD, Uhl TL, Kibler WB. More elevated fastballs associated with placement on the injured list due to shoulder injury. Arthrosc Sports Med Rehabil. 2022;4:e623–8.
73. Michener LA, Abrams JS, Huxel Bliven KC, et al. National athletic trainers' association position statement: evaluation, management, and outcomes of and return-to—play criteria for overhead athletes with superior labral anterior-posterior injuries. J Athl Train. 2018;53:209–29.
74. Pozzi F, Plummer HA, Shanley E, et al. Preseason shoulder range of motion screening and in-season risk of shoulder and elbow injuries in overhead athletes: systematic review and meta-analysis. Br J Sports Med. 2020;54:1019–27.
75. Agresta CE, Krieg K, Freehill MT. Risk factors for baseball-related arm injuries: a systematic review. Orthop J Sports Med. 2019;7:2325967119825557.
76. Manske R, Wilk KE, Davies G, Ellenbecker T, Reinold M. Glenohumeral motion deficits: friend or foe? Int J Sports Phys Ther. 2013;8:537–53.
77. Wilk KE, Macrina LC, Fleisig GS, et al. Deficits in glenohumeral passive range of motion increase risk of shoulder injury in professional baseball pitchers: a prospective study. Am J Sports Med. 2015;43(10):2379–85.
78. Shanley E, Rauh MJ, Michener L, Ellenbecker TS, Garrison JC, Thigpen CA. Shoulder range of motion measures as risk factors for shoulder and elbow injuries in high school softball and baseball players. Am J Sports Med. 2006;39:1997–2006.
79. Crenshaw AH, Kilgore WE. Surgical treatment of bicipital tenosynovitis. J Bone Joint Surg Am. 1966;48A(8):1496–502.
80. O'Brien SJ, Pagnani MJ, Fealy S, McGlynn SR, Wilson JB. The active compression test: a new and effective test for diagnosing labral tears and acromioclavicular joint abnormality. Am J Sports Med. 1998;26(5):610–3.
81. Kibler WB, Sciascia AD, Dome DC, Hester PW, Jacobs C. Clinical utility of new and traditional exam tests for biceps and superior glenoid labral injuries. Am J Sports Med. 2009;37(9):1840–7.
82. Kim SH, Ha KI, Han KY. Biceps load test: a clinical test for superior labrum anterior and posterior lesions in shoulders with recurrent anterior dislocations. Am J Sports Med. 1999;27(3):300–3.
83. Kibler WB. Specificity and sensitivity of the anterior slide test in throwing athletes with superior glenoid labral tears. Arthroscopy. 1995;11(3):296–300.
84. Hegedus EJ, Goode A, Campbell S, et al. Physical examination tests of the shoulder: a systematic review with meta-analysis of individual tests. Br J Sports Med. 2008;42:80–92.
85. Hegedus EJ, Goode AP, Cook CE, et al. Which physical examination tests provide clinicians with the most value when examining the shoulder? Update of a systematic review with meta-analysis of individual tests. Br J Sports Med. 2012;46:964–78.
86. Walsworth MK, Doukas WC, Murphy KP, Mielcarek BJ, Michener LA. Reliability and diagnostic accuracy of history and physical examination for diagnosing glenoid labral tears. Am J Sports Med. 2008;36(1):162–8.
87. Schlechter JA, Summa S, Rubin BD. The passive distraction test: a new diagnostic aid for clinically significant superior labral pathology. Arthroscopy. 2009;25:1374–9.
88. Oh JH, Kim JY, Kim WS, Gong HS, Lee JH. The evaluation of various physical examinations for the diagnosis of type II superior labrum anterior and posterior lesion. Am J Sports Med. 2008;36(2):353–9.
89. Parentis MA, Glousman RE, Mohr KS, Yocum LA. An evaluation of the provocative tests for superior labral anterior posterior lesions. Am J Sports Med. 2006;34(2):265–8.
90. McFarland EG, Kim TK, Savino RM. Clinical assessment of three common tests for superior labral anterior-posterior lesions. Am J Sports Med. 2002;30(6):810–5.
91. Mimori K, Muneta T, Nakagawa T, Shinomiya K. A new pain provocation test for superior labral tears of the shoulder. Am J Sports Med. 1999;27(2):137–42.
92. Nakagawa S, Yoneda M, Hayashida K, Obata M, Fukushima S, Miyazaki Y. Forced shoulder abduction and elbow flexion test: a new simple clinical test to detect superior labral injury in the throwing shoulder. Arthroscopy. 2005;21(11):1290–5.
93. Guanche CA, Jones DC. Clinical testing for tears of the glenoid labrum. Arthroscopy. 2003;19(5):517–23.
94. Myers TH, Zemanovic JR, Andrews JR. The resisted supination external rotation test: a new test for the diagnosis of superior labral anterior posterior lesions. Am J Sports Med. 2005;33(9):1315–20.
95. Ebinger N, Magosch P, Lichtenberg S, Habermeyer P. A new SLAP test: the supine flexion resistance test. Arthroscopy. 2008;24:500–5.
96. Cook C, Beaty S, Kissenberth MJ, Siffri P, Pill SG, Hawkins RJ. Diagnostic accuracy of five orthopedic clinical tests for diagnosis of superior labrum anterior posterior (SLAP) lesions. J Shoulder Elb Surg. 2012;21:13–22.
97. Fowler EM, Horsley IG, Rolf CG. Clinical and arthroscopic findings in recreationally active patients. Sports Med Arthrosc Rehabil Ther Technol. 2010;2(2):1–8.
98. Liu SH, Henry MH, Nuccion SL. A prospective evaluation of a new physical examination in predicting glenoid labral tears. Am J Sports Med. 1996;24(6):721–5.
99. Kim SH, Ha KI, Ahn JH, Kim SH, Choi HJ. Biceps load test II: a clinical test for SLAP lesions of the shoulder. Arthroscopy. 2001;17:160–4.
100. Jia X, Peterson SA, Khosravi AH, Almareddi V, Pannirselvam V, McFarland EG. Examination of the shoulder: the past, the present, and the future. J Bone Joint Surg Am. 2009;91(Suppl 6):10–8.
101. McClure PW, Tate AR, Kareha S, Irwin D, Zlupko E. A clinical method for identifying scapular

dyskinesis: part 1: reliability. J Athl Train. 2009;44(2):160–4.
102. Tate AR, McClure PW, Kareha S, Irwin D, Barbe MF. A clinical method for identifying scapular dyskinesis: part 2: validity. J Athl Train. 2009;44(2):165–73.
103. Sciascia A, Kibler WB. Current views of scapular dyskinesis and its possible clinical relevance. Int J Sports Phys Ther. 2022;17:117–30.
104. Lesniak BP, Baraga MG, Jose J, Smith MK, Cunningham S, Kaplan LD. Glenohumeral findings on magnetic resonance imaging correlate with innings pitched in asymptomatic pitchers. Am J Sports Med. 2013;41:2022–7.
105. Miniaci A, Mascia AT, Salonen DC, Becker EJ. Magnetic resonance imaging of the shoulder in asymptomatic professional baseball players. Am J Sports Med. 2002;30(1):66–73.
106. McCulloch PC, Andrews WJ, Alexander J, Brekke A, Duwani S, Noble P. The effect on external rotation of an anchor placed anterior to the biceps in type 2 SLAP repairs in a cadaveric throwing model. Arthroscopy. 2013;29(1):18–24.
107. Lee SJ, Kim JH, Gwak HC, et al. Influence of glenoid labral bumper height and capsular volume on clinical outcomes after arthroscopic Bankart repair as assessed with serial CT arthrogram: can anterior-inferior volume fraction be a prognostic factor? Am J Sports Med. 2020;48:1846–56.
108. Dines JS, ElAttrache NS. Horizontal mattress with a knotless anchor to better recreate the normal superior labrum anatomy. Arthroscopy. 2008;24:1422–5.
109. McGarry MH, Nguyen ML, Quigley RJ, Hanypsiak B, Gupta R, Lee TQ. The effect of long and short head biceps loading on glenohumeral joint rotational range of motion and humeral head position. Knee Surg Sports Traumatol Arthrosc. 2016;24:1979–87.
110. Fedoriw WW, Ramkumar P, McCulloch PC, Lintner DM. Return to play after treatment of superior labral tears in professional baseball players. Am J Sports Med. 2014;42(5):1155–60.
111. Hashiguchi H, Iwashita S, Yoneda M, Takai S. Factors influencing outcomes of nonsurgical treatment for baseball players with SLAP lesion. Asia Pac J Sports Med Arthrosc Rehabil Technol. 2018;14:6–9.
112. Yoon JH, Song KJ, Ji MY, Lee BS, Oh JK. Effect of a 12 week rehabilitation exercise program on shoulder proprioception, instability and pain in baseball players with shoulder instability. Iran J Public Health. 2020;49:1467–75.
113. Edwards SL, Lee JA, Bell JE, et al. Nonoperative treatment of superior labrum anterior posterior tears: improvements in pain, function, and quality of life. Am J Sports Med. 2010;38(7):1456–61.
114. Shin JS, Lee J, Jeon YS, Ko YW, Kim RG. Clinical outcomes of non-operative treatment for patients presenting SLAP lesions in diagnostic provocative tests and MR arthrography. Knee Surg Sports Traumatol Arthrosc. 2017;25:3296–302.
115. Jang SH, Seo JG, Jang HS, Jung JE, Kim JG. Predictive factors associated with failure of nonoperative treatment of superior labrum anterior-posterior tears. J Shoulder Elb Surg. 2016;25:428–34.
116. Sciascia A. Rehabilitation of the painful shoulder. J Shoulder Elb Surg. 2024;33:494–506.
117. Lukasiewicz AC, McClure P, Michener L, Pratt N, Sennett B. Comparison of 3-dimensional scapular position and orientation between subjects with and without shoulder impingement. J Orthop Sports Phys Ther. 1999;29(10):574–86.
118. Kebaetse M, McClure PW, Pratt N. Thoracic position effect on shoulder range of motion, strength, and three-dimensional scapular kinematics. Arch Phys Med Rehabil. 1999;80:945–50.
119. Borstad JD, Ludewig PM. The effect of long versus short pectoralis minor resting length on scapular kinematics in healthy individuals. J Orthop Sports Phys Ther. 2005;35(4):227–38.
120. Thigpen CA, Padua DA, Michener LA, et al. Head and shoulder posture affect scapular mechanics and muscle activity in overhead tasks. J Electromyogr Kinesiol. 2010;20(4):701–9.
121. Shiravi S, Letafatkar A, Bertozzi L, Pillastrini P, Tazji MK. Efficacy of abdominal control feedback and scapula stabilization exercises in participants with forward head, round shoulder postures and neck movement impairment. Sports Health. 2019;11:272–9.
122. Weon JH, Oh JS, Cynn HS, Kim YW, Kwon OY, Yi CH. Influence of forward head posture on scapular upward rotators during isometric shoulder flexion. J Bodyw Mov Ther. 2010;14:367–74.
123. Kang JI, Choi HH, Jeong DK, Choi H, Moon YJ, Park JS. Effect of scapular stabilization exercise on neck alignment and muscle activity in patients with forward head posture. J Phys Ther Sci. 2018;30:804–8.
124. Reuther KE, Thomas SJ, Tucker JJ, et al. Scapular dyskinesis is detrimental to shoulder tendon properties and joint mechanics in a rat model. J Orthop Res. 2014;32(11):1436–43.
125. Kibler WB, Sennett B, Sciascia A. New paradigms for the throwing shoulder: pathophysiology and examination. In: Huddleston JI, Lieberman JR, editors. Instructional course lectures, vol. 68. Rosemont: American Academy of Orthopaedic Surgeons/Wolters Kluwer; 2019. p. 491–8.
126. Sciascia A. Evaluating scapular dyskinesis. Athl Train Sports Healthcare. 2020;12:6–10.
127. Dines JS, Frank JB, Akerman M, Yocum LA. Glenohumeral internal rotation deficits in baseball players with ulnar collateral ligament insufficiency. Am J Sports Med. 2009;37(3):566–70.
128. Wilk KE, Macrina LC, Fleisig GS, et al. Correlation of glenohumeral internal rotation deficit and total rotational motion to shoulder injuries in professional baseball pitchers. Am J Sports Med. 2011;39(2):329–35.
129. Wilk KE, Macrina LC, Fleisig GS, et al. Deficits in glenohumeral passive range of motion increase

risk of elbow injury in professional baseball pitchers: a prospective study. Am J Sports Med. 2014;42:2075–81.
130. Shanley E, Rauh MJ, Michener LA, Ellenbecker TS. Incidence of injuries in high school softball and baseball players. J Athl Train. 2011;46:648–54.
131. Garrison JC, Cole MA, Conway JE, Macko MJ, Thigpen C, Shanley E. Shoulder range of motion deficits in baseball players with an ulnar collateral ligament tear. Am J Sports Med. 2012;40(11):2597–603.
132. Lee BJS, Garrison JC, Conway JE, Pollard K, Aryal S. The relationship between humeral retrotorsion and shoulder range of motion in baseball players with an ulnar collateral ligament tear. Orthop J Sports Med. 2016;4(10):2325967116667497.
133. Camp CL, Zajac JM, Pearson DB, et al. Decreased shoulder external rotation and flexion are greater predictors of injury than internal rotation deficits: analysis of 132 pitcher seasons in professional baseball. Arthroscopy. 2017;33:1629–36.
134. Kalo K, Vogt L, Sieland J, Banzer W, Niederer D. Injury and training history are associated with glenohumeral internal rotation deficit in youth tennis athletes. BMC Musculoskelet Disord. 2020;21:553.
135. Hayes K, Walton JR, Szomor ZL, Murrell GAC. Reliability of 3 methods of assessing shoulder strength. J Shoulder Elb Surg. 2002;11:33–9.
136. Ziegler P, Kuhle L, Stockle U, et al. Evaluation of the constant score: which is the method to assess the objective strength? BMC Musculoskelet Dis. 2019;20:403.
137. Dvir Z. Grade 4 in manual muscle testing: the problem with submaximal strength assessment. Clin Rehabil. 1997;11:36–41.
138. Schrama PPM, Stenneberg MS, Lucas C, van Trijffel E. Intraexaminer reliability of hand-held dynamometry in the upper extremity: a systematic review. Arch Phys Med Rehabil. 2014;95:2444–69.
139. Ellenbecker TS, Roetert EP. Age specific isokinetic glenohumeral internal and external rotation strength in elite junior tennis players. J Sci Med Sport. 2003;6(1):63–70.
140. Cools AM, Witvrouw EE, DeClercq GA, Vanderstraeten GG, Cambier DC. Evaluation of isokinetic force production and associated muscle activity in the scapular rotators during a protraction-retraction movement in overhead athletes with impingement symptoms. Br J Sports Med. 2004;38:64–8.
141. Mulligan IJ, Biddington WB, Barnhart BD, Ellenbecker TS. Isokinetic profile of shoulder internal and external rotators of high school aged baseball pitchers. J Strength Cond Res. 2004;18:861–6.
142. Cools AM, Witvrouw EE, Mahieu NN, Danneels LA. Isokinetic scapular muscle performance in overhead athletes with and without impingement symptoms. J Athl Train. 2005;40(2):104–10.
143. Cools AM, Geerooms E, Van den Berghe DF, Cambier DC, Witvrouw EE. Isokinetic scapular muscle performance in young elite gymnasts. J Athl Train. 2007;42:458–63.
144. Jones PA, Bampouras TM. A comparison of isokinetic and functional methods of assessing bilateral strength imbalance. J Strength Cond Res. 2010;24(6):1553–8.
145. Papotto BM, Rice T, Malone T, Butterfield T, Uhl TL. Reliability of isometric and eccentric isokinetic shoulder external rotation. J Sport Rehabil. 2016;25:1–7.
146. Kibler WB, Sciascia AD, Dome DC. Evaluation of apparent and absolute supraspinatus strength in patients with shoulder injury using the scapular retraction test. Am J Sports Med. 2006;34(10):1643–7.
147. Smith J, Kotajarvi BR, Padgett DJ, Eischen JJ. Effect of scapular protraction and retraction on isometric shoulder elevation strength. Arch Phys Med Rehabil. 2002;83:367–70.
148. Smith J, Dietrich CT, Kotajarvi BR, Kaufman KR. The effect of scapular protraction on isometric shoulder rotation strength in normal subjects. J Shoulder Elb Surg. 2006;15:339–43.
149. Tate AR, McClure P, Kareha S, Irwin D. Effect of the scapula reposition test on shoulder impingement symptoms and elevation strength in overhead athletes. J Orthop Sports Phys Ther. 2008;38(1):4–11.
150. Custodio GAP, Terroni EC, Martins J, Gobatto CF, de Oliveira AS. Intra—and interrater reliability of belt-stabilized hand-held dynamometer in scapular protraction strength tests in individuals with shoulder pain. Phys Ther Sport. 2023;61:51–6.
151. Karagiannopoulos C, Griech S, Leggin B. Reliability and validity of the active force digital dynamometer in assessing shoulder muscle force across different user experience levels. Int J Sports Phys Ther. 2022;17:669–76.
152. Li L, McGuinness BK, Layer JS, Song Y, Jensen MA, Dai B. Longitudinal assessments of strength and dynamic balance from pre-injury baseline to 3 and 4 months after labrum repairs in collegiate athletes. Physiother Theory Pract. 2022;38:2505–13.
153. Suprak DN, Sahlberg JD, Chalmers GR, Cunningham W. Shoulder elevation affects joint position sense and muscle activation differently in upright and supine body orientations. Hum Mov Sci. 2016;46:148–58.
154. Hirashima M, Kadota H, Sakurai S, Kudo K, Ohtsuki T. Sequential muscle activity and its functional role in the upper extremity and trunk during overarm throwing. J Sports Sci. 2002;20:301–10.
155. Hirashima M, Kudo K, Watarai K, Ohtsuki T. Control of 3D limb dynamics in unconstrained overarm throws of different speeds performed by skilled baseball players. J Neurophysiol. 2007;97(1):680–91.
156. Hirashima M, Yamane K, Nakamura Y, Ohtsuki T. Kinetic chain of overarm throwing in terms of joint rotations revealed by induced acceleration analysis. J Biomech. 2008;41:2874–83.
157. Toyoshima S, Miyashita M. Force-velocity relation in throwing. Res Q. 1973;44(1):86–95.

158. Toyoshima S, Hoshikawa T, Miyashita M. Contributions of body parts to throwing performance. In: Nelson RC, Morehouse CA, editors. Biomechanics IV. Baltimore: University Park Press; 1974. p. 169–74.
159. Bouisset S, Zattara M. A sequence of postural movements precedes voluntary movement. Neurosci Lett. 1981;22:263–70.
160. Zattara M, Bouisset S. Posturo-kinetic organisation during the early phase of voluntary upper limb movement. 1 Normal subjects. J Neurol Neurosurg Psychiatry. 1988;51:956–65.
161. Marshall R, Elliott BC. Long axis rotation: the missing link in proximal to distal segment sequencing. J Sports Sci. 2000;18(4):247–54.
162. Kenny IC, McCloy AJ, Wallace ES, Otto SR. Segmental sequencing of kinetic energy in a computer-simulated golf swing. Sports Eng. 2008;11:37–45.
163. Cordo PJ, Nashner LM. Properties of postural adjustments associated with rapid arm movements. J Neurophysiol. 1982;47(2):287–308.
164. Hodges PW, Richardson CA. Feedforward contraction of transversus abdominus is not influenced by the direction of arm movement. Exp Brain Res. 1997;114:362–70.
165. Hodges PW, Richardson CA. Relationship between limb movement and associated contraction of the trunk muscles. Ergonomics. 1997;40:1220–30.
166. Hodges P, Cresswell A, Thorstensson A. Preparatory trunk motion accompanies rapid upper limb movement. Exp Brain Res. 1999;124(1):69–79.
167. Reinold MM, Escamilla R, Wilk KE. Current concepts in the scientific and clinical rationale behind exercises for glenohumeral and scapulothoracic musculature. J Orthop Sports Phys Ther. 2009;39:105–17.
168. Kibler WB, Sciascia AD, Uhl TL, Tambay N, Cunningham T. Electromyographic analysis of specific exercises for scapular control in early phases of shoulder rehabilitation. Am J Sports Med. 2008;36(9):1789–98.
169. De May K, Daneels L, Cagnie B, Van den Bosch L, Flier J, Cools AM. Kinetic chain influences on upper and lower trapezius muscle activation during eight variations of a scapular retraction exercise in overhead athletes. J Sci Med Sport. 2013;16:65–70.
170. Cools AM, Borms D, Cottens S, Himpe M, Meersdom S, Cagnie B. Rehabilitation exercises for athletes with biceps disorders and slap lesions: a continuum of exercises with increasing loads on the biceps. Am J Sports Med. 2014;42:1315–22.
171. De May K, Danneels L, Cagnie B, Huyghe L, Seyns E, Cools AM. Conscious correction of scapular orientation in overhead athletes performing selected shoulder rehabilitation exercises: the effect on trapezius muscle activation measured by surface electromyography. J Orthop Sports Phys Ther. 2013;43(1):3–10.
172. Ou HL, Huang TS, Chen YT, et al. Alterations of scapular kinematics and associated muscle activation specific to symptomatic dyskinesis type after conscious control. Man Ther. 2016;26:97–103.
173. Huang TS, Du WY, Wang TG, et al. Progressive conscious control of scapular orientation with video feedback has improvement in muscle balance ratio in patients with scapular dyskinesis: a randomized controlled trial. J Shoulder Elb Surg. 2018;27:1407–14.
174. Mottram SL, Woledge RC, Morrissey D. Motion analysis study of a scapular orientation exercise and subjects' ability to learn the exercise. Man Ther. 2009;14:13–8.
175. Worsley P, Warner M, Mottram S, et al. Motor control retraining exercises for shoulder impingement: effects on function, muscle activation, and biomechanics in young adults. J Shoulder Elb Surg. 2013;22:e11–9.
176. Du WY, Huang TS, Chiu YC, et al. Single-session video and electromyography feedback in overhead athletes with scapular dyskinesis and impingement syndrome. J Athl Train. 2020;55:265–73.
177. Antunes A, Carnide F, Matias R. Real-time kinematic biofeedback improves scapulothoracic control and performance during scapular-focused exercises: a single-blind randomized controlled laboratory study. Hum Mov Sci. 2016;48:44–53.
178. Weon JH, Kwon OY, Cynn HS, Lee WH, Kim TH, Yi CH. Real-time visual feedback can be used to activate scapular upward rotators in people with scapular winging: an experimental study. J Physiother. 2011;57:101–7.
179. Oliver GD, Plummer HA, Gascon SS. Electromyographic analysis of traditional and kinetic chain exercises for dynamic shoulder movements. J Strength Cond Res. 2016;30:3146–54.
180. Oliver GD, Washington JK, Barfield JW, Gascon SS, Gilmer G. Quantitative analysis of proximal and distal kinetic chain musculature during dynamic exercises. J Strength Cond Res. 2018;32:1545–53.
181. Wasserberger KW, Downs JL, Barfield JW, Williams TK, Oliver GD. Lumbopelvic-hip complex and scapular stabilizing muscle activations during full-body exercises with and without resistance bands. J Strength Cond Res. 2020;34:2840–8.
182. De May K, Danneels L, Cagnie B, Cools A. Are kinetic chain rowing exercises relevant in shoulder and trunk injury prevention training? Br J Sports Med. 2011;45(4):320.
183. Sciascia A, Cromwell R. Kinetic chain rehabilitation: a theoretical framework. Rehabil Res Pract. 2012;2012:1–9.
184. Sciascia A. Managing scapular dyskinesis. Athl Train Sports Healthcare. 2020;12:102–7.
185. McMullen J, Uhl TL. A kinetic chain approach for shoulder rehabilitation. J Athl Train. 2000;35(3):329–37.
186. Ellenbecker TS, Roetert EP, Kibler WB, Kovacs MS. Applied biomechanics of tennis. In: Magee DJ, Manske RC, Zachazewski JE, Quillen WS, editors.

Athletic and sport issues in musculoskeletal rehabilitation. St. Louis: Elsevier; 2011. p. 265–86.

187. Kibler WB, Wilkes T, Sciascia A. Mechanics and pathomechanics in the overhead athlete. Clin Sports Med. 2013;32(4):637–51.
188. Fleisig GS, Andrews JR, Dillman CJ, Escamilla RF. Kinetics of baseball pitching with implications about injury mechanisms. Am J Sports Med. 1995;23(2):233–9.
189. Dias T, Lerch BG, Slowik JS, et al. Biomechanical basis of interval throwing programs for baseball pitchers: a systematic review. Int J Sports Phys Ther. 2023;18:1036–53.
190. Myers NL, Kibler WB, Lamborn L, et al. Reliability and validity of a biomechanically based analysis method for the tennis serve. Int J Sports Phys Ther. 2017;12:437–49.
191. Sutter EG, Orenduff J, Fox WJ, Myers J, Garrigues GE. Predicting injury in professional baseball pitchers from delivery mechanics: a statistical model using quantitative video analysis. Orthopedics. 2018;41:43–53.
192. Davis JT, Limpisvasti O, Fluhme D, et al. The effect of pitching biomechanics on the upper extremity in youth and adolescent baseball pitchers. Am J Sports Med. 2009;37(8):1484–91.
193. Kibler WB. Biomechanical analysis of the shoulder during tennis activities. Clin Sports Med. 1995;14:79–85.
194. Wilk KE, Macrina LC. Nonoperative and postoperative rehabilitation for glenohumeral instability. Clin Sports Med. 2013;32:865–914.
195. Hermanns CA, Coda RG, Cheema S, et al. Variability in rehabilitation protocols after superior labrum anterior posterior surgical repair. Kans J Med. 2021;11:243–8.

Part III

Shoulder Instability and Sports

Shoulder Instability in Throwing Athletes

16

Teruhisa Mihata

16.1 Characteristics and Pathomechanics in Throwing Athletes with Shoulder Instability

During arm-cocking to the acceleration phase of a throwing motion, 380 N of anterior force is generated on the glenohumeral joint [1]. To prevent excessive anterior translation with such a large anterior force applied during the throwing motion, the anterior capsular ligaments, including the anterior band of the inferior glenohumeral ligament (AIGHL) and middle glenohumeral ligament, need to function very well. Once the anterior capsular ligaments loosen because of an anterior labral tear, anterior capsular tear, or humeral avulsion of the glenohumeral ligament (HAGL) lesion after anterior shoulder subluxation or dislocation, most throwing athletes can no longer throw a ball at the maximum velocity and consequently cannot play in the game. Even though throwing athletes can have severe shoulder pain during throwing, most do not have any problem during daily life because the amount of increased anterior laxity is small. In most throwing athletes, the bone defect in the glenoid or humeral head is not severe (Fig. 16.1), because they often come to the clinic only after a couple of shoulder subluxations or dislocations.

T. Mihata (✉)
Department of Orthopedic Surgery, Osaka Medical and Pharmaceutical University, Takatsuki, Osaka, Japan

First Towakai Hospital, Takatsuki, Osaka, Japan

Katsuragi Hospital, Kishiwada, Osaka, Japan
e-mail: tmihata@ompu.ac.jp

E. Calvo et al. (eds.), *Complex and Revision Problems in Shoulder Instability*,
https://doi.org/10.1007/978-3-031-81389-4_16

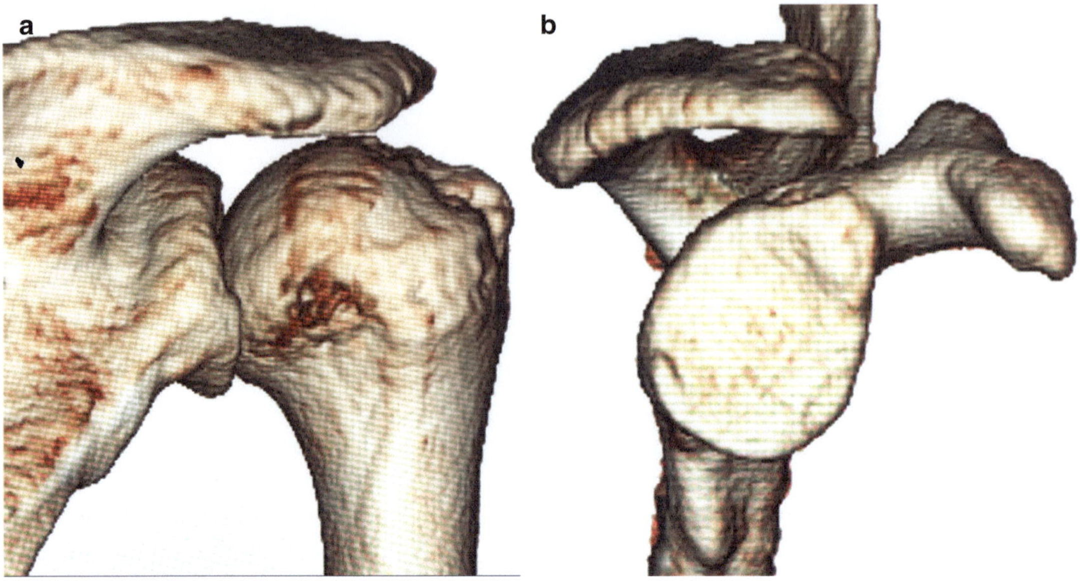

Fig. 16.1 Three-dimensional computed tomography in a professional baseball pitcher after shoulder dislocation showed a minimal bone defect in the glenoid and humeral head

16.2 Why the Rate of Return to Sports After Surgical Treatment Is Low

Nonsurgical treatment does not work in most overhead throwing athletes with anterior shoulder instability after a traumatic shoulder dislocation. If the athletes want to return to their overhead throwing sports, surgical management is essential. Coracoid transfer and the remplissage technique are not indicated for anterior shoulder instability in throwing athletes because of the minimal bone defect in the glenoid and humeral head. Anatomical repair of the torn labrum or capsular ligaments is the best surgical option to improve shoulder function in these athletes. However, the shoulder external rotation angle is decreased after anterior labral repair. In our previous study, mean loss of shoulder external rotation angle at 90° of shoulder abduction was 10°, compared with the contralateral shoulder, at 1 year after antero-inferior labral repair (Bankart repair) [2]. Ball velocity is affected by maximum shoulder external rotation angle in throwing athletes [3]. Therefore, these athletes—especially baseball pitchers—have difficulty returning to their previous performance level owing to decreased ball velocity, even though they usually don't feel any pain or instability after anterior labral repair [4].

16.3 AIGHL Reconstruction: Our Solution to Maximize the External Rotation Angle with Anterior Stabilization

For anterior shoulder instability, Bankart repair is a reliable technique for preventing shoulder dislocation. However, a biomechanical study showed that anteroinferior labral repair decreases anterior glenohumeral translation and external rotation [5], because both anterior glenohumeral translation and external rotation are correlated with the length of the AIGHL (Fig. 16.2) [6]. The decrease in external rotation after anteroinferior labral repair was 12.5° in a biomechanical study [5] and 10° in a clinical study [2]. For overhead throwing athletes, a reduction of around 10° makes a return to previous performance levels difficult [4].

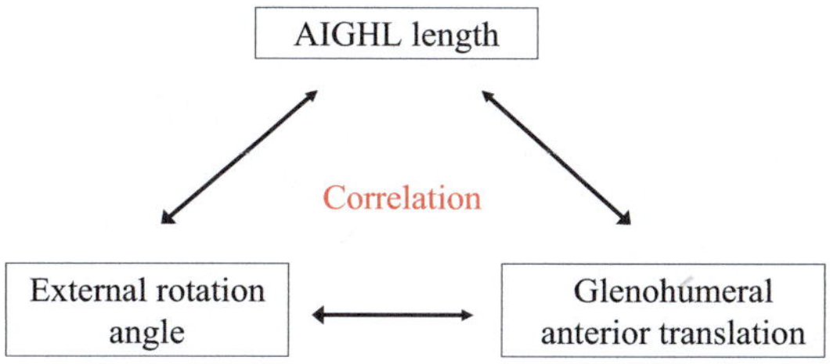

Fig. 16.2 Correlation between AIGHL length, shoulder external rotation angle, and glenohumeral anterior translation

In the suture-repair technique, the repaired tissue, including the capsule, ligament, and tendon, is shortened because the tissue on the wound sides of the suture bites overlaps after knot tying. Even though surgeons can repair the anteroinferior capsular ligament with small suture bites, shortening of the capsular ligament cannot be avoided, resulting in decreased anterior glenohumeral translation and external rotation after anteroinferior labral repair than in intact shoulders [5]. To prevent this overtightening of the anteroinferior capsular ligament, we developed an AIGHL reconstruction technique that uses a fascia lata graft. In this surgery, a fascia lata graft is attached between the AIGHL and glenoid to maintain the original length of the AIGHL after suturing. Our biomechanical study (unpublished data) showed that AIGHL reconstruction completely restored anterior stability while maintaining the maximum shoulder external rotation angle after surgery, in contrast to Bankart repair, which decreases external rotation substantially. Our preliminary clinical results (unpublished data) show that, with complete restoration of shoulder external rotation, elite throwing athletes could resume their throwing programs as early as 3 or 4 months after AIGHL reconstruction and were able to return to their previous levels at 6–8 months postoperatively.

16.4 Shoulder Dislocation During Throwing Motion in the Game

Although shoulder dislocation during throwing motion in the game is very rare, we saw two patients of professional baseball pitchers. Just after injury, orthopedic surgeons recommended nonoperative treatment for more than 3 months for all of the players. However, their shoulder instability and pain did not improve at all. MRI showed severe AIGHL defect, Bankart lesion, and HAGL lesion (Fig. 16.3) with severe articular-sided partial-thickness rotator cuff tears in the supraspinatus and infraspinatus tendons (Fig. 16.4). Therefore, I performed arthroscopic AIGHL reconstruction for the severe AIGHL defect (Fig. 16.5) and arthroscopic superior capsule reconstruction (SCR) with rotator cuff repair (SCR for Reinforcement of rotator cuff repair: SCR-R) (Fig. 16.6). Fascia lata grafts for AIGHL reconstruction and SCR were fixed at the maximum shoulder external rotation position and 90° of shoulder abduction. At 3 months after surgery, both players could achieve the maximum shoulder external rotation angle at 90° of shoulder abduction, and they were able to return to the game without shoulder instability by 8 months after surgery.

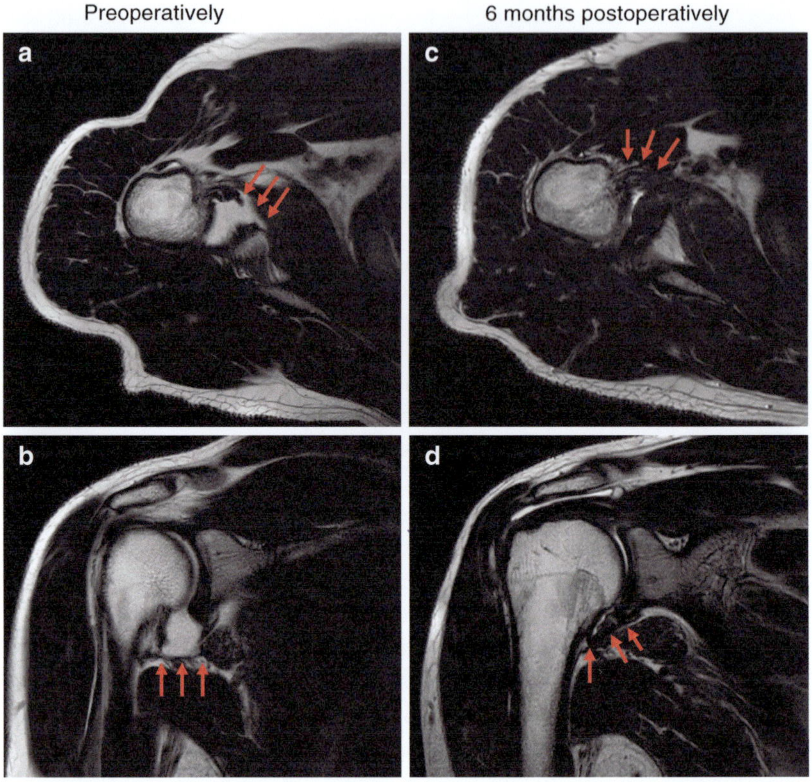

Fig. 16.3 Magnetic resonance imaging after shoulder dislocation during throwing motion (**a, b**) and at 6 months after AIGHL reconstruction (**c, d**). Red arrows show the AIGHL defect in (**a**) and (**b**) and the reconstructed AIGHL in (**c**) and (**d**)

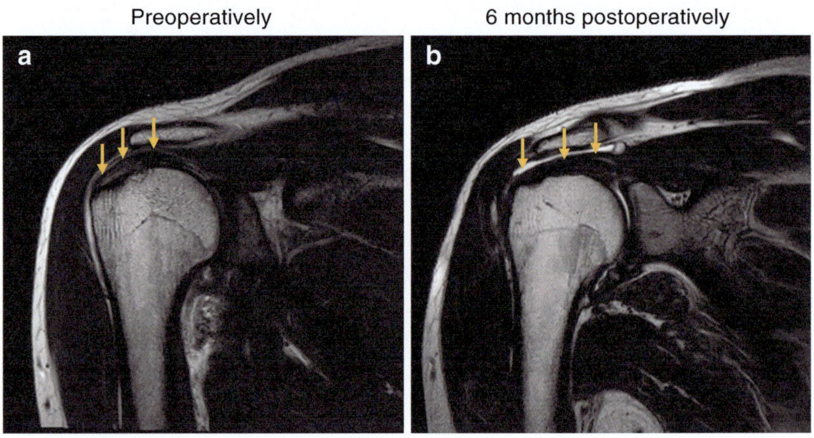

Fig. 16.4 Magnetic resonance imaging of severe partial-thickness articular-sided rotator cuff tear (**a**, arrows) and superior capsule reconstruction with rotator cuff repair (**b**, arrows)

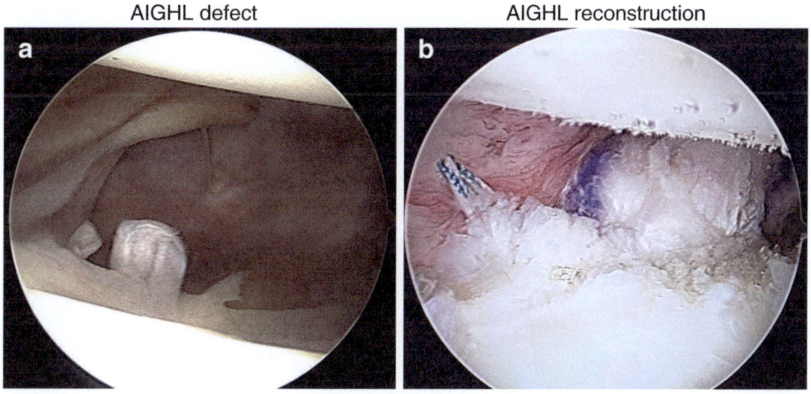

Fig. 16.5 Arthroscopic findings in AIGHL defect (**a**), and AIGHL reconstructed by using fascia lata (**b**)

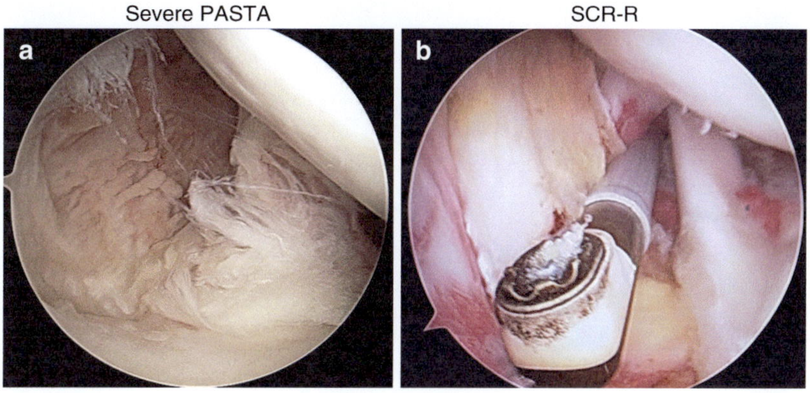

Fig. 16.6 Arthroscopic findings in partial-thickness articular-sided rotator cuff tear (**a**), and superior capsule reconstruction using fascia lata with rotator cuff repair (SCR-R; **b**). PASTA, partial articular supraspinatus tendon avulsion

16.5 Conclusion

After shoulder dislocation during throwing, AIGHL reconstruction by using a fascia lata autograft is a reliable surgical option to stabilize the shoulder joint while maintaining the maximum shoulder external rotation angle at 90° of shoulder abduction, allowing even elite athletes to return to throwing at a high-performance level.

References

1. Fleisig GS, Andrews JR, Dillman CJ, Escamilla RF. Kinetics of baseball pitching with implications about injury mechanisms. Am J Sports Med. 1995;23(2):233–9. https://doi.org/10.1177/036354659502300218.
2. Tanaka H, Mihata T, Hasegawa A, Neo M. Clinical outcome after arthroscopic surgeries in baseball players with traumatic anterior shoulder instability. Katakansetsu. 2022;46:22–5.
3. Werner SL, Suri M, Guido JA Jr, Meister K, Jones DG. Relationships between ball velocity and throwing mechanics in collegiate baseball pitchers. J Shoulder Elb Surg. 2008;17(6):905–8. https://doi.org/10.1016/j.jse.2008.04.002.
4. Park JY, Lee JH, Oh KS, Chung SW, Lim JJ, Noh YM. Return to play after arthroscopic treatment for shoulder instability in elite and professional baseball players. J Shoulder Elb Surg. 2019;28(1):77–81. https://doi.org/10.1016/j.jse.2018.07.006.
5. Alberta FG, Elattrache NS, Mihata T, McGarry MH, Tibone JE, Lee TQ. Arthroscopic anteroinferior suture plication resulting in decreased glenohumeral translation and external rotation. Study of a cadaver model. J Bone Joint Surg Am. 2006;88(1):179–87. https://doi.org/10.2106/JBJS.D.02974.
6. Mihata T, Lee Y, McGarry MH, Abe M, Lee TQ. Excessive humeral external rotation results in increased shoulder laxity. Am J Sports Med. 2004;32(5):1278–85. https://doi.org/10.1177/0363546503262188.

Shoulder Instability in the Collision Athlete

17

Liam A. Peebles, Nigel O. Blackwood, Matthew J. Kraeutler, and Mary K. Mulcahey

17.1 Incidence and Epidemiology of Shoulder Instability in Collision Athletes

17.1.1 Incidence

Glenohumeral instability is a common injury among athletes, namely in those participating in contact and collision sports. Aside from anterior cruciate ligament tears, anterior shoulder instability results in more time away from play than any other injury in young collision athletes [1–3]. More than half (52.5%) of the shoulder dislocations presenting to emergency departments (ED) in the United States are sports-related, with American football being the most common contact sport resulting in shoulder instability (15.2% of all dislocations) [4]. Males comprise the vast majority of patients with sports-related shoulder dislocations, accounting for 86.1% of instability events [4]. In collegiate athletes, the estimated incidence of glenohumeral instability has been reported to be 0.12 per 1000 athlete exposures (AEs) [3]. A similar disparity between sexes in rates of shoulder dislocation is also seen in athletic populations, as the incidence in males and females is 0.15 and 0.06 per 1000 athletes, respectively. These rates are considerably higher for contact sport athletes, with the most common collegiate sports including men's spring football (0.4/1000 AEs), men's wrestling (0.21/1000 AEs), women's ice hockey (0.18/1000 AEs), men's fall football (0.18/1000 AEs), and men's ice hockey (0.17/1000 AEs). Men's football (spring and fall) has been reported to account for 76% of all shoulder dislocations in National Collegiate Athletic Association (NCAA) athletes. Although there is limited data available regarding the incidence of shoulder instability in professional athletes, a previous study reporting on 336 college football players entering the National Football League combine found that 14% of players had a history of shoulder instability and 10% had prior shoulder stabilization surgery [5]. Professional athletes competing in contact sports have also been found to have shorter careers compared to noncontact athletes following anterior shoulder stabilization, and although there is no statistically significant difference in duration of play after surgery (3.8 years versus 5.8 years, $p > 0.05$), this carries

L. A. Peebles
Department of Orthopaedic Surgery, University of Michigan Medical Center, Ann Arbor, MI, USA

N. O. Blackwood
Tulane University School of Medicine, New Orleans, LA, USA

M. J. Kraeutler
Department of Orthopaedic Surgery & Rehabilitation, Texas Tech University Health Sciences Center, Lubbock, TX, USA

M. K. Mulcahey (✉)
Department of Orthopaedic Surgery and Rehabilitation, Loyola University Medical Center, Maywood, IL, USA

E. Calvo et al. (eds.), *Complex and Revision Problems in Shoulder Instability*,
https://doi.org/10.1007/978-3-031-81389-4_17

an undeniable clinical significance when considering the 2 years of lost compensation at the professional level [6].

In a multicenter study of 45 contact intercollegiate athletes with in-season anterior shoulder instability events managed nonoperatively, Dickens et al. [7] reported that 73.3% (33/45) were able to return to play (RTP) after a median of 5 days lost from competition. However, it should be noted that more than half (21/33, 63.6%) of these athletes reported episodes of recurrent instability following RTP in the form of frank dislocation (11/33, 33.3%) or subluxation (10/33, 30.3%) and only 66.7% (22/33) were able to complete the season. These rates of recurrent instability in contact or collision athletes are similar to those reported by Sachs et al. [8], who found that younger athletes participating in such sports were at the greatest risk of recurrence compared to all other patients studied. The authors reported that this subgroup of athletes had a 55% (17/31) redislocation rate following RTP at a mean follow-up of 4 years.

17.1.2 Mechanism of Injury and Associated Injuries

Regardless of sports participation, anterior glenohumeral instability can be caused by both direct and indirect forces [9]. Indirect mechanisms of injury result from falling onto an outstretched arm with the shoulder in an abducted and externally rotated position, as is seen when making a tackle in football or the follow-through of a strike when a boxer misses their opponent. A more direct mechanism of injury occurs when an anteriorly directed blow is delivered to the back of the shoulder, as may be seen in a rugby tackle or scrum. Younger athletes participating in contact or collision sports are particularly susceptible to such forces on the shoulder, and the majority of anterior shoulder instability episodes occur secondary to traumatic events. Athletes may present with a range of pathology, including microinstability, subluxation, or dislocation, and these episodes of instability most commonly result from contact with another player or object [3, 6, 10].

Table 17.1 Incidence of associated injuries following events of primary or recurrent shoulder instability

Associated injury	Incidence following anterior instability event
1. Bankart lesion	87–100% of first-time dislocations
2. Bony Bankart lesion	11–73%, 20% in contact athletes
3. Rotator cuff injury	13–14%, increases with age from 40 to 60 years old
4. SLAP tear	10–20%, up to 30% in NFL combine athletes
5. Hill-Sachs lesion	67–93% in primary cases, up to 100% in recurrent cases

SLAP superior labrum anterior to posterior, *NFL* National Football League

Following anterior shoulder dislocation or subluxation, damage to the surrounding soft tissue and bony architecture is nearly inevitable. Associated injuries to the dynamic and static soft tissue stabilizers of the glenohumeral joint may include Bankart lesions, bony Bankart lesions, rotator cuff injuries, and superior labrum anterior to posterior (SLAP) tears (Table 17.1). In the setting of recurrent anterior instability, progressive damage to the anteroinferior glenohumeral capsule results in capsular attenuation. Laxity of the glenohumeral capsule has been noted in up to 30% of patients with chronic instability, with magnetic resonance imaging (MRI) studies demonstrating an average elongation of 19% to the anteroinferior capsule and corresponding glenohumeral ligaments [11, 12]. Defined as an avulsion of the anterior shoulder capsule and glenoid labrum from the glenoid rim, Bankart lesions are the most common soft tissue injury following anterior shoulder dislocation and have been reported in 87–100% of first-time dislocations [11, 13, 14]. Although the Bankart lesion has previously been described as the “essential lesion” of recurrent anterior instability and is by far the most important, there is likely a range of soft tissue pathology that may need to be addressed at the time of surgery. A bony Bankart lesion describes a fracture of the anterior-inferior glenoid. Although the incidence is variable, bony Bankart lesions have been observed in 11–73% of patients with anterior instability and in approximately 20% of contact (rugby) athletes [11, 15,

16]. The rotator cuff complex is an important dynamic stabilizer of the shoulder, and injuries may range from partial undersurface tears to complete, full-thickness tears. The incidence of rotator cuff injury following primary episodes of instability ranges from 13% to 14%, and although less of a concern in younger athletes, this rate increases with advancing age and episodes of recurrence in patients 40–60 years old [11, 14, 17, 18]. Although less common, SLAP tears have been reported to occur in 10–20% of patients with recurrent anterior instability and may be more symptomatic in overhead or contact athletes [11, 19]. In an analysis of 340 American football players at the NFL combine with confirmed labral pathology on MRI, Mannava and colleagues [20] identified SLAP tears in more than 30% of athletes and reported that linebackers and linemen were at the highest risk for labral injury.

It is well documented that glenoid bone loss (GBL) most commonly results from recurrent damage to the anterior glenoid rim by the humeral head upon dislocation or subluxation. Although GBL > 20–25% has historically been accepted as the cutoff for shoulder stabilization with bony augmentation, multiple studies have since demonstrated that this value is likely lower than previously reported [21–24]. In a variety of higher risk populations, including collegiate contact athletes and young military personnel, subcritical GBL ranging from 13.5–15% has been identified as a significant risk factor for inferior outcomes and recurrent instability following arthroscopic Bankart repair (ABR) and thus should be considered an indication for anterior glenoid bone grafting [25–27]. Shaha and colleagues [25] were the first to define a subcritical level of GBL, noting that >13.5% was associated with significantly lower Western Ontario Shoulder Instability (WOSI) scores and unacceptable outcomes in 72 highly active military personnel at a mean follow-up of 4 years. Similarly, in a cohort of 405 patients followed for an average of 5 years, Dekker et al. [26] reported that patients with any GBL have over a four-times greater risk of recurrence following arthroscopic stabilization, while those with >15% GBL are at a nearly three-times greater risk of recurrence compared to those with <15% GBL. Specifically in contact and collision athletes with recurrent anterior shoulder instability undergoing anterior shoulder stabilization, average preoperative GBL has been reported to range from 10.6% to 13% [28–31]. It has also been reported that contact athletes with GBL > 20% are at a considerably higher risk (OR = 9.8) of poor functional outcomes following anterior shoulder stabilization with a coracoid transfer procedure compared to those with GBL < 20% [29].

Recurrent anterior instability also results in damage to the humeral head, creating an impaction fracture to the posterolateral aspect of the humeral head as it translates across the anterior glenoid rim (Hill-Sachs Lesion [HSL]). HSLs are common in the setting of primary shoulder instability, with a reported incidence of 67–93% in primary cases and approaching 100% in cases of recurrent instability [11, 32–35]. Contact and collision athletes have been reported to have a significantly higher risk of recurrent instability when treated with ABR alone versus ABR with remplissage [36]. HSLs are described as engaging or nonengaging in relation to their mechanical behavior relative to the glenoid. Nonengaging HSLs are oriented parallel to the humeral shaft and diagonally to the anterior margin of the glenoid when the arm is abducted and externally rotated; however, they do not contact the anterior glenoid rim. In contrast, engaging HSLs typically present with the long axis of the defect parallel to the anterior glenoid and obliquely to the humeral shaft with the shoulder in a functional position [37]. With this in mind, it is imperative to consider the overall size of the HSL and its relationship to the glenoid track, as massive, large volume HSLs will likely engage regardless of orientation. The glenoid track, as first described by DiGiacomo et al. [38], is defined as the contact zone between the humeral head and glenoid with the shoulder positioned in abduction and external rotation. "Off-track" HSLs are those that extend beyond the glenoid track and engage with the anterior glenoid rim, while "on-track" lesions are contained within the glenoid track and do not engage. Utilizing three-dimensional (3-D) CT imaging, the glenoid track instability management score (GTIMS) incorporates these principles and has been shown to more conservatively delineate anterior instability treatment with promising postoperative patient outcomes compared to previously proposed treatment algorithms [39–41].

Engaging HSLs have been identified as a risk factor for recurrence following ABR, and HSLs created with the arm in an abducted position will have a higher Hill-Sachs angle and an increased risk of engagement [38, 42]. Additionally, increasing amounts of bipolar bone loss (GBL defect and HSL size) has been identified as a significant risk factor for recurrent instability following ABR in male contact athletes [43]. In the setting of bipolar bone loss, GBL severity has been found to directly influence multiple aspects of HSL morphology. Peebles et al. [44] demonstrated that patients presenting with smaller glenoid defects have significantly narrower and deeper HSLs with less humeral head surface area loss, while more extensive GBL is associated with wider yet shallower HSLs. It has also been reported that more medialized HSLs have a significantly larger volume, greater width, more surface area loss, and higher lesion angles while being located more inferiorly on the humeral head [45]. A 2020 study by Yamamoto et al. [46] assessed the effect of more medially extending HSLs on postoperative outcomes, characterizing them as either "peripheral" or "central-track" lesions relative to the width of the glenoid track. The authors reported significantly worse clinical outcomes following ABR in patients with "peripheral-track" HSLs occupying ≥75% of the glenoid track. With the aforementioned findings in mind, surgeons should expect patients presenting with more extensive GBL to have wider HSLs occupying a greater proportion of the glenoid track and ultimately an increased risk of inferior outcomes following ABR.

17.2 Management of Shoulder Instability in Collision Athletes

17.2.1 Nonoperative

The primary relative indications for nonoperative management with immobilization and physical therapy include patients with a low risk of recurrence, low functional demand, events of primary instability, no GBL, age >30 years old or <14 years old, and in-season athletes seeking to RTP during their respective season [47]. A prospective study by Hovelius et al. [48] reported recurrence rates for primary dislocations treated nonoperatively after 25 years. Forty-three percent of patients did not dislocate again, 7% redislocated once, 35% required surgery or remained unstable, and 14% redislocated multiple times but eventually became stable without surgery. Arciero et al. [49] reported in 1994 that ABR significantly reduced the recurrence rate in young athletes who sustained an acute, initial anterior dislocation of the shoulder. Buss et al. [50] reported in 2004 that most athletes were able to complete the remainder of their season when treated nonoperatively after a dislocation, but 37% experienced another dislocation.

Recent studies have reported worse outcomes with initial nonoperative management of a first-time anterior shoulder dislocation. Belk et al. [51] performed a systematic review of 259 patients and reported that patients, namely active males in their 20s and 30s, treated surgically for primary anterior dislocation have lower rates of recurrence and decreased need for future surgery compared to patients treated nonoperatively. Similarly, a systematic review by Kraeutler et al. [52] reported operative management significantly reduces recurrence rates in young and active first-time dislocators. Fox et al. [53] reported patients who underwent ABR after the initial dislocation had decreased risk of recurrent dislocation compared to patients treated surgically after the second dislocation.

17.2.2 Arthroscopic Bankart Repair

Arthroscopic or open Bankart repair is indicated for patients with a primary anterior instability event, failed nonoperative measures, high risk of recurrence but minimal GBL, an on-track Hill-Sachs Lesion (HSL), symptomatic instability on exam, or a labral tear/Bankart lesion on MRI. With these relative indications in mind, it is important to note that there is a growing body of literature supporting operative management of first-time dislocations in young, active patients [54–57]. In a randomized controlled trial of patients under 25 years old with a first-time anterior dislocation, Pougès et al. [55] reported significantly lower rates of recurrent instability (10% vs. 70%, $p = 0.0001$) and significantly better clinical outcomes at 2 years in patients treated with ABR versus those managed nonoperatively. Saper et al. [58] reported ABR effectively restored stability in 90% of cases, and 80% returned to their preinjury level of sport. Studies by Domos et al. [59] and Tasaki et al. [60] reported good outcomes and low recurrence rates in high-risk collision athletes treated with ABR with adjunct remplissage or Bristow procedure, respectively. Shah et al. [61] reported that all rugby players treated with ABR returned to preinjury level of sport, and 91% remained stable.

Yamamoto et al. [62] reported the shoulder instability recurrence rate following Bankart repair was three-times higher in contact athletes than in noncontact athletes. Alkaduhimi et al. [63] found that collision athletes have an increased risk for redislocation in comparison to non-collision athletes after an ABR, although there were no differences in return to sport. Pasqualini et al. [64] reported that collision/contact athletes had higher recurrence rates after ABR when compared with non-collision athletes. The authors emphasized that the variability in recurrence rate is influenced by the type of sport. Rossi et al. [65] found that there is great variability in the rate of return to sport at the same level, in shoulder performance after returning to competition, and in the postoperative recurrence rates based on the sport. Nakagawa et al. [66] reported lower rates of recurrent instability in collision athletes without preoperative glenoid defects (7.1%) compared to those who had preoperative glenoid defects (43.6%). The authors also noted recurrent instability in 33.3% of rugby players, 17.2% of American football players, and 17.9% of other collision/contact sport athletes.

17.2.3 Open Bankart Repair

A recent consensus statement by Hurley et al. [47] and The Anterior Shoulder Instability International Consensus Group noted that Bankart repair should be performed arthroscopically in most patient populations, though open Bankart repair may be indicated in patients with a high risk of recurrence and minimal GBL. Monk et al. [67] reported 92% return to sport and a low revision rate among young collision athletes who underwent open Bankart repair. Hickey et al. [68] found high rates of patient-reported satisfaction, excellent functional outcomes, and high rates of return to play at mid-term follow-up among collision athletes aged 18 years or under who underwent open Bankart repair. However, they also reported high rates of recurrence and revision surgical stabilization. In a cohort of 130 contact athletes with recurrent anterior instability, Bitar et al. [69] found no differences in outcomes or rates of recurrent instability in those who underwent open Bankart repair with inferior capsular shift compared to patients undergoing the Latarjet procedure. It is important to note that all patients in this prospective cohort study had minimal to no GBL and only on-track HSLs, with the authors stating that open Bankart repair is contraindicated in patients with considerable GBL. Bonnevialle et al. [16] reported the open Latarjet procedure outperformed open Bankart repair in terms of stability, time to return to play, and radiological outcomes at long-term follow-up in competitive rugby players.

17.2.4 Latarjet Procedure

Shoulder instability associated with critical GBL is commonly treated with the Latarjet procedure, which involves transfer of a coracoid autograft to the anterior glenoid rim to extend the glenoid articular surface ("bone-block" effect) while simultaneously providing stability in abduction through the "sling effect" provided by the transposed conjoint tendon [70, 71]. Indications for anterior shoulder stabilization with the Latarjet procedure include recurrent instability, failed prior surgery, collision sport participation, critical glenoid bone loss (>15–20%), and bipolar bone loss resulting in an "off-track" lesion [70, 72]. Bony augmentation with coracoid autograft is needed when GBL is severe enough such that soft tissue repair alone is unlikely to definitively stabilize the shoulder (Figs. 17.1 and 17.2). The Latarjet procedure may be performed traditionally or with a modified congruent arc technique [73]. A systematic review by Mengers et al. [74] reported that the traditional Latarjet had lower incidence of fibrous union or nonunion and broken, loose, or improperly placed screws, and the congruent arc modification had superior rates of return to sport, incidence of subluxation or positive apprehension, and revision for recurrence. Brzoska et al. [75] reported 95% RTP and 21% complication rates in professional athletes after arthroscopic Latarjet. Paulino et al. [76] found no difference in recurrence after open Latarjet in collision and non-collision athletes.

Privitera et al. [28] performed open Latarjet on collision athletes and reported 8% recurrence rate and 14% subjective instability. Forty-nine percent returned to their prior level of sport, 14% returned to a lower level, 12% changed sports, and 25% changed sports and decreased activity level or quit sports. Patients with more dislocations before surgery were less likely to return to their previous level of sport. The percent GBL was not associated with RTP rate, averaging 10.4% (range, 3.8–22.5%) in cases without previous stabilization surgery and 11.0% (range, 1.6–30.3%) in cases with previous stabilization surgery [28]. Neyton et al. [77] reported no recurrence and 65% RTP in rugby players treated with Latarjet. Hurley et al. [78] noted that the open Latarjet procedure in young collision athletes resulted in high rates of RTP, excellent functional outcomes, and low recurrence and complication rates at mid-term follow-up. Patients who did not RTP after open Latarjet exhibited poor psychological readiness to RTP and worse pain scores compared with patients who did RTP. Hurley et al. [79, 80] performed a retrospective review and a systematic review of young contact athletes

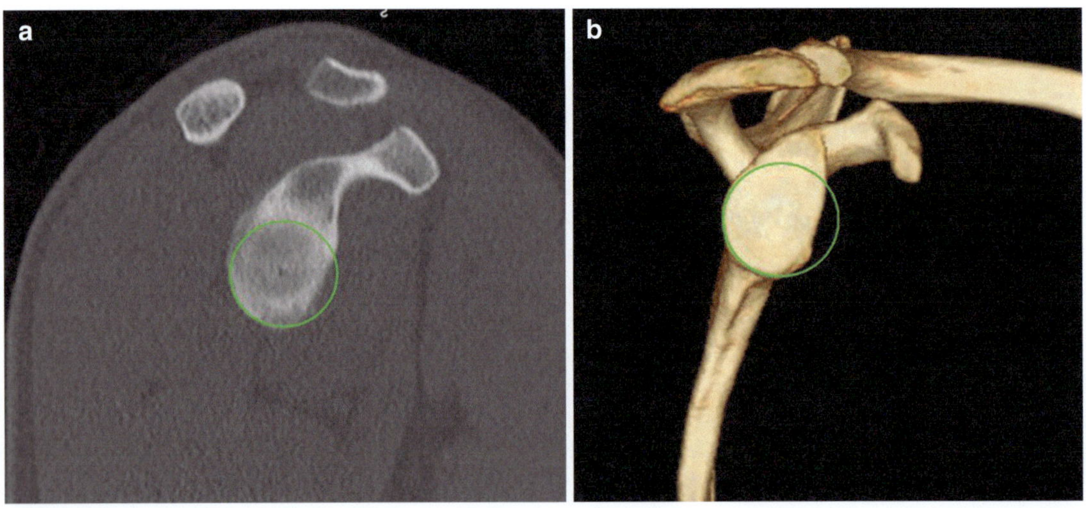

Fig. 17.1 Right shoulder with preoperative (**a**) 2D axial computed tomography (CT) and (**b**) en-face view 3D CT imaging with best-fit circle in place to estimate preoperative glenoid bone loss. (Images courtesy of Dr. Matthew T. Provencher, MD, MBA)

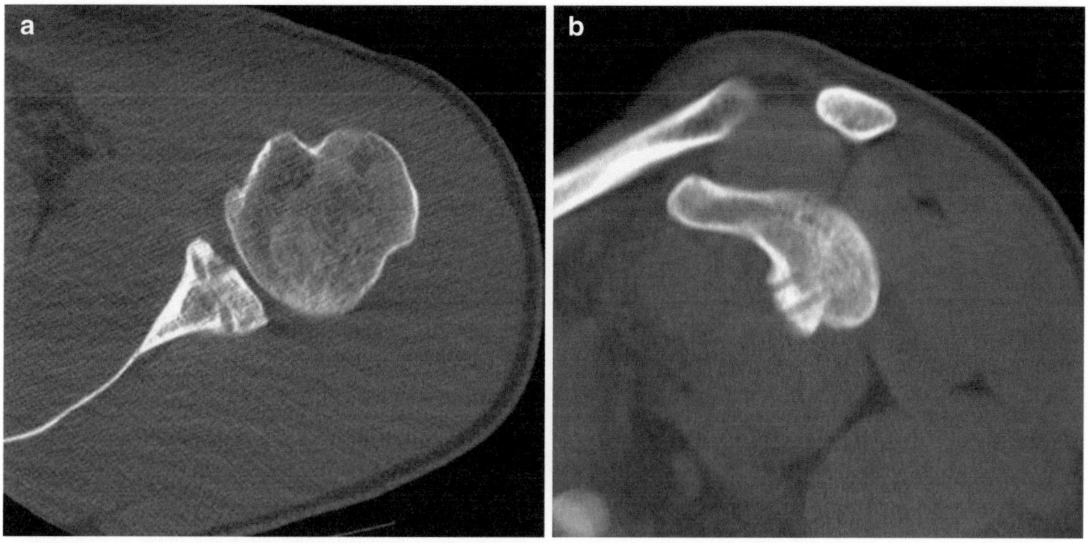

Fig. 17.2 Postoperative (**a**) axial and (**b**) sagittal 2D CT scans of left shoulder after undergoing anterior shoulder stabilization with open Latarjet. (Images courtesy of Dr. Matthew T. Provencher, MD, MBA)

and reported no significant difference in rates or timing of RTP following ABR or open Latarjet procedure. The authors found no studies reporting a significant difference in rate of RTP at preinjury level or among collision athletes.

17.2.5 Iliac Crest Bone Graft (ICBG) or Distal Tibia Allograft (DTA)

The indications for anterior glenoid bone grafting may include >20% GBL, failed prior Latarjet procedure, and epilepsy. Relative indications for glenoid bone grafting (with iliac crest bone graft [ICBG], distal tibia allograft [DTA], or distal clavicular autograft [DCA]) over a Latarjet are GBL greater than can be treated with available coracoid graft size, surgeon preference, and failed prior Latarjet or glenoid bone-grafting procedure [70, 81]. Moroder et al. [82] reported ICBG for recurrent anterior shoulder instability showed excellent results regarding stability and function after a mean follow-up period of 18 years. In a separate study, Moroder and colleagues [83] found no difference in clinical or radiologic outcomes between patients undergoing anterior stabilization with Latarjet or ICBG, though complications included decreased postoperative internal rotation in the Latarjet group and donor-site paresthesia in the ICBG group. Ayramidis et al. [84] reported excellent clinical and radiological midterm outcomes after arthroscopic ICBG. Giannakos et al. [85] found a 67% success rate in patients who underwent revision shoulder stabilization with arthroscopic Eden-Hybinette procedure following prior failed open Latarjet or open/arthroscopic Bankart repair. Fifty-eight percent returned to sport and 17% had recurrent subluxations. Litchfield et al. [86] reported ICBG and the Latarjet procedure did not differ in instability outcomes at 6, 12, and 24 months. Ortmaier et al. [87] performed ICBG on athletes and reported 100% of athletes RTP, but 41% changed sports. In the same cohort, 15% of patients cited their shoulder as the reason for the change, but all returned to the same level in their new sport.

In the setting of a failed Latarjet secondary to subluxation or dislocation, Ernstbrunner et al. [88] performed salvage stabilization procedures with ICBG with mixed results at a mean follow-up of 4.5 years. Nearly half of the patients (7/16, 43.4%) reported recurrent instability following management with ICBG, with the authors noting that patients with unclear instability etiology, subscapularis insufficiency, inferior subluxation, uncontrolled seizures, or psychological disorders

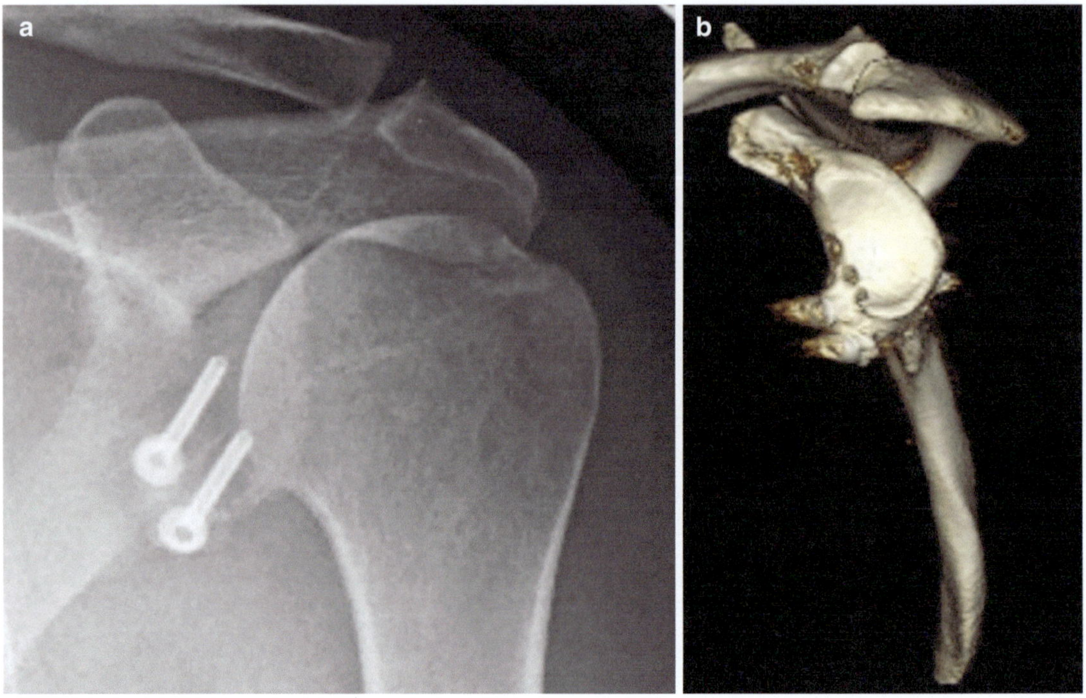

Fig. 17.3 Postoperative imaging of a left shoulder on (**a**) anterior-posterior (AP) radiograph and (**b**) en-face view 3D CT demonstrating a failed Latarjet procedure with massive graft resorption and intact hardware. (Images courtesy of Dr. Matthew T. Provencher, MD, MBA)

had inferior outcomes. Provencher et al. [81] reported that young, physically active military patients who underwent DTA after failed Latarjet demonstrated excellent clinical outcomes and near-complete osseous union at the glenoid-allograft interface (Figs. 17.3 and 17.4). Martinez-Catalan et al. [89] reported arthroscopic ICBG leads to satisfactory clinical outcomes and a low recurrence rate after failed Latarjet.

17.2.6 In-Season Athletes

Management of anterior shoulder instability for in-season athletes is a decision between the athlete and physician, which depends on a variety of factors, including timing in the season, the specific sport and position, year in school, and contract status. Most athletes will be able to return to play during the same season, albeit with a higher risk of recurrence [7, 48, 50, 90, 91]. The Nonoperative Instability Severity Index Score was developed by Tokish et al. [92] to assist in determining which athletes have a high probability of successful return to play. Bony Bankart and Hill-Sachs lesions as well as GBL are important indicators of poor prognosis with nonoperative management. In any scenario, the management of the in-season athlete requires careful balance of physical and psychological demands of sport and the goals of the athlete. Proper counseling of expected risks and benefits of all treatment options are paramount to success.

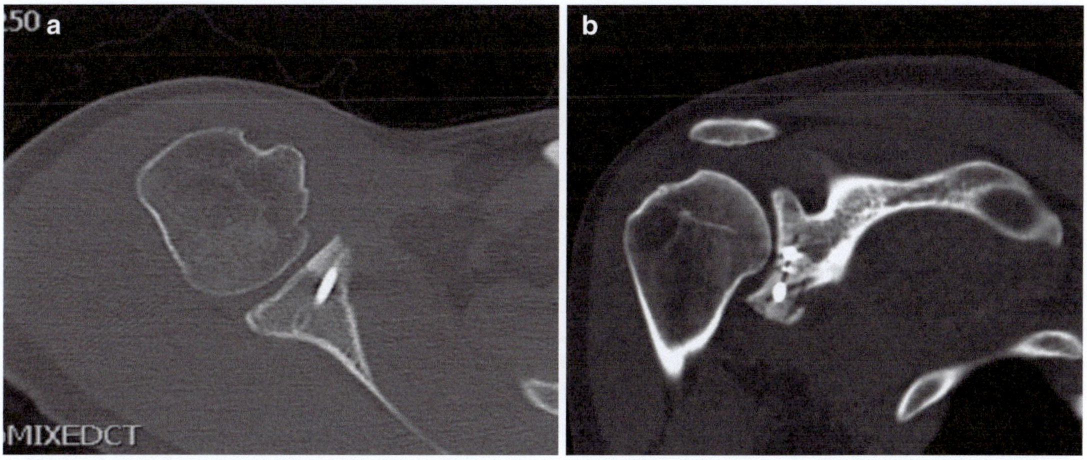

Fig. 17.4 Postoperative imaging of left shoulder on (**a**) axial and (**b**) coronal 2D CT imaging after undergoing free glenoid bone grafting with distal tibia allograft. (Images courtesy of Dr. Matthew T. Provencher, MD, MBA)

17.3 Conclusion

In the setting of acute or recurrent anterior shoulder instability, contact and collision athletes remain a challenging subset of patients to treat and have a greater risk of recurrent instability following both operative and nonoperative management. Although most athletes may be able to return to play during the same season, the elevated risk of recurrent instability and further damage to the osseous and soft tissue stabilizers of the shoulder must be strongly considered and thoroughly discussed with the patient and their families. In contact athletes presenting with acute or recurrent anterior instability and minimal GBL, surgical treatment options may include open or arthroscopic Bankart repair and Latarjet. Athletes with a history of previously failed open or arthroscopic Bankart repair or those with evidence of significant GBL (>15–20%) should be managed with Latarjet or free glenoid bone grafting with ICBG or DTA. Finally, patients returning to contact and collision sports who have recurrent instability following Latarjet or athletes with extensive GBL (>25%) should be considered for free glenoid bone grafting (Table 17.2).

Table 17.2 Treatment recommendations for management of shoulder instability in contact athletes

Indication	Treatment recommendation
1. In-season primary instability event	Nonoperative vs. arthroscopic Bankart
2. Recurrent instability, no GBL	Arthroscopic Bankart vs. open Bankart vs. Latarjet
3. Recurrent instability, GBL > 15–20%	Latarjet vs. free glenoid bone grafting[a]
4. Failed Latarjet or GBL > 25%	Free glenoid bone grafting[a]
5. On-track (nonengaging) HSL	Bankart repair + Remplissage
6. Off-track (engaging) HSL	Bankart repair + HSL grafting

GBL glenoid bone loss, *HSL* Hill-Sachs Lesion
[a] Iliac crest bone graft, distal tibia allograft, or distal clavicle autograft

Acknowledgements The authors would like to extend their deep gratitude to CAPT Matthew T. Provencher MD, MBA, USNR (Ret.) for contributing the patient cases used for figures in this manuscript. Your expertise and mentorship have greatly enriched the scope and clarity of this chapter, thank you for your contributions.

References

1. Dumont GD, Russell RD, Robertson WJ. Anterior shoulder instability: a review of pathoanatomy, diagnosis and treatment. Curr Rev Musculoskelet Med. 2011;4(4):200–7. https://doi.org/10.1007/s12178-011-9092-9.
2. Headey J, Brooks JH, Kemp SP. The epidemiology of shoulder injuries in English professional rugby union. Am J Sports Med. 2007;35(9):1537–43. https://doi.org/10.1177/0363546507300691.
3. Owens BD, Agel J, Mountcastle SB, Cameron KL, Nelson BJ. Incidence of glenohumeral instability in collegiate athletics. Am J Sports Med. 2009;37(9):1750–4. https://doi.org/10.1177/0363546509334591.
4. Becker B, Spadafore S, Oberle L, Spittler J, Khodaee M. Epidemiology of shoulder dislocation treated at emergency departments in the United States between 1997 and 2021. Orthop J Sports Med. 2024;12(3):23259671241234930. https://doi.org/10.1177/23259671241234930.
5. Kaplan LD, Flanigan DC, Norwig J, Jost P, Bradley J. Prevalence and variance of shoulder injuries in elite collegiate football players. Am J Sports Med. 2005;33(8):1142–6. https://doi.org/10.1177/0363546505274718.
6. Dekker TJ, Goldenberg B, Lacheta L, Horan MP, Millett PJ. Anterior shoulder instability in the professional athlete: return to competition, time to return, and career length. Orthop J Sports Med. 2020;8(11):2325967120959728. https://doi.org/10.1177/2325967120959728.
7. Dickens JF, Owens BD, Cameron KL, Kilcoyne K, Allred CD, Svoboda SJ, et al. Return to play and recurrent instability after in-season anterior shoulder instability: a prospective multicenter study. Am J Sports Med. 2014;42(12):2842–50. https://doi.org/10.1177/0363546514553181.
8. Sachs RA, Lin D, Stone ML, Paxton E, Kuney M. Can the need for future surgery for acute traumatic anterior shoulder dislocation be predicted? J Bone Joint Surg Am. 2007;89(8):1665–74. https://doi.org/10.2106/JBJS.F.00261.
9. Burra G, Andrews JR. Acute shoulder and elbow dislocations in the athlete. Orthop Clin North Am. 2002;33(3):479–95. https://doi.org/10.1016/s0030-5898(01)00005-0.
10. Owens BD, Duffey ML, Nelson BJ, DeBerardino TM, Taylor DC, Mountcastle SB. The incidence and characteristics of shoulder instability at the United States military academy. Am J Sports Med. 2007;35(7):1168–73. https://doi.org/10.1177/0363546506295179.
11. Yiannakopoulos CK, Mataragas E, Antonogiannakis E. A comparison of the spectrum of intra-articular lesions in acute and chronic anterior shoulder instability. Arthroscopy. 2007;23(9):985–90. https://doi.org/10.1016/j.arthro.2007.05.009.
12. Urayama M, Itoi E, Sashi R, Minagawa H, Sato K. Capsular elongation in shoulders with recurrent anterior dislocation. Quantitative assessment with magnetic resonance arthrography. Am J Sports Med. 2003;31(1):64–7. https://doi.org/10.1177/03635465030310012201.
13. Robinson CM, Jenkins PJ, White TO, Ker A, Will E. Primary arthroscopic stabilization for a first-time anterior dislocation of the shoulder. A randomized, double-blind trial. J Bone Joint Surg Am. 2008;90(4):708–21. https://doi.org/10.2106/JBJS.G.00679.
14. Gill TJ, Micheli LJ, Gebhard F, Binder C. Bankart repair for anterior instability of the shoulder. Long-term outcome. J Bone Joint Surg Am. 1997;79(6):850–7. https://doi.org/10.2106/00004623-199706000-00008.
15. Gill TJ, Zarins B. Open repairs for the treatment of anterior shoulder instability. Am J Sports Med. 2003;31(1):142–53. https://doi.org/10.1177/03635465030310011001.
16. Bonnevialle N, Mattesi L, Martinel V, Letartre R, Barret H, Mansat P. Outcomes at long-term follow-up after open Latarjet versus open Bankart repair in Rugby players. Orthop J Sports Med. 2023;11(8):23259671231184394. https://doi.org/10.1177/23259671231184394.
17. Imhoff AB, Ansah P, Tischer T, Reiter C, Bartl C, Hench M, et al. Arthroscopic repair of anterior-inferior glenohumeral instability using a portal at the 5:30-o'clock position: analysis of the effects of age, fixation method, and concomitant shoulder injury on surgical outcomes. Am J Sports Med. 2010;38(9):1795–803. https://doi.org/10.1177/0363546510370199.
18. Hintermann B, Gachter A. Arthroscopic findings after shoulder dislocation. Am J Sports Med. 1995;23(5):545–51. https://doi.org/10.1177/036354659502300505.
19. Weber SC, Martin DF, Seiler JG 3rd, Harrast JJ. Superior labrum anterior and posterior lesions of the shoulder: incidence rates, complications, and outcomes as reported by American Board of Orthopedic Surgery. Part II candidates. Am J Sports Med. 2012;40(7):1538–43. https://doi.org/10.1177/0363546512447785.
20. Mannava S, Frangiamore SJ, Murphy CP, Sanchez A, Sanchez G, Dornan GJ, et al. Prevalence of shoulder labral injury in collegiate football players at the National Football League Scouting Combine. Orthop J Sports Med. 2018;6(7):2325967118783982. https://doi.org/10.1177/2325967118783982.

21. Boileau P, Villalba M, Hery JY, Balg F, Ahrens P, Neyton L. Risk factors for recurrence of shoulder instability after arthroscopic Bankart repair. J Bone Joint Surg Am. 2006;88(8):1755–63. https://doi.org/10.2106/JBJS.E.00817.
22. Mologne TS, Provencher MT, Menzel KA, Vachon TA, Dewing CB. Arthroscopic stabilization in patients with an inverted pear glenoid: results in patients with bone loss of the anterior glenoid. Am J Sports Med. 2007;35(8):1276–83. https://doi.org/10.1177/0363546507300262.
23. Provencher MT, Bhatia S, Ghodadra NS, Grumet RC, Bach BR Jr, Dewing CB, et al. Recurrent shoulder instability: current concepts for evaluation and management of glenoid bone loss. J Bone Joint Surg Am. 2010;92(Suppl 2):133–51. https://doi.org/10.2106/JBJS.J.00906.
24. Bigliani LU, Newton PM, Steinmann SP, Connor PM, McLlveen SJ. Glenoid rim lesions associated with recurrent anterior dislocation of the shoulder. Am J Sports Med. 1998;26(1):41–5. https://doi.org/10.1177/03635465980260012301.
25. Shaha JS, Cook JB, Song DJ, Rowles DJ, Bottoni CR, Shaha SH, et al. Redefining "critical" bone loss in shoulder instability: functional outcomes worsen with "subcritical" bone loss. Am J Sports Med. 2015;43(7):1719–25. https://doi.org/10.1177/0363546515578250.
26. Dekker TJ, Peebles LA, Bernhardson AS, Rosenberg SI, Murphy CP, Golijanin P, et al. Risk factors for recurrence after arthroscopic instability repair-the importance of glenoid bone loss >15%, patient age, and duration of symptoms: a matched cohort analysis. Am J Sports Med. 2020;48(12):3036–41. https://doi.org/10.1177/0363546520949840.
27. Dickens JF, Owens BD, Cameron KL, DeBerardino TM, Masini BD, Peck KY, et al. The effect of subcritical bone loss and exposure on recurrent instability after arthroscopic Bankart repair in intercollegiate American football. Am J Sports Med. 2017;45(8):1769–75. https://doi.org/10.1177/0363546517704184.
28. Privitera DM, Sinz NJ, Miller LR, Siegel EJ, Solberg MJ, Daniels SD, et al. Clinical outcomes following the Latarjet procedure in contact and collision athletes. J Bone Joint Surg Am. 2018;100(6):459–65. https://doi.org/10.2106/JBJS.17.00566.
29. Shibuya K, Kawasaki T, Hasegawa Y, Gonda Y, Itoigawa Y, Sobue S, et al. Glenoid bone loss is a risk factor for poor clinical results after coracoid transfer in Rugby players with shoulder dislocations. Orthop J Sports Med. 2021;9(3):2325967121993233. https://doi.org/10.1177/2325967121993233.
30. Hurley ET, Moore TK, Kilkenny C, Khan S, White-Gibson A, Dickens JF, et al. Young collision athletes have high rate of return to play and good clinical outcomes following open Latarjet procedure. Arthroscopy. 2024;40(4):1075–80. https://doi.org/10.1016/j.arthro.2023.09.007.
31. Rossi LA, Gorodischer T, Brandariz R, Tanoira I, Pasqualini I, Ranalletta M. High rate of return to sports and low recurrences with the Latarjet procedure in high-risk competitive athletes with Glenohumeral instability and a glenoid bone loss <20. Arthrosc Sports Med Rehabil. 2020;2(6):e735–42. https://doi.org/10.1016/j.asmr.2020.06.004.
32. Rowe CR, Zarins B, Ciullo JV. Recurrent anterior dislocation of the shoulder after surgical repair. Apparent causes of failure and treatment. J Bone Joint Surg Am. 1984;66(2):159–68.
33. Widjaja AB, Tran A, Bailey M, Proper S. Correlation between Bankart and Hill-Sachs lesions in anterior shoulder dislocation. ANZ J Surg. 2006;76(6):436–8. https://doi.org/10.1111/j.1445-2197.2006.03760.x.
34. Welsh MF, Willing RT, Giles JW, Athwal GS, Johnson JA. A rigid body model for the assessment of glenohumeral joint mechanics: influence of osseous defects on range of motion and dislocation. J Biomech. 2016;49(4):514–9. https://doi.org/10.1016/j.jbiomech.2015.11.001.
35. Provencher MT, Frank RM, Leclere LE, Metzger PD, Ryu JJ, Bernhardson A, et al. The Hill-Sachs lesion: diagnosis, classification, and management. J Am Acad Orthop Surg. 2012;20(4):242–52. https://doi.org/10.5435/JAAOS-20-04-242.
36. Lin A, Barrow AE, Charles S, Shannon M, Fox MA, Herman ZJ, et al. Remplissage reduces recurrent instability in high-risk patients with on-track Hill-Sachs lesions. J Shoulder Elb Surg. 2023;32(6S):S99–S105. https://doi.org/10.1016/j.jse.2023.02.011.
37. Di Giacomo G, Golijanin P, Sanchez G, Provencher MT. Radiographic analysis of the Hill-Sachs lesion in anteroinferior shoulder instability after first-time dislocations. Arthroscopy. 2016;32(8):1509–14. https://doi.org/10.1016/j.arthro.2016.01.022.
38. Di Giacomo G, Itoi E, Burkhart SS. Evolving concept of bipolar bone loss and the Hill-Sachs lesion: from "engaging/non-engaging" lesion to "on-track/off-track" lesion. Arthroscopy. 2014;30(1):90–8. https://doi.org/10.1016/j.arthro.2013.10.004.
39. Balg F, Boileau P. The instability severity index score. A simple pre-operative score to select patients for arthroscopic or open shoulder stabilisation. J Bone Joint Surg Br. 2007;89(11):1470–7. https://doi.org/10.1302/0301-620X.89B11.18962.
40. Di Giacomo G, Peebles LA, Pugliese M, Dekker TJ, Golijanin P, Sanchez A, et al. Glenoid track instability management score: radiographic modification of the instability severity index score. Arthroscopy. 2020;36(1):56–67. https://doi.org/10.1016/j.arthro.2019.07.020.
41. Dekker TJ, Peebles LA, Bernhardson AS, Golijanin P, Di Giacomo G, Hackett TR, et al. Limited predictive value of the instability severity index score: evaluation of 217 consecutive cases of recurrent anterior shoulder instability. Arthroscopy. 2021;37(5):1381–91. https://doi.org/10.1016/j.arthro.2020.12.185.
42. Burkhart SS, De Beer JF. Traumatic glenohumeral bone defects and their relationship to failure of arthroscopic Bankart repairs: significance of the inverted-pear glenoid and the humeral engaging

Hill-Sachs lesion. Arthroscopy. 2000;16(7):677–94. https://doi.org/10.1053/jars.2000.17715.
43. Nakagawa S, Hanai H, Mae T, Hayashida K, Yoneda M. Bipolar bone loss in male athletes with traumatic anterior shoulder instability: an evaluation using a new scoring system. Orthop J Sports Med. 2018;6(7):2325967118782420. https://doi.org/10.1177/2325967118782420.
44. Peebles LA, Golijanin P, Peebles AM, Douglass BW, Arner JW, Provencher MT. Glenoid bone loss directly affects Hill-Sachs morphology: an advanced 3-dimensional analysis. Am J Sports Med. 2022;50(9):2469–75. https://doi.org/10.1177/03635465221101016.
45. Golijanin P, Peebles L, Arner JW, Douglass B, Peebles A, Rider D, et al. Advanced 3-dimensional characterization of Hill-Sachs lesions in 100 anterior shoulder instability patients. Arthroscopy. 2021;37(11):3255–61. https://doi.org/10.1016/j.arthro.2021.05.015.
46. Yamamoto N, Shinagawa K, Hatta T, Itoi E. Peripheral-track and central-Track Hill-Sachs lesions: a new concept of assessing an on-track lesion. Am J Sports Med. 2020;48(1):33–8. https://doi.org/10.1177/0363546519886319.
47. Hurley ET, Matache BA, Wong I, Itoi E, Strauss EJ, Delaney RA, et al. Anterior shoulder instability part I-diagnosis, nonoperative management, and Bankart repair—an international consensus statement. Arthroscopy. 2022;38(2):214–23.e7. https://doi.org/10.1016/j.arthro.2021.07.022.
48. Hovelius L, Olofsson A, Sandstrom B, Augustini BG, Krantz L, Fredin H, et al. Nonoperative treatment of primary anterior shoulder dislocation in patients forty years of age and younger. A prospective twenty-five-year follow-up. J Bone Joint Surg Am. 2008;90(5):945–52. https://doi.org/10.2106/JBJS.G.00070.
49. Arciero RA, Wheeler JH, Ryan JB, McBride JT. Arthroscopic Bankart repair versus nonoperative treatment for acute, initial anterior shoulder dislocations. Am J Sports Med. 1994;22(5):589–94. https://doi.org/10.1177/036354659402200504.
50. Buss DD, Lynch GP, Meyer CP, Huber SM, Freehill MQ. Nonoperative management for in-season athletes with anterior shoulder instability. Am J Sports Med. 2004;32(6):1430–3. https://doi.org/10.1177/0363546503262069.
51. Belk JW, Wharton BR, Houck DA, Bravman JT, Kraeutler MJ, Mayer B, et al. Shoulder stabilization versus immobilization for first-time anterior shoulder dislocation: a systematic review and meta-analysis of level 1 randomized controlled trials. Am J Sports Med. 2023;51(6):1634–43. https://doi.org/10.1177/03635465211065403.
52. Kraeutler MJ, Belk JW, Carver TJ, McCarty EC, Khodaee M. Traumatic primary anterior glenohumeral joint dislocation in sports: a systematic review of operative versus nonoperative management. Curr Sports Med Rep. 2020;19(11):468–78. https://doi.org/10.1249/JSR.0000000000000772.
53. Fox MA, Drain NP, Rai A, Zheng A, Carlos NB, Serrano Riera R, et al. Increased failure rates after arthroscopic Bankart repair after second dislocation compared to primary dislocation with comparable clinical outcomes. Arthroscopy. 2023;39(3):682–8. https://doi.org/10.1016/j.arthro.2022.10.012.
54. Bottoni CR, Wilckens JH, DeBerardino TM, D'Alleyrand JC, Rooney RC, Harpstrite JK, et al. A prospective, randomized evaluation of arthroscopic stabilization versus nonoperative treatment in patients with acute, traumatic, first-time shoulder dislocations. Am J Sports Med. 2002;30(4):576–80. https://doi.org/10.1177/03635465020300041801.
55. Pouges C, Hardy A, Vervoort T, Amouyel T, Duriez P, Lalanne C, et al. Arthroscopic Bankart repair versus immobilization for first episode of anterior shoulder dislocation before the age of 25: a randomized controlled trial. Am J Sports Med. 2021;49(5):1166–74. https://doi.org/10.1177/0363546521996381.
56. Kirkley A, Werstine R, Ratjek A, Griffin S. Prospective randomized clinical trial comparing the effectiveness of immediate arthroscopic stabilization versus immobilization and rehabilitation in first traumatic anterior dislocations of the shoulder: long-term evaluation. Arthroscopy. 2005;21(1):55–63. https://doi.org/10.1016/j.arthro.2004.09.018.
57. Uhring J, Rey PB, Rochet S, Obert L. Interest of emergency arthroscopic stabilization in primary shoulder dislocation in young athletes. Orthop Traumatol Surg Res. 2014;100(8 Suppl):S401–8. https://doi.org/10.1016/j.otsr.2014.09.008.
58. Saper MG, Milchteim C, Zondervan RL, Andrews JR, Ostrander RV 3rd. Outcomes after arthroscopic Bankart repair in adolescent athletes participating in collision and contact sports. Orthop J Sports Med. 2017;5(3):2325967117697950. https://doi.org/10.1177/2325967117697950.
59. Domos P, Ascione F, Wallace AL. Arthroscopic Bankart repair with remplissage for non-engaging Hill-Sachs lesion in professional collision athletes. Shoulder Elbow. 2019;11(1):17–25. https://doi.org/10.1177/1758573217728414.
60. Tasaki A, Morita W, Nozaki T, Yonekura Y, Saito M, Phillips BB, et al. Arthroscopic Bankart repair and open Bristow procedure in the treatment of anterior shoulder instability with osseous glenoid lesions in collision athletes. Orthop J Sports Med. 2021;9(5):23259671211008274. https://doi.org/10.1177/23259671211008274.
61. Shah N, Nadiri MN, Torrance E, Funk L. Arthroscopic repair of bony Bankart lesions in collision athletes. Shoulder Elbow. 2018;10(3):201–6. https://doi.org/10.1177/1758573217717102.
62. Yamamoto N, Kijima H, Nagamoto H, Kurokawa D, Takahashi H, Sano H, et al. Outcome of Bankart repair in contact versus non-contact athletes. Orthop

Traumatol Surg Res. 2015;101(4):415–9. https://doi.org/10.1016/j.otsr.2015.03.008.
63. Alkaduhimi H, van der Linde JA, Willigenburg NW, Paulino Pereira NR, van Deurzen DF, van den Bekerom MP. Redislocation risk after an arthroscopic Bankart procedure in collision athletes: a systematic review. J Shoulder Elb Surg. 2016;25(9):1549–58. https://doi.org/10.1016/j.jse.2016.05.002.
64. Pasqualini I, Rossi LA, Franco JVA, Denard PJ, Fieiras C, Escobar Liquitay C, et al. Results after arthroscopic Bankart repair in contact athletes should not be reported globally because of the high variability in recurrences among the different contact or collision sports: a systematic review. Arthroscopy. 2024;40(2):523–39.e2. https://doi.org/10.1016/j.arthro.2023.06.037.
65. Rossi LA, Tanoira I, Gorodischer T, Pasqualini I, Ranalletta M. High variability in functional outcomes and recurrences between contact sports after arthroscopic Bankart repair: a comparative study of 351 patients with a minimum 3-year follow-up. Arthrosc Sports Med Rehabil. 2020;2(5):e575–81. https://doi.org/10.1016/j.asmr.2020.07.004.
66. Nakagawa S, Mae T, Yoneda K, Kinugasa K, Nakamura H. Influence of glenoid defect size and bone fragment size on the clinical outcome after arthroscopic Bankart repair in male collision/contact athletes. Am J Sports Med. 2017;45(9):1967–74. https://doi.org/10.1177/0363546517700864.
67. Monk AP, Crua E, Gatenby GC, Walsh AJ, Stanley JC, Rosenfeldt MP, et al. Clinical outcomes following open anterior shoulder stabilization for glenohumeral instability in the young collision athlete. J Shoulder Elb Surg. 2022;31(7):1474–8. https://doi.org/10.1016/j.jse.2021.12.013.
68. Hickey IPM, Davey MS, Hurley ET, Gaafar M, Delaney RA, Mullett H. Return to play following open Bankart repair in collision athletes aged 18 years or less. J Shoulder Elb Surg. 2022;31(6S):S8–S12. https://doi.org/10.1016/j.jse.2021.11.001.
69. Bitar IJ, Bustos DG, Marangoni LD, Robles C, Gentile L, Bertiche P. Outcomes of open Bankart repair plus inferior capsular shift compared with Latarjet procedure in contact athletes with recurrent anterior shoulder instability. Arch Bone Joint Surg. 2023;11(1):39–46. https://doi.org/10.22038/ABJS.2022.60208.2974.
70. Hurley ET, Matache BA, Wong I, Itoi E, Strauss EJ, Delaney RA, et al. Anterior shoulder instability part II-Latarjet, remplissage, and glenoid bone-grafting—an international consensus statement. Arthroscopy. 2022;38(2):224–33.e6. https://doi.org/10.1016/j.arthro.2021.07.023.
71. Yamamoto N, Muraki T, An KN, Sperling JW, Cofield RH, Itoi E, et al. The stabilizing mechanism of the Latarjet procedure: a cadaveric study. J Bone Joint Surg Am. 2013;95(15):1390–7. https://doi.org/10.2106/JBJS.L.00777.
72. Tanghe KK, Peebles LA, Ridley TJ, Provencher MT. Latarjet procedure with coracoclavicular ligament augmentation for traumatic coracoid fracture and recurrent anterior glenohumeral instability in an elite contact athlete. Arthrosc Tech. 2020;9(11):e1689–96. https://doi.org/10.1016/j.eats.2020.07.010.
73. Pasqualini I, De Cicco FL, Tanoira I, Ranalletta M, Rossi LA. Classic versus congruent-arc Latarjet procedures. Arthroscopy. 2023;39(1):8–10. https://doi.org/10.1016/j.arthro.2022.08.016.
74. Mengers SRP, Knapik DM, Kaufman MW, Edwards G, Voos JE, Gillespie RJ, et al. Clinical outcomes of the traditional Latarjet versus the congruent arc modification for the treatment of recurrent anterior shoulder instability: a meta-analysis. Orthop J Sports Med. 2021;9(10):23259671211030204. https://doi.org/10.1177/23259671211030204.
75. Brzoska R, Laprus H, Malik SS, Solecki W, Juszczak B, Blasiak A. Return to preinjury-level sports after arthroscopic Latarjet for recurrent anterior shoulder instability in professional athletes. Orthop J Sports Med. 2023;11(5):23259671231166371. https://doi.org/10.1177/23259671231166371.
76. Paulino Pereira NR, van der Linde JA, Alkaduhimi H, Longo UG, van den Bekerom MPJ. Are collision athletes at a higher risk of re-dislocation after an open Bristow-Latarjet procedure? A systematic review and meta-analysis. Shoulder Elbow. 2018;10(2):75–86. https://doi.org/10.1177/1758573217728290.
77. Neyton L, Young A, Dawidziak B, Visona E, Hager JP, Fournier Y, et al. Surgical treatment of anterior instability in rugby union players: clinical and radiographic results of the Latarjet-Patte procedure with minimum 5-year follow-up. J Shoulder Elb Surg. 2012;21(12):1721–7. https://doi.org/10.1016/j.jse.2012.01.023.
78. Hurley ET, Davey MS, Montgomery C, Moore DM, Mojica ES, Gaafar M, et al. Analysis of athletes who did not return to play after open Latarjet. Orthop J Sports Med. 2022;10(2):23259671211071082. https://doi.org/10.1177/23259671211071082.
79. Hurley ET, Davey MS, Montgomery C, O'Doherty R, Gaafar M, Pauzenberger L, et al. Arthroscopic Bankart repair versus open Latarjet for first-time dislocators in athletes. Orthop J Sports Med. 2021;9(8):23259671211023803. https://doi.org/10.1177/23259671211023803.
80. Hurley ET, Danilkowicz RM, Paul AV, Myers H, Anakwenze OA, Klifto CS, et al. Majority of studies show similar rates of return to play after arthroscopic Bankart repair or Latarjet procedure: a systematic review. Arthroscopy. 2024;40(2):515–22. https://doi.org/10.1016/j.arthro.2023.04.017.
81. Provencher MT, Peebles LA, Aman ZS, Bernhardson AS, Murphy CP, Sanchez A, et al. Management of the failed Latarjet procedure: outcomes of revision surgery with fresh distal tibial allograft. Am J Sports Med. 2019;47(12):2795–802. https://doi.org/10.1177/0363546519871896.

82. Moroder P, Plachel F, Becker J, Schulz E, Abdic S, Haas M, et al. Clinical and radiological long-term results after implant-free, autologous, iliac crest bone graft procedure for the treatment of anterior shoulder instability. Am J Sports Med. 2018;46(12):2975–80. https://doi.org/10.1177/0363546518795165.
83. Moroder P, Schulz E, Wierer G, Auffarth A, Habermeyer P, Resch H, et al. Neer award 2019: Latarjet procedure vs. iliac crest bone graft transfer for treatment of anterior shoulder instability with glenoid bone loss: a prospective randomized trial. J Shoulder Elb Surg. 2019;28(7):1298–307. https://doi.org/10.1016/j.jse.2019.03.035.
84. Avramidis G, Kokkineli S, Trellopoulos A, Tsiogka A, Natsika M, Brilakis E, et al. Excellent clinical and radiological midterm outcomes for the management of recurrent anterior shoulder instability by all-arthroscopic modified eden-hybinette procedure using iliac crest autograft and double-pair button fixation system: 3-year clinical case series with no loss to follow-up. Arthroscopy. 2021;37(3):795–803. https://doi.org/10.1016/j.arthro.2020.10.036.
85. Giannakos A, Vezeridis PS, Schwartz DG, Jany R, Lafosse L. All-arthroscopic revision Eden-Hybinette procedure for failed instability surgery: technique and preliminary results. Arthroscopy. 2017;33(1):39–48. https://doi.org/10.1016/j.arthro.2016.05.021.
86. Litchfield R. In anterior shoulder instability with glenoid bone loss, iliac crest bone graft transfer and the Latarjet procedure did not differ for instability measures at 6, 12, and 24 months. J Bone Joint Surg Am. 2020;102(4):340. https://doi.org/10.2106/JBJS.19.01329.
87. Ortmaier R, Fink C, Schobersberger W, Kindermann H, Mattiassich G, Hochreiter J, et al. Return to sports after glenoid reconstruction using an implant-free iliac crest bone graft. Orthop Traumatol Surg Res. 2019;105(8):1471–9. https://doi.org/10.1016/j.otsr.2019.07.012.
88. Ernstbrunner L, Pastor T, Waltenspul M, Gerber C, Wieser K. Salvage iliac crest bone grafting for a failed Latarjet procedure: analysis of failed and successful procedures. Am J Sports Med. 2021;49(13):3620–7. https://doi.org/10.1177/03635465211040468.
89. Martinez-Catalan N, Werthel JD, Kazum E, Valenti P. Failed Latarjet treated with full arthroscopic Eden-Hybinette procedure using two cortical suture buttons leads to satisfactory clinical outcomes and low recurrence rate. Arthroscopy. 2022;38(4):1126–33. https://doi.org/10.1016/j.arthro.2021.10.026.
90. Robinson CM, Howes J, Murdoch H, Will E, Graham C. Functional outcome and risk of recurrent instability after primary traumatic anterior shoulder dislocation in young patients. J Bone Joint Surg Am. 2006;88(11):2326–36. https://doi.org/10.2106/JBJS.E.01327.
91. Wheeler JH, Ryan JB, Arciero RA, Molinari RN. Arthroscopic versus nonoperative treatment of acute shoulder dislocations in young athletes. Arthroscopy. 1989;5(3):213–7. https://doi.org/10.1016/0749-8063(89)90174-6.
92. Tokish JM, Thigpen CA, Kissenberth MJ, Tolan SJ, Lonergan KT, Tokish JM Jr, et al. The nonoperative instability severity index score (NISIS): a simple tool to guide operative versus nonoperative treatment of the unstable shoulder. Sports Health. 2020;12(6):598–602. https://doi.org/10.1177/1941738120925738.

18 Shoulder Instability in the Teenage Athlete

Cristina Delgado, Jose María Martínez, and Emilio Calvo

18.1 Introduction

Glenohumeral instability is a very common condition, especially among young active patients. With increasing teenage participation in competitive contact sports over the past decade, traumatic anterior shoulder instability is becoming even more prevalent.

Teenage athletes present with many of the same complaints as adults, but differences in anatomy often lead to age-specific issues. On the one hand, adolescent patients have shown the higher risk of recurrence [1]. Recurrent instability compromises soft-tissue stabilizers, increases the risk of developing bone loss and off-track Hill-Sachs (HS) lesions and may cause articular cartilage damage in the glenohumeral joint [2, 3]. Furthermore, persistent instability may interfere with sports practice and impairs quality of life. On the other hand, specific anatomy features should be considered when diagnosing and treating these patients (i.e., open physis, ossification centers, soft-tissue elasticity) [3]. Improving our knowledge of this condition is crucial to help drive targeted evidence-based treatment algorithms.

To date, no consensus exists on the treatment of instability in teenagers. Given the high risk of recurrence, surgical stabilization following the first episodes is typically recommended [4]. The arthroscopic Bankart repair is, as in adults, the most common procedure for the treatment of anterior glenohumeral instability, especially in first dislocation episodes. However, high rates of recurrence have been reported in the long run, especially in young athletes [5]. The high rate of recurrent dislocation following the Bankart repair has led to combine *remplissage* with Bankart repair and to increase of bone-block procedures such as the Latarjet for the young active patients. While the literature concerning adult patients shows good short—and long-term outcomes, with a low recurrence and complication rate, little is known about this procedure in young patients.

In this chapter, we focus on anterior glenohumeral instability in the adolescent athlete. The epidemiology, natural history including risk of recurrence and risk of bone loss development, and treatment options are discussed.

C. Delgado (✉) · J. M. Martínez
Shoulder and Elbow Reconstructive Surgery Unit, Department of Orthopedic Surgery and Traumatology, Fundación Jiménez Diaz, Madrid, Spain
e-mail: cristina.delgadoc@quironsalud.es

E. Calvo
Department of Orthopedic Surgery and Traumatology, Hospital Universitario Fundacion Jimenez, Universidad Autonoma, Madrid, Spain
e-mail: ecalvo@fjd.es

E. Calvo et al. (eds.), *Complex and Revision Problems in Shoulder Instability*,
https://doi.org/10.1007/978-3-031-81389-4_18

18.2 Epidemiology

Shoulder dislocations are becoming increasingly common among pediatric and adolescent patients as enrollment of this subjects in competitive competitions begin earlier.

Young patients have shown the greatest risk of suffering anterior glenohumeral instability. Literature shows that the proportion of patients who redislocate is inversely related to the age at the time of primary dislocation [6]. However, when analyzing adolescents with shoulder instability it is important to distinguish two different groups: those aged 14–17 years at the time of primary dislocation and those less than 14 years of age at the time of the primary dislocation. Zachilli et al. revealed an overall dislocation rate among all ages of 23.9/100.000 person-years. Interestingly this incidence was of 0.92/100.000 person-years among patients 0–9 years rising to 39.71 among patients 10–19 years old [7]. These results were later supported by Leroux. et al., who found in a 1937 series of patients with glenohumeral instability, a higher instability rate in patients aged 16 years than those between 10–12 years [6].

Similar to that reported in the adult population, male sex has been proposed as a risk factor for dislocation but discrepancies between studies exist [1]. Hyperlaxity and sports activities have also been described as risk factors for instability recurrence [8, 9]. More specifically, young collision athletes are particularly high-risk group for instability with an estimated incidence of 15% [1].

18.3 Natural History

18.3.1 Risk Factors for Recurrence

According to literature, rates of recurrent instability after a first episode of dislocation can reach 96% in young patients [1]. During the last years, many papers dealing with risk factors of recurrence have been written. Olds et al. specifically analyzed risk factors predisposing to recurrent shoulder instability in children 18 years and under [1]. Their systematic review, encompassing six studies, identified several risk factors: age, gender, shoulder dominance and injury side, mechanism of injury, state of physis closure, and bony lesions (HS and glenoid bone loss).

Young age has been proposed to be the most predictable risk factor for recurrence. Hovelius et al. in a large cohort prospective study found that 2 years after the first dislocation, 51% of patients younger than 22 years had recurred and a further 16% regarded their shoulders as unstable although they had no recurrence [3]. Failure rates kept increasing with time: at 5-years follow-up the percentage of shoulders with no redislocation or surgical stabilization procedure was as low as 29%. Roberts et al. confirmed the poor prognosis at young age [10]. The authors analyzed 133 patients aged 14–18 years old and found a recurrent dislocation rate of 76.7%, with recurrences occurring most commonly within 2 years of their initial injury. Moreover, only 7% remained stable 10 years after the initial dislocation. Interestingly, no correlation between age and redislocation was found. On the latter, it is important to note that patients aged 14–18 have shown the greatest risk of recurrence following first dislocation whereas those patients under 14 years old were at lower risk of recurrence [11]. This subgroup of patients, in whom the proximal humeral physis remains open, are more likely to suffer a greater tuberosity or metaphyseal fracture rather than a dislocation [3]. Other suggested reason for patients younger than 14 years being at lower risk of recurrence is a softer tissue elasticity of the capsulolabral complex in skeletally immature patients because of a higher ratio of type III to type I collagen [12].Discrepancy in the literature exists on whether gender is a specific risk factor for recurrent shoulder instability or not. Recent studies suggest that recurrences may not be related to gender itself, but to the sports in which patients are enrolled or a more traumatic mechanism of injury [2].Other risk factors for recurrence include practice of sports, more specifically, young collision athletes, and presence of bone loss [8].

18.3.2 Bone Loss

Glenoid and humerus bone loss has been reported in up to 22% and 32% after the initial dislocation and in 86–100% of cases in recurrent instability in adults [13]. Glenoid bone loss seems particularly common in the adolescent population, with 48.2% of patients having at least mild bone loss and 13% having bone loss of >20% according to Ellis et al. [14]. The incidence of bone loss seems particularly high in adolescents who suffered the primary dislocation while playing sports [14].

While the literature concerning adult patients show that glenoid bone loss greater than 13.5–15% of the articular surface predispose patients to recurrence and worse outcomes, little is known on the amount of glenoid defect considered critical in adolescent population [9, 15]. Dickens et al. specifically evaluated the influence of bone loss in patients between 18–23 years old practicing American football treated with an arthroscopic Bankart repair. The authors stablished at 13.5% the threshold of Bankart repair obtaining satisfactory results. Conversely, according to Nakagawa et al. in teenage competitive athlete shoulders with a glenoid defect and bone fragment, bone union after arthroscopic Bankart repair is the factor most affecting postoperative stability regardless of the preoperative glenoid defect size [16]. This lack of agreement may be because of the paucity of studies specifically analyzing the influence of bone loss in adolescents, but also because mimics with normal glenoid ossification makes sometimes difficult to identify bone defects [17].

Young age has also been identified as an independent factor for the development of an off-track HS lesion. Lau et al. reported a 9.38-fold higher risk to develop an off-track HS lesion in adolescent patients [18]. These results have been recently supported by Delgado et al. who found that young age and variables related to persistent instability (higher number of instability episodes, increased time from first instability episode and surgery) predisposed to off-track HS lesions [2]. Also, enrollment in overhead activities was a predictor of off-track HS lesions.

18.4 Diagnosis

18.4.1 History and Physical Evaluation

As in the adult population, a complete physical examination and anamnesis is mandatory. The history should address number of dislocations, mechanism of injury and age at first dislocation, subjective feeling of instability or apprehension arm's positioning, participation on sports, assessing both type of sport and level of competition and future plans in that sport. Physical exam should document any asymmetry, if present, and range of movement. Neurovascular status and signs of hyperlaxity should be carefully assessed. Specific anterior instability maneuvers are identical to those used in the adult population, including the load and shift test, hyperabduction test, anterior apprehension sign, relocation, and releases tests.

18.4.2 Imaging

Imaging evaluation begins with standard shoulder x-ray views. Special attention should be paid on open physis and possible physeal injuries (Fig. 18.1) [19]. Also, one should be aware of glenoid ossification centers being unfused, especially with the anterior secondary ossification center which can mimic an anterior bony Bankart lesion in males 11–17 and females 11–12 years old in whom the ossification center remains unfused [17].

Preoperative magnetic resonance imaging (MRI) or computed tomography (CT) scan are routinely requested in the adult population. MRI can help in distinguishing glenoid ossification centers and is essential for soft tissue most common lesions evaluation, including anteroinferior labral lesion (Bankart), anterior labral periosteal sleeve avulsion (ALPSA), or less frequently a humeral avulsion of the glenohumeral ligament (HAGL lesion). The CT scan is considered the gold-standard for bone loss diagnosis. However, the use of CT scan in the pediatric population should be balanced

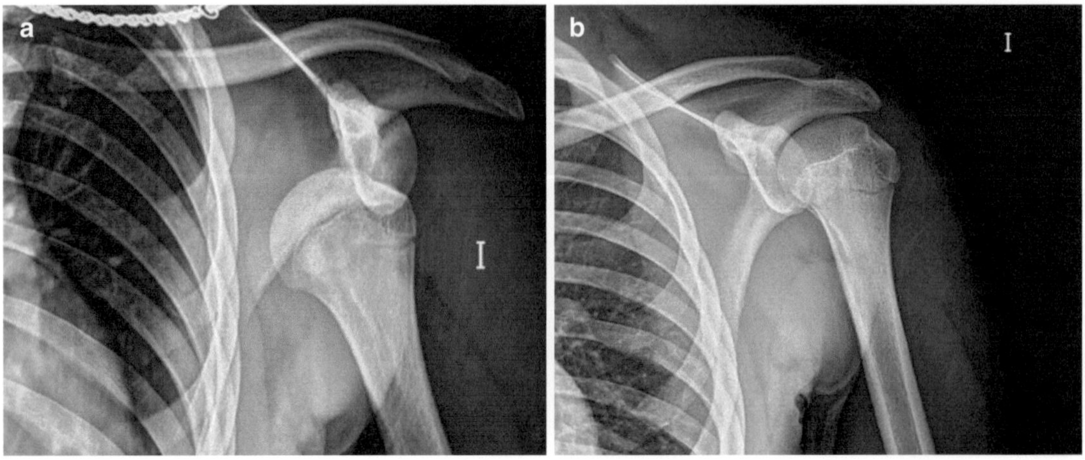

Fig. 18.1 Conventional AP X-ray AP views of a left shoulder showing an anterior shoulder dislocation (**a**) and reduction (**b**) in a skeletally immature patient

against the potential effects of radiation. According to Gyftopoulos et al. [20], glenoid track can accurately be assessed with MRI, whereas Chalmers et al. and Bishop et al. showed, respectively, less accuracy and reliability when using MRI for bone loss assessment [21, 22]. Therefore, the role of MRI in evaluating bone loss, especially in the adolescent population, is yet to be stablished and CT-scan is still the standard of care when suspecting bone loss.

18.5 Management

18.5.1 Initial Management: Acute Dislocation

In acute dislocation gentle reduction maneuvers should be performed in order to avoid increasing HS lesion size during the reduction [23]. After reduction, there is still no consensus on both the position and length of immobilization, with no clear benefit for immobilizations longer than 1 week or with the use of external rotation slings [24]. Following immobilization period a physiotherapy program involving periscapular and rotator cuff muscle strengthening is encouraged [25].

18.5.2 Management in First-Time Dislocators

Historically, the more widespread practice was to delay surgical intervention until there are two or further episodes of instability [26]. However, over the past years there has been a trend toward shoulder stabilization in first-time dislocators, especially in the teenage athlete population [27].

As stated previously, young age has been identified as an independent risk factor for recurrent instability [8], development of glenoid defects, and off-track HS lesions [2]. These lesions have shown not only higher risk of recurrence and failure of soft tissue procedures but also an impact on shoulder function and an impairment of quality of life. More specifically, patients with off-track lesions have shown a higher degree of instability and worse preoperative [2] and postoperative scores [28]. Therefore, recurrent instability results in persistent symptoms that interfere daily living activities and sports participation [11]. On the latter, sports participation is an important issue in the treatment of shoulder instability; it is both a well-known risk factor for recurrence and an important outcome commonly disturbed in recurrent instability [2, 29]. Since this population is the one most commonly enrolled in sports activities, limitation of sports participation may highly impair their quality of life. On the other hand, repeat dislocations may cause articular damage to the glenohumeral joint and subsequent glenohumeral arthropathy [3]. Hovelius et al. found that as the number of episodes of dislocation increase, the incidence of osteoarthritis rises [3]. Interestingly patients younger than 25 years when primary dislocation occurred developed less osteoarthritis than patients aged 26–40 years at first dislocation. Finally, repeated dislocations have been identified in the adult population as risk factors for failure of soft-tissue procedures [30]. Therefore, an early surgical intervention in young patients may avoid, on the one hand, development of more severe bony lesions and, on the other hand, the need of more complex surgeries like *remplissage* or bone block procedures, and also function impairment, osteoarthritis development, and surgery failures.

Several studies have shown that early arthroscopic stabilization results in a decrease in recurrent instability, better function, and quality of life. Gigis et al. prospectively analyzed two cohorts of adolescent patients (15–18 years old): a group of 38 patients treated surgically after a first dislocation episode and a second group of 29 patients treated conservatively [4]. At the last follow-up, a significantly higher recurrence rate, noted at 70.3%, was found in the conservative treatment compared with the surgical group in which the recurrence rate was set at 13.1%. Lower recurrence rates in patients treated with surgery after first instability episode were further supported by the systematic review performed by Longo et al., including 15 studies, 705 shoulders, of patients up to 18 years old [27]. The authors found an overall recurrence rate of 17.5% (55/134) in patients undergoing surgery after a first dislocation episode, whereas the recurrence rate in those treated operatively after two or more dislocations reached 71.3% (293/411). In addition, patients undergoing surgery after a first dislocation episode perform better at sports and have better functional status.

However, long-term outcome studies have demonstrated that not all adolescent patients with first-time dislocations treated nonoperatively will develop repeat instability [31]. Hence, when considering surgery after single dislocation different factors need to be taken into consideration, especially age and patient's sports practice and future plans in that sport. Regarding age, skeletally immature patients who are managed nonoperatively have similar outcomes than those undergoing surgery, and therefore, nonoperative treatment should be considered for first-time dislocations [19]. Thus, for clinical decision-making, young population should be divided into two subgroups: skeletally mature adolescents (around age 14 or greater) and pediatric patients with open proximal humerus physes. The first group should be managed surgically, whereas the latter advocate nonsurgical management for first dislocation [4]. With regards to sport practice, as return to sport may be higher in patients treated operatively than those managed nonoperatively, desire to return to high-level contact sports may be considered as a relative surgical indication [27]. Therefore, considering literature, patients between 14–20 years enrolled in high-level contact sports would benefit from an early surgical intervention.

18.5.3 Bankart Repair

The arthroscopic Bankart repair, as in adult population, is the most common technique for the treatment of anterior glenohumeral instability. Satisfactory short-term outcomes but unacceptable high long-term recurrence rates have been reported in adults [32]. Since adolescents have itself a higher risk of recurrence and are most commonly involved in contact sports, higher risk of recurrence is expected in this population. Yet, the results in the teenagers are limited.

Ozturk et al. reported on a series of 53 patients aged younger than 25 years who underwent an arthroscopic capsulolabral repair. Of those, 26 patients were younger than 20 years and showed a surgical failure rate close to 12%, being 87% of athletes able to play their previous sport at a mean follow-up of 27 months [33]. Interestingly, the authors did not find statically difference in rates of recurrence between patients younger and older than 20 years. Similarly, Jones et al. reported on a series of 30 patients aged 11–18 years old surgically treated with an arthroscopic Bankart procedure, with 82% of patients being free of recurrence. All these studies concluded that arthroscopic stabilization should be considered an effective surgical option in the young population. It is interesting to note that, despite the failure rate following Bankart repair in the adolescent population, the overall reported return-to-sport rate is almost constantly satisfactory as confirmed in the systematic review performed by Kasik et al. [34]. After the analysis of 11 studies, 426 adolescent athletes [34], the authors revealed that at a mean follow-up of 48.8 months following an anterior stabilization procedure, 81.5% of patients had returned to sports at preinjury level. Of the remaining, 11.5% were able to return to a lower level of competition and 7% were unable to return to any athletic competition.

In contrast, Kramer et al. reported a failure rate up to 33.3% at a mean of 20.7 months postoperatively and a trend toward recurrent instability in those patients involved in contact sports [5]. These results were further supported by Ayeni's systematic review. Patients undergoing an arthroscopic Bankart repair experienced a recurrence rate of 24%, achieving in 77% of the cases pre-injury level of sport. Nevertheless, athletes, especially collision athletes, have been reported to be at an increased risk of redislocation after soft-tissue stabilization procedures. Torrance et al. and Nixon et al. showed recurrences rates as high as 51% and 31% in contact players younger than 18 years [35, 36]. In contrast, Saper et al. showed the arthroscopic Bankart repair as an effective technique in adolescents participating in collision and contact sports at a minimum 4 years follow-up with recurrence rates noted at 10% and 80% of patients achieving pre-injury level of sport [37]. Besides practicing contact sports, Cheng et al. found that adolescents with more than one dislocation episode before surgery and those with glenoid retroversion less than 6° had a higher risk of recurrent instability postoperatively [38]. Hyperlaxity, presence of bone loss, and off-track HS lesion have also been identified as risk factors for failure of soft-tissue procedures and should be taken into account when indicating a Bankart procedure in teenage athletes [5]. In addition, better results have been observed when indicating this procedure after a first dislocation [39]. Therefore, when evaluating the possibility of performing a Bankart repair, all these risk factors should be taken into account considering that teenagers are indeed at higher risk of failure.

18.5.4 Remplissage

The efficacy of *remplissage* in reducing the recurrence in patients undergoing an arthroscopic Bankart repair is well stablished in adult population, especially in the setting of a Bankart repair with an engaging HS lesion [40], but outcomes in teenagers have only been reported by Hughes et al. [41]. Their results strongly support the use of remplissage in adolescents with recurrent anterior shoulder dislocations and a HS lesion without significant glenoid loss [41] (Fig. 18.2). They matched, based on preoperative features including HS lesion length, 20 subjects treated with an isolated Bankart procedure with 21 patients in whom a *remplissage* was added to the Bankart repair. At a minimum 2 years follow-up the recurrence rate strongly favored adding the remplissage procedure (13.3% vs. 47.1% recurrence rate) without apparent deleterious effects of the associated procedure. In terms of return to sports, 47.1% (8/17) and 60% (9/15) and regarding return to sport rates in the *remplissage* and isolated Bankart respectively. Overall return to sports rates were better in Garcia et al. [42] and Lazarides et al. [43] series, with rates noted at 95.5% and 90.7% respectively, but data concerning adolescents was not specifically provided.

The complication rate of this procedure is very low [43], but concern exists regarding the loss of external rotation [44]. Boileau et al. [44] reported a 10° decrease on external rotation after a remplissage procedure at 12 months but found no clinical implication of this limitation. A similar restriction occurred in the adolescent population analyzed by Hughes, with loss of external rotation observed in 57% of patients undergoing a remplissage versus 20% in whom an isolated Bankart was performed [41].

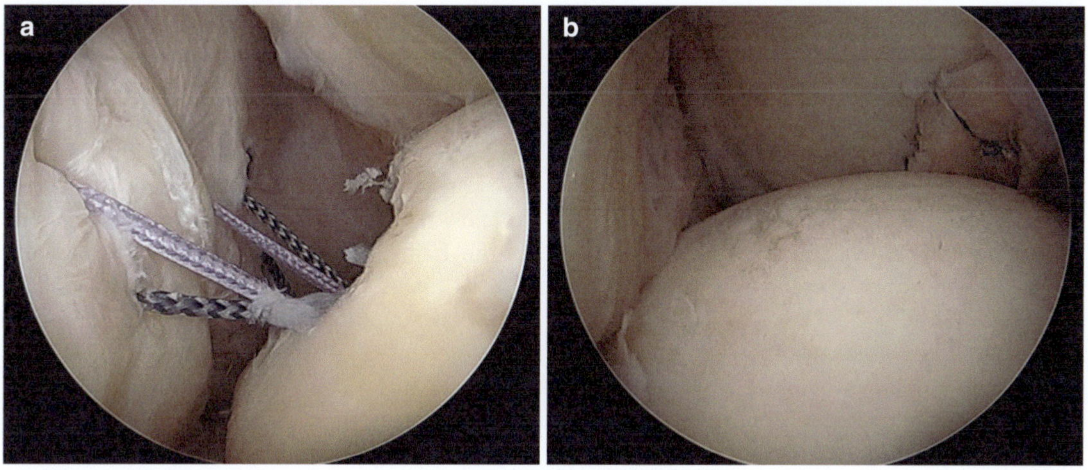

Fig. 18.2 Right shoulder, intraoperative images of an 18-year-old male treated with an arthroscopic remplissage. (**a**) Sutures passed; (**b**) capsulotenodesis completed

18.6 Bone-Block Procedures

18.6.1 Latarjet

The Latarjet procedure, both open and arthroscopic, has demonstrated to be a reliable and effective technique with good clinical outcomes and low recurrence rates [45–47]. However, there is limited evidence with regard to the Latarjet procedure in adolescent and skeletally immature patients. Since anterior shoulder instability commonly affects young patients, many studies do include adolescents even skeletally immature patients in their series, but there is paucity of studies specifically analyzing the results on this population [48–51].

Overall, studies that examine the outcomes of the Latarjet procedure have reported good to excellent outcomes in both the open and arthroscopic approaches, in terms of recurrence, with recurrence rates noted at 0–8% and 2% respectively [45, 46], patient reported outcomes and radiological outcomes [47, 52]. Shoulder instability is also restored in teenager's series. Domos et al. in their series of 45 patients aged 13–17 years old, found a recurrence rate of 4% and 24% of persistent apprehension [48]. Kahn et al. and Rossi et al. reported a similar recurrence and apprehension rates, noted at 7%/25% and 3.3%/0% respectively [50]. In addition, satisfactory clinical and functional status, with increasing outcomes from preoperative to postoperative, and excellent radiological results were obtained [51]. According to literature, these satisfactory results maintained over time. A recent systematic review, including 13 studies evaluating the Latarjet with more than 10 years follow-up, found that the Latarjet resulted in low recurrent instability rates (8.5%) and excellent functional outcomes [53]. However, none of the included studies evaluated patients younger than 20 years.

On the other hand, return to sports is considered to be one of the greatest concerns in patients undergoing surgery for anterior shoulder instability, especially in young and active patients [54]. Recent systematic reviews reported high rates of return to previous sports after the Latarjet procedure. Hurley et al. in a systematic review evolving 36 studies, 2134 shoulders, found at mean 5.8 months postoperative a return to play rate of 88.8%, with 72.6% returning to the same level of play [55]. Similarly, Abdul-Rassoul found a return to sport rate of 83.6% among patients undergoing and open Latarjet and 94.0% after an arthroscopic Latarjet. However, none of the included studies specifically evaluated patients younger than 20 years. When analyzing this specific population high return to sports rates have also been reported. In Domos et al. series 75% of patients were able to return to previous sport after the Latarjet procedure [48]. Interestingly, competitive young athletes also obtained high return to play rates achieving the same preoperative level according to Rossi et al., who found that, of 60 teenage competitive athletes, 93% returned to sports, 84% of whom returned to the same preoperative level [56].

Despite these satisfactory results, it is important to note that this technique is not devoid of complications, such as coracoid fracture, glenohumeral arthrosis, restricted shoulder range of movement, infections, and neurological or vascular lesions, most commonly axillary, musculocutaneous, or suprascapular nerve [46, 57]. Also, subscapularis function has shown to be diminished at 1 year postoperative [58]. According to Griesser et al. [57] systematic review, complication rate following the Latarjet procedure can be as high as 30%. Lower rates of complications have recently been reported following the arthroscopic Latarjet technique [46]. No complications but recurrences were reported in Domos et al. and Rossi et al. adolescent series [48, 51]. Nevertheless, there are specific potential complications related to this group to be account. Firstly, concern exists on the possibility of growth disturbances or glenoid deformities, especially in those aged 15 years or younger who presented incomplete ossification of the scapula. Rossi et al. did not find these complications at a mean follow-up of 58 months [51]. Similarly, Domos et al. in their series of patients ranged 13–17 years old did not observe growth disturbances or glenoid deformities after 6.6 years postoperative [48]. On the other hand, screws related complications including irritation, intraarticular penetration, breakage, should be considered, especially in those active competing patients which are more likely to suffer a trauma, and consequent screw breakage. Finally, potential risk of developing osteoarthritis should be considered when performing this technique. Hurley et al. in their systematic review found at a 16.6 years follow-up after a Latarjet procedure grade I arthritic changes in 26.5% of patients, whereas 12.3% showed grade II-IV arthritic changes. Progression of osteoarthritis was observed in 22.6% of patients without previous osteoarthritis and 23.5% of those with preoperative osteoarthritis signs. However, it is difficult to know if these osteoarthritis changes were due to the Latarjet procedure or were part of the natural history. Moreover, it should be considered that nonoperative treatment itself risks the development of osteoarthritis. Only Domos et al. and Rossi et al. have evaluated arthritis in young patients undergoing a Latarjet procedure. Signs of osteoarthritis were found in only 4 (9%/7%) of the patients in both series [48, 51]. It is important to note that mean follow-up was set just at 79 and 58 months respectively. Thus, longer follow-up series are needed to determine the real influence of Latarjet on osteoarthritis development.

Given the high risk of developing large off-track HS lesions [2] and risk of recurrence [10] in young patients, the Latarjet procedure seems the ideal technique for managing glenohumeral instability in adolescents, especially in those with bone defects and recurrent episodes of dislocation (Fig. 18.3). This hypothesis has recently been proved by Wieser et al. in their comparative study of 41 teenagers treated with an arthroscopic Bankart and 37 teenagers undergoing an open Latarjet. The authors found a treatment failure rate of 57% (20/41) in the Bankart repair group and 6% (2/37) in the Latarjet meaning significantly higher revision rate for instability in the Bankart group.

18.6.2 Free Graft Bone-Block Procedures

Glenoid bone augmentation using free bone grafts, such as iliac crest, distal tibia allograft, distal clavicle, or scapular spine autograft, has recently emerged as an alternative for the management of patients with subcritical bone loss and reparable soft-tissue injuries [13] and for those patients in whom the coracoid graft is

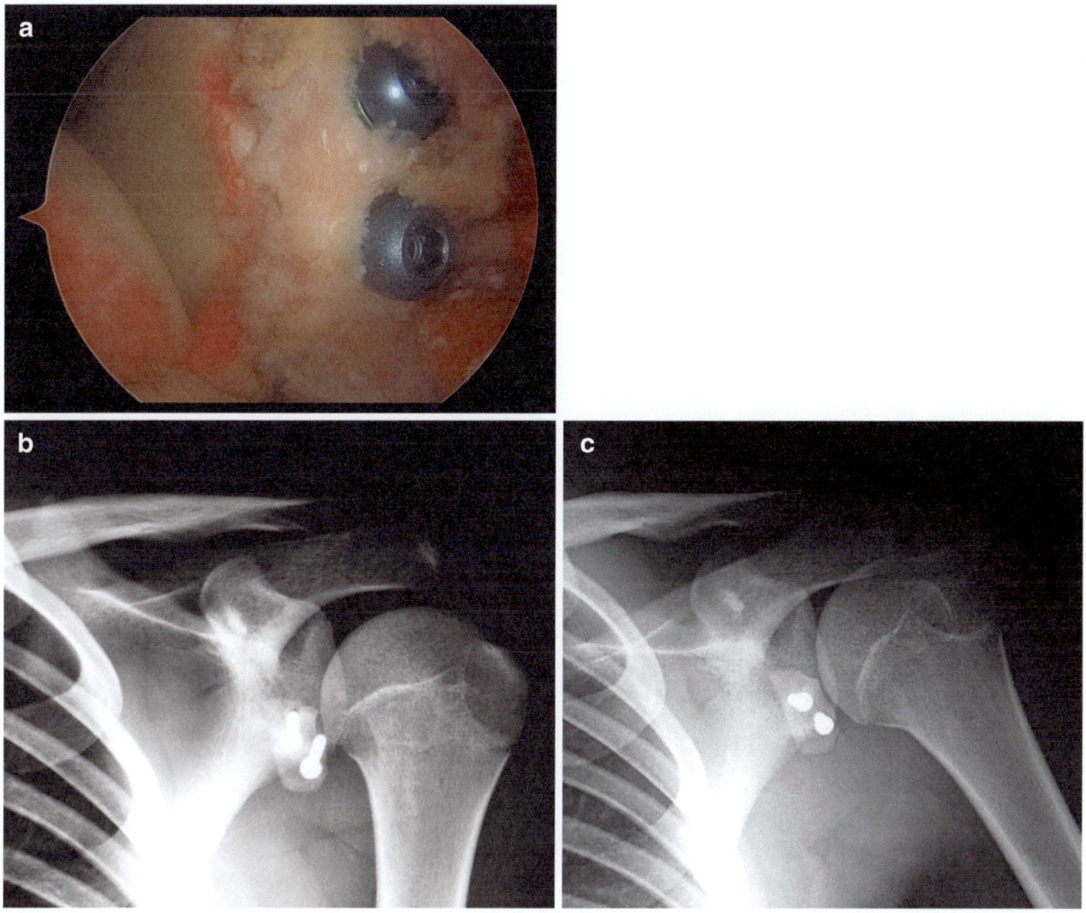

Fig. 18.3 Left shoulder, intraoperative and postoperative images of a 16-year-old male treated with an arthroscopic Latarjet. (**a**) intraoperative (**b** and **c**) postoperative x-rays

enough to restore the glenoid track [59]. Iliac crest and distal tibia allograft have shown excellent results in adult populations, but never have been used in children [13]. Distal clavicle autograft is not desirable in adolescents since distal clavicular physes are still open [60].

18.7 Conclusion

Teenage athletes are the group at greatest risk of recurrence and development of off-track HS lesions. As the number of young, adolescent patients enrolled in sports activities is increasing, an increase in glenohumeral instability prevalence is expected, and, with that, the number of stabilization procedures.

Bankart repair results in good short-term clinical and functional outcomes, but its high failures rates have led to a shift of increasing Latarjet in the adolescent athlete. This technique provides excellent clinical and radiological outcomes with a low complication rate and may be considered as primary surgery in those teenage athletes with off-track HS lesions or significant bone loss.

Key Points

- Patients aged 14–17 years enrolled in contact sports are those at higher risk of suffering an anterior glenohumeral dislocation.
- With the rise of adolescent sports participation, there has been an increase in the incidence of anterior glenohumeral instability.
- When interpreting young shoulder imaging, attention should be paid to the presence of open physes and normal glenoid ossification centers which can mimic bony-Bankart lesions.
- Teenage athletes are the group at greatest risk of recurrence and development of off-track Hill-Sachs lesions and may better benefit from a surgical stabilization procedure after the first dislocation episode.
- The arthroscopic Bankart repair yields good clinical results and return to sports rates, but high rates of recurrence are a matter of concern.
- The remplissage procedure has shown to reduce the recurrence rate without no deleterious effect in adolescents with recurrent anterior shoulder dislocations and a Hill-Sachs lesion without significant glenoid loss.
- Considering the high risk of failure of the Bankart repair in this population performing a Latarjet procedure should be strongly considered as a primary procedure for recurrent anterior shoulder instability.
- The Latarjet procedure provides in teenage athletes excellent clinical and functional results, and high return to sport rates with a low complication rate.
- Although bone-block procedures using free grafts have shown excellent results in adults, there is a further lack of information evaluating these techniques in teenagers.

References

1. Olds M, Donaldson K, Ellis R, Kersten P. In children 18 years and under, what promotes recurrent shoulder instability after traumatic anterior shoulder dislocation? A systematic review and meta-analysis of risk factors. Br J Sports Med. 2016;50(18):1135–41. https://doi.org/10.1136/bjsports-2015-095149.
2. Delgado C, Luengo-Alonso G, Valencia M, Martinez-Catalan N, Calvo E. Association of instability history and off-track hill-Sachs lesions in anterior shoulder instability. Orthop J Sports Med. 2023;11:23259671231213858. https://doi.org/10.1177/23259671231213858.
3. Hovelius L, Rahme H. Primary anterior dislocation of the shoulder: long-term prognosis at the age of 40 years or younger. Knee Surg Sports Traumatol Arthrosc. 2016;24(2):330–42. https://doi.org/10.1007/s00167-015-3980-2.
4. Gigis I, Heikenfeld R, Kapinas A, Listringhaus R, Godolias G. Arthroscopic versus conservative treatment of first anterior dislocation of the shoulder in adolescents. J Pediatr Orthop. 2014;34(4):421–5. https://doi.org/10.1097/bpo.0000000000000108.
5. Kramer J, Gajudo G, Pandya NK. Risk of recurrent instability after arthroscopic stabilization for shoulder instability in adolescent patients. Orthop J Sports Med. 2019;7(9):2325967119868995. https://doi.org/10.1177/2325967119868995.
6. Leroux T, Ogilvie-Harris D, Veillette C, Chahal J, Dwyer T, Khoshbin A, et al. The epidemiology of primary anterior shoulder dislocations in patients aged 10 to 16 years. Am J Sports Med. 2015;43(9):2111–7. https://doi.org/10.1177/0363546515591996.
7. Zacchilli MA, Owens BD. Epidemiology of shoulder dislocations presenting to emergency departments in the United States. J Bone Joint Surg Am. 2010;92(3):542–9. https://doi.org/10.2106/jbjs.i.00450.
8. Olds M, Ellis R, Donaldson K, Parmar P, Kersten P. Risk factors which predispose first-time traumatic anterior shoulder dislocations to recurrent instability in adults: a systematic review and meta-analysis. Br J Sports Med. 2015;49(14):913–22. https://doi.org/10.1136/bjsports-2014-094342.
9. Calvo E, Granizo JJ, Fernandez-Yruegas D. Criteria for arthroscopic treatment of anterior instability of the shoulder: a prospective study. J Bone Joint Surg Br. 2005;87(5):677–83. https://doi.org/10.1302/0301-620x.87b5.15794.
10. Roberts SB, Beattie N, McNiven ND, Robinson CM. The natural history of primary anterior dislocation of the glenohumeral joint in adolescence. Bone Joint J. 2015;97-b(4):520–6. https://doi.org/10.1302/0301-620x.97b4.34989.
11. Cordischi K, Li X, Busconi B. Intermediate outcomes after primary traumatic anterior shoulder dislocation in skeletally immature patients aged 10 to 13

years. Orthopedics. 2009;32(9):686–90. https://doi.org/10.3928/01477447-20090728-34.
12. Rong YH, Zhang GA, Wang C, Ning FG. Quantification of type I and III collagen content in normal human skin in different age groups. Zhonghua Shao Shang Za Zhi. 2008;24(1):51–3.
13. Calvo E, Delgado C. Management of off-track Hill-Sachs lesions in anterior glenohumeral instability. J Exp Orthop. 2023;10(1):30. https://doi.org/10.1186/s40634-023-00588-x.
14. Ellis HB Jr, Seiter M, Wise K, Wilson P. Glenoid bone loss in traumatic glenohumeral instability in the adolescent population. J Pediatr Orthop. 2017;37(1):30–5. https://doi.org/10.1097/bpo.0000000000000586.
15. Shaha JS, Cook JB, Song DJ, Rowles DJ, Bottoni CR, Shaha SH, Tokish JM. Redefining "critical" bone loss in shoulder instability: functional outcomes worsen with "subcritical" bone loss. Am J Sports Med. 2015;43(7):1719–25. https://doi.org/10.1177/0363546515578250.
16. Nakagawa S, Hirose T, Tsunematsu T, Ohori T, Yokoi H, Mae T, Yoneda M. Is preoperative glenoid defect size a reliable indicator of postoperative recurrence after arthroscopic Bankart repair in teenage competitive athletes? J Shoulder Elb Surg. 2023;32(6):1165–73. https://doi.org/10.1016/j.jse.2022.11.026.
17. Sidharthan S, Greditzer HG, Heath MR, Suryavanshi JR, Green DW, Fabricant PD. Normal glenoid ossification in pediatric and adolescent shoulders mimics bankart lesions: a magnetic resonance imaging-based study. Arthroscopy. 2020;36(2):336–44. https://doi.org/10.1016/j.arthro.2019.08.011.
18. Lau BC, Conway D, Curran PF, Feeley BT, Pandya NK. Bipolar bone loss in patients with anterior shoulder dislocation: a comparison of adolescents versus adult patients. Arthroscopy. 2017;33(10):1755–61. https://doi.org/10.1016/j.arthro.2017.04.004.
19. Parvaresh KC, Vargas-Vila M, Bomar JD, Pennock AT. Anterior glenohumeral instability in the adolescent athlete. JBJS Rev. 2020;8(2):e0080. https://doi.org/10.2106/jbjs.rvw.19.00080.
20. Gyftopoulos S, Hasan S, Bencardino J, Mayo J, Nayyar S, Babb J, Jazrawi L. Diagnostic accuracy of MRI in the measurement of glenoid bone loss. AJR Am J Roentgenol. 2012;199(4):873–8. https://doi.org/10.2214/ajr.11.7639.
21. Chalmers PN, Christensen G, O'Neill D, Tashjian RZ. Does bone loss imaging modality, measurement methodology, and interobserver reliability alter treatment in glenohumeral instability? Arthroscopy. 2020;36(1):12–9. https://doi.org/10.1016/j.arthro.2019.06.025.
22. Bishop JY, Jones GL, Rerko MA, Donaldson C. 3-D CT is the most reliable imaging modality when quantifying glenoid bone loss. Clin Orthop Relat Res. 2013;471(4):1251–6. https://doi.org/10.1007/s11999-012-2607-x.
23. Ruiz Ibán MA, Pérez Expósito R, Vicente Bártulos A, Vega Rodriguez R, Ruiz Díaz R, Diaz Heredia J. The size of the Hill Sachs defect increases during reduction of a first time shoulder dislocation in older adults: a pilot study in 20 cases. J Exp Orthop. 2023;10(1):143. https://doi.org/10.1186/s40634-023-00667-z.
24. Galvin JW, Ernat JJ, Waterman BR, Stadecker MJ, Parada SA. The epidemiology and natural history of anterior shoulder instability. Curr Rev Musculoskelet Med. 2017;4:411–24.
25. Watson S, Allen B, Grant JA. A clinical review of return-to-play considerations after anterior shoulder dislocation. Sports Health. 2016;8(4):336–41. https://doi.org/10.1177/1941738116651956.
26. Rugg CM, Hettrich CM, Ortiz S, Wolf BR, Zhang AL. Surgical stabilization for first-time shoulder dislocators: a multicenter analysis. J Shoulder Elb Surg. 2018;27(4):674–85. https://doi.org/10.1016/j.jse.2017.10.041.
27. Longo UG, van der Linde JA, Loppini M, Coco V, Poolman RW, Denaro V. Surgical versus nonoperative treatment in patients up to 18 years old with traumatic shoulder instability: a systematic review and quantitative synthesis of the literature. Arthroscopy. 2016;32(5):944–52. https://doi.org/10.1016/j.arthro.2015.10.020.
28. Shaha JS, Cook JB, Rowles DJ, Bottoni CR, Shaha SH, Tokish JM. Clinical validation of the glenoid track concept in anterior glenohumeral instability. J Bone Joint Surg Am. 2016;98(22):1918–23. https://doi.org/10.2106/jbjs.15.01099.
29. Nakagawa S, Ozaki R, Take Y, Iuchi R, Mae T. Relationship between glenoid defects and Hill-Sachs lesions in shoulders with traumatic anterior instability. Am J Sports Med. 2015;43(11):2763–73. https://doi.org/10.1177/0363546515597668.
30. Fox MA, Drain NP, Rai A, Zheng A, Carlos NB, Serrano Riera R, et al. Increased failure rates after arthroscopic Bankart repair after second dislocation compared to primary dislocation with comparable clinical outcomes. Arthroscopy. 2023;39(3):682–8. https://doi.org/10.1016/j.arthro.2022.10.012.
31. Hovelius L, Augustini BG, Fredin H, Johansson O, Norlin R, Thorling J. Primary anterior dislocation of the shoulder in young patients. A ten-year prospective study. J Bone Joint Surg Am. 1996;78(11):1677–84. https://doi.org/10.2106/00004623-199611000-00006.
32. Murphy AI, Hurley ET, Hurley DJ, Pauzenberger L, Mullett H. Long-term outcomes of the arthroscopic Bankart repair: a systematic review of studies at 10-year follow-up. J Shoulder Elb Surg. 2019;28(11):2084–9. https://doi.org/10.1016/j.jse.2019.04.057.
33. Ozturk BY, Maak TG, Fabricant P, Altchek DW, Williams RJ, Warren RF, et al. Return to sports after arthroscopic anterior stabilization in patients aged younger than 25 years. Arthroscopy. 2013;29(12):1922–31. https://doi.org/10.1016/j.arthro.2013.09.008.
34. Kasik CS, Rosen MR, Saper MG, Zondervan RL. High rate of return to sport in adolescent athletes following anterior shoulder stabilisation: a system-

atic review. J ISAKOS. 2019;4(1):33–40. https://doi.org/10.1136/jisakos-2018-000224.
35. Torrance E, Clarke CJ, Monga P, Funk L, Walton MJ. Recurrence after arthroscopic labral repair for traumatic anterior instability in adolescent rugby and contact athletes. Am J Sports Med. 2018;46(12):2969–74. https://doi.org/10.1177/0363546518794673.
36. Nixon MF, Keenan O, Funk L. High recurrence of instability in adolescents playing contact sports after arthroscopic shoulder stabilization. J Pediatr Orthop B. 2015;24(3):173–7. https://doi.org/10.1097/bpb.0000000000000135.
37. Saper MG, Milchteim C, Zondervan RL, Andrews JR, Ostrander RV 3rd. Outcomes after arthroscopic Bankart repair in adolescent athletes participating in collision and contact sports. Orthop J Sports Med. 2017;5(3):2325967117697950. https://doi.org/10.1177/2325967117697950.
38. Cheng TT, Edmonds EW, Bastrom TP, Pennock AT. Glenoid pathology, skeletal immaturity, and multiple preoperative instability events are risk factors for recurrent anterior shoulder instability after arthroscopic stabilization in adolescent athletes. Arthroscopy. 2021;37(5):1427–33. https://doi.org/10.1016/j.arthro.2020.12.211.
39. Owens BD, DeBerardino TM, Nelson BJ, Thurman J, Cameron KL, Taylor DC, et al. Long-term follow-up of acute arthroscopic Bankart repair for initial anterior shoulder dislocations in young athletes. Am J Sports Med. 2009;37(4):669–73. https://doi.org/10.1177/0363546508328416.
40. MacDonald P, McRae S, Old J, Marsh J, Dubberley J, Stranges G, et al. Arthroscopic Bankart repair with and without arthroscopic infraspinatus remplissage in anterior shoulder instability with a Hill-Sachs defect: a randomized controlled trial. J Shoulder Elb Surg. 2021;30(6):1288–98. https://doi.org/10.1016/j.jse.2020.11.013.
41. Hughes JL, Bastrom T, Pennock AT, Edmonds EW. Arthroscopic Bankart repairs with and without remplissage in recurrent adolescent anterior shoulder instability with Hill-Sachs deformity. Orthop J Sports Med. 2018;6(12):2325967118813981. https://doi.org/10.1177/2325967118813981.
42. Garcia GH, Wu HH, Liu JN, Huffman GR, Kelly JDt. Outcomes of the remplissage procedure and its effects on return to sports: average 5-year follow-up. Am J Sports Med. 2016;44(5):1124–30. https://doi.org/10.1177/0363546515626199.
43. Lazarides AL, Duchman KR, Ledbetter L, Riboh JC, Garrigues GE. Arthroscopic remplissage for anterior shoulder instability: a systematic review of clinical and biomechanical studies. Arthroscopy. 2019;35(2):617–28. https://doi.org/10.1016/j.arthro.2018.09.029.
44. Boileau P, O'Shea K, Vargas P, Pinedo M, Old J, Zumstein M. Anatomical and functional results after arthroscopic Hill-Sachs remplissage. J Bone Joint Surg Am. 2012;94(7):618–26. https://doi.org/10.2106/jbjs.k.00101.
45. Bhatia S, Frank RM, Ghodadra NS, Hsu AR, Romeo AA, Bach BR Jr, et al. The outcomes and surgical techniques of the Latarjet procedure. Arthroscopy. 2014;30(2):227–35. https://doi.org/10.1016/j.arthro.2013.10.013.
46. Gupta A, Delaney R, Petkin K, Lafosse L. Complications of the Latarjet procedure. Curr Rev Musculoskelet Med. 2015;8(1):59–66. https://doi.org/10.1007/s12178-015-9258-y.
47. Boileau P, Saliken D, Gendre P, Seeto BL, d'Ollonne T, Gonzalez JF, Bronsard N. Arthroscopic Latarjet: suture-button fixation is a safe and reliable alternative to screw fixation. Arthroscopy. 2019;35(4):1050–61. https://doi.org/10.1016/j.arthro.2018.11.012.
48. Domos P, Chelli M, Lunini E, Ascione F, Bercik MJ, Neyton L, et al. Clinical and radiographic outcomes of the open Latarjet procedure in skeletally immature patients. J Shoulder Elb Surg. 2020;29(6):1206–13. https://doi.org/10.1016/j.jse.2019.09.039.
49. Waltenspül M, Ernstbrunner L, Ackermann J, Thiel K, Galvin JW, Wieser K. Long-term results and failure analysis of the open Latarjet procedure and arthroscopic Bankart repair in adolescents. JBJS. 2022;104(12):1046–54. https://doi.org/10.2106/jbjs.21.01050.
50. Khan A, Samba A, Pereira B, Canavese F. Anterior dislocation of the shoulder in skeletally immature patients: comparison between non-operative treatment versus open Latarjet's procedure. Bone Joint J. 2014;96-b(3):354–9. https://doi.org/10.1302/0301-620x.96b3.32167.
51. Rossi LA, Tanoira I, Bruchmann MG, Pasqualini I, Ranalletta M. The Latarjet procedure in competitive athletes younger than 20 years old with a significant glenoid bone loss. Shoulder Elbow. 2020;14:21–8. https://doi.org/10.1177/1758573220944166.
52. Delgado C, Calvo E, Diaz Heredia J, Cañete San Pastor P, Garcia Navlet M, Ruiz Ibán MA. Graft position, healing, and resorption in anterior glenohumeral instability. A comparison of four glenoid augmentation techniques. Orthop J Sports Med. 2023;12(6):23259671241253163.
53. Hurley ET, Jamal MS, Ali ZS, Montgomery C, Pauzenberger L, Mullett H. Long-term outcomes of the Latarjet procedure for anterior shoulder instability: a systematic review of studies at 10-year follow-up. J Shoulder Elb Surg. 2019;28(2):e33–9. https://doi.org/10.1016/j.jse.2018.08.028.
54. Warth RJ, Briggs KK, Dornan GJ, Horan MP, Millett PJ. Patient expectations before arthroscopic shoulder surgery: correlation with patients' reasons for seeking treatment. J Shoulder Elb Surg. 2013;22(12):1676–81. https://doi.org/10.1016/j.jse.2013.05.003.
55. Hurley ET, Montgomery C, Jamal MS, Shimozono Y, Ali Z, Pauzenberger L, Mullett H. Return to play after the Latarjet procedure for anterior shoulder instability: a systematic review. Am J Sports Med. 2019;47(12):3002–8. https://doi.org/10.1177/0363546519831005.

56. Rossi LA, Gorodischer T, Brandariz R, Tanoira I, Pasqualini I, Ranalletta M. High rate of return to sports and low recurrences with the Latarjet procedure in high risk competitive athletes with glenohumeral instability and a glenoid bone loss <20. Arthrosc Sports Med Rehabil. 2020;2(6):e735–42. https://doi.org/10.1016/j.asmr.2020.06.004.
57. Griesser MJ, Harris JD, McCoy BW, Hussain WM, Jones MH, Bishop JY, Miniaci A. Complications and re-operations after Bristow-Latarjet shoulder stabilization: a systematic review. J Shoulder Elb Surg. 2013;22(2):286–92. https://doi.org/10.1016/j.jse.2012.09.009.
58. Valencia M, Fernández-Bermejo G, Martín-Ríos MD, Fernández-Jara J, Morcillo-Barrenechea D, Coifman-Lucena I, et al. Subscapularis structural integrity and function after arthroscopic Latarjet procedure at a minimum 2-year follow-up. J Shoulder Elb Surg. 2020;29(1):104–12. https://doi.org/10.1016/j.jse.2019.05.027.
59. Calvo C, Calvo J, Rojas D, Valencia M, Calvo E. Clinical relevance of persistent off-track hill-Sachs lesion after arthroscopic Latarjet procedure. Am J Sports Med. 2021;49(8):2006–12. https://doi.org/10.1177/03635465211019979.
60. Bonazza NA, Riboh JC. Management of recurrent anterior shoulder instability after surgical stabilization in children and adolescents. Curr Rev Musculoskelet Med. 2020;13(2):164–72. https://doi.org/10.1007/s12178-020-09612-4.

Shoulder Dislocation in the Mid-Season Athlete

19

Joseph P. DeAngelis

19.1 Introduction

Shoulder instability is a common and difficult problem for athletes of all ages. In this volume, the management of the unstable shoulder is examined by acknowledging all of the pathologic changes that can occur because of instability—Bankart lesions, bone loss on the glenoid and humeral head, injury to the humeral insertion of the anterior-inferior glenohumeral ligament (HAGL), superior labrum (SLAP tear), and even the rotator cuff. Additionally, the authors have examined how individual athletes may face unique risks for shoulder instability because of a soft tissue disorder resulting in hypermobility or a medical condition that can result in a convulsion (epilepsy). Specific sports may also pose a discrete challenge because of athlete's position (overhead thrower) or because of their sport's competitive design (collision). In the setting of the many factors that contribute to the etiology and effect of shoulder instability on the injured athlete, the commonality among all competitive athletes is the seasonal nature of competition. This chapter focuses on the management of a shoulder instability event that occurs during the athlete's season, and builds on the concepts presented in this volume to offer a framework for clinicians and athletes managing a shoulder dislocation after a mid-season (in-season) event.

The treatment of mid-season shoulder instability is controversial. There is no established consensus to indicate the singular, best way to treat an athlete with a shoulder dislocation during the season. Each athlete's treatment should be individualized in order to strike a careful balance between the opportunities afforded to them by the current season and the long-term health of the athlete and their shoulder. For this reason, shared decision-making is essential to a successful collaboration among the essential parties, and a rigorous dialogue should, at a minimum, include the athlete (and their family), physician, coach, athletic trainer, and other key stakeholders (agent/representation).

Importantly, it is possible to return to sport participation following a shoulder dislocation. However, the nonoperative treatment of shoulder instability is associated with both a faster return to play and a higher rate of recurrent instability. By comparison, the operative treatment of shoulder instability is likely to represent a season-ending event. It is associated with high rates of return-to-sport with significantly lower rates of recurrent instability.

In making this difficult choice, clinicians can serve as a guide to the decision-making process, helping to gather the essential elements of the athlete's history, physical examination, and imag-

J. P. DeAngelis (✉)
Department of Orthopaedics, Beth Israel Deaconess Medical Center, Harvard Medical School, Boston, MA, USA
e-mail: jpdeange@bidmc.harvard.edu

E. Calvo et al. (eds.), *Complex and Revision Problems in Shoulder Instability*,
https://doi.org/10.1007/978-3-031-81389-4_19

ing studies, and combine them with a realistic assessment of their impact on the athlete's opportunity in the current season.

19.2 History and Physical Examination

The shoulder is the most commonly dislocated joint in the human body [1], and collision athletes experience a high rate of shoulder instability [2, 3]. In athletes with a history of shoulder instability, a recurrent instability event should be treated with careful consideration [4]. Similarly, for an individual that may have a predisposition towards ligamentous laxity or hypermobility, shoulder instability needs to be thoughtfully factored into the context of their baseline physical function and contralateral shoulder's clinical examination [5]. The third most impactful consideration is the timing of the instability event, as a function of the relative duration of the season, the expected outcome of the season, and the athlete's recruitment prospects [6].

A late-season injury is more easily managed if the team's post-season prospects are limited. Similarly, more senior athletes can be more comfortable in their decision-making, if their clinical outcome is not likely to influence their prospects for subsequent selection. The greatest challenge faces a younger athlete, with a first-time instability event, early in the season. In this scenario, the clinician's recommendation regarding the course and timing of treatment has the most influence, supporting both the athlete and the coaching staff in setting expectations [7].

Following an in-season shoulder dislocation, the acute management of an injured athlete should include the precise execution of Basic Life Support (BLS) and Advanced Trauma Life Support (ATLS) protocols. When appropriate, the careful examination of the injured shoulder should include a thorough neurovascular examination at the time of the injury, prior to the shoulder's reduction, and following the shoulder's reduction. This physical examination needs to confirm the absence of any associated pathology. Brachial plexus and axillary nerve injuries can occur in up to 55% of all shoulder dislocations, and the majority will resolve in time [8]. Until the neurologic sequelae of the event are resolved, the athlete cannot return to sport safely.

19.3 Imaging

The initial assessment of a shoulder dislocation should include plain radiographs. When possible, pre-reduction x-rays help to document the shoulder dislocation and exclude any additional pathology. A fracture can occur in up to 25% of anterior shoulder dislocations [9, 10]. Subsequent, post-reduction imaging serves to document the successful reduction of the glenohumeral joint and assess the shoulder for any unintended effects of the manipulation. The accurate completion of orthogonal images is essential to the assessment of the shoulder girdle. It is important to obtain images that are perpendicular to fully characterize the shoulder. The x-rays must include either a true anterior-posterior (AP) view of the glenohumeral joint (Grashey) and a scapular Y view, or any AP view and an axillary lateral view.

Three-dimensional imaging can be employed, if necessary, to minimize the manipulation of the injured shoulder and to better assess any irregularity seen on the plain films. In the acute setting, computed tomography (CT) is an efficient and accurate modality. It will quantify the presence or absence of bony sequelae, and represents the gold standard when measuring the size of a defect on the glenoid and/or the humeral head [11].

For in-season athletes, bipolar bone loss needs to be carefully assessed and may represent a surgical indication. An acute fracture of the glenoid as well as glenoid bone loss involving greater than 15% of the articular surface warrants surgical consideration. Similarly, humeral impaction fractures (Hill-Sachs lesions) that are medial to the width of the glenoid tract will engage the anterior glenoid and dislocate the shoulder. As a result, these Off-Tract lesions represent a surgical indication in the in-season athlete. Any other fracture involving the shoulder girdle should be carefully considered, as it may prevent them from returning during the season.

For patients seen in follow-up, magnetic resonance imaging (MRI) is routinely performed to examine the unstable shoulder for both osseous and soft-tissue pathology. Specific sequela need to be treated in accordance with their known natural history. A humeral avulsion of the anterior-inferior glenohumeral ligament (HAGL) has a high-rate of recurrent instability, unless it is repaired surgically [12, 13]. Similarly, glenolabral articular disruptions (GLAD) and anterior labral periosteal sleeve avulsions (ALPSA) have worse outcomes if they are not recognized and appropriately addressed [14–16]. Acute rotator cuff tears, involving more than 50% of the tendon's thickness, as a well as superior labral pathology, with or without biceps involvement, may represent a different degree of injury severity. When identified, these sequelae of shoulder instability need to be factored into a comprehensive treatment plan.

19.4 Decision Framework

For the mid-season athletes who sustain a shoulder dislocation, it is possible to return-to-sports participation during the same season, if they meet all the correct diagnostic criteria and are able to successfully rehabilitate the injured shoulder in anticipation of their return. Because the nonoperative treatment of shoulder instability carries a higher rate of recurrent instability, careful consideration should be used to determine if the injured mid-season athlete can be safely treated without surgery.

To be eligible for an attempt at nonoperative management, the athlete should not have an acute neurologic injury (brachial plexopathy or axillary nerve palsy), a displaced fracture of the glenoid (Bony Bankart lesions) or critical glenoid bone loss (>15%), an Off-Tract Hill-Sachs impaction fracture, a history of shoulder instability (recurrent instability), or any other pathologic sequelae of their instability event (HAGL, ALPSA, rotator cuff tear, SLAP tear, or other fracture) (Table 19.1).

If the mid-season athlete meets these criteria, nonoperative management may afford them an opportunity to return to sport participation during the index season. The conversation surrounding this decision should include the athlete (and their family), the treating orthopaedic surgeon, coach, athletic trainer, and other key stakeholders (agent/representation), and needs to acknowledge that the nonoperative option has a higher rate of recurrent instability and a risk of increased glenoid bone loss [17].

Table 19.1 Exclusion criteria for nonoperative treatment

Mid-season athletes who have had a shoulder dislocation should NOT attempt a nonoperative plan of care, if they have any of these diagnoses
Acute neurologic injury (brachial plexus or axillary nerve palsy)
Displaced acute fracture of the glenoid (Bony Bankart)
Glenoid bone loss >15%
Off-track humeral bone loss
Recurrent shoulder instability
HAGL or ALPSA lesion
Other displaced fracture
Acute rotator cuff tear
Displaced SLAP tear

If selected, the nonoperative plan of care will have the athlete work with a rehabilitation specialist (athletic trainer, physical therapist, or the equivalent) to achieve the full strength (symmetric with the contralateral shoulder), full range of motion (symmetric with their contralateral shoulder), and complete relief of pain. Once achieved, the athlete will begin a return-to-sport program to reestablish the sport-specific skills required for competition, and then introduce a graduated return-to-play. If the athlete experiences recurrent instability during their rehabilitation, they should consider operative treatment. If they are unable to achieve a complete recovery, their return-to-sport should be delayed, accordingly.

19.5 Other Considerations

While the traditional assessment of an athlete's readiness to play has emphasized their physical performance (range of motion, strength, sport-specific skills), the athlete's psychological readiness warrants consideration. The Shoulder Instability Return to Sport after Injury (SIRSI)

score was developed to quantify the psychological domain [18]. The athlete's ability to return to sport has been shown to correlate with an increase in their SIRSI score. A threshold of 55 points has been suggested as a criterion for readiness [19].

19.6 Conclusion

Mid-season shoulder instability represents a difficult problem for athletes and their medical providers. Because there is no established consensus to indicate the best way to treat an athlete with a shoulder dislocation during the season, the choice of treatment for each athlete is individualized in an attempt to balance their goals for the current season and their long-term health and performance.

The nonoperative treatment of shoulder instability is associated with a faster return to play and a higher rate of recurrent instability. The operative treatment of shoulder instability represents a season-ending event. In making this difficult choice, clinicians can guide the decision-making process by gathering the essential elements of the athlete's history, physical examination, and imaging studies, to identify a plan of care that best supports the athlete's successful return to sport.

References

1. Ward JP, Bradley JP. Decision making in the in-season athlete with shoulder instability. Clin Sports Med. 2013;32(4):685–96. https://doi.org/10.1016/j.csm.2013.07.005.
2. Hovelius L, Augustini BG, Fredin H, Johansson O, Norlin R, Thorling J. Primary anterior dislocation of the shoulder in young patients. A ten-year prospective study. J Bone Joint Surg Am. 1996;78(11):1677–84. https://doi.org/10.2106/00004623-199611000-00006.
3. Owens BD, Agel J, Mountcastle SB, Cameron KL, Nelson BJ. Incidence of glenohumeral instability in collegiate athletics. Am J Sports Med. 2009;37(9):1750–4. https://doi.org/10.1177/0363546509334591.
4. Lau BC, Hutyra CA, Gonzalez JM, Mather RC 3rd, Owens BD, Levine WN, Garrigues GE, Kelly JD, Kovacevic D, Abrams JS, Cuomo F, McMahon PJ, Kaar S, Dines JS, Miniaci A, Nagda S, Braman JP, Harrison AK, MacDonald P, Riboh JC. Surgical treatment for recurrent shoulder instability: factors influencing surgeon decision making. J Shoulder Elb Surg. 2021;30(3):e85–102. https://doi.org/10.1016/j.jse.2020.07.003.
5. Rupp MC, Rutledge JC, Quinn PM, Millett PJ. Management of shoulder instability in patients with underlying hyperlaxity. Curr Rev Musculoskelet Med. 2023;16(4):123–44. https://doi.org/10.1007/s12178-023-09822-6.
6. Wolf BR, Tranovich MA, Marcussen B, Powell KJ, Fleming JA, Shaffer MA. Team approach: treatment of shoulder instability in athletes. JBJS Rev. 2021;9(11) https://doi.org/10.2106/JBJS.RVW.21.00087.
7. Fink Barnes LA, Jobin CM, Popkin CA, Ahmad CS. Athletes with anterior shoulder instability: a prospective study on player perceptions of injury and treatment. Orthop J Sports Med. 2021;9(9):23259671211032239. https://doi.org/10.1177/23259671211032239.
8. Gutkowska O, Martynkiewicz J, Urban M, Gosk J. Brachial plexus injury after shoulder dislocation: a literature review. Neurosurg Rev. 2020;43(2):407–23. https://doi.org/10.1007/s10143-018-1001-x.
9. Emond M, Le Sage N, Lavoie A, Rochette L. Clinical factors predicting fractures associated with an anterior shoulder dislocation. Acad Emerg Med. 2004;11(8):853–8. https://doi.org/10.1111/j.1553-2712.2004.tb00768.x.
10. Oldrini I, Coventry L, Novak A, Gwilym S, Metcalfe D. Clinical predictors of fracture in patients with shoulder dislocation: systematic review of diagnostic test accuracy studies. Emerg Med J. 2023;40(5):379–84. https://doi.org/10.1136/emermed-2022-212696.
11. Friedman LG, Ulloa SA, Braun DT, Saad HA, Jones MH, Miniaci AA. Glenoid bone loss measurement in recurrent shoulder dislocation: assessment of measurement agreement between CT and MRI. Orthop J Sports Med. 2014;2(9):2325967114549541. https://doi.org/10.1177/2325967114549541.
12. Longo UG, Rizzello G, Ciuffreda M, Locher J, Berton A, Salvatore G, Denaro V. Humeral avulsion of the glenohumeral ligaments: a systematic review. Arthroscopy. 2016;32(9):1868–76. https://doi.org/10.1016/j.arthro.2016.03.009.
13. Freshman RD, Zhang AL, Benjamin Ma C, Feeley BT, Ortiz S, Patel J, Dunn W, Wolf BR, Hettrich C, Lansdown D, et al. Factors associated with humeral avulsion of Glenohumeral ligament lesions in patients with anterior shoulder instability: an analysis of the MOON shoulder instability cohort. Orthop J Sports Med. 2023;11(10):23259671231206757. https://doi.org/10.1177/23259671231206757.
14. Orner CA, Bastrom TP, Pennock AT, Edmonds EW. Clinical outcomes of adolescents with anterior shoulder instability and glenolabral articular disruption lesions compared with isolated Bankart lesions. Orthop J Sports Med. 2023;11(11):23259671231214007. https://doi.org/10.1177/23259671231214007.
15. Ernat JJ, Rakowski DR, Ruzbarsky JJ, Johnson DW, Casp AJ, Peebles AM, Hanson J, Katthagan JC,

Horan MP, Provencher CMT, Millett PJ. Arthroscopic characterization, treatment, and outcomes of glenoid labral articular disruption lesions. Am J Sports Med. 2022;50(5):1328–35. https://doi.org/10.1177/03635465221076854.

16. Arner JW, Cooper JD, Elrick BP, Rakowski DR, Ruzbarsky JJ, Horan MP, Millett PJ. Outcomes of arthroscopic anterior labroligamentous periosteal sleeve avulsion lesions: a minimum 2-year follow-up. Am J Sports Med. 2022;50(6):1512–9. https://doi.org/10.1177/03635465221090902.
17. Dickens JF, Slaven SE, Cameron KL, Pickett AM, Posner M, Campbell SE, Owens BD. Prospective evaluation of glenoid bone loss after first-time and recurrent anterior glenohumeral instability events. Am J Sports Med. 2019;47(5):1082–9. https://doi.org/10.1177/0363546519831286.
18. Gerometta A, Klouche S, Herman S, Lefevre N, Bohu Y. The shoulder instability-return to sport after injury (SIRSI): a valid and reproducible scale to quantify psychological readiness to return to sport after traumatic shoulder instability. Knee Surg Sports Traumatol Arthrosc. 2018;26(1):203–11. https://doi.org/10.1007/s00167-017-4645-0.
19. Rossi LA, Pasqualini I, Brandariz R, Fuentes N, Fieiras C, Tanoira I, Ranalletta M. Relationship of the SIRSI score to return to sports after surgical stabilization of glenohumeral instability. Am J Sports Med. 2022;50(12):3318–25. https://doi.org/10.1177/03635465221118369.

Return to Sport After Shoulder Stabilization

20

Zachary J. Herman, Fritz Steuer,
Gillian M. Ahrendt, Sophia McMahon,
and Albert Lin

20.1 Introduction

Return to sport after injury is a continuum with shared decision-making between physician and athlete. The return to sport decision is multifactorial, involving physical, psychological, sport-related, and social factors. Ultimately, returning to sport requires balancing the risk of an undesired outcome, such as reinjury, and the risk tolerance of provider and athlete [1]. While many factors can confound this paradigm, objective and robust assessments of return to sport readiness are necessary to accurately determine risk and guide decision-making. This chapter focuses on return to sport specifically after shoulder stabilization, with an emphasis on postoperative healing, rehabilitation, criteria-based functional testing, psychological readiness assessments, and procedure-specific and sport-specific considerations.

Glenohumeral instability is a common pathology among athletes with 0.12 injuries per 1000 athlete exposures [2]. Injury rates are higher among contact and collision athletes, approaching 15% with anterior dislocation as the most common pattern [3, 4]. While controversy exists regarding operative versus nonoperative management after first-time dislocation, operative management confers lower recurrence rates [5–7]. Surgical management of glenohumeral joint instability includes soft tissue stabilization with or without bony augmentation. Soft tissue stabilization, now largely performed arthroscopically, involves Bankart repair to secure the injured labrum to the glenoid rim, and capsular plication to reduce capsular redundancy due to permanent deformation [8, 9]. These procedures can be performed with or without remplissage, which can augment soft tissue stabilization in the setting of a high risk or off-track Hill-Sachs lesion [10]. Bony augmentation, namely the Latarjet procedure, is indicated in the setting of critical glenoid bone loss (>20–25%) or for patients at high risk for recurrence due to age, level of competition, and collision sport athletes [5]. Surgical stabilization aims to restore glenohumeral joint function, minimize recurrence, and maximize return to activity.

Returning to sport is an important preoperative expectation among athletes seeking treatment for shoulder injury and postoperative expectations remain high [11]. Plath et al. reported 92% of patients expected to return to sport at their pre-injury level of play with no restrictions, 79% expected no recurrent instability, and 71% expected no pain, independent of activity [12]. As can often be the case, expecta-

Z. J. Herman · F. Steuer · G. M. Ahrendt ·
S. McMahon · A. Lin (✉)
Department of Orthopaedic Surgery, University of Pittsburgh, Pittsburgh, PA, USA
e-mail: hermanz@upmc.edu; steuerf@upmc.edu; ahrendtgm2@upmc.edu; mcmahonsi@upmc.edu; lina2@upmc.edu; hammerstrommm@upmc.edu

E. Calvo et al. (eds.), *Complex and Revision Problems in Shoulder Instability*,
https://doi.org/10.1007/978-3-031-81389-4_20

tions may not match reality with reported rates of return to sport varying widely, ranging from 47–97.5%, with the proportion of athletes who return to pre-injury level of play after arthroscopic Bankart repair or Latarjet ranging from 71–77% [13–15]. Recurrent instability and redislocation rates are also variable and partially depend on surgical procedure. At long-term follow-up after primary arthroscopic Bankart repair, 16% of patients experienced redislocation and 31.2% experienced recurrent instability [4]. In a population of competitive collision athletes, Latarjet repair has been shown to have a 2-year redislocation rate of 0.8% and 3-year redislocation rate of 4.8% [16, 17]. Return to play rates among competitive collision athletes after open Latarjet repair were 88.6% with return to pre-injury level in 69.5% [17]. Therefore, it is essential to appropriately counsel patients preoperatively based on their individual risk factors, surgical indications, and expectations.

Postoperatively, rehabilitation focuses on restoration of muscle strength, function, and dynamic stability while balancing sufficient repair healing with progressive return to increasingly intensive activity [18]. Multiple rehabilitation models are described with differential emphasis on the physical domains of strength, range of motion, neuromuscular control, and apprehension, while more recently, cognitive and psychological aspects of recovery have received increased attention and are incorporated [19]. Time from surgery and subjective assessments provide the traditional framework for return to sport clearance decisions; however, objective criteria-based protocols show promising results for predicting return to play and pre-injury level of play, particularly in anterior instability. The outcomes and merits of these protocols, in addition to functional testing for shoulder instability, will be discussed in detail in subsequent sections.

Understanding the factors that affect athletes' return to play decisions can aid providers in tailoring rehabilitation to patient-specific needs. A qualitative study investigating return to sport after arthroscopic Bankart repair cited fear of reinjury, shifts in priority, mood, social support, and self-motivation as influential to athletes' decision-making [20]. This underscores the weight that psychological and psychosocial factors have regarding the rehabilitation and return to play process. Evaluating psychological readiness and knowing which factors impact an athlete's return to sport decision can help physicians identify patients at risk for not returning to sport and guide rehabilitation to improve outcomes after surgery.

20.2 Domains for Return to Sport

When considering postoperative recovery in shoulder injuries it is essential to define the criteria that constitute ideal recovery and failed recovery. Most recently, the 2022 Bern Consensus Statement detailed prevention, rehabilitation, and return to sports guidelines after shoulder injury [21]. Specifically, the consensus statement defined six domains that clinicians should consider in evaluating an athlete prior to returning to sports. These domains, with weighting of importance based on the individual athlete, were defined as (1) pain, (2) active shoulder joint range of motion (ROM), (3) strength, power, and endurance, (4) kinetic chain, (5) psychological readiness, and (6) sports-specific demands [21]. The priority of domains shift based on individual athlete needs and sport requirements, for example, while it is suggested that contact athletes return pain-free, it is debated if overhead/throwing athletes require complete absence of pain prior to return [21]. Return to participation with pain is an option included in the consensus; however, achieving pain-free activity prior to performance level participation is recommended [21]. This differentiation between overhead and contact athletes continues with achieving a full ROM, where the sports-specific requirements of throwers require full ROM far more than some contact athletes [21]. As with many of these domains the relative weight placed on each depends on the individual. These sports-specific requirements naturally were extended to the third domain - strength, power, and endurance; where it is important that clinician and physical therapist assess the strength and power requirements of a weightlifter differently than a tennis player, for example [21]. Interwoven with this was the fourth domain, kinetic chain, which identified how characteristics of the sport could dictate specific measures to assess function [21]. The fifth domain, psychological readiness, is a critical component for nearly all athletes, thus we dedicated a section to further explore this domain [21]. The last domain, sport specific, supports a requirement for clinicians to understand the demands of their patient's sport and position [21]. This sixth domain is an overarching theme of the previous five domains to ensure that a patient's rehabilitation plan is appropriately balanced and tailored to their needs to maximize the likelihood of successful RTS [21]. Consideration of these six domains can aid in determining key criteria to balance when evaluating the progress of a recovery athlete.

20.3 Timing of Rehabilitation: Accelerated Vs. Conventional Postoperative Protocols

The overall purpose of rehabilitation is to progressively regain shoulder function, strength, and range of motion while also protecting the operative site. Although rehabilitation protocols are heterogeneous, a relatively constant feature is an initial period of immobilization to allow tissue healing, then progression of both passive and active range of motion, followed by an increase in strength and endurance, and finally return to sport. Protocols vary between different surgical procedures, such as arthroscopic versus open Bankart repair, for example, mainly in the timing of this progression. As many athletes hope to return to sport as soon as possible, designing protocols that allow them to return quickly without jeopardizing the surgical site is an area of clinical interest.

Conventional rehabilitation protocols typically call for a long period of complete immobilization after surgical repair, with some extending to 6 weeks. However, common outcomes following prolonged periods of immobilization include stiffness and reduction in strength [22]. For this reason, there has been an increase in studies that seek to analyze the effects of accelerated rehabilitation protocols, and, more specifically, how the outcomes differ from conventional programs. A more accelerated protocol may entail a progression from complete immobilization to moderate stress to light passive and active range of motion activities such as pendulum exercises, rope and pulley exercises, and wand exercises in weeks 0–4 postoperatively [18]. Recently, a systematic review by Lloyd et al. in 2021 analyzed 14 articles and found that accelerated physical therapy programs may lead to similar functional outcomes as conservative protocols [23]. In a level 1 randomized study, 62 patients with recurrent shoulder instability were randomized to accelerated rehabilitation versus conventional rehabilitation timelines following Arthroscopic Bankart Repair [24]. The results supported that recurrence did not increase, and postoperative patient reported outcomes were comparable to those who underwent conventional rehabilitation protocols [25].

The rehabilitation protocol after anterior surgical shoulder stabilization (Fig. 20.1) follows a system of four phases, which include a period of immobilization (weeks 0–4), progressive recovery of passive and active range of motion (weeks 5–20), a strengthening program beginning at week 6, and progression to returning to sports and work activities between months 4–6 [26]. During the immobilization phase, emphasis is placed on tissue healing and small introductions to active assisted range of motion (AAROM) forward elevation and external rotations beginning at week 2, such as rope and pulley-assisted elevation, and other similar passive activities [26]. Stress is also added in the forms of controlled submaximal tissue loading and dynamic stabilization [18]. These exercises proceed with the goal of obtaining passive and assisted-active range of motion of forward flexion (FF) to 90°, external rotation (ER) to 30°, and internal rotation (IR) to 45° [18].

Phase II (weeks 4–6) continues to emphasize surgical repair, in addition to a gradual increase in submaximal tissue loading,

Anterior Shoulder Rehabilitation Protocol	Time	Goals
Phase I (Immobilization)	**0 to 4 weeks**	• Allow time for tissue healing • Active assisted & passive FF to 90° • Active assisted & passive ER to 30° • Active assisted & passive IR to 45°
Focus on tissue healing	0 to 2 weeks	
Active-assisted range of motion forward elevation and external rotation	2 to 4 weeks	
Phase II (AROM)	**4 to 6 weeks**	• Full AROM • Except ER at 90° abduction to protect repair
Continued passive FF, ER, and IR exercises	4 to 6 weeks	
Introduction active range of motion	4 to 6 weeks	
Phase III (Strengthening)	**12 to 24 weeks**	• Normalize strength, proprioception, endurance, and dynamic stability for desired activity and level of competition desired
Gradual increase in stresses on shoulder	12 to 24 weeks	
Customization based on athlete	12 to 24 weeks	
Phase IV (Return to sport)	**4 to 6 months**	• Utilize CBRTS to identify functional deficits • Sport specific exercises • Achieve CBRTS
Criteria based return to sport testing (CBRTS)	4 to 6 months	

Fig. 20.1 Rehabilitation protocol and goals after anterior shoulder stabilization. *FF* forward flexion, *ER* external rotation, *IR* internal rotation, *AROM* active range of motion

dynamic stabilization, and ROM with continuation of passive FF, ER, and IR exercises, and an introduction to active range of motion exercises. The goal at the end of this phase is to achieve full AROM, except external rotation at 90° abduction where anterior repair sites will experience the greatest strain [18, 26]. Isometric strengthening activities continue, and there is an introduction to isotonic strengthening exercises [18, 23].

Phase III of rehabilitation (weeks 12–24 postoperatively) aims to normalize strength, proprioception, endurance, and dynamic stability of the glenohumeral joint, with an added goal of developing the skills and power required for higher level activities [18]. Similar to the other phases, these are achieved through a gradual increase in stress. During this phase, it is important to customize the protocol for each patient based on the type of activity and level of competition to which they strive to return. For example, the protocol for an elite contact athlete will differ from that of a recreational athlete [18, 26]. This phase is considered complete when the patient achieves comparable strength to the uninjured side and can perform active range of motion exercises without pain [23].

Phase IV focuses on return to sport or activity level and requires that the athlete achieve full AROM/PROM with the appropriate strength and endurance. This phase is often unique to the athlete and the determination can be time or criteria based. Given its importance we have dedicated the next section this final phase.

20.4 Return to Sport Considerations: Timing, Objective Criteria, and Functional Testing

Based on the 2022 International Consensus Statement, general criteria for return to sport include restoration of strength, range of motion, and proprioception; apprehension- and pain-free activity, and sport-specific skills, with the recommendation for particular attention to overhead, collision, and elite athletes [27]. As previously described, time from surgery is traditionally implemented as a metric to guide return to sport with 5–6 months generally accepted. A systematic review including 58 studies regarding criteria for return to sport after anterior shoulder stabilization reported 52% of studies used 6 months as the cutoff; however, this ranged widely from 1.5 to 12 months [28]. Multiple studies have demonstrated shortcomings of utilizing time as an independent parameter to guide return to sport decisions as it is arbitrary and subjective. A multicenter study found that only 55% of patients achieved baseline strength and a <20° side-to-side difference in range of motion at 6 months postoperatively [29]. Furthermore, a functional, objective, and criteria-based protocol to determine return to sport readiness revealed 88% of patients had significant deficits at 6 months postoperatively [30]. Therefore, it is important to incorporate objective metrics to assess athletes prior to their return to sport.

Testing batteries have been developed to comprehensively evaluate shoulder strength and function with varying measurement reliability [30, 31]. Parameters include isokinetic internal and external strength, external rotation endurance testing, Closed Kinetic Chain Upper Extremity Stability test (CKCUES) and the unilateral seated shot-put test. Validity and reliability testing demonstrated good to excellent intra-rater reliability for all isokinetic, isometric, and functional assessments. Endurance testing was more challenging to evaluate with only poor to moderate intra-rater reliability. While the minimal detectable change for all testing parameters ranged from 20–69%, overall, the testing battery demonstrates promising results of an objective method to assess return to sport readiness that can aid clinical decision-making [31]. An alternative commonly studied and implemented functional test is the Upper Quarter Y-Balance test, which can be objectively assessed [32–34].

Further evidence supporting the use of objective criteria-based return to sport testing (CBRTS) emerged from a retrospective case control study of 36 high-risk patients following arthroscopic Bankart repair. Return to sport clearance required achieving 90% of contralateral extremity internal rotation and external rotation strength, 90% distance of contralateral extremity for unilateral seated shot put, and above the 75th percentile (female reference) or 85th percentile (male reference) on CKCUES [35]. Only six patients passed all metrics at 6-months postoperatively and 84% failed at least one component of the testing protocol. Patients who were not cleared to return to sport at 6 months continued structured rehabilitation tailored to their specific deficits identified from the CBRTS. Compared to a control group who was cleared to return to sport based on range of motion and strength assessed on physical exam 5–6 months postoperatively, patients who passed the CBRTS testing had a reduced rate of recurrent instability (5% vs. 22%, OR 4.85; $p < 0.001$) [35]. Furthermore, the redislocation rate at 2 years after arthroscopic Bankart repair was 6.5% among competitive overhead and contact athletes who were required to complete a functional testing protocol prior to return to sport [36]. In a smaller study on CBRTS in open Latarjet, authors concluded that CBRTS may be useful in identifying functional deficits, but could not make conclusions on recurrent instability [37]. Overall, these findings support that objective return to sport testing metrics may identify range of motion and strength deficits with the opportunity to target improvement through more focused rehabilitation before returning to sport, resulting in lower recurrence rates.

Functional return to sport testing measures patients' performance and capabilities after a period of rehabilitation. As shoulder demands vary between sports, further studies are needed to design the optimal sport-specific combinations of tests to evaluate athletes' readiness; however, tests should evaluate strength, range of motion, stability, endurance, proprioception, and neuromuscular coordination. Based on a 2024 modified-Delphi consensus study by the International Shoulder Instability Group, a rehabilitation guide composed of 27 interventions deemed critical to shoulder instability rehabilitation, with a particular emphasis on diminishing apprehension, was designed [19]. Regarding range of motion, wand-assisted exercise, wall slides, active assisted internal/external rotation, and end range exercises were included. Neuromuscular ball exercises, weightbearing proprioceptive activities, performing exercises without visual input, neuromuscular stimulation of the scapula and rotator cuff, and task-specific activities were recommended. Sport-specific overhead and non-overhead activities, neurocognitive reactive multitasking activities, plyometrics, and high-speed multiplanar activities were also critical to include. Gradual exposure to apprehension-provoking positions and training in these positions were incorporated as part of a cognitive-behavioral approach to target patients' fear of apprehension [19]. This approach exemplifies bridging the gap between restoring physical function and the psychological aspects of recovery after injury.

20.5 Assessing Psychological Readiness to Return to Sport

In addition to assessing an athlete's progress in physical recovery towards return to sport with objective criteria, it is important to also assess psychological readiness. Tjong et al. found that fear of reinjury, shifts in priority, mood, social support, and self-motivation strongly influenced athletes' decision to return to sport after arthroscopic Bankart repair independent of their functional recovery [20]. Patients with poor psychological readiness have been shown to report higher pain scores and lower satisfaction than athletes who returned to sport [38]. Monitoring athletes' mental and emotional preparedness through the return to sport process is therefore essential to gauging timing for return to sport and clinical outcomes.

The Return to Sport after Injury scale was initially developed to measure athletes' psychological state after anterior cruciate ligament injury (ACL-RSI) [39]. Further studies have demonstrated that psychological outcomes did not correlate with patients' physical recovery after ACL injury when assessed at 9 months postoperatively, the expected time to return to sport [40]. More recently, the Shoulder Instability-Return to Sport after Injury (SIRSI) questionnaire was modified from the ACL-RSI to evaluate four elements of psychological readiness: performance confidence, reinjury risk and fear, emotions, and rehabilitation and surgery [41]. The assessment tool is a 12-item questionnaire with each item graded on a 10-point scale with a maximum score of 100 points [41]. Higher SIRSI scores indicate more positive psychological responses with a cutoff score of 55 points indicating psychological readiness [14, 42].

A prospective study of 104 athletes after arthroscopic Bankart repair or Latarjet implemented SIRSI to assess psychological readiness. All athletes participated in the same structured rehabilitation protocol and were cleared to return to sport when they achieved pre-injury strength and range of motion without pain or apprehension. Of the 88 athletes who returned to sport, 76.8% were psychologically ready, whereas only 4.5% of patients who did not return to sport achieved psychological readiness based on achieving the SIRSI cutoff score [14]. The SIRSI score demonstrated strong predictive ability for returning to pre-injury level of play. The odds of returning to pre-injury level of play increases 11.7 times for every 10-point increase in SIRSI score, and 100% of athletes who returned to pre-injury level of play achieved SIRSI score greater than the threshold value [14]. Importantly, SIRSI scores were significantly associated with return to sport outcomes compared to functional outcomes [14].

A similar proportion of athletes achieved psychological readiness in a retrospective matched-cohort study of athletes 12 months after open Latarjet. Only 20% of patients in the cohort who did not return to sport passed the SIRSI cutoff score compared to 81.4% in the cohort who returned to sport. This study highlighted an important distinction, where 95.7% of athletes who returned to sport were more willing to undergo future surgery again if required compared to only 68.6% of athletes who did not return to sport [38]. A low score response to the "willingness to undergo future surgery" item on the SIRSI questionnaire was the only independent factor associated with lower return to play. Interestingly, responses to items assessing athlete confidence to perform at previous level of sport, confidence in shoulder stability, and fear of reinjuring shoulder were not significantly different between cohorts [38]. These findings provide insight into athletes' values and priorities in their personal return to sport risk-assessment.

The SIRSI questionnaire has been incorporated into comprehensive protocols alongside criteria-based return to sport testing batteries. The S-STARTS test combines SIRSI with four physical performance tests to provide a composite score with a maximum of 21 points with promising internal validity [43]. Additionally, a short-form SIRSI questionnaire was developed to shorten the 12-item questionnaire to 5 items, offering decreased patient burden and increased efficiency in the clinical setting. The short-form assessment was shown to effectively distinguish between patients who returned to sport compared to those who did not, and athletes who returned to pre-injury play levels [44]. Notably, the benchmark scores to determine psychological readiness were greater on the short form: cutoff values of 54 to return to play and 59 to return to pre-injury level were identified for the short form versus 52 and 55, respectively, on the original SIRSI questionnaire [44]. However, the short form also demonstrated strong predictive ability and an alternative, convenient assessment for patients and providers.

20.6 Author's Algorithm for Return to Sport After Anterior Stabilization

For patients' status post arthroscopic anterior labral repair with capsulorrhaphy or open Latarjet, the senior author's general postoperative management begins with 4 weeks of sling immobilization for the first phase. Elbow range of motion begins after the first postoperative clinic evaluation, which occurs 2 weeks postoperatively. At this 2-week point, formal physical therapy with passive range of motion exercises, closed kinetic chain motion with use of a home-based Shoulder Strengthening and Stabilization System, and pendulum exercises are also initiated. To protect the Bankart repair and healing, external rotation is limited to 30° at the side for the first 6 weeks. Active range of motion begins at 8 weeks postoperatively and strengthening begins at 12 weeks postoperatively. Interval clinic evaluations occur at 3 and 5 months postoperatively where patient reported outcome measures including Subjective Shoulder Value (SSV), pain via the visual analog scale (VAS), and the American Shoulder and Elbow Surgeons (ASES) score. Return to sport testing is performed at approximately 5 months postoperatively to guide return to sport decision-making.

The return to sport testing protocol is performed by licensed physical therapists and includes range of motion, strength, and functional testing. All parameters are objectively evaluated with specific criteria set to determine test passage or failure. Patients are required to pass all test elements for return to sport clearance. The total arc of external rotation (ER)—internal rotation (IR) motion is assessed; with the goal of a total ROM difference less than 5° and an internal rotation deficit less than 15° on the involved side. Strength testing involves unilateral ER-IR at 0° abduction while patient positioned supine, unilateral ER-IR at 90° abduction while patient positioned prone, unilateral ER and IR isokinetically measured at 60°/s, and unilateral ER and IR isokinetically measured at 180°/s. This portion of the return to sport test is modified for overhead throwing athletes, where ER and IR are isokinetically measured at 300°/s. Achieving greater than 90% of the uninvolved shoulder is required to pass the return to sport test. Finally, the Closed Kinetic Chain Upper Extremity Test (CKC UE), Unilateral Seated Shot-Put Test, and Y-Balance Test are incorporated in the testing protocol. On the CKC UE, the goal is to achieve more than 21 touches to the contralateral wrist without apprehension. Successfully passing the Unilateral Seated Shot-Put Test requires 95–100% of the uninvolved shoulder when the involved shoulder is dominant, or 80% of the uninvolved shoulder when the involved shoulder is nondominant. The goal on the Y-Balance test is to reach 90% of the contralateral limb in all directions. Patients continue tailored physical therapy based on deficits identified through the return to sport test when not all components are passed. In general, if the athlete does not pass one component, specific therapy is directed at the deficit over 4–6 weeks with eventual clearance after the directed therapy. If the athlete does not pass two or more components, a return to sport test is often repeated 4–6 weeks after continued therapy with clearance contingent on passing the repeat test.

20.7 Return to Sport after Posterior Stabilization

As a much less common procedure than anterior shoulder stabilization, rehabilitation and RTS in posterior shoulder instability (PSI) is less understood and more heterogenous than anterior stabilization. One of the largest epidemiological studies, the MOON study, only found 23% of patients presenting for shoulder instability presented with posterior instability which is still a substantial increase over the small earlier studies of incidence [45]. Importantly, the rate of surgical intervention for posterior instability has been increasing over the past few decades from 53.1% in the early 2000s to 87.5% in the 2010's, thus highlighting a growing need for understanding rehabilitation and RTS in patients after posterior instability surgical intervention [46]. This increase in posterior instability cases comprised largely of arthroscopic repairs with studies looking at the latter half of the 2010's showing greater than 90% of repairs were performed arthroscopically [47]. This is likely due to literature showing better outcomes and higher RTS with lower recurrence of instability or need for revision than open procedures [48].

Given the recent increase and shifts in PSI management, it is not surprising that studies looking at posterior instability rehabilitation and RTS have found heterogeneity and lack of consensus. Fortunately, following surgical stabilization, cases of PSI still have a high RTS at any level with systematic reviews showing a pooled average of 86.9% RTS with 74.9% achieving the same level of play as pre-injury [49, 50]. Some studies that break down RTS by type of athlete have demonstrated lower rates with throwing athletes than non-throwing athletes [49, 50].

Rehabilitation protocols vary widely following surgical stabilization for PSI. The most recent systematic review investigating 204 ACGME-accredited programs was able to identify 39 post-operative protocols, while the immediate postoperative phase was similar across protocols (94.9% in postoperative sling), the protocols deviated significantly in the active and passive range of motion phases [51]. While active range of motion of hand, wrist, and elbow was almost always initiated (92.3%), shoulder active range of motion with supine forward elevation and external rotation was less common (64.1% and 61.5%) [51]. Passive range of motion guidance varied substantially with a 90° passive external rotation starting from 0 to 12-weeks postoperatively [51]. Later progression in active range of motion varied substantially as well, with the goal to achieve full active range of motion at 9–12 weeks postoperatively [51]. RTS, often the primary goal for recovering athletes, was only identified in 56.4% of these studies, with most protocols utilizing a time-based criteria for return to sports at 16–28 weeks postoperatively [51]. While decreased recurrent instability has been demonstrated in anterior instability for athletes undergoing CBRTS testing following surgical stabilization, its utility in posterior instability is less clear [35, 52]. Recent literature has shown CBRTS testing did not reduce recurrent instability following stabilization for PSI, however, two-thirds of athletes failed at least one section of testing with authors suggesting its utility in guiding targeted rehabilitation [52].

Overall, posterior instability has a high rate of return to sports; however, the determination of when to return to play remains unclear with studies on CBRTS testing as a possible under-utilized and poorly understood clinical tool compared to anterior shoulder instability [50]. A combination of time-based and CBRTS will likely be the best path forward for clinicians though future studies will be necessary to determine the ideal protocol for directing RTP following surgical stabilization for PSI.

20.8 Conclusion

The primary goal of most athletes is return to play, with most carrying high expectations of meeting this goal. Further improvements in RTS rates are necessary to meet these goals and expectations. Postoperative rehabilitation strategies that are sports and goals specific are necessary, and can be guided by the domains discussed above, which maximize the chances of RTS. Criteria-based testing for RTS has been shown to be particularly valuable for reducing dislocations and recurrent instability following anterior surgical stabilization and at a minimum, can be used to inform targeted rehabilitation following posterior surgical stabilization. Regardless of surgical intervention, rehabilitation ideally achieves a pain-free shoulder with the ROM and strength that the athlete requires. Surgeons must also consider the psyche of the athlete and ensure both physically and psychologically readiness for return to their sport. An individualized treatment algorithm that balances all of these factors is necessary to optimize outcomes.

References

1. Shrier I. Strategic Assessment of Risk and Risk Tolerance (StARRT) framework for return-to-play decision-making. Br J Sports Med. 2015;49:1311–5.
2. Owens BD, Agel J, Mountcastle SB, Cameron KL, Nelson BJ. Incidence of glenohumeral instability in collegiate athletics. Am J Sports Med. 2009;37:1750–4.
3. Kawasaki T, Ota C, Urayama S, Maki N, Nagayama M, Kaketa T, et al. Incidence of and risk factors for traumatic anterior shoulder dislocation: an epidemiologic study in high-school rugby players. J Shoulder Elb Surg. 2014;23:1624–30.
4. Murphy AI, Hurley ET, Hurley DJ, Pauzenberger L, Mullett H. Long-term outcomes of the arthroscopic Bankart repair: a systematic review of studies at 10-year follow-up. J Shoulder Elb Surg. 2019;28:2084–9.
5. Nazzal EM, Herman ZJ, Engler ID, Dalton JF, Freehill MT, Lin A. First-time traumatic anterior shoulder dislocation: current concepts. J ISAKOS. 2023;8:101–7.
6. Novakofski KD, Melugin HP, Leland DP, Bernard CD, Krych AJ, Camp CL. Nonoperative management of anterior shoulder instability can result in high rates of recurrent instability and pain at long-term follow-up. J Shoulder Elb Surg. 2022;31:352–8.
7. Van Spanning SH, Verweij LPE, Priester-Vink S, Van Deurzen DFP, Van Den Bekerom MPJ. Operative versus nonoperative treatment following first-time anterior shoulder dislocation: a systematic review and meta-analysis. JBJS Rev. 2021;9(9) https://doi.org/10.2106/JBJS.RVW.20.00232.
8. Bigliani LU, Pollock RG, Soslowsky LJ, Flatow EL, Pawluk RJ, Mow VC. Tensile properties of the inferior glenohumeral ligament. J Orthop Res. 1992;10:187–97.
9. Higgins LD, Warner JJP. Arthroscopic Bankart repair. Clin Sports Med. 2000;19:49–62.
10. Lin A, Barrow AE, Charles S, Shannon M, Fox MA, Herman ZJ, et al. Remplissage reduces recurrent instability in high-risk patients with on-track Hill-Sachs lesions. J Shoulder Elb Surg. 2023;32:S99–105.
11. Warth RJ, Briggs KK, Dornan GJ, Horan MP, Millett PJ. Patient expectations before arthroscopic shoulder surgery: correlation with patients' reasons for seeking treatment. J Shoulder Elb Surg. 2013;22:1676–81.
12. Plath JE, Saier T, Feucht MJ, Minzlaff P, Seppel G, Braun S, et al. Patients' expectations of shoulder instability repair. Knee Surg Sports Traumatol Arthrosc. 2018;26:15–23.
13. Abdul-Rassoul H, Galvin JW, Curry EJ, Simon J, Li X. Return to sport after surgical treatment for anterior shoulder instability: a systematic review: response. Am J Sports Med. 2019;47:NP24–7.
14. Rossi LA, Pasqualini I, Brandariz R, Fuentes N, Fieiras C, Tanoira I, et al. Relationship of the SIRSI score to return to sports after surgical stabilization of glenohumeral instability. Am J Sports Med. 2022;50:3318–25.
15. Ialenti MN, Mulvihill JD, Feinstein M, Zhang AL, Feeley BT. Return to play following shoulder stabilization: a systematic review and meta-analysis. Orthop J Sports Med. 2017;5:232596711772605.
16. Hovelius L, Sandström B, Sundgren K, Saebö M. One hundred eighteen Bristow-Latarjet repairs for recurrent anterior dislocation of the shoulder prospectively followed for fifteen years: study I—clinical results. J Shoulder Elb Surg. 2004;13:509–16.
17. Hurley ET, Moore TK, Kilkenny C, Khan S, White-Gibson A, Dickens JF, et al. Young Collision athletes have high rate of return to play and good clinical outcomes following open Latarjet procedure. Arthroscopy. 2024;40:1075–80.
18. Popchak A, Patterson-Lynch B, Christain H, Irrgang JJ. Rehabilitation and return to sports after anterior shoulder stabilization. Ann Joint. 2017;2:62.
19. van Gastel ML, van Iersel TP, Tutuhatunewa ED, Cools AM, van den Bekerom MPJ, Hekman KMC, et al. Development of a rehabilitation guideline for patients undergoing an arthroscopic Bankart repair after traumatic anterior shoulder dislocation, focusing on diminishing apprehension: an international Delphi-based consensus study. J Orthop Sports Phys Ther. 2024;54:289–301.
20. Tjong VK, Devitt BM, Murnaghan ML, Ogilvie-Harris DJ, Theodoropoulos JS. A qualitative investigation of return to sport after arthroscopic Bankart repair: beyond stability. Am J Sports Med. 2015;43:2005–11.
21. Schwank A, Blazey P, Asker M, Møller M, Hägglund M, Gard S, et al. 2022 Bern consensus statement on shoulder injury prevention, rehabilitation, and return

to sport for athletes at all participation levels. J Orthop Sports Phys Ther. 2022;52:11–28.

22. Littlewood C, Bateman M, Clark D, Selfe J, Watkinson D, Walton M, et al. Rehabilitation following rotator cuff repair: a systematic review. Should Elb. 2015;7:115–24.
23. Lloyd G, Day J, Lu J, Lincoln A, Attanasio S, Svoboda S. Postoperative rehabilitation of anterior glenohumeral joint instability surgery: a systematic review. Sports Med Arthrosc Rev. 2021;29:54.
24. Kim S-H, Ha K-I, Jung M-W, Lim M-S, Kim Y-M, Park J-H. Accelerated rehabilitation after arthroscopic Bankart repair for selected cases: a prospective randomized clinical study. Arthroscopy. 2003;19:722–31.
25. Kim S-H, Ha K-I, Cho Y-B, Ryu B-D, Oh I. Arthroscopic anterior stabilization of the shoulder: two to six-year follow-up. JBJS. 2003;85:1511.
26. Gaunt BW, Shaffer MA, Sauers EL, Michener LA, McCluskey GM, Thigpen C, et al. The American Society of Shoulder and Elbow Therapists' consensus rehabilitation guideline for arthroscopic anterior capsulolabral repair of the shoulder. J Orthop Sports Phys Ther. 2010;40:155–68.
27. Matache BA, Hurley ET, Wong I, Itoi E, Strauss EJ, Delaney RA, et al. Anterior shoulder instability part III—revision surgery, rehabilitation and return to play, and clinical follow-up—an international consensus statement. Arthroscopy. 2022;38:234–42.e6.
28. Ciccotti MC, Syed U, Hoffman R, Abboud JA, Ciccotti MG, Freedman KB. Return to play criteria following surgical stabilization for traumatic anterior shoulder instability: a systematic review. Arthroscopy. 2018;34:903–13.
29. Frantz TL, Everhart JS, Cvetanovich GL, Neviaser A, Jones GL, Hettrich CM, et al. Are patients who undergo the Latarjet procedure ready to return to play at 6 months? A Multicenter Orthopaedic Outcomes Network (MOON) Shoulder Group cohort study. Am J Sports Med. 2020;48:923–30.
30. Wilson KW, Popchak A, Li RT, Kane G, Lin A. Return to sport testing at 6 months after arthroscopic shoulder stabilization reveals residual strength and functional deficits. J Shoulder Elb Surg. 2020;29:S107–14.
31. Popchak A, Poploski K, Patterson-Lynch B, Nigolian J, Lin A. Reliability and validity of a return to sports testing battery for the shoulder. Phys Ther Sport. 2021;48:1–11.
32. Taylor JB, Wright AA, Smoliga JM, DePew JT, Hegedus EJ. Upper-extremity physical-performance tests in college athletes. J Sport Rehabil. 2016;25:146–54.
33. Gorman PP, Butler RJ, Plisky PJ, Kiesel KB. Upper quarter Y balance test: reliability and performance comparison between genders in active adults. J Strength Cond Res. 2012;26:3043–8.
34. Westrick RB, Miller JM, Carow SD, Gerber JP. Exploration of the y-balance test for assessment of upper quarter closed kinetic chain performance. Int J Sports Phys Ther. 2012;7:139–47.
35. Drummond Junior M, Popchak A, Wilson K, Kane G, Lin A. Criteria-based return-to-sport testing is associated with lower recurrence rates following arthroscopic Bankart repair. J Shoulder Elb Surg. 2021;30:S14–20.
36. Kelley TD, Clegg S, Rodenhouse P, Hinz J, Busconi BD. Functional rehabilitation and return to play after arthroscopic surgical stabilization for anterior shoulder instability. Sports Health. 2022;14:733–9.
37. Reddy RP, Como M, Charles S, Herman ZJ, Nazzal EM, Como CJ, et al. Criteria-based return to sport testing after open Latarjet reveals residual deficits and can be utilized for sports clearance with excellent outcomes at mean 3.6 year follow-up: a small case series of competitive athletes. Phys Ther Sport. 2024;65:23–9.
38. Hurley ET, Davey MS, Montgomery C, Moore DM, Mojica ES, Gaafar M, et al. Analysis of athletes who did not return to play after open Latarjet. Orthop J Sports Med. 2022;10:232596712110710.
39. Webster KE, Feller JA, Lambros C. Development and preliminary validation of a scale to measure the psychological impact of returning to sport following anterior cruciate ligament reconstruction surgery. Phys Ther Sport. 2008;9:9–15.
40. O'Connor RF, King E, Richter C, Webster KE, Falvey ÉC. No relationship between strength and power scores and anterior cruciate ligament return to sport after injury scale 9 months after anterior cruciate ligament reconstruction. Am J Sports Med. 2020;48:78–84.
41. Olds M, Webster KE. Factor structure of the shoulder instability return to sport after injury scale: performance confidence, reinjury fear and risk, emotions, rehabilitation and surgery. Am J Sports Med. 2021;49:2737–42.
42. Gerometta A, Klouche S, Herman S, Lefevre N, Bohu Y. The Shoulder Instability-Return to Sport after Injury (SIRSI): a valid and reproducible scale to quantify psychological readiness to return to sport after traumatic shoulder instability. Knee Surg Sports Traumatol Arthrosc. 2018;26:203–11.
43. Juré D, Blache Y, Degot M, Vigne G, Nové-Josserand L, Godenèche A, et al. The S-STARTS test: validation of a composite test for the assessment of readiness to return to sport after shoulder stabilization surgery. Sports Health. 2022;14:254–61.
44. Pasqualini I, Rossi LA, Brandariz R, Tanoira I, Fuentes N, Ranalletta M. The short, 5-item shoulder instability–return to sport after injury score performs as well as the longer version in predicting psychological readiness to return to sport. Arthroscopy. 2023;39:1131–8.e1.
45. Kraeutler MJ, McCarty EC, Belk JW, Wolf BR, Hettrich CM, Ortiz SF, et al. Descriptive epidemiology of the MOON shoulder instability cohort. Am J Sports Med. 2018;46:1064–9.
46. Woodmass JM, Lee J, Wu IT, Desai VS, Camp CL, Dahm DL, et al. Incidence of posterior shoulder instability and trends in surgical reconstruction: a

22-year population-based study. J Shoulder Elb Surg. 2019;28:611–6.
47. Lemme NJ, Bokshan SL, Yang D, Meghani O, Alsoof D, Lau BC, et al. Trends in the surgical treatment of posterior shoulder instability in the United States from 2016 to 2020. Should Elb. 2023;15:405–10.
48. DeLong JM, Jiang K, Bradley JP. Posterior instability of the shoulder: a systematic review and meta-analysis of clinical outcomes. Am J Sports Med. 2015;43:1805–17.
49. Matar RN, Shah NS, Gardner TJ, Grawe BM. Return to sport after surgical treatment for posterior shoulder instability: a systematic review. JSES Int. 2020;4:797–802.
50. Fried JW, Hurley ET, Duenes ML, Manjunath AK, Virk M, Gonzalez-Lomas G, et al. Return to play after arthroscopic stabilization for posterior shoulder instability—a systematic review. Arthrosc Sports Med Rehabil. 2021;3:e249–56.
51. Dacey S, Meghani O, Dove JH, Lemme NJ, Byrne RA, Owens BD. Lack of consensus in rehabilitation protocols after posterior shoulder stabilization. Orthop J Sports Med. 2023;11(5):23259671231161589. https://doi.org/10.1177/23259671231161589.
52. Reddy RP, Rai A, Como M, Sebastiani R, Como C, Hyre N, et al. Criteria-based return-to-sport testing helps identify functional deficits in young athletes following posterior labral repair but may not reduce recurrence or increase return to play. JSES Int. 2023;7:385–92.

Part IV

Posterior Shoulder Instability

Posterior Shoulder Instability

21

Teo Shao Jin, Bryan Loh, Tay Hui Wen, and T. T. Denny Lie

21.1 Introduction and Epidemiology

The glenohumeral joint is known to be the most mobile joint in the human body. As an inherent trade-off, it is also the most unstable, with only 1/3 of the humeral head articulating with the glenoid at any one point in time [1]. Yet, Posterior Shoulder Instability (PSI) is a relatively rare condition, with an incidence of only 4.64 per 100,000 person-years in the general population and accounting for less than 3% of all glenohumeral instability [2]. Peak incidence occurs in the 14–19 year old age group, with a significant predilection for males. It tends to affect high-level athletes participating in collision or overhead sports.

Structures contributing to shoulder joint stability can be broadly divided into static and dynamic stabilizers. Static stabilizers include the bony anatomy and capsulolabral complex. With little bony congruence, the capsulolabral complex performs a critical role in shoulder joint stability. However, the posterior capsule has been found to be thinner compared to the anterior capsule, with a lower failure strain [3]. In particular, the posterior band of the inferior glenohumeral ligament (IGHL) provides primary anteroposterior stability with the arm in flexion and internal rotation, with other ligaments playing a secondary role. The labrum increases the depth of the shallow glenoid concavity, increases joint congruence, and enhances the concavity compression mechanism to keep the humeral head centred in the glenoid [4].

The main dynamic stabilizers of the shoulder are the rotator cuff group of muscles. Of these, the subscapularis has been identified as the most important dynamic stabilizer in preventing PSI [5]. However, the dynamic stabilizers, including the deltoid and biceps, work in a synchronous manner to produce a balanced force couple to keep the humeral head enlocated. The restoration of this force couple is a major focus of rehabilitative programs in treating PSI.

21.2 Pathomechanism

Rather than being a single well-defined clinical entity, PSI exists on a spectrum with varying presentation and severity. Three broad etiological categories have been proposed for PSI: acute traumatic, recurrent microtraumatic, and atraumatic [6].

T. S. Jin (✉) · B. Loh · T. H. Wen · T. T. Denny Lie
Department of Orthopaedic Surgery, Singapore General Hospital, Singapore, Singapore
e-mail: shaojin.teo@mohh.com.sg; bryan.loh@mohh.com.sg; huiwen.tay@mohh.com.sg; denny.lie.t.t@singhealth.com.sg

E. Calvo et al. (eds.), *Complex and Revision Problems in Shoulder Instability*,
https://doi.org/10.1007/978-3-031-81389-4_21

21.2.1 Acute Traumatic

This commonly refers to traumatic posterior dislocation that occurs as a result of a posteriorly directed force on the shoulder when the arm is in a forward flexed, adduction and internally rotated position. Such a mechanism is often associated with bony fractures on the anterior humeral head or posterior glenoid rim or soft tissue injuries of the rotator cuff and capsulolabral complex. This is seen in contact sports athletes such as rugby and football players.

In addition, posterior shoulder dislocations associated with epileptic seizures, electrocution, and electroconvulsive therapy also have a similar pattern of injury. Activation of the stronger internal rotators overpower the weaker external rotators, resulting in internal rotation and posterior dislocation. Most bilateral posterior dislocations are the result of such a mechanism.

21.2.2 Recurrent Microtraumatic

This occurs with repeated episodes of microtrauma to the posterior capsulolabral complex, each insufficient to cause frank dislocation the glenohumeral joint. However, with time there is attenuation of the posterior capsule and increasing PSI. This is classically observed in overhead throwing athletes. In the follow-through phase of a throw, the shoulder transits into an adducted, flexed, and internally rotated position, placing the posterior capsulolabral complex under strain. In addition, the peelback mechanism that occurs in the late cocking phase has been linked to posterior SLAP tears, which can propagate further posteriorly into the posterior labrum.

21.2.3 Atraumatic

Atraumatic PSI usually is seen in patients with underlying connective tissue abnormalities. This can be unidirectional or multidirectional in nature. Some studies have reported additional bony factors, such as excessive glenoid retroversion or shallow glenoid cavity, that predispose to atraumatic instability [7].

21.3 Clinical Presentation and Physical Examination

Unlike the more commonly seen anterior shoulder instability, symptoms reported by PSI patients tend to be vague, with posterior shoulder pain being the most common rather than frank instability. Other symptoms include general shoulder pain, weakness of the arm after overhead activity to generalized instability [8, 9]. Patients may report position-specific symptoms, often when the shoulder is in flexion, adduction, and internal rotation.

In suspected cases of posterior shoulder instability, a thorough physical examination is important. Examination may reveal the presence of posterior glenohumeral joint line tenderness or the loss of internal rotation with a concomitant increase in external rotation on ROM testing.

In addition, the following special tests for PSI have been reported: Jerk test [10], Kim test [11], Posterior Apprehension Test, and the Load and Shift test [6]. More recently, the Dynamic Posterior Instability Test (DPIT) has been introduced [12]. Unlike its anterior counterpart, the posterior apprehension test is not as sensitive in detecting PSI [13]. Kim et al. found that a combination of the Kim test and Jerk test showed a 97% sensitivity in detecting posterior shoulder instability [11].

21.3.1 Kim Test

First reported by Kim et al. in 2005, the Kim test has been found to have a sensitivity of 80% and specificity of 94% [14]. The patient is first placed in a seated position and the arm abducted to 90°. The examiner cups the elbow with one hand while stabilizing the arm with the other. The patient's arm is elevated an additional 45° while an axial force is applied to the elbow and a down-

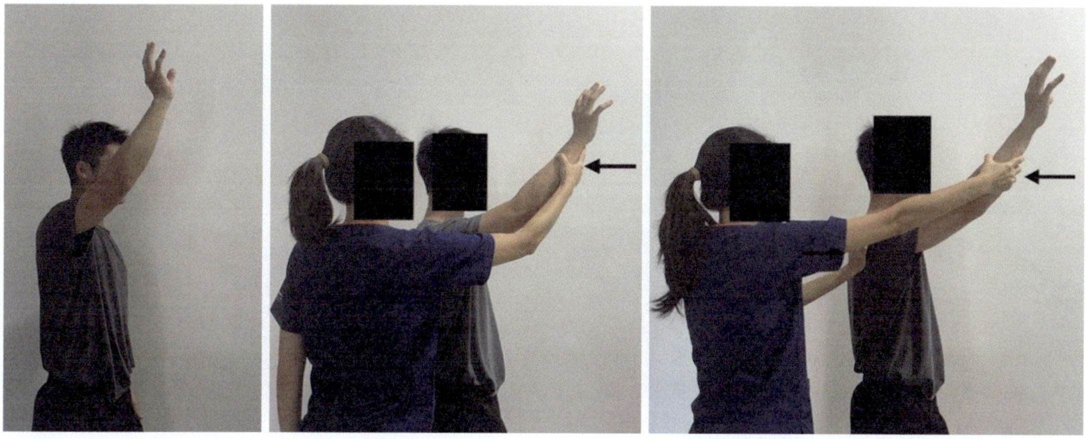

Fig. 21.1 Kim test for posteroinferior instability

ward and posterior force is applied to the arm (Fig. 21.1). The sudden onset of pain signifies a positive test.

21.3.2 Jerk Test

The Jerk test has been found to have a sensitivity of 90% and specificity of 85%. The patient is first placed in a seated position with the arm in 90° of forward flexion, adduction, and internal rotation. The examiner's stabilizes the shoulder girdle with one hand, while the other hand cups the elbow and applies axial loading along the humerus. This results in a posteriorly directed force on the shoulder and a clunk may be felt as the humeral head subluxes posteriorly. The arm is then moved horizontally across the body, bringing it into abduction. This produces a perceptible and more prominent second clunk as the humeral head is reduced (Fig. 21.2). A positive Jerk test has been reported to be associated with failure of conservative treatment [15].

21.3.3 Load and Shift Test

The sensitivity and specificity of the Load and Shift test has not been previously reported in the context of PSI. The patient is first placed in a seated position with the arm hanging by the side. The shoulder girdle is stabilized with one hand while the humeral head is held in the other hand with the thumb posteriorly and the other fingers anteriorly. The head is loaded by firmly pushing it into the glenoid. A posteriorly directed force is applied to the humeral head and the amount of translation noted. Posterior translation greater than 50% of the humeral head diameter is generally recognized as a positive test.

21.3.4 Dynamic Posterior Instability Test (DPIT)

First described in 2022 and designed for overhead athletes, the DPIT has a sensitivity of 94% and specificity of 95% [12]. The patient is asked to simulate a ball throwing motion and to freeze at the ball release position. The examiner then flexes the shoulder to approximately 140° of forward flexion. The patient is then asked to actively flex the shoulder against the examiner's hand (Fig. 21.3). Sudden onset of posterior shoulder pain or a sensation of instability is considered a positive result. As a follow-up, the humeral head can be stabilized posteriorly with the examiner's thumb, preventing posterior subluxation. Improvement of symptom with this stabilization is a further positive sign (Table 21.1).

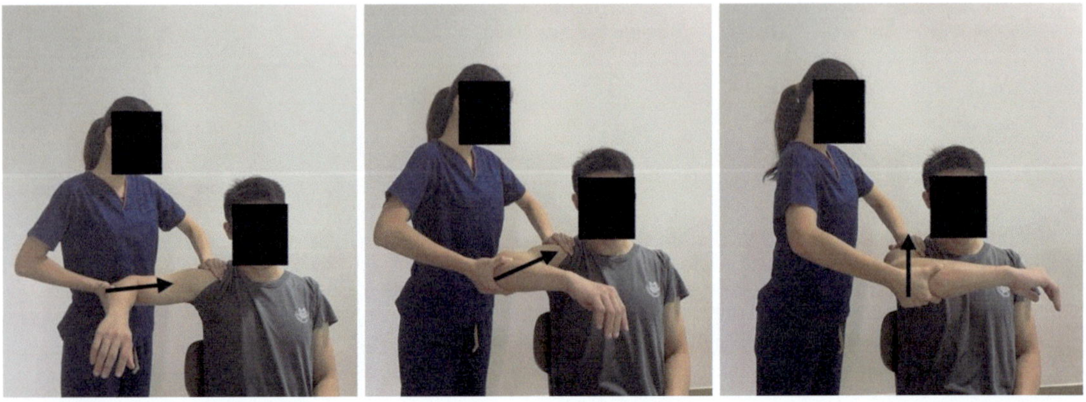

Fig. 21.2 Jerk test for posteroinferior instability

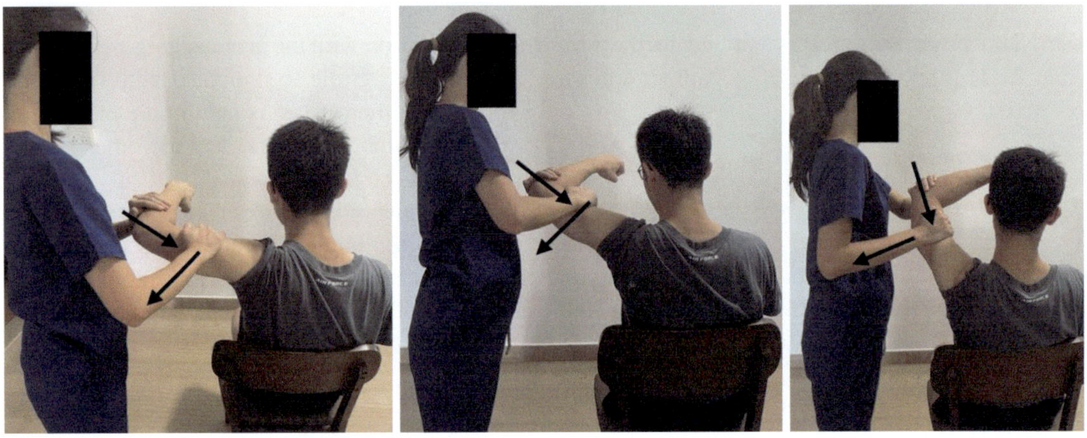

Fig. 21.3 Dynamic posterior instability test

Table 21.1 Special tests for PSI

Test	Sensitivity	Specificity
Kim test	80%	94%
Jerk test	90%	85%
Load & shift test	–[a]	–[a]
Dynamic posterior instability test	94%	95%

[a] Not previously reported

21.4 Imaging and Radiographic Assessment

21.4.1 Radiographs

While initial radiographs are often normal, it is important to obtain standard anteroposterior (AP), Y-scapular, and axillary radiographs of the shoulder. Possible radiographic findings include:

21.4.1.1 Light Bulb Sign

Classically seen on the AP view of a posteriorly dislocated shoulder, the light bulb shaped appearance of the humeral head results from excessive internal rotation of the shoulder that brings the greater and lesser tuberosity out of view.

21.4.1.2 Reverse Hill-Sachs lesion (RHSL)

This is an impaction fracture of the anteromedial humeral head best appreciated on the axillary view (Figs. 21.4 and 21.5). It results from contact between the humeral head and the posterior glenoid during a dislocation event.

21.4.1.3 Posterior Glenoid Fracture

This can occur when the humeral head impacts the posterior glenoid rim during a dislocation event, and is best appreciated on the axillary view.

21.4.2 Magnetic Resonance Imaging (MRI)

MRI is often the imaging modality of choice in the evaluation of shoulder pathologies, especially when no obvious bony injury is appreciated on initial radiographs. It has high sensitivity in detecting soft tissue injuries, especially in the posterior capsulolabral complex in the context of PSI [16].

21.4.2.1 Reverse Bankart

A common finding is a reverse Bankart lesion, where the posteroinferior labrum is detached from its glenoid attachment (Fig. 21.6). As the posterior band of the IGHL is attached to the posteroinferior labrum, this results in posterior laxity and increased posterior translation of the humeral head. When a tear occurs between the posterior labrum and articular cartilage without detachment of the labrum, it is known as a Kim lesion. Kim lesions are easily missed and can result in persistent instability if not treated [17]. Other patterns of injury include posterior labrocapsular periosteal sleeve avulsion (POLPSA) where the posterior scapular periosteum is stripped along with the labrum and humeral avulsion of the posterior glenohumeral ligament [18]. Injuries to the rotator cuff, especially in the teres minor or infraspinatus tendon or insertional avulsion, may also be seen.

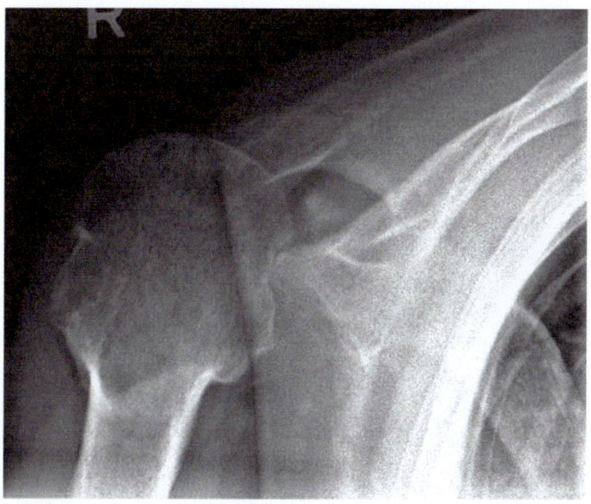

Fig. 21.4 Reverse Hill-Sach lesion on the anterior humeral head engaging the posterior glenoid (Valpeau view)

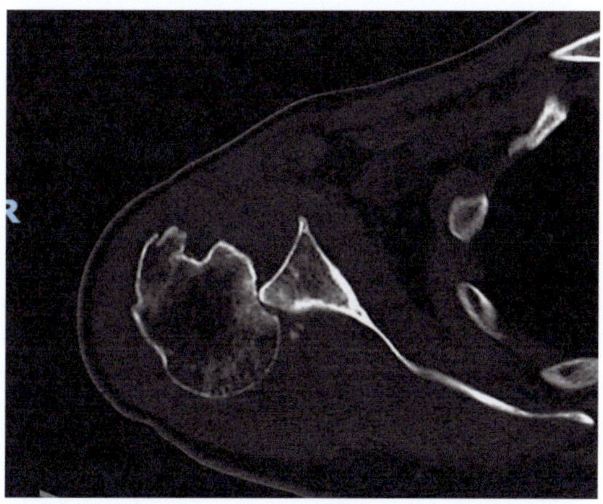

Fig. 21.5 Axial slice from a CT scan of the same patient in Fig. 21.3. Reverse Hill-Sach lesion engaging the posterior glenoid visible

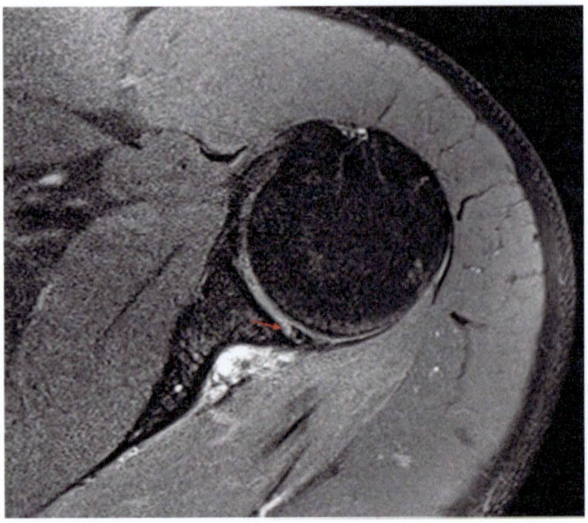

Fig. 21.6 Axial T2 slice showing the presence of a posterior labral tear (red arrow)

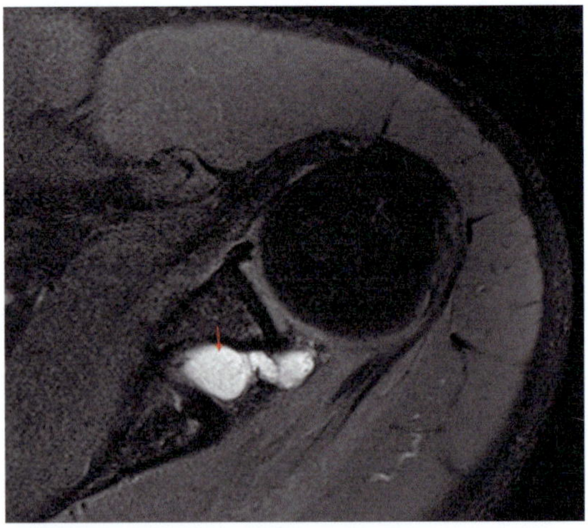

Fig. 21.7 Axial T2 slice of the same patient showing the presence of a posterior paralabral cyst (red arrow)

21.4.2.2 Paralabral Cyst

Paralabral cysts are ganglion cysts formed from the seepage of joint fluid through preexisting labral tears (Fig. 21.7). In the context of posterior labral tears, posterior para-labral cysts can form and cause compression neuropathy of the suprascapular nerve at the spinoglenoid notch resulting in infraspinatus weakness. Paralabral cysts can also form superiorly due to SLAP tears, resulting in suprascapular nerve compression at the suprascapular notch and causing both supraspinatus and infraspinatus weakness [19]. Inferiorly, paralabral cyst can press on the axillary nerve in the quadrilateral space, causing teres minor weakness.

21.4.3 Computed Tomography (CT)

CT scans are useful in assessing bony anatomy and pathology, including fractures, version, and bone loss. They also allow 3D reconstruction to be performed to facilitate surgical planning.

21.4.3.1 Glenoid Retroversion

Excessive glenoid retroversion has been suggested to be a significant risk factor for PSI in some studies but its exact role remains controversial [20, 21]. Case series of version correction glenoid osteotomies have been described in literature, albeit with mixed result and small cohort size.

Partially accounting for the variability in result is the variability in measuring glenoid version. Two methods of measurement have been popularized—the Friedman method and the Poon and Ting (PT) method.

In the Friedman method, on an axial slice at the mid-glenoid level, a first line is drawn down the long axis of the scapular, connecting the medial border of the scapular to the centre of the glenoid. A second line is drawn connecting the anterior and posterior border of the glenoid (Fig. 21.8) [22]. A study utilizing the Friedman

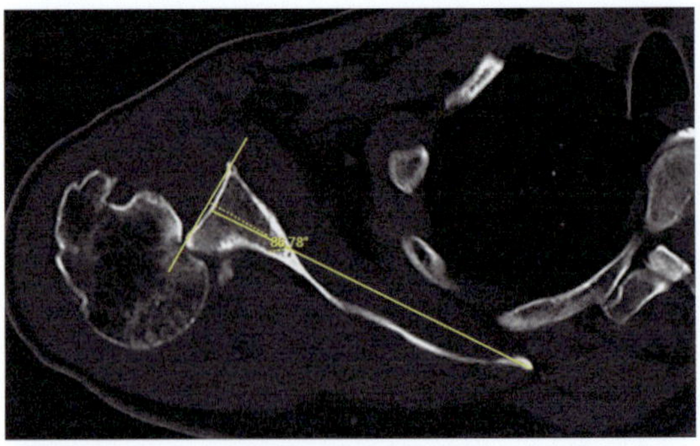

Fig. 21.8 Friedman's method of measuring glenoid version illustrated on this mid-coronal axial slice of the scapula

method found a significantly increased glenoid retroversion of −9.0 in 31 patients with PSI, when comparted to a mean version of −4.0 in a group of 30 control individuals [20].

The PT method was suggested more recently, and measures glenoid version based on the glenoid vault without consideration of the scapular body [23]. This removes the influence of the glenoid body, which has large variation in morphology between individuals. With the PT method, on a mid-glenoid axial cut, an isosceles triangle is drawn in the medial end of the glenoid endosteal vault. A line is drawn through the medial end of the vault, bisecting the isosceles triangle. A second line is drawn connecting the anterior and posterior glenoid rim (Fig. 21.9). Higher interobserver reliability of 0.96 and intra-observer reliability of 0.97 have been reported with PT method.

Nonetheless, concerns have also been raised with the intrinsic variability in measuring version on two-dimensional imaging due to differences in scapular rotation, patient positioning, and axis of the scanner [24, 25]. A recent study found that every one additional degree of scapular abduction increased the measured glenoid anteversion by 0.42° [26]. Hence, the use of three-dimensional imaging has been suggested for more accurate and objective measurement of glenoid version. However, it remains to be seen if this will translate into improved surgical outcome.

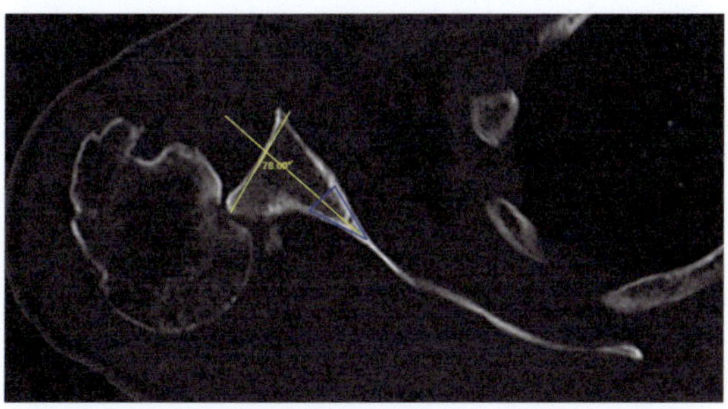

Fig. 21.9 Poon and Ting's method illustrated. An isosceles triangle is drawn into the glenoid vault (blue triangle). A line bisecting this triangle is used to measure the glenoid version

21.4.3.2 Reverse Hill Sach Lesion

The size of a RHSL can be expressed as a percentage of the articular surface, or with the gamma angle, which is formed between the bicipital groove and posterior margin of the RHSL (Fig. 21.10) [27]. In isolated RHSL, a gamma angle >90° has been shown to result in engagement and posterior instability. With concomitant glenoid bone loss, an additional 2° can be added to the gamma angle for every mm of bone loss [28]. When measured as a percentage of the articular surface, a threshold of 25% has been suggested to define critical bone loss.

21.4.3.3 Glenoid Bone Loss

Glenoid bone loss is best measured on a 3D reconstructed en face view of the glenoid. The amount of bone loss is expressed as a percentage of a best fit circle. This circle is constructed by modelling the inferior two-thirds of the glenoid as a true circle, as the glenoid itself is not a perfect circle (Fig. 21.11) [29]. Increasing amount of glenoid bone loss has been shown to be correlated with increasing failure rate after soft tissue

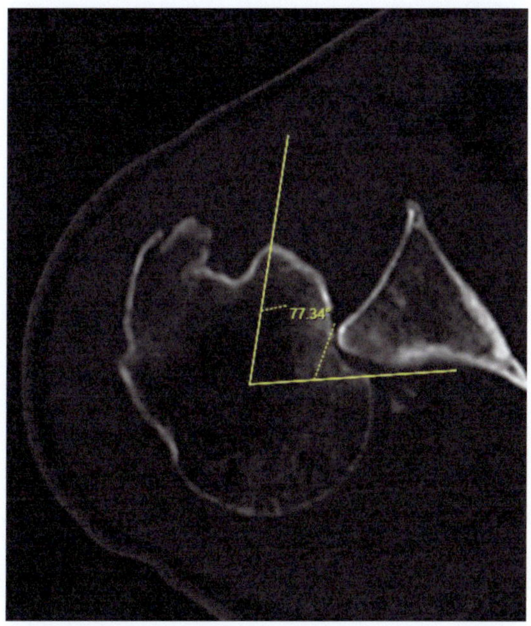

Fig. 21.10 Gamma angle is measured between the posterior aspect of the RHSL and the medial wall of the bicipital groove

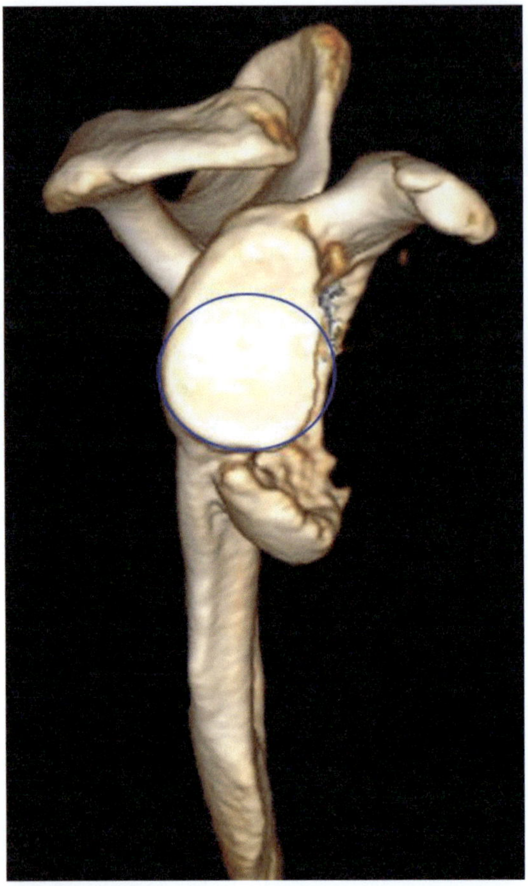

Fig. 21.11 En face view of the glenoid in a 3D scapular reconstruction. A best fit circle (blue circle) is fitted onto the inferior two-thirds of the glenoid to estimate bone loss

procedure. The threshold of critical glenoid bone loss has been estimated to be around 15% [30].

21.5 Treatment Algorithm

There is currently a lack of large, high quality prospective trials evaluating the optimal treatment algorithm of PSI. The majority of existing literature consist of retrospective case series that often lack statistical power.

Regardless, it is generally recognized that most patients would benefit from a course of conservative treatment with structured physiotherapy for a period of 6 months. This is further detailed in the following section on nonoperative treatment. However, it has been observed that patients with an acute traumatic aetiology have significantly higher rates of failure with conservative treatment. Burkhead et al. found good outcome, as measured with the Rowe and Zarin score, in 94% of atraumatic PSI compared to only 36% in traumatic PSI [31]. A separate study on the epidemiology of PSI in a young athletic population found that 77% of cases eventually required surgical intervention [32]. Hence, it is reasonable that patients with acute traumatic PSI be counselled for surgical treatment on presentation, especially in young and high functioning candidates. In addition, patients with large bony injuries visible on initial radiographs are also unlikely to do well with conservative management.

Once a decision is made for surgical treatment, a choice has to be made between soft tissue and bony procedures. Advanced imaging, ideally a CT scan, is helpful in determining the presence and degree of bone loss. In the absence of significant bone loss, a posterior labral stabilization with capsular plication is commonly done with widely reported outcomes. When significant glenoid retroversion is present, isolated labral repair may not provide sufficient stability and a posterior glenoid opening osteotomy can be considered to improve version.

When there is significant bone loss, isolated soft tissue procedures often result in high failure rates. Critical bone loss in the humeral head has been described as 25% of the articular surface. With HH bone loss involving 25–40% of the articular surface, surgical options include anatomical options such as allograft bone grafting and nonanatomical options such as transfer of the subscapularis tendon into the HH defect (McLaughlin procedure). With HH bone loss greater than 40%, replacement of the HH has been advocated, due to high rates of osteoarthritis and recurrent instability with preservation.

The critical threshold for glenoid bone loss has been generally reported to be in the range of 15% [33]. A case-control study of 75 patients found 10.4 times higher rates of failure of posterior capsulolabral repair with 11% bone loss, and this increased to 24.4 times with 15% bone loss [30]. In a different cadaveric study, glenoid bone defect greater than 15% resulted in failure of the

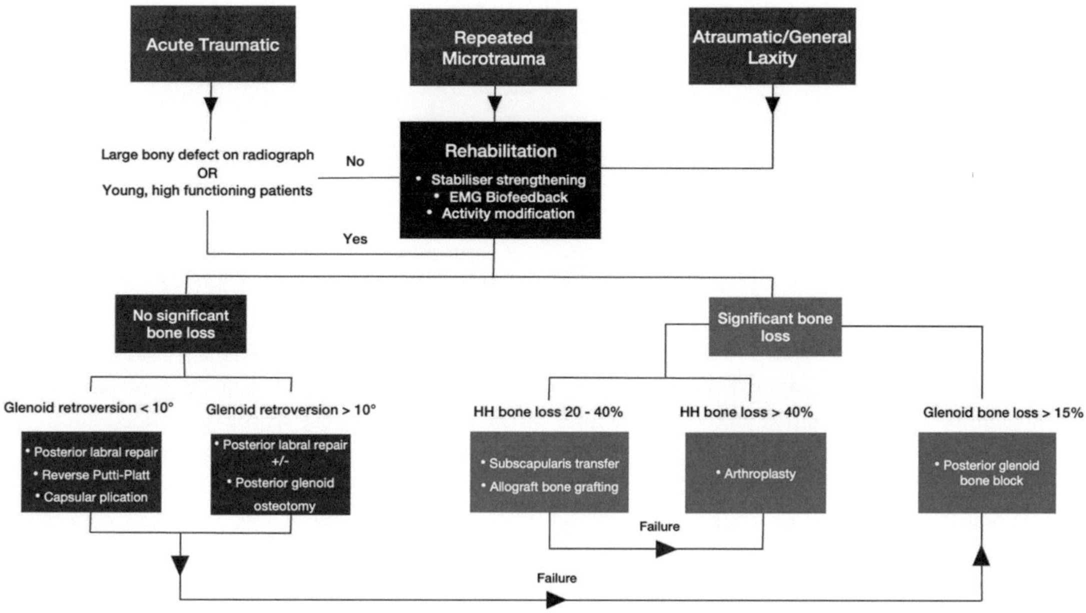

Fig. 21.12 Suggested treatment algorithm

capsulolabral repair to restore glenohumeral stability and humeral head position [33]. When glenoid bone loss is critical, a posterior bone block procedure is necessary. The source of this bone block has traditionally been iliac crest autograft, but distal tibial allograft has been described [34].

A suggested algorithm is presented in Fig. 21.12.

21.6 Conservative Treatment

A trial of nonsurgical treatment is an acceptable and recommended first line option for most patients with PSI. However, the rate of success is dependent on the underlying aetiology and acute traumatic aetiology is associated with higher failure rates.

The cornerstone of nonsurgical treatment is rehabilitation. Rehabilitation relies on strengthening of the posterior dynamic stabilizers, primarily the subscapularis, as well as the external rotators of the humerus including teres minor and infraspinatus to prevent excessive internal rotation. Together, this also increases the anteroposterior force couple and further reinforces glenohumeral joint stability [35]. In addition, biofeedback with electromyogram monitoring has been described to improve muscle coordination and firing pattern. A cases series described the use of such a technique to correct abnormally relaxed posterior deltoid with good outcomes in PSI [36].

21.7 Surgical Treatment

21.7.1 Indications for Surgery (After a Period of Failed Conservative Management)

- Symptomatic patients with isolated posterior shoulder instability.
- Posttraumatic posterior dislocations.
- Multidirectional instability patients with predominant posterior instability.
- Posterior shoulder instability post epilepsy (relative).

21.7.2 Arthroscopic Posterolabral Capsular Repair

Arthroscopic posterior capsulolabral repair is the mainstay of treatment for the above indications. Conventionally posterior labral repairs are performed with the patient in the lateral decubitus position. This technique is done in the beach chair position and increasingly more common and popular, as it enables anterior labral repair and conversion to open surgery.

After creation of the diagnostic and working portals, the posterior labrum is then debrided and its attachment to the glenoid rasped and roughened. A low posterior double-loaded suture anchor is inserted at the 7 or 7:30 o'clock position (right shoulder). The first pair of sutures is used to catch both the labrum and the posterior inferior capsule and used to pull the inferior capsule superiorly. The second pair of sutures catches both the labrum and the posterolateral capsule and results in a significant medial shift. Knots are then tied with the arm in neutral rotation. This will not only create a significant medial-lateral capsular shift but will also close the posterior portal (Figs. 21.13a–m) [37].

In terms of clinical outcome, many studies report high rates of patient satisfaction with low recurrence rates [38]. However, some studies suggest overhead throwers may not necessarily return to a preinjury level of performance. McClincy et al. performed an analysis of 48 overhead throwing athletes matched to non-throwing athletes who all underwent an arthroscopic posterior capsulolabral reconstruction [39]. While no significant difference in patient reported outcomes scores were noted at a mean follow up of 37 months, only 60% of throwers were able to return to their preinjury level of competitive throwing.

21.7.3 Para Labral Cyst Decompression

Paralabral cysts are swellings that arise around the glenoid and are associated with labral tears. They may occur as an extravasation of joint fluid after a labral tear into the spinoglenoid notch. These cysts occur more frequently in the spinoglenoid notch due to absence of any muscle of tendon directly over this space. Compression of the suprascapular nerve may result and the patient may present with weakness on external rotation (Infraspinatus).

Management of such cysts include ultrasound-guided percutaneous aspiration and arthroscopic decompression. Ultrasound-guided aspirations may be offered as the first line of treatment but they have a high recurrence rate and may lead to an overall lower patient satisfaction rate.

The example below is a 28-year-old young male gym enthusiast who experienced shoulder pain and weakness in external rotation without any specific history of trauma. MRI revealed a posterior labral tear which extended superiorly and inferiorly, associated with mutliloculated paralabral cyst formation posterior to the posterior labrum that extended into the spinoglenoid notch measuring 2.7 × 1.5 × 1.1 cm (Fig. 21.14). The patient then underwent a posterior labral repair with decompression of the cyst that was achieved during mobilization of the posterior labrum as shown in (Fig. 21.15) [40, 41].

21.7.4 McLaughlin Procedure

The McLaughlin procedure was first described in 1952, and it involves the filling of the RHSL with the subscapularis tendon, which is detached from its insertion and re-attached into the lesser tuberosity (Fig. 21.16) [42]. This has the effect of filling the humeral head defect and converting any remaining defect to an extra-articular one. Various modifications of this procedure have been made since its description, including the transfer of the lesser tuberosity into the defect (Modified McLaughlin) and fixation of the subscapularis tendon into the RHSL without detachment of its insertion (Reverse Remplissage). Augmentation of the transfer with extracellular matrix has been further described [43].

Literature on outcome remains scarce and limited to small cohorts. A recent meta-analysis found nine studies with a total of only 97 shoulders. The recurrent instability rate was low at 2.1% and both occurred in patients with epileptic seizures [44].

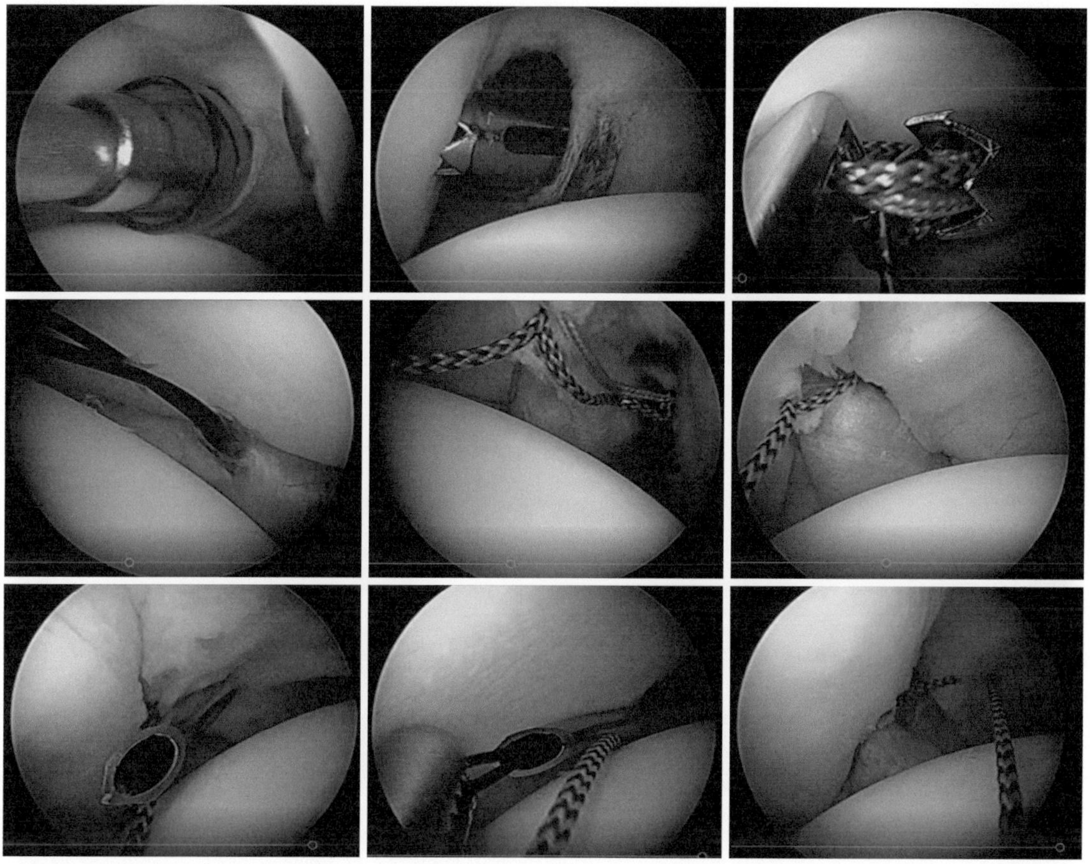

Fig. 21.13 (**a**) Viewed from anterolateral portal, a cannula is inserted into the main working posterior portal. (**b**) A drill guide is placed at the posterior glenoid edge, at about 45° to the surface. (**c**) One limb from each suture pair is retrieved to the antero-inferior portal. (**d**) A suture passer takes a bite of the labrum and the posteroinferior capsule. (**e**) The purple suture is shuttled through to tent and pull the inferior capsule upwards. (**f**) Tying the purple suture achieves a significant inferior capsular shift upwards. (**g**) The suture passer then takes a bite of the posterolateral capsule. (**h**) The monofilament is retrieved to the anterosuperior portal. (**i**) The blue suture is then shuttled through. (**j**) Tying the blue suture tightens the posterolateral capsule medially, effecting a significant medial shift. (**k**) The labral repair and a significant inferior and lateral capsular shift are achieved. (**l**) Preparation of Posterior labral tear in the lateral decubitus position (Viewing portal: ant-superior, Working portal: mid-anterior). (**m**) Posterior labrum repair with a double-loaded suture anchor

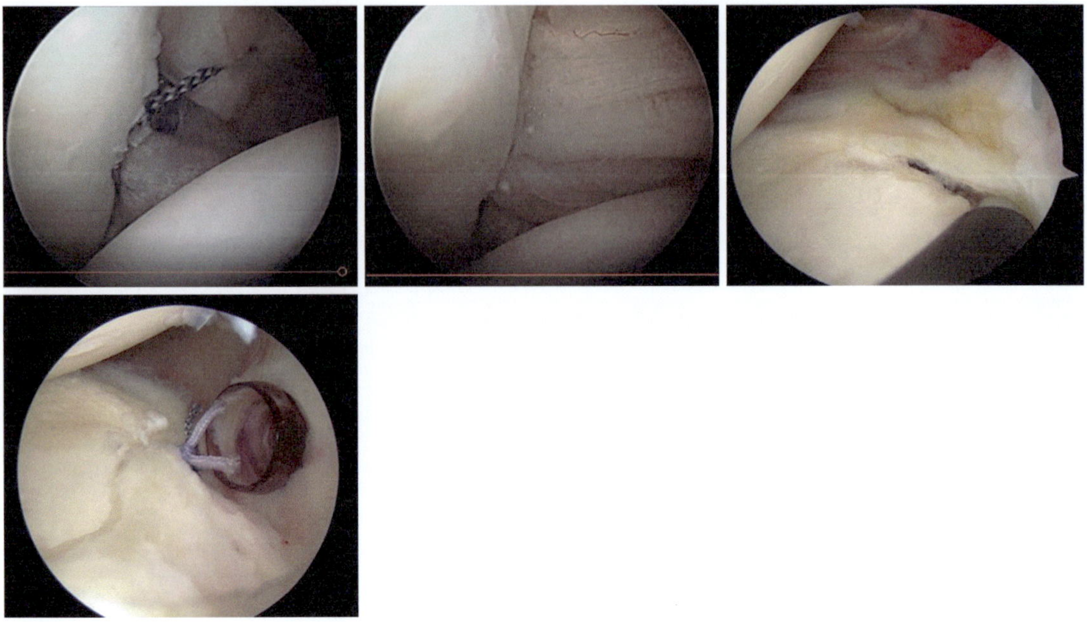

Fig. 21.13 (continued)

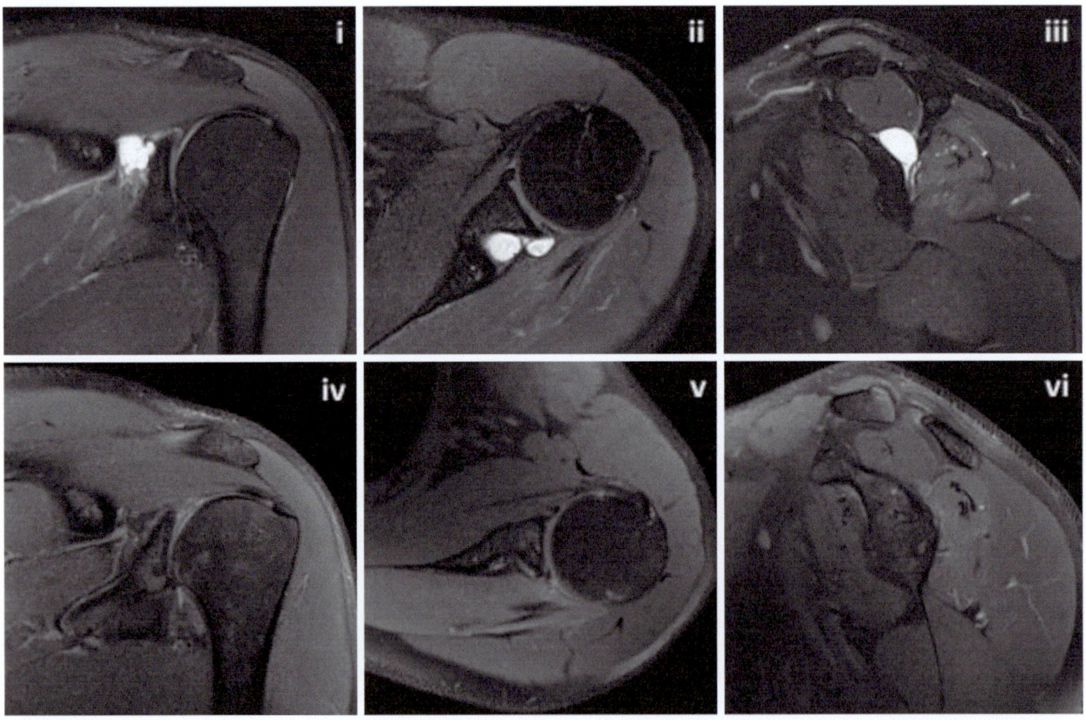

Fig. 21.14 MRI T2-weighted cuts of the right shoulder showing the spinoglenoid notch cyst and posterior labral tear

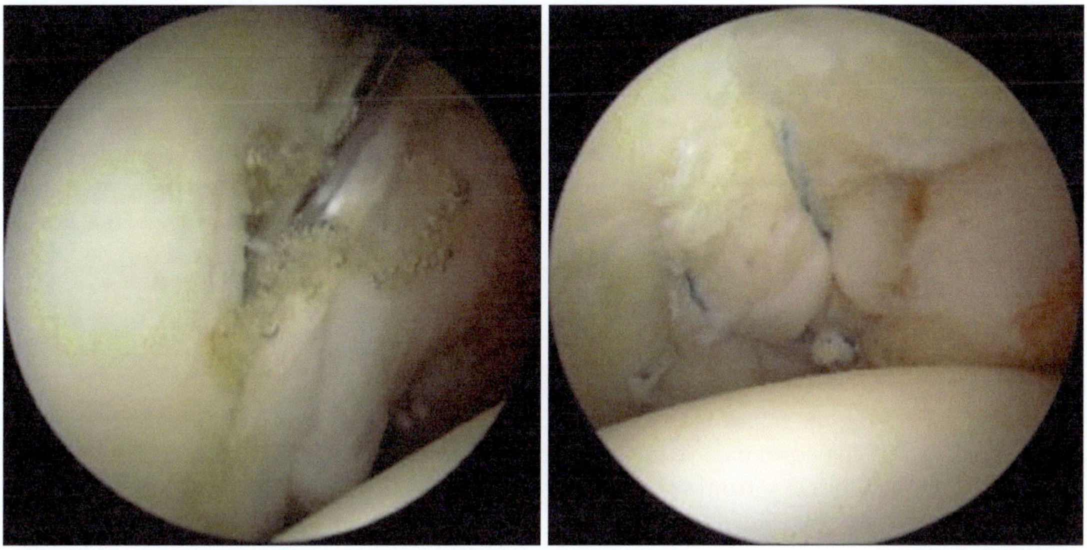

Fig. 21.15 Arthroscopic photos showing mobilization of posterior labrum with outflow of cystic material (left) and repair of posterior labrum using suture anchors with additional posterior capsular shift (right)

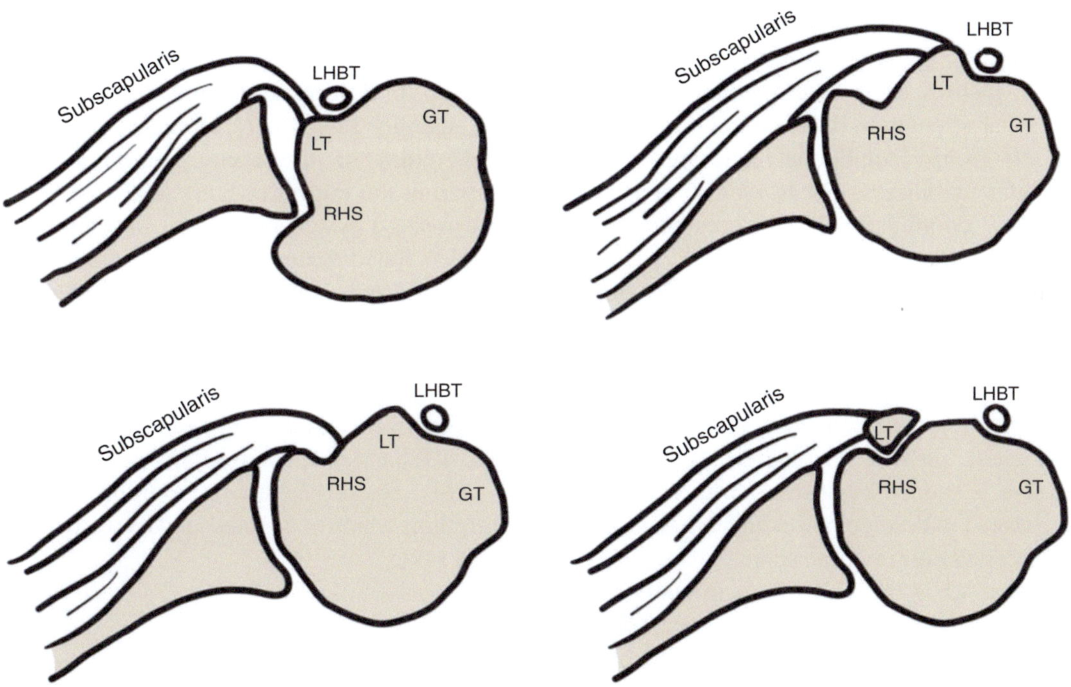

Fig. 21.16 Illustrated McLaughlin procedure

21.8 Postoperative Rehabilitation

There is currently very limited literature on rehabilitation after surgical treatment of PSI. However, common principles apply—including the importance of communication and collaboration between surgeon and physiotherapist. Goldenberg et al. published a detailed review of current best practices that can be used as a guide [45].

Broadly, post-operative rehabilitation can be divided into phases.

Phase I covers the immediate postoperative period up to the fourth week where the surgical repair has to be protected. The senior author's preference is the use of a gunslinger brace to prevent internal rotation. Pendular exercises is encouraged. Limited passive ROM can be started, with the extent depending on tissue quality and strength of construct. Excessive internal rotation is avoided to prevent stressing the posterior capsule.

Phase II starts from the fourth post-operative week. The patient is started on passive full ROM exercises to prevent stiffness. However, internal rotation can continue to be limited if there are concerns regarding healing.

Phase III starts from the seventh post-operative week and the patient is allowed active full ROM and the sling can be removed. Concurrently, isometric exercises can be started.

Phase IV starts when full ROM is regained and it focuses on resistance training to regain muscular strength in the shoulder girdle. Target muscle groups include the rotator cuff and the scapular stabilizers. Focus is also placed on muscle coordination and scapulohumeral control.

Phase V usually starts 3 months after surgery when the surgical repair is thought to be healed. The shoulder can be further loaded and strengthened in position of stress on the posterior capsule. Such exercises include push-ups, planks, and chest presses. Plyometric exercises that involve a sudden explosive movement can be introduced to develop power and dynamic stability necessary for return to sport.

Phase VI is the safe return to sport or/and work for the patient, usually occurring at 6 months after surgery. There should be full recovery of strength in external rotation. Functional testing relevant to the specific sport and patient's level of play should be conducted before return to sport. Thereafter, a gradual progression to premorbid baseline is recommended.

21.9 Outcomes of Treatment

Outcomes of surgical treatment of PSI have historically been considered inferior to anterior instability, although results have improved with time. Existing studies have mostly examined only soft tissue procedures, largely due to the relative rarity of bony procedures.

21.9.1 Recurrent Instability

The rates of recurrent instability after surgical treatment have ranged between 7–20%, depending on the severity of injury and surgical treatment. Multicentre registry data from Norway found 1-year recurrent instability rate after arthroscopic labral repair of 16% in posterior instability, as compared to only 10% in anterior instability [46]. In the largest prospective study to date, 200 shoulders in athletes underwent arthroscopic capsulolabral stabilization were followed up for 3 years and only 9% had less than good stability scores [47]. However, only 64% could return to the same premorbid level. Illustrating the impact of bony injury on recurrence rates, a systematic review including 847 shoulders found recurrent instability rate of 7.5% in cases of only soft tissue abnormalities and 8.5% in shoulders with additional bony abnormalities [48].

In a series of 14 patients with recurrent PSI who underwent posterior bone block with autograft, 4 (28.6%) experienced recurrent instability. This could be due to significant graft resorption, which was noted in 62% of patients on CT [49].

21.9.2 Return to Sport

The rate of return to sports has been reported to be in the range of 60–90%. However, the proportion that is able to achieve pre-morbid level of play is significantly lower, particularly in overhead throwing athletes [50]. When compared to anterior instability, lower rates of return to sport have also been noted [51].

A systematic review by DeLong reported return to sports of 91.8% in 611 shoulders, but only 67.4% were able to achieve the pre-morbid level of play. This dropped further to 58.1% in overhead throwing atheletes [38]. In the prospective study of 200 shoulders in an atheletic population described earlier, 90% returned to sports but only 64% managed to return to pre-morbid level [47].

21.10 The Locked Posterior-Dislocation

A locked posterior dislocation of the shoulder is an uncommon but challenging condition. Often, it results from a posterior dislocation that was missed on presentation. This can happen when clinical attention is directed towards concomitant medical conditions, such as a seizure, and subtle radiographic signs are not detected. Up to 79% of posterior dislocations are missed on initial presentation [52]. The delay in recognition has been associated with poorer outcomes even after surgical treatment [53]. This is postulated to result from progression of the RHSL with increasing amount of time the shoulder is dislocated. When closed reduction fails, the shoulder is "locked." Conservative treatment is rarely acceptable with the shoulder locked in dislocation.

Surgical treatment depends on the size of the RHSL. In RHSL involving less than 40% of the articular surface, a variety of joint preserving options have been recommended. McLaughlin suggested utilizing the subscapularis tendon to fill the RHSL and converting the intra-articular defect into an extra-articular defect. Subsequent popular modifications of this technique have filled the RHSL with either the lesser tuberosity or allograft. Good results have been reported with these techniques [53–56]. In addition, elevation of the articular depression and filling of the subchondral defect with allograft or bone cement has been described, but long-term outcomes are unclear. A case report described the use of femoral head allograft to fill the RHSL in a patient with chronic locked posterior shoulder dislocation and 40% involvement of the humeral head articular surface [57]. Good outcome was reported at 1 year post-surgery.

When more than 40% of the articular surface is involved, replacement of the humeral head is often necessary, with poor outcomes reported with joint preserving options due to onset of osteoarthritis and recurrent instability [58].

References

1. Doehrmann R, Frush TJ. Posterior shoulder instability. In: StatPearls. Treasure Island, FL: StatPearls Publishing; 2024.
2. Woodmass JM, Lee J, Wu IT, Desai VS, Camp CL, Dahm DL, Krych AJ. Incidence of posterior shoulder instability and trends in surgical reconstruction: a 22-year population-based study. J Shoulder Elb Surg. 2019;28:611–6.
3. Bey MJ, Hunter SA, Kilambi N, Butler DL, Lindenfeld TN. Structural and mechanical properties of the glenohumeral joint posterior capsule. J Shoulder Elb Surg. 2005;14:201–6.
4. Lippitt SB, Vanderhooft JE, Harris SL, Sidles JA, Harryman DT, Matsen FA. Glenohumeral stability from concavity-compression: a quantitative analysis. J Shoulder Elb Surg. 1993;2:27–35.
5. Blasier RB, Soslowsky LJ, Malicky DM, Palmer ML. Posterior glenohumeral subluxation: active and passive stabilization in a biomechanical model. J Bone Joint Surg Am. 1997;79:433–40.
6. Millett PJ, Clavert P, Hatch GFR, Warner JJP. Recurrent posterior shoulder instability. J Am Acad Orthop Surg. 2006;14:464–76.
7. Kim S-H, Noh K-C, Park J-S, Ryu B-D, Oh I. Loss of chondrolabral containment of the glenohumeral joint in atraumatic posteroinferior multidirectional instability. J Bone Joint Surg. 2005;87:92–8.
8. Provencher MT, Bhatia S, Ghodadra NS, Grumet RC, Bach BR, Dewing CB, LeClere L, Romeo AA. Recurrent shoulder instability: current concepts for evaluation and management of glenoid bone loss. J Bone Joint Surg Am. 2010;92(Suppl 2):133–51.
9. Neer CS. Involuntary inferior and multidirectional instability of the shoulder: etiology, recognition, and treatment. Instr Course Lect. 1985;34:232–8.
10. Kim SH, Park JC, Park JS, Oh I. Painful jerk test: a predictor of success in nonoperative treatment of posteroinferior instability of the shoulder. Am J Sports Med. 2004;32:1849–55.
11. Kim SH, Park JS, Jeong WK, Shin SK. The Kim test: a novel test for posteroinferior labral lesion of the shoulder—a comparison to the Jerk test. Am J Sports Med. 2005;33:1188–92.

12. Arner JW, Nickoli MS, Lawyer TJ, Conway JE, Bradley JP. Dynamic posterior instability test: a new test for posterior glenohumeral instability. Indian J Orthop. 2022;56:2022–7.
13. Schwartz E, Warren RF, O'Brien SJ, Fronek J. Posterior shoulder instability. Orthop Clin North Am. 1987;18:409–19.
14. Kim S-H, Park J-S, Jeong W-K, Shin S-K. The Kim test. Am J Sports Med. 2005;33:1188–92.
15. Kim S-H, Park J-C, Park J-S, Oh I. Painful jerk test: a predictor of success in nonoperative treatment of posteroinferior instability of the shoulder. Am J Sports Med. 2004;32:1849–55.
16. Liu F, Cheng X, Dong J, Zhou D, Sun Q, Bai X, Wang D. Imaging modality for measuring the presence and extent of the labral lesions of the shoulder: a systematic review and meta-analysis. BMC Musculoskelet Disord. 2019;20:487.
17. Kim S-H, Ha K-I, Yoo J-C, Noh K-C. Kim's lesion: an incomplete and concealed avulsion of the posteroinferior labrum in posterior or multidirectional posteroinferior instability of the shoulder. Arthroscopy. 2004;20:712–20.
18. Yu J, Ashman C, Jones G. The POLPSA lesion: MR imaging findings with arthroscopic correlation in patients with posterior instability. Skeletal Radiol. 2002;31:396–9.
19. Boykin RE, Friedman DJ, Higgins LD, Warner JJP. Suprascapular neuropathy. J Bone Joint Surg. 2010;92:2348–64.
20. Privitera DM, Siegel EJ, Miller LR, Sinz NJ, Higgins LD. Glenoid version and its relationship to glenohumeral instability and labral tears. J Shoulder Elb Surg. 2016;25:1056–63.
21. Gottschalk MB, Ghasem A, Todd D, Daruwalla J, Xerogeanes J, Karas S. Posterior shoulder instability: does glenoid retroversion predict recurrence and contralateral instability? Arthroscopy. 2015;31:488–93.
22. Friedman RJ, Hawthorne KB, Genez BM. The use of computerized tomography in the measurement of glenoid version. J Bone Joint Surg Am. 1992;74:1032–7.
23. Poon PC, Ting FSH. A 2-dimensional glenoid vault method for measuring glenoid version on computed tomography. J Shoulder Elb Surg. 2012;21:329–35.
24. Bokor DJ, O'Sullivan MD, Hazan GJ. Variability of measurement of glenoid version on computed tomography scan. J Shoulder Elb Surg. 1999;8:595–8.
25. Budge MD, Lewis GS, Schaefer E, Coquia S, Flemming DJ, Armstrong AD. Comparison of standard two-dimensional and three-dimensional corrected glenoid version measurements. J Shoulder Elb Surg. 2011;20:577–83.
26. Bryce CD, Davison AC, Lewis GS, Wang L, Flemming DJ, Armstrong AD. Two-dimensional glenoid version measurements vary with coronal and sagittal scapular rotation. J Bone Joint Surg Am Vol. 2010;92:692–9.
27. Moroder P, Runer A, Kraemer M, et al. Influence of defect size and localization on the engagement of reverse Hill-Sachs lesions. Am J Sports Med. 2015;43:542–8.
28. Moroder P, Plachel F, Tauber M, Habermeyer P, Imhoff A, Liem D, Lill H, Resch H, Gerhardt C, Scheibel M. Risk of engagement of bipolar bone defects in posterior shoulder instability. Am J Sports Med. 2017;45:2835–9.
29. Sugaya H, Moriishi J, Dohi M, Kon Y, Tsuchiya A. Glenoid rim morphology in recurrent anterior glenohumeral instability. J Bone Joint Surg Am. 2003;85:878–84.
30. Arner JW, Ruzbarsky JJ, Midtgaard K, Peebles L, Bradley JP, Provencher MT. Defining critical glenoid bone loss in posterior shoulder capsulolabral repair. Am J Sports Med. 2021;49:2013–9.
31. Burkhead WZ, Rockwood CA. Treatment of instability of the shoulder with an exercise program. J Bone Joint Surg Am. 1992;74:890–6.
32. Lanzi JT, Chandler PJ, Cameron KL, Bader JM, Owens BD. Epidemiology of posterior glenohumeral instability in a young athletic population. Am J Sports Med. 2017;45:3315–21.
33. Shin S-J, Koh YW, Bui C, Jeong WK, Akeda M, Cho NS, McGarry MH, Lee TQ. What is the critical value of glenoid bone loss at which soft tissue Bankart repair does not restore glenohumeral translation, restricts range of motion, and leads to abnormal humeral head position? Am J Sports Med. 2016;44:2784–91.
34. Millett PJ, Schoenahl J-Y, Register B, Gaskill TR, van Deurzen Derek FP, Martetschläger F. Reconstruction of posterior glenoid deficiency using distal tibial osteoarticular allograft. Knee Surg Sports Traumatol Arthrosc. 2013;21:445–9.
35. Tibone JE, Bradley JP. The treatment of posterior subluxation in athletes. Clin Orthop Relat Res. 1993;291:124–37.
36. Beall MS, Diefenbach G, Allen A. Electromyographic biofeedback in the treatment of voluntary posterior instability of the shoulder. Am J Sports Med. 1987;15:175–8.
37. Lie DTT. Shoulder surgery made easy! World Scientific; 2023. https://doi.org/10.1142/12657.
38. DeLong JM, Jiang K, Bradley JP. Posterior instability of the shoulder. Am J Sports Med. 2015;43:1805–17.
39. McClincy MP, Arner JW, Bradley JP. Posterior shoulder instability in throwing athletes: a case-matched comparison of throwers and non-throwers. Arthroscopy. 2015;31:1041–51.
40. Sim DS, Lie DTT. Suprascapular nerve compression by spinoglenoid cysts arising from posterior labral tears: Unusual presentation in young male gym enthusiasts—Case report. J Orthop Rep. 2023;2:100147.
41. Memon M, Kay J, Ginsberg L, Simunovic N, Bak K, Lapner P, Ayeni OR. Arthroscopic management of suprascapular neuropathy of the shoulder improves pain and functional outcomes with minimal complication rates. Knee Surg Sports Traumatol Arthrosc. 2018;26:240–66.
42. McLaughlin HL. Posterior dislocation of the shoulder. J Bone Joint Surg Am. 1952;24A:584–90.
43. Dimock R, Memon K, Consigliere P, Polyzois I, Imam MA, Narvani AA. Posterior shoulder instabil-

ity: the augmented McLaughlin procedure. Arch Bone Jt Surg. 2020;8:729–33.
44. Berk AN, Rao AJ, Hysong AA, Ifarraguerri AM, Trofa DP, Schiffern SC, Connor PM, Hamid N, Saltzman BM. Clinical and radiographic outcomes of the modified McLaughlin procedure for locked posterior dislocation of the shoulder: a systematic review. JSES Rev Rep Tech. 2024;4:8–14.
45. Goldenberg BT, Goldsten P, Lacheta L, Arner JW, Provencher MT, Millett PJ. Rehabilitation following posterior shoulder stabilization. Int J Sports Phys Ther. 2021;16(3):930–40. https://doi.org/10.26603/001c.22501.
46. Blomquist J, Solheim E, Liavaag S, Schroder CP, Espehaug B, Havelin LI. Shoulder instability surgery in Norway. Acta Orthop. 2012;83:165–70.
47. Bradley JP, McClincy MP, Arner JW, Tejwani SG. Arthroscopic capsulolabral reconstruction for posterior instability of the shoulder. Am J Sports Med. 2013;41:2005–14.
48. Longo UG, Ciuffreda M, Locher J, Casciaro C, Mannering N, Maffulli N, Denaro V. Posterior shoulder instability: a systematic review. Br Med Bull. 2020;134:34–53.
49. Villefort C, Stern C, Gerber C, Wyss S, Ernstbrunner L, Wieser K. Mid-term to long-term results of open posterior bone block grafting in recurrent posterior shoulder instability: a clinical and CT-based analysis. JSES Int. 2023;7:211–7.
50. Fried JW, Hurley ET, Duenes ML, Manjunath AK, Virk M, Gonzalez-Lomas G, Campbell KA. Return to play after arthroscopic stabilization for posterior shoulder instability—a systematic review. Arthrosc Sports Med Rehabil. 2021;3:e249–56.
51. Vopat ML, Coda RG, Giusti NE, Baker J, Tarakemeh A, Schroeppel JP, Mullen S, Randall J, Provencher MT, Vopat BG. Differences in outcomes between anterior and posterior shoulder instability after arthroscopic Bankart repair: a systematic review and meta-analysis. Orthop J Sports Med. 2021;9:232596712110064.
52. Kelly MJ, Holton AE, Cassar-Gheiti AJ, Hanna SA, Quinlan JF, Molony DC. The aetiology of posterior glenohumeral dislocations and occurrence of associated injuries. Bone Joint J. 2019;101-B:15–21.
53. Cohen M, Fonseca R, Galvão Amaral MV, Monteiro MT, Motta Filho GR. Treatment of chronic locked posterior dislocation of the shoulder with the modified McLaughlin procedure. J Shoulder Elb Surg. 2022;31:100–6.
54. Haritinian EG, Stoica IC, Popescu R, Gheorghievici GL, Nové-Josserand L. Treatment and outcomes of chronic locked posterior shoulder dislocations: a retrospective case series. BMC Musculoskelet Disord. 2023;24:82.
55. Guehring M, Lambert S, Stoeckle U, Ziegler P. Posterior shoulder dislocation with associated reverse Hill-Sachs lesion: treatment options and functional outcome after a 5-year follow up. BMC Musculoskelet Disord. 2017;18:442.
56. Konrads C, Konrads MI, Döbele S, Histing T, Ziegler P. Posterior shoulder dislocation with associated reverse Hill–Sachs lesion: clinical outcome 10 years after joint-preserving surgery. Arch Orthop Trauma Surg. 2022;143:2503–7.
57. Junwei S. Allograft reconstruction of humeral head defect in treatment of chronic locked posterior shoulder dislocation: a case report. Int J Clin Stud Med Case Rep. 2021; https://doi.org/10.46998/IJCMCR.2021.12.000285.
58. Sperling JW, Pring M, Antuna SA, Cofield RH. Shoulder arthroplasty for locked posterior dislocation of the shoulder. J Shoulder Elb Surg. 2004;13:522–7.

Bone Defects in Posterior Instability

22

Gregory Hoy, Michael Blaser,
and Lukas Ernstbrunner

22.1 Introduction

The incidence of posterior shoulder instability was historically underestimated. This is mainly due to the fact that symptoms and clinical examination are less clear than in anterior shoulder instability [1]. With the improvement of contemporary imaging modalities and a better understanding of the underlying pathology, current evidence numbers of posterior shoulder instability lie around 10–18% [2–6]. The numbers of patients diagnosed with posterior shoulder instability are rising and at the same time it has been reported that 77% of these patients with posterior instability require surgical stabilization eventually [4]. Considering that surgical management of symptomatic posterior shoulder instability is challenging, these numbers are alarming.

Posterior shoulder instability is multifactorial and in most of the cases involves some extent of bony defect/deficiency. While in traumatic posterior instability structural damage usually results from a single traumatic event leading to postero-inferior labral tear, glenoid bone loss and or antero-medial humeral head bone loss (reverse Hill-Sachs lesion). In atraumatic or micro-traumatic posterior instability, the underlying pathology can be a spectrum of developmental postero-inferior glenoid bony deficiency, glenoid dysplasia with excessive glenoid retroversion, and more recently identified in patients with posterior acromial pathology [7–10].

Failing non-operative management, a variety of surgical treatment options for posterior instability have been described including posterior soft tissue reconstruction, glenoid bone grafting and glenoid osteotomy [8, 10–17]. Recurrent instability following these procedures can be challenging to manage, with some of the techniques reporting recurrence in up to 73% [18].

This book chapter aims to outline how to assess bony pathologies encountered in posterior shoulder instability, as well as the respective treatment options and their outcome.

G. Hoy (✉)
Melbourne Orthopaedic Group, Monash University, Melbourne, VIC, Australia
e-mail: gahoy@mog.com.au

M. Blaser
Austin Hospital, Melbourne, VIC, Australia

L. Ernstbrunner
Reconstructive Orthopaedics Melbourne (ROM) & Box Hill Hospital, Eastern Health & University of Melbourne, Melbourne, VIC, Australia

22.2 Assessment of Bony Pathology

22.2.1 Glenoid and Humeral Bone Loss

While MRI and CT scans are known to be equally effective in evaluating glenohumeral bone loss in

E. Calvo et al. (eds.), *Complex and Revision Problems in Shoulder Instability*,
https://doi.org/10.1007/978-3-031-81389-4_22

cases of anterior shoulder instability, there is a lack of similar confirmatory data for posterior instability [19]. The "perfect circle" technique is the most frequently used method for measuring posterior glenoid bone loss and can be applied to both 2D sagittal reconstructions and 3D imaging. This technique follows the concepts used for quantifying glenoid bone loss in anterior instability [20–24]. It involves viewing the glenoid in an en-face 2D or 3D reconstruction image with a best-fit circle placed on the lower two-thirds of the glenoid. The width of the posterior bone defect is divided by the circle's diameter to calculate the percentage of bone loss. The significance of preoperative glenoid bone loss on failure rates following soft tissue reconstruction procedures is well understood in anterior shoulder instability. A clinically significant threshold for posterior glenoid bone loss has yet to be defined.

There is also a difference in orientation of bone loss comparing anterior instability with posterior instability. While anterior bone loss tends to be parallel to the long axis of the glenoid, posterior bone loss is more oblique. Dekker et al. [25] analysed 3D CT scans of 71 patients with recurrent posterior shoulder instability, revealing that the mean total arc of bone loss was most commonly located in the posterior-inferior quadrant (6:44 to 9:28 o'clock in a right shoulder), which is about 30° off the long axis of the glenoid. Recognizing this orientation is crucial for identifying lesions on imaging and during arthroscopy.

Similar to the glenoid track concept in anterior shoulder instability [26], it is important to acknowledge that in traumatic posterior instability bony pathology can be bipolar, i.e. involving both the postero-inferior glenoid and antero-medial surface of the humeral head. These so-called reverse Hill-Sachs lesions pose a risk of re-engagement with the posterior glenoid rim during internal rotation. The size and location of a reverse Hill-Sachs lesion can be measured on CT by calculating the gamma angle [27]. It was determined that the critical gamma angle is approximately 90°. Engagement of "sub-critical" reverse Hill-Sachs lesions may occur when the patient's internal rotation capacity is increased or when there is a bipolar bone defect [28].

22.2.2 Glenoid Retroversion and Dysplasia

Excessive glenoid retroversion is a commonly overlooked (concomitant) pathology in posterior shoulder instability. Retroversion greater than 10° has been associated with contributing to posterior instability [29]. As such, it should be routine practice measuring glenoid retroversion as part of the assessment in patients with posterior instability. Multiple methods have been described to measure glenoid version and can be done on axial CT or MRI images. The Friedman technique is the most commonly used method and is easy to perform but requires the whole scapula to be imaged [30]. It calculates the angle between a line connecting the medial scapular body and the midpoint of the glenoid fossa and a line connecting the anterior and posterior glenoid edges in the axial plane.

Further comprehensive evaluation of advanced imaging for atraumatic posterior glenohumeral instability must include an analysis of posterior humeral head subluxation and the consideration of glenoid dysplasia. Glenoid dysplasia is thought to be a result of scapular developmental anomalies [7, 31]. It is associated with a deficiency of the postero-inferior bony glenoid, increased glenoid retroversion, increased capsular volume and hyperplasia of the posterior labrum and cartilage [7, 32, 33]. Each of these potential pathologies in patients with atraumatic posterior shoulder instability should be worked up with CT and MRI scans. Posterior humeral head subluxation is another pathology seen in patients with glenoid dysplasia. It can be measured on axial CT slices and is defined as more than 65% of humeral-head subluxation according to the modified subluxation index [34].

22.2.3 Acromial Pathology

Recent studies have shown that acromial morphology is linked to posterior instability [9]. Patients with posterior instability have an acromion that is high-riding and oriented more horizontally in the sagittal plane, thus providing less osseous restraint against posterior translation of the humeral head. Measurement of posterior acromial morphology was initially described using plain X-rays and includes quantifying posterior acromial tilt, anterior and posterior acromial coverage and posterior acromial height. Posterior acromial height is the most distinctive measurement for posterior instability and a cut-off value of more than 23 mm is considered abnormal [9]. It is measured on true lateral radiographs with the coracoid process and scapular spine forming symmetric upper limbs of a "Y". A reference line is drawn connecting the inferior angle of the scapula with the centre of the intersection of the small arms of the "Y". A second line, perpendicular from the reference line to the most posterior point of the inferior aspect of the acromion, is drawn and the distance from the centre of the intersection of the small arms of the "Y" to this perpendicular line determines the posterior acromial height.

22.3 Treatment Options and Outcome

22.3.1 Non-operative Management

Posterior instability is most commonly atraumatic and as such may benefit from a physiotherapy focusing on scapular control, subscapularis-predominant strengthening exercises, proprioception and activity modification [35]. However, non-operative management has shown to have a high failure rate specifically in young, highly active patients or athletes, as these patients usually recall a distinct initial traumatic event leading to recurrent posterior instability symptoms. As such, in military personnel or collegiate athletes, the non-operative to operative conversion rate is roughly 50% [36, 37]. Whether early surgical intervention in this high-risk population is beneficial in order to prevent early onset of dislocation arthropathy remains controversial, although there is clear evidence in anterior shoulder instability that recurrence is the main trigger of arthropathy [38, 39].

22.3.2 Posterior Labral Reconstruction

Arthroscopic posterior labral reconstruction with suture anchors with or without capsular plication is still the gold-standard surgical technique for patients with posterior shoulder instability. Most recent pooled data and meta-analysis suggests at short-term follow-up that around 90% patients following posterior labral reconstruction are satisfied with their outcome, less than 10% experience recurrence and 5% require revision surgery [40]. However, similar to anterior labral reconstruction [41–43], recurrence rates increase significantly over time, most likely resulting from micro-instability leading to fatigue failure of the repair or the failure in recognizing concomitant pathology such as glenoid bone loss or excessive glenoid retroversion [29, 44, 45].

An analysis by Arner et al. [44] looked at the relationship between posterior glenoid bone loss and failure rates following posterior capsulolabral reconstruction. They found that the average posterior glenoid bone loss in patients who failed treatment was 6.8% vs. 4.6% in the successfully treated group. More importantly, with 11% posterior glenoid bone loss a 10 times higher surgical failure rate was observed, while 15% bone loss resulted in a 24 times higher failure rate. Similarly, Wolfe et al. [45] noted a 44% failure rate of arthroscopic repair when posterior glenoid bone loss exceeded 14%. Further research is required to define a threshold of posterior glenoid bone loss contraindicating a posterior labral reconstruction but based on the current literature it is likely to be below the 10% mark.

22.3.3 Posterior Glenoid Bone Grafting

The use of a posterior glenoid bone block has gained popularity over the last year besides the fact that its indication is still lacking a consensus. It is usually used in traumatic posterior shoulder instability associated with glenoid bone loss or a reverse Hill-Sachs lesion due to its ability to extend the glenoid track and in these patients, outcome is usually predictable, however outcome studies for posterior glenoid bone block procedures usually lack power. Gilat et al. [46] reported in a series of 10 patients treated with distal tibial allograft stabilization for an average posterior glenoid bone loss of 26% a 10% recurrence rate and a 20% revision rate due to symptomatic or intra-articular implants. Provencher et al. [47] observed in a series of 27 patients treated with distal tibial allograft stabilization no recurrences despite a similar average posterior glenoid bone loss of 24% and a 4% revision rate due to deep infection. Camenzind et al. [48] showed in a series of 18 patients treated with arthroscopically assisted iliac crest bone grafting a high patients' satisfaction rate but also a 37% revision rate for symptomatic hardware at long-term follow-up.

Posterior glenoid bone grafting may also have a role in patients with (minimally) increased glenoid retroversion or mild glenoid dysplasia [49]. However, certain studies report that posterior glenoid bone block procedures are associated with a recurrent instability rate as high as 73% [18]. The exact failure mechanism associated with this procedure is unclear; however, excessive glenoid retroversion or significant postero-inferior glenoid deficiency associated with glenoid dysplasia cannot be addressed with isolated glenoid bone grafting procedures and may explain the high failure rate in these particular patients [50].

Posterior glenoid bone procedures can be performed through an open posterior approach or arthroscopically assisted. The arthroscopic techniques have gained popularity due to their known advantages such as improved intra-articular visibility and the ability to address concomitant pathologies, and a less invasive and muscle-sparing approach with better cosmesis. In both approaches, the capsule is opened, the labrum is elevated, and the bone block is secured with screws or transglenoid suspensory fixation. The capsule and labrum are repaired either intra-articularly or extra-articularly. Graft options for posterior glenoid bone grafting include tricortical iliac crest autograft, scapular spine autograft, distal clavicle autograft and distal tibia allograft. Autografts have their known advantages, namely ready availability, higher bony incorporation, lower costs and no immunogenic risks as compared with allografts. The disadvantages are donor side morbidity, especially when then bone graft is harvested from the iliac crest. In contrast, distal tibial allograft has shown similar biomechanical properties to iliac crest and scapular spine autograft while avoiding donor side morbidity [51, 52].

22.3.4 Reverse Hill-Sachs Lesion

Traditionally, rotational humeral osteotomies or the so-called Weber-osteotomy was performed to derotate a large, engaging reverse Hill-Sachs lesion away from the glenoid track. However, outcome following this procedure is unpredictable and associated with a high complication rate [53, 54].

More contemporary options treating large reverse Hill-Sachs lesions include resurfacing the defect or creating a barrier using subscapularis tenodesis (i.e. McLaughlin procedure) or a lesser tuberosity osteotomy (i.e. modified McLaughlin procedure) into the defect to prevent engagement. Hawkins et al. [55] described the modified McLaughlin procedure which comprises osteotomy and transfer of the lesser tuberosity into the defect. Pooled data of the modified McLaughlin procedure in 96 patients suggest that it results in good range of motion, 100% osseointegration, recurrent instability of 2% and revision surgery of 1% for irritating hardware [56].

If the reverse Hill-Sachs lesion involves more than 30% of the humeral head articular surface, humeral head allograft reconstruction has been described. Gerber et al. [57] reported on a series of 19 patients with a 5-year follow-up after reconstruction with humeral or femoral head allografts for locked posterior shoulder dislocations involving more than 30% humeral head articular surface. While such injury is severely debilitating, 18 patients rated their outcome as excellent (one as fair), the Subjective Shoulder Value averaged at 88% and active anterior elevations ranged 145° and active external rotation 42°. Only two patients required arthroplasty and four patients showed radiographic signs of advanced osteoarthritis.

22.3.5 Glenoid Osteotomy

Excessive glenoid retroversion is frequently observed in patients with posterior shoulder instability, and a higher degree of retroversion usually indicates a greater risk of recurrence or contralateral posterior instability [5, 58]. It is also a major factor in humeral head decentration within the glenoid concavity. A cadaveric study by Imhoff et al. [29] demonstrated that posterior humeral head translation increased by 2 mm for every 5° increment of glenoid retroversion. They found that posterior labral reconstruction helped restore humeral head centration as long as glenoid version did not exceed 10° of retroversion. This is in line with clinical data, showing that posterior humeral head subluxation frequently persists postoperatively, and as such, it is still an unrecognized entity responsible for glenohumeral osteoarthritis in young adults [59–61].

Some authors have therefore focused on correcting glenoid retroversion with an opening-wedge osteotomy as described in detail by Scott [16]. The reported results of such osteotomies in patients with glenoid dysplasia vary [62, 63], with studies reporting substantial complications [64, 65]. There is limited follow-up and numbers but in a series of seven patients 15 years after glenoid osteotomy, Waltenspül et al. [10] noted that instability persisted in 86% with similar pain levels as preoperatively, and that glenohumeral degeneration was established in all patients included. It was also observed that in five out of seven patients the humeral head remained decentered besides good radiographic correction of glenoid retroversion.

22.3.6 Posterior J-Graft (Author's Preferred Technique)

The author's preferred technique is a recently introduced surgical technique which combines a posterior opening-wedge osteotomy with glenoid concavity reconstruction using an implant-free, J-shaped autograft iliac crest bone graft [14]. The surgical technique involves a unicortical glenoid osteotomy roughly 2 cm medial to the posterior glenoid rim. The osteotomy is carefully opened until neutral glenoid version is achieved as per preoperative planning. A bicortical iliac crest bone graft is molded into a J-shaped graft, which has the following typical measurements: 25 mm in width (superoinferior dimension of graft surface area that faces the humeral head (a glenoid in the en-face view)), 10 mm in height (anteroposterior graft surface area that faces the humeral head), and 30 mm in length (part of the graft that is impacted into the osteotomy; long leg of the J). The part of the graft that faces the humeral head (short leg of the J) is used to reconstruct the postero-inferior glenoid concavity and usually needs to be molded until flush with the native glenoid cartilage.

The preliminary short-term results of 7 patients with atraumatic posterior shoulder instability associated with excessive glenoid retroversion and postero-inferior glenoid deficiency revealed that the posterior J-graft is able to reconstruct posteroinferior glenoid morphology, correct glenoid retroversion and improve posterior shoulder instability [14]. At 2 years follow-up, mean Subjective Shoulder Value was 90% and the Constant pain scores 15 points (i.e. no pain). There was no progression in radiographic signs of osteoarthritis and the median humeral-head subluxation index decreased from 69% preoperatively to 55% postoperatively ($p = 0.02$), and in two patients posterior humeral head subluxation was reversed to a centred humeral head. Union of the implant-free J-graft was achieved in all patients, preoperative glenoid retroversion was corrected from 16° to 0° postoperatively and the preoperative glenoid surface area was increased by an average of 20%. Biomechanical analysis of the posterior

J-graft in a cadaver model confirmed the promising preliminary results and demonstrated reliable restoration of initial glenohumeral joint stability, normalization of contact patterns comparable to that of an intact shoulder joint with neutral retroversion, and secure initial graft fixation in the cadaver model [13]. The authors of this chapter have expanded their indications for the posterior J-graft and have started using it in athletes with posterior glenoid bone loss and minimally increased glenoid retroversion. First clinical results of this cohort are yet to be published.

22.3.7 Acromial Osteotomy

Posterior shoulder instability has been linked to patients with an acromion that is high-riding and flat in the sagittal plane, thus lacking osseous restraint against posterior humeral head translation [9]. Gerber et al. [66] were the first to address this lack of posterior humeral head restraint in a 40-year-old patient with static posterior humeral head subluxation by performing a 3D planned acromial and glenoid osteotomy, which resulted in recentering of the humeral head and full shoulder function at 2 years follow-up. Further research is needed to determine whether surgical interventions that address abnormal acromial morphology associated with posterior shoulder instability and/or posterior humeral head subluxation can result in a stable, centred, functional and pain-free shoulder.

References

1. Pollock RG, Bigliani LU. Recurrent posterior shoulder instability. Diagnosis and treatment. Clin Orthop Relat Res. 1993;291:85–96.
2. Arner JW, McClincy MP, Bradley JP. Arthroscopic stabilization of posterior shoulder instability is successful in American football players. Arthroscopy. 2015;31(8):1466–71.
3. Bokshan SL, Kotchman HM, Li LT, et al. Incidence of posterior shoulder instability in the United States military: demographic considerations from a high-risk population. Am J Sports Med. 2021;49(2):340–5.
4. Lanzi JT Jr, Chandler PJ, Cameron KL, Bader JM, Owens BD. Epidemiology of posterior glenohumeral instability in a young athletic population. Am J Sports Med. 2017;45(14):3315–21.
5. Owens BD, Campbell SE, Cameron KL. Risk factors for posterior shoulder instability in young athletes. Am J Sports Med. 2013;41(11):2645–9.
6. Owens BD, Duffey ML, Nelson BJ, et al. The incidence and characteristics of shoulder instability at the United States military academy. Am J Sports Med. 2007;35(7):1168–73.
7. Eichinger JK, Galvin JW, Grassbaugh JA, Parada SA, Li X. Glenoid dysplasia: pathophysiology, diagnosis, and management. J Bone Joint Surg Am. 2016;98(11):958–68.
8. Galvin JW, Morte DR, Grassbaugh JA, et al. Arthroscopic treatment of posterior shoulder instability in patients with and without glenoid dysplasia: a comparative outcomes analysis. J Shoulder Elb Surg. 2017;26(12):2103–9.
9. Meyer DC, Ernstbrunner L, Boyce G, et al. Posterior acromial morphology is significantly associated with posterior shoulder instability. J Bone Joint Surg Am. 2019;101(14):1253–60.
10. Waltenspul M, Haller T, Ernstbrunner L, et al. Long-term outcome after posterior opening glenoid wedge osteotomy for posterior shoulder instability associated with excessive glenoid retroversion. J Shoulder Elb Surg. 2022;31(1):81–9.
11. Camenzind RS, Gossing L, Martin Becerra J, et al. Restoration of the posterior glenoid in recurrent posterior shoulder instability using an arthroscopically placed iliac crest bone graft: a computed tomography-based analysis. Orthop J Sports Med. 2021;9(1):2325967120976378.
12. DiMaria S, Bokshan SL, Nacca C, Owens B. History of surgical stabilization for posterior shoulder instability. JSES Open Access. 2019;3(4):350–6.
13. Ernstbrunner L, Borbas P, Ker AM, et al. Biomechanical analysis of posterior open-wedge osteotomy and glenoid concavity reconstruction using an implant-free, J-shaped iliac crest bone graft. Am J Sports Med. 2022;50(14):3889–96.
14. Ernstbrunner L, Haller T, Waltenspul M, Wieser K, Gerber C. Posterior open-wedge osteotomy and glenoid concavity reconstruction using an implant-free, J-shaped iliac crest bone graft in atraumatic posterior instability with pathologic glenoid retroversion and dysplasia: a preliminary report. Clin Orthop Relat Res. 2022;479(9):1995–2005.
15. Fuchs B, Jost B, Gerber C. Posterior-inferior capsular shift for the treatment of recurrent, voluntary posterior subluxation of the shoulder. J Bone Joint Surg Am. 2000;82(1):16–25.
16. Scott DJ Jr. Treatment of recurrent posterior dislocations of the shoulder by glenoplasty. Report of three cases. J Bone Joint Surg Am. 1967;49(3):471–6.
17. Villefort C, Stern C, Gerber C, et al. Mid-term to long-term results of open posterior bone block grafting in

recurrent posterior shoulder instability: a clinical and CT-based analysis. JSES Int. 2023;7(2):211–7.
18. Cognetti DJ, Hughes JD, Kay J, et al. Bone block augmentation of the posterior glenoid for recurrent posterior shoulder instability is associated with high rates of clinical failure: a systematic review. Arthroscopy. 2022;38(2):551–63. e555
19. Hines A, Cook JB, Shaha JS, et al. Glenoid bone loss in posterior shoulder instability: prevalence and outcomes in arthroscopic treatment. Am J Sports Med. 2018;46(5):1053–7.
20. Ernstbrunner L, De Nard B, Olthof M, et al. Long-term results of the arthroscopic Bankart repair for recurrent anterior shoulder instability in patients older than 40 years: a comparison with the open Latarjet procedure. Am J Sports Med. 2020;48(9):2090–6.
21. Ernstbrunner L, Pastor T, Waltenspul M, Gerber C, Wieser K. Salvage iliac crest bone grafting for a failed Latarjet procedure: analysis of failed and successful procedures. Am J Sports Med. 2021;49(13):3620–7.
22. Ernstbrunner L, Plachel F, Heuberer P, et al. Arthroscopic versus open iliac crest bone grafting in recurrent anterior shoulder instability with glenoid bone loss: a computed tomography-based quantitative assessment. Arthroscopy. 2018;34(2):352–9.
23. Ernstbrunner L, Wartmann L, Zimmermann SM, et al. Long-term results of the open Latarjet procedure for recurrent anterior shoulder instability in patients older than 40 years. Am J Sports Med. 2019;47:3057–64.
24. Magarelli N, Milano G, Sergio P, et al. Intra-observer and interobserver reliability of the 'Pico' computed tomography method for quantification of glenoid bone defect in anterior shoulder instability. Skelet Radiol. 2009;38(11):1071–5.
25. Dekker TJ, Peebles LA, Goldenberg BT, et al. Location of the glenoid defect in shoulders with recurrent posterior glenohumeral instability. Am J Sports Med. 2019;47(13):3051–6.
26. Yamamoto N, Itoi E, Abe H, et al. Contact between the glenoid and the humeral head in abduction, external rotation, and horizontal extension: a new concept of glenoid track. J Shoulder Elb Surg. 2007;16(5):649–56.
27. Moroder P, Runer A, Kraemer M, et al. Influence of defect size and localization on the engagement of reverse Hill-Sachs lesions. Am J Sports Med. 2015;43(3):542–8.
28. Moroder P, Plachel F, Tauber M, et al. Risk of engagement of bipolar bone defects in posterior shoulder instability. Am J Sports Med. 2017;45(12):2835–9.
29. Imhoff FB, Camenzind RS, Obopilwe E, et al. Glenoid retroversion is an important factor for humeral head centration and the biomechanics of posterior shoulder stability. Knee Surg Sports Traumatol Arthrosc. 2019;27(12):3952–61.
30. Friedman RJ, Hawthorne KB, Genez BM. The use of computerized tomography in the measurement of glenoid version. J Bone Joint Surg Am. 1992;74(7):1032–7.
31. Landau JP, Hoenecke HR. Genetic and biomechanical determinants of glenoid version: implications for glenoid implant placement in shoulder arthroplasty. J Shoulder Elb Surg. 2009;18(4):661–7.
32. Harper KW, Helms CA, Haystead CM, Higgins LD. Glenoid dysplasia: incidence and association with posterior labral tears as evaluated on MRI. AJR Am J Roentgenol. 2005;184(3):984–8.
33. Weishaupt D, Zanetti M, Nyffeler RW, Gerber C, Hodler J. Posterior glenoid rim deficiency in recurrent (atraumatic) posterior shoulder instability. Skelet Radiol. 2000;29(4):204–10.
34. Walch G, Boulahia A, Boileau P, Kempf JF. Primary glenohumeral osteoarthritis: clinical and radiographic classification. The Aequalis Group. Acta Orthop Belgica. 1998;64(Suppl 2):46–52.
35. Watson L, Balster S, Lenssen R, Hoy G, Pizzari T. The effects of a conservative rehabilitation program for multidirectional instability of the shoulder. J Shoulder Elb Surg. 2018;27(1):104–11.
36. Christensen DL, Elsenbeck MJ, Wolfe JA, et al. Risk factors for failure of nonoperative treatment of posterior shoulder labral tears on magnetic resonance imaging. Mil Med. 2020;185(9–10):e1556–61.
37. Woodmass JM, Lee J, Johnson NR, et al. Nonoperative management of posterior shoulder instability: an assessment of survival and predictors for conversion to surgery at 1 to 10 years after diagnosis. Arthroscopy. 2019;35(7):1964–70.
38. Ernstbrunner L, Robinson DL, Huang Y, et al. The influence of glenoid bone loss and graft positioning on graft and cartilage contact pressures after the Latarjet procedure. Am J Sports Med. 2023;51(9):2454–64.
39. Hovelius L, Saeboe M. Neer Award 2008: arthropathy after primary anterior shoulder dislocation—223 shoulders prospectively followed up for twenty-five years. J Shoulder Elb Surg. 2009;18(3):339–47.
40. Ralph J, Hurley E, Lunn K, et al. Outcomes of arthroscopic stabilization for posterior shoulder instability—a systematic review. J Shoulder Elb Surg. 2024;33(11):2530–8.
41. Castagna A, Markopoulos N, Conti M, et al. Arthroscopic bankart suture-anchor repair: radiological and clinical outcome at minimum 10 years of follow-up. Am J Sports Med. 2010;38(10):2012–6.
42. van der Linde JA, van Kampen DA, Terwee CB, et al. Long-term results after arthroscopic shoulder stabilization using suture anchors: an 8- to 10-year follow-up. Am J Sports Med. 2011;39(11):2396–403.
43. Vermeulen AE, Landman EBM, Veen EJD, Nienhuis S, Koorevaar CT. Long-term clinical outcome of arthroscopic Bankart repair with suture anchors. J Shoulder Elb Surg. 2019;28(5):e137–43.
44. Arner JW, Ruzbarsky JJ, Midtgaard K, et al. Defining critical glenoid bone loss in posterior shoulder capsulolabral repair. Am J Sports Med. 2021;49(8):2013–9.
45. Wolfe JA, Elsenbeck M, Nappo K, et al. Effect of posterior glenoid bone loss and retroversion on arthroscopic posterior glenohumeral stabilization. Am J Sports Med. 2020;48(11):2621–7.

46. Gilat R, Haunschild ED, Tauro T, et al. Distal Tibial allograft augmentation for posterior shoulder instability associated with glenoid bony deficiency: a case series. Arthrosc Sports Med Rehabil. 2020;2(6):e743–52.
47. Provencher MT, Frank RM, Golijanin P, et al. Distal tibia allograft glenoid reconstruction in recurrent anterior shoulder instability: clinical and radiographic outcomes. Arthroscopy. 2017;33(5):891–7.
48. Camenzind RS, Martin Becerra J, Gossing L, et al. Acceptable long-term outcomes of arthroscopic bone grafting for recurrent posterior shoulder instability: minimum follow-up of 5 years. Arthroscopy. 2021;37(3):816–23.
49. Wellmann M, Pastor MF, Ettinger M, Koester K, Smith T. Arthroscopic posterior bone block stabilization-early results of an effective procedure for the recurrent posterior instability. Knee Surg Sports Traumatol Arthrosc. 2018;26(1):292–8.
50. Ernstbrunner L, Loucas R, Ker A, et al. Biomechanics of posterior glenoid bone block procedures for posterior instability with and without correction of glenoid retroversion. J Shoulder Elb Surg. 2021;30(7):e444.
51. Frank RM, Shin J, Saccomanno MF, et al. Comparison of glenohumeral contact pressures and contact areas after posterior glenoid reconstruction with an iliac crest bone graft or distal tibial osteochondral allograft. Am J Sports Med. 2014;42(11):2574–82.
52. Nacca C, Gil JA, DeFroda SF, Badida R, Owens BD. Comparison of a distal tibial allograft and scapular spinal autograft for posterior shoulder instability with glenoid bone loss. Orthop J Sports Med. 2018;6(7):2325967118786697.
53. Brooks-Hill AL, Forster BB, van Wyngaarden C, Hawkins R, Regan WD. Weber osteotomy for large Hill-Sachs defects: clinical and CT assessments. Clin Orthop Relat Res. 2013;471(8):2548–55.
54. Keppler P, Holz U, Thielemann FW, Meinig R. Locked posterior dislocation of the shoulder: treatment using rotational osteotomy of the humerus. J Orthop Trauma. 1994;8(4):286–92.
55. Hawkins RJ, Neer CS 2nd, Pianta RM, Mendoza FX. Locked posterior dislocation of the shoulder. J Bone Joint Surg Am. 1987;69(1):9–18.
56. Berk AN, Rao AJ, Hysong AA, et al. Clinical and radiographic outcomes of the modified McLaughlin procedure for locked posterior dislocation of the shoulder: a systematic review. JSES Rev Rep Tech. 2024;4(1):8–14.
57. Gerber C, Catanzaro S, Jundt-Ecker M, Farshad M. Long-term outcome of segmental reconstruction of the humeral head for the treatment of locked posterior dislocation of the shoulder. J Shoulder Elb Surg. 2014;23(11):1682–90.
58. Gottschalk MB, Ghasem A, Todd D, et al. Posterior shoulder instability: does glenoid retroversion predict recurrence and contralateral instability? Arthroscopy. 2015;31(3):488–93.
59. Domos P, Checchia CS, Walch G. Walch B0 glenoid: pre-osteoarthritic posterior subluxation of the humeral head. J Shoulder Elb Surg. 2018;27(1):181–8.
60. Walch G, Ascani C, Boulahia A, Nove-Josserand L, Edwards TB. Static posterior subluxation of the humeral head: an unrecognized entity responsible for glenohumeral osteoarthritis in the young adult. J Shoulder Elb Surg. 2002;11(4):309–14.
61. Walch G, Badet R, Boulahia A, Khoury A. Morphologic study of the glenoid in primary glenohumeral osteoarthritis. J Arthroplast. 1999;14(6):756–60.
62. Inui H, Nobuhara K. Glenoid osteotomy for atraumatic posteroinferior shoulder instability associated with glenoid dysplasia. Bone Joint J. 2018;100-B(3):331–7.
63. Lacheta L, Singh TSP, Hovsepian JM, et al. Posterior open wedge glenoid osteotomy provides reliable results in young patients with increased glenoid retroversion and posterior shoulder instability. Knee Surg Sports Traumatol Arthrosc. 2019;27(1):299–304.
64. Hawkins RH. Glenoid osteotomy for recurrent posterior subluxation of the shoulder: assessment by computed axial tomography. J Shoulder Elb Surg. 1996;5(5):393–400.
65. Johnston GH, Hawkins RJ, Haddad R, Fowler PJ. A complication of posterior glenoid osteotomy for recurrent posterior shoulder instability. Clin Orthop Relat Res. 1984;187:147–9.
66. Gerber C, Sigrist B, Hochreiter B. Correction of static posterior shoulder subluxation by restoring normal scapular anatomy using acromion and glenoid osteotomies: a case report. JBJS Case Connect. 2023;13(2):e23.00060. https://doi.org/10.2106/JBJS.CC.23.00060.

Part V

Complications After Shoulder Stabilization

The Failed Soft Tissue Repair in Anterior Shoulder Instability

23

Deepak N. Bhatia

23.1 Introduction

Soft tissue repair for management of anterior shoulder instability is one of the most frequently performed procedures in the shoulder. The spectrum of soft tissue repair procedures includes the classic arthroscopic/open Bankart repair and capsular shift, and the more recent augmented repairs that involve transfer of the long biceps tendon (dynamic anterior stabilization) and Hill-Sachs remplissage procedures. Soft tissue repairs are reliable when performed using the correct technique and for the optimal indications. However, high failure rates of approximately 30% have been reported in soft tissue repairs over a long-term follow-up, and approximately 15% of athletes are unable to return to sports after an arthroscopic stabilization procedure [1, 2]. This chapter presents an analysis of the etiological factors and treatment strategies for revision of soft tissue repair failures in anterior shoulder instability.

D. N. Bhatia (✉)
SportsDocs®, Mumbai, Maharashtra, India

Sir HN Reliance Foundation Hospital and Research Centre, Mumbai, Maharashtra, India

23.2 Causative Factors for Failures

Failure of a soft tissue stabilization procedure can be defined as recurrent instability after surgery, persistent apprehension that interferes with sports or other activities, and/or pain or stiffness that prevents full functional use of the arm. Failure of the shoulder to achieve optimal stability after surgery is multifactorial, and the etiological factors that predispose a soft tissue repair to failure can be broadly classified under: (a) Patho-anatomical factors, (b) variability in assessment methods, and (c) technical failures. Compounding factors like age at first dislocation, joint hypermobility, type and level of sporting activity, and arm dominance further add to the predisposition for post-operative recurrence of instability.

(a) **Patho-anatomical Factors:** Pathological variations in soft tissues or bony morphology of the glenohumeral joint can impact the stability of the joint.
   (i) Ligament laxity and labral tissue quality: Hyperlaxity generally coexists with a thinner and more elastic capsule. Additionally, labral tissue is often deficient or attenuated in hyperlax individuals. Radiologically, these shoulders are usually in the on-track zone; however, dynamic assessment will often demonstrate excessive translation that may be

E. Calvo et al. (eds.), *Complex and Revision Problems in Shoulder Instability*,
https://doi.org/10.1007/978-3-031-81389-4_23

interpreted as peripheral-tracking [3, 4]. This lack of capsulo-labral robustness and laxity-induced excessive translation results in a repair that is structurally suboptimal, and/or may be predisposed to stretching out to the presurgical level of hypermobility; any subsequent trauma can thereafter cause a subluxation or dislocation, and thereby result in failure of soft tissue repair. Boden et al. reported that capsuloligamentous shoulder laxity was a significant independent risk factor for failure after primary arthroscopic Bankart repair; patients with hyperlaxity and near-track lesions had a recurrent instability rate almost double that of patients without hyperlaxity [5].

(ii) Glenoid osseous geometry: The bony geometry of the glenohumeral joint is complex and even small variations in glenoid morphometry can impact shoulder stability [6, 7]. Concavity compression is the main stabilizing mechanism of the glenohumeral joint; this compression mechanism is altered by any factor that changes the glenoid concavity (glenoid depth, curvature length, and radius of curvature) and can be measured as the bony shoulder stability ratio (BSSR) [8]. The BSSR shows a significant reduction with mild bone loss (0–10%) and with constitutional flattening of glenoid curvature [6–8]. A recent clinical study suggests that glenoid concavity measured as BSSR is strongly correlated with surgical failure after arthroscopic soft tissue stabilization procedures, and may reflect shoulder instability caused by glenoid bone morphology more accurately than glenoid bone defect size [9].

(iii) Glenohumeral bone loss: Glenoid and humeral bone defects can independently affect anterior shoulder stability. The exact quantification of a significant glenoid defect is controversial and ranges from 7% to 25% on the glenoid side [10]. Humeral defects are more difficult to quantify precisely and hence this parameter is not used in routine practice. The radiologically measured glenoid track concept proposed by Itoi and DiGiacomo is the current gold standard method to assess the severity of instability, and soft tissue repairs performed for "off-track" lesions are at high-risk of failure [11]. Recent studies have identified a high-risk group (peripheral track, near-track) within the on-track morphology, and it is likely that these radiologically measured peripheral lesions may mimic an off-track morphology under dynamic conditions [3–5, 12].

(iv) Associated soft tissue lesions: Specific soft tissue lesions have been identified as higher-risk pathology that may predispose a Bankart repair to failure; these include Anterior Labroligamentous Periosteal Sleeve Avulsion Lesions (ALPSA), Glenolabral Articular Disruption Lesion (GLAD), humeral avulsion of glenohumeral ligament (HAGL), and isolated subscapularis tears [13–15].

(b) **Variability in Assessment Methods:** Decision-making in anterior shoulder instability can affect postoperative recurrence of instability after soft tissue repairs. Current algorithms are based on radiological measurements of bone loss for assessment of glenoid bone defect size and magnitude of Hill-Sach's interval, and these values are then used to classify the morphology in on- or off-track [12]. However, several recent studies have suggested that radiological measurements may be inaccurate for quantification of bone defects, and high interobserver variability and moderate reliability has been reported for classification of lesion morphology using radiological methods [3, 16–18]. Instability scoring systems rely greatly on presence of significant bone defects; variability in measurement may therefore underestimate the need for a bone grafting procedure and result in failure of soft tissue repairs [19].

(c) **Technical Failures:** With increasing expertise and experience in arthroscopic shoulder stabilization, technical failures are infrequent. With newer anchor designs, anchor pull-out or anchor-induced osteolysis is rare. Newer techniques using multiple anchors or double-row repairs may cause glenoid rim fractures (postage-stamp fractures), and this is a reported cause of soft tissue repair failure in anterior instability [20].

23.3 Management

Prior to formulating a treatment plan, a meticulous evaluation is necessary to understand the predisposing and compounding factors that have led to postoperative instability recurrence after soft tissue repair.

23.3.1 Clinical Assessment

Clinical evaluation involves a detailed history of the current and presurgery symptoms and the severity of trauma that led to the initial and subsequent episodes. A history suggestive of past voluntary or habitual instability episodes indicates an incorrect indication for initial stabilization surgery; similarly, history of sleep episodes prior to surgery, or epilepsy, may point towards initial bony instability that could have required a bony reconstructive procedure. An inquiry into current symptoms will differentiate recurrent instability failures from the functional failures due to stiffness or persistent disabling apprehension. Details of current sports activities are important to understand the type and level of sport (contact/collision sports) and the desire to return to pre-injury sporting level is crucial in planning revision surgery.

Physical examination is necessary to confirm the presence and direction of instability (anterior apprehension test) and should include documentation of range of motion and strength in different muscle groups. A reduction in subscapularis strength (lift-off and bear-hug tests) may indicate subscapularis failure from a previous open repair, and external rotation weakness may indicate infraspinatus function impairment from a previous remplissage procedure [21]. Evaluation of laxity is performed using the sulcus test and O'Gagey's hyperabduction test and can be scored using the criteria described by Beighton et al. [22, 23].

23.3.2 Radiological Imaging

Radiological imaging is necessary to understand the predisposing cause of repair failure and to assess the pathology that needs to be addressed in revision surgery (Fig. 23.1). Additional assessment of imaging that was performed prior to the initial failed procedure should be performed if available. Radiological imaging is also useful for instability scores; radiographs (true anteroposterior and external rotation views) are necessary for instability severity index score (ISIS), and CT scans are needed to calculate the glenoid track for Glenoid Track Instability Management Score (GTIMS) [19]. Assessment of glenoid bone loss is performed using the best-fit circle or the contralateral glenoid (Pico method), and the glenoid track is calculated as described by DiGiacomo et al. [19, 24]. Concavity parameters may be used to calculate the BSSR, however, the exact role of this parameter in treatment algorithms remains undefined [6, 8].

23.3.3 Arthroscopic Evaluation

Intraoperative diagnostic arthroscopy is a valuable adjunct to radiology for surgery planning. Initial diagnostic assessment helps determine the type of soft tissue disruption (ALPSA, Bankart tear), and the robustness of the capsulolabral tissue can be evaluated (Figs. 23.2, 23.3, and 23.4). Anchors from previous repair may be proud and

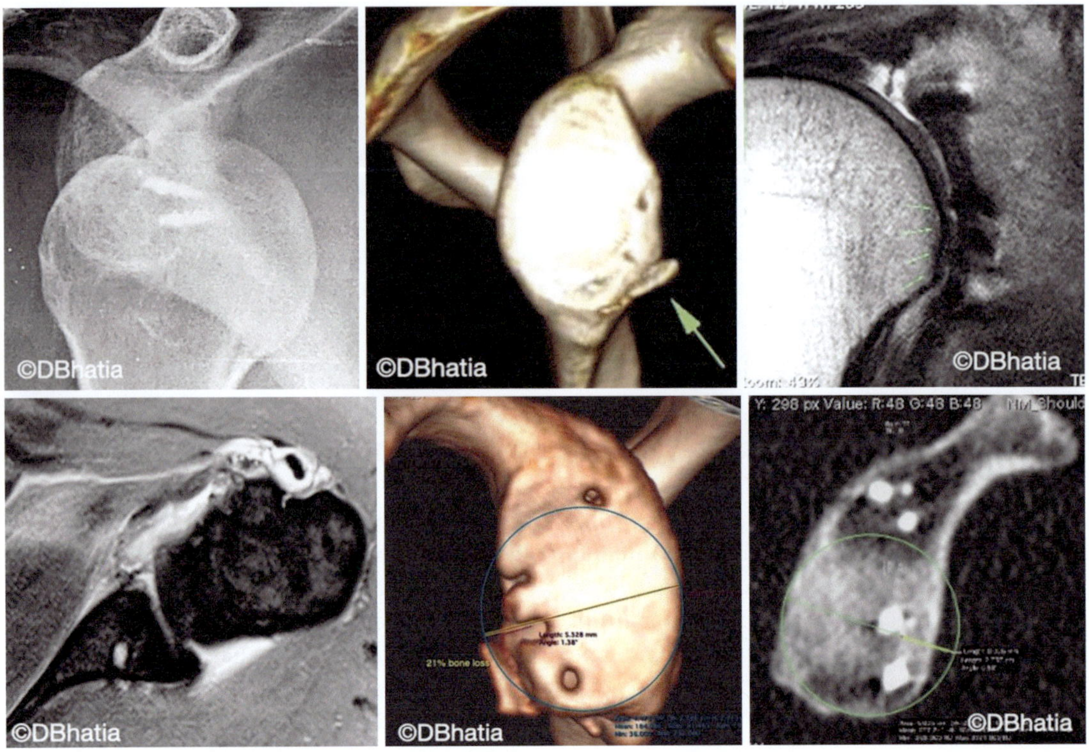

Fig. 23.1 Radiological imaging in different cases in failures of soft tissue repair are shown. Radiograph of a dislocated shoulder shows the remplissage anchors in-situ (top left). MRI image shows disruption of the repaired capsule-labral tissue with chondral injuryover anterior glenoid (bottom left). CT scan images show subcritical glenoid bone loss with an avulsed bony fragment (top middle) and osteolysis around anchor sites (bottom middle). Prominent metal anchors and associated chondral changes are shown in top and bottom right images

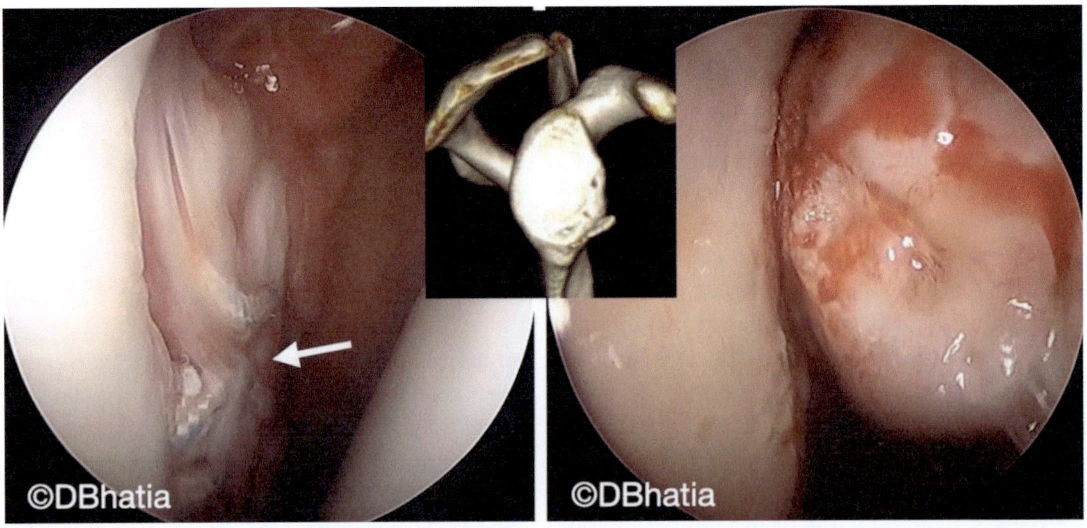

Fig. 23.2 Pathology in a failed Bankart repair is demonstrated. Labral tissue is disrupted and suture remnants are visualized (arrow, Left image). Associated glenoid bone loss appears subcritical (Inset image) and a bone avulsion fragment is seen. Dynamic arthroscopic standardized tracking (DAST) demonstrates an off-track Hill-Sach's lesion (Right image)

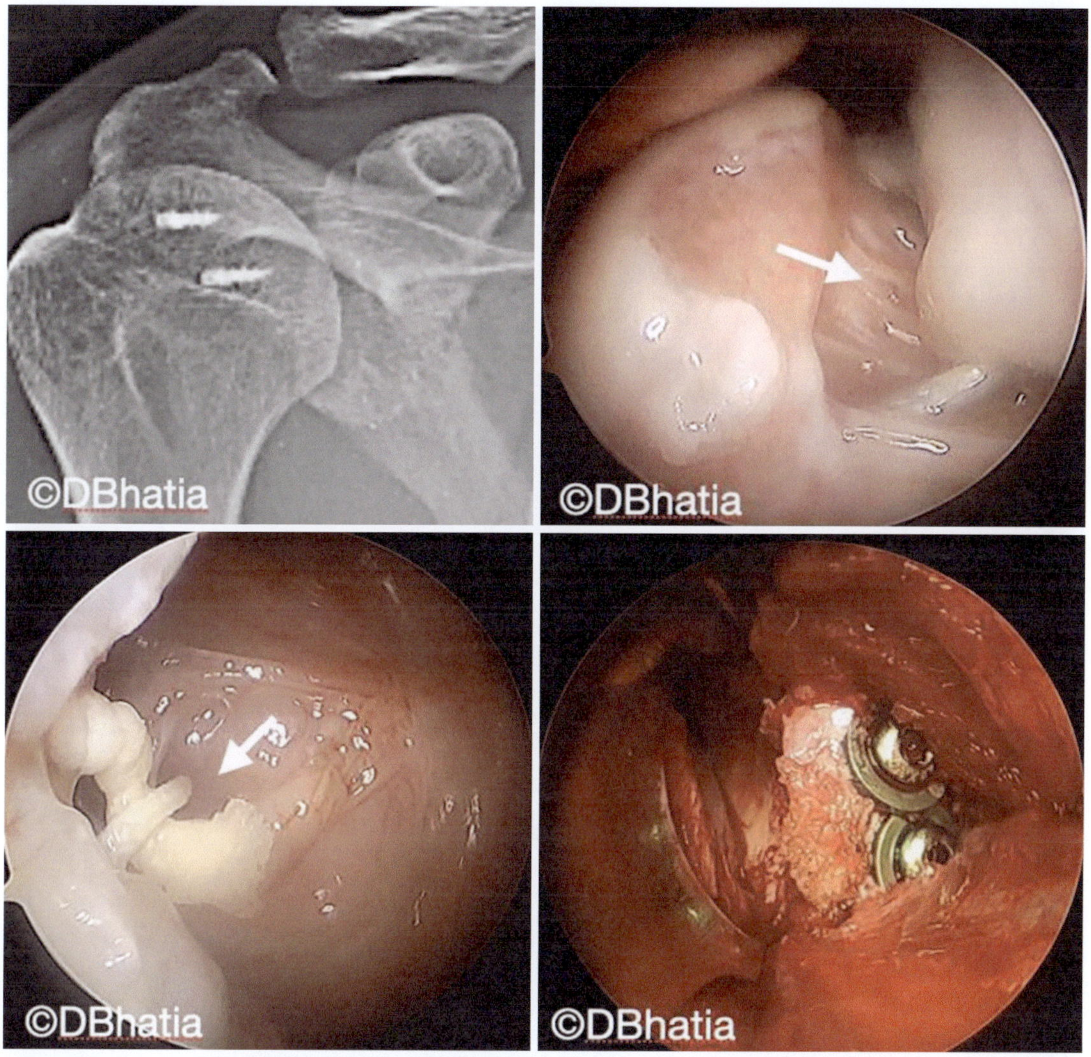

Fig. 23.3 Pathology in a failed labral repair augmented with remplissage (top left image) is demonstrated. Labral tissue is attenuated and only remnant sutures from anchors are seen (arrow, bottom Left image). Failure of remplissage is seen and a gap between the tendon and humeral head bone is visualized (top right). Revision surgery was performed with a classic Latarjet procedure (bottom right)

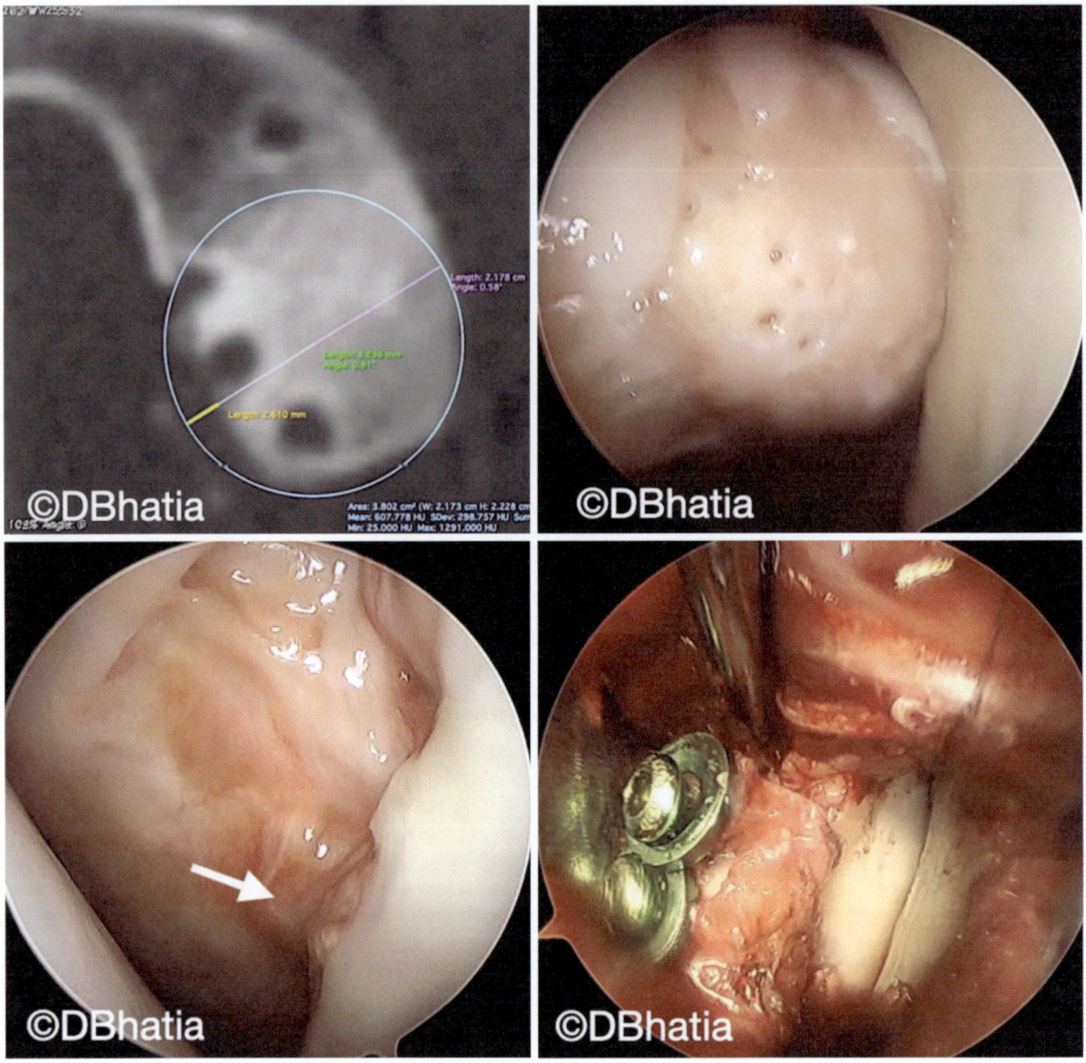

Fig. 23.4 Pathology in a failed labral repair with severe osteolysis around anchor sites (top and bottom left images) is demonstrated. Labral tissue is attenuated and anterior glenoid erosion from anchor site osteolysis is visualized (arrow, bottom left image). Dynamic arthroscopic standardized tracking (DAST) demonstrates an off-track Hill-Sach's lesion (top right) and revision surgery was performed with a classic Latarjet procedure (bottom right)

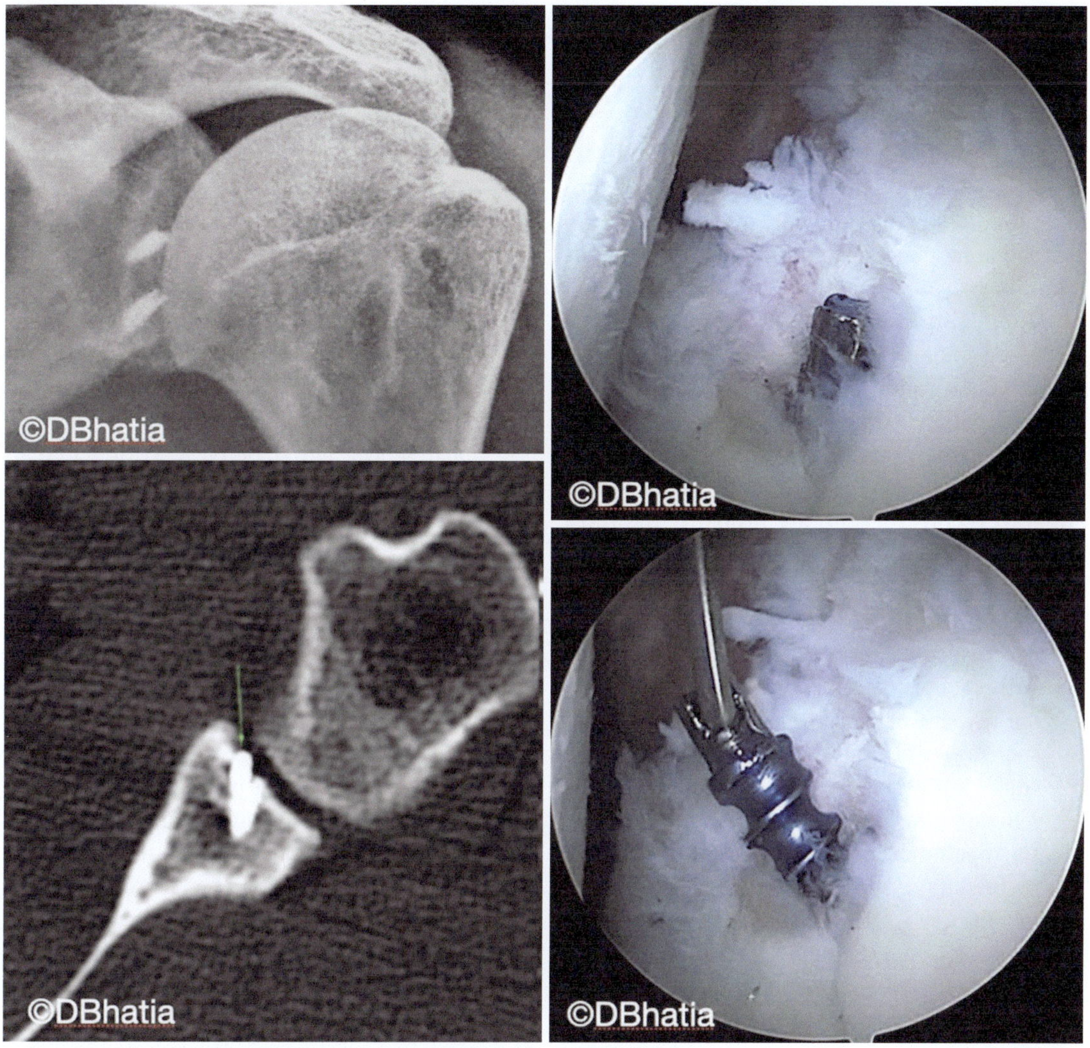

Fig. 23.5 Prominent metal anchors can be identified on CT scans (top and bottom left). Associated chondral injury may be visualized on arthroscopy (top right) and impinging anchors must be removed prior to reconstruction (bottom right)

necessitate removal (Fig. 23.5). Preexisting chondral damage should be documented and any cartilage fragments/flaps (GLAF lesions) and osseous loose bodies should be excised. The axillary pouch should be visualized to identify HAGL lesions that may coexist with significant bone defects [25]. Dynamic tracking is useful as it documents the glenoid track under dynamic conditions, and the effect of laxity-induced translation on the radiologically measured glenoid track can be assessed (Figs. 23.2 and 23.4). Dynamic arthroscopic standardized tracking (DAST) is performed by first aligning the Hill-Sachs lesion parallel with the anterior glenoid rim by arm abduction and forward flexion; thereafter an anteriorly directed force using thumb pressure is applied, and Hill-Sachs lesions are classified into on- or off-track, and peripheral track [3].

23.4 Treatment

23.4.1 Surgical Options

Surgery is indicated in postoperative recurrent anterior instability (recurrent episodes of subluxation/dislocation) and may also be offered in cases where persistent apprehension prevents return to pre-injury sporting or functional level. Revision surgical options that have been described include arthroscopic/open capsulolabral repair and augmentation of capsulolabral repair with a remplissage procedure; however, bone graft reconstruction techniques (Latarjet, Eden-Hybinette, and distal tibial allograft reconstruction) are probably the most reliable revision procedures for failed soft tissue repairs.

(a) *Arthroscopic Capsule-Labral Repair:* Arthroscopic repair may be considered during revision surgery in a low-demand (non-sporting) and non-hyperlax individual with small bone lesions [26]. Moreover, labral remnant tissue after a previous failed soft tissue repair must be sufficiently robust to allow mobilization and reattachment, and glenohumeral bone defects should be within the on-track morphology (radiological and DAST). Repair augmentation with remplissage may be performed for additional stability; however, the risk of loss of range of motion is a possibility. Lee and Shin reported satisfactory 2-year clinical outcomes in 82% of patients without recurrent shoulder instability after failed arthroscopic Bankart repair [27]. However, Slaven et al. reported a high failure rate of 44% in a young military population with <20% glenoid bone loss. In another systematic review [28], Hong et al. reported a failure rate between 6% and 47%, and return to sports rate between 26% and 88%, in patients with <20% glenoid bone loss [29].

(b) *Bone Reconstructive Procedures:* Most soft tissue repair failures occur in the presence of glenohumeral bone defects ranging between 7% and 25% or more. Bone graft reconstruction of the anterior glenoid, with or without capsulo-labral repair, can predictably restore glenoid osseous geometry and stability. Both arthroscopic and open Latarjet procedures are effective in stabilizing the recurrent instability after a soft tissue repair failure. Lho et al. compared revision Bankart repair and Latarjet procedure for failed Bankart repair; they suggested that Latarjet procedure was superior for functional scores and stability, and for return to preinjury level of sports [30]. However, they found that postoperative pain and the limitation of external rotation at side were worse with higher complications. In another study, Calvo et al. reported that the arthroscopic Latarjet as a revision surgery provides comparable clinical outcomes to the primary Latarjet procedure with a low postoperative recurrence rate. These authors suggested a decreased level of postoperative sports participation and external rotation with the arm by the side in their patients [31]. Şahin et al. reported that previous arthroscopic Bankart repair did not significantly influence coracoid graft osteolysis, and both primary and revision Latarjet procedures showed satisfactory clinical outcomes [32]. In contrast, Flinkkilä et al. reported that a previous failed arthroscopic Bankart repair was a significant independent risk factor for inferior outcome. In their study, 4 patients in the primary surgery group and 13 patients in the revision group had at least one subluxation or instability perception after Latarjet procedure, and had worse functional scores as compared to those who underwent Latarjet as the primary surgery [33]. Similarly, in a systematic review, Karavan et al. concluded that the revision Latarjet procedure for a failed Bankart repair resulted in higher rates of complications, recurrent instability, and revisions in comparison with the Latarjet procedure performed as a primary procedure [34]. Besides the Latarjet procedure, other autografts (iliac crest, scapula spine, distal clavicle) or allografts (distal tibia, distal radius) can be used for bony glenoid reconstruction and these procedures are performed either open or arthroscopic with similar outcomes. The magnitude of glenoid bone defect may have a role in the choice of surgical bone grafting procedure. The classic Latarjet procedure completely reconstructs the osseous geometry in a glenoid defect size of 20–25%; however, larger defects (>30%) are best reconstructed with grafts that provide a larger surface area (congruent-arc Latarjet modification, iliac crest autografts, and distal tibia allografts) [7].

23.4.2 Rehabilitation

Surgical revision repair (soft tissue or bony) carries the risk of postoperative stiffness, and this can vary depending upon the chondral wear and extent of repair. Early rehab is necessary, and it should begin as soon as the patient is comfortable after surgery. External rotation in arm adducted position and active forward flexion are commenced in the first postoperative week after bony procedures and may be delayed to 3 weeks in soft tissue repairs. Full range of motion and strength should be achieved within 8–12 weeks; thereafter sport-specific conditioning is commenced in preparation for return to play, and unrestricted return to contact sports may take 8–9 months (Table 23.1).

Conflict of Interest The author(s) declare that they have no competing interests. All authors, their immediate family, and any research foundation with which they are affiliated did not receive any financial payments or other benefits from any commercial entity related to the subject of this article. The author retains the copyright to images, videos, and content in the manuscript.

Table 23.1 Key steps in management of a failed soft tissue repair for anterior shoulder instability

Identify the predisposing and compounding factors that resulted in recurrence of instability after a soft tissue repair.
A thorough clinical evaluation and examination involves detailed documentation of presurgical and current symptoms (pain, weakness, stiffness, and instability episodes) and mechanisms of dislocation. Inquire into medical history for voluntary instability, inherited collagen disorders, and epilepsy.
Radiological series for evaluation should include radiographs (true AP and external rotation views), CT scans with 3D reconstruction, and MRI images. Images prior to first surgery must be reviewed if available.
Arthroscopic evaluation is necessary to assess soft tissue lesion, tissue quality, chondral damage, loose bodies, and coexisting lesions (HAGL, SLAP). Dynamic arthroscopic standardized test (DAST) is useful to classify glenohumeral defects into on- and off-track, and peripheral track.
Arthroscopic removal of loose bodies and proud sutures or anchors is performed and associated lesions like SLAP tears and posterior labral tears are addressed.
Arthroscopic capsulolabral repair is performed in a low-demand (non-sporting) and non-hyperlax individual, and in cases where glenohumeral bone defects are within the on-track morphology and labral remnant is sufficient and robust to allow mobilization and reattachment.
Additional arthroscopic hill-Sachs remplissage may be performed to augment the revision capsulolabral repair. This increases the risk of postoperative stiffness, especially in external rotation and may affect return to play in athletes.
Bone grafting procedures (Latarjet, allografts) provide consistent and predictably good outcomes. These can be performed arthroscopic or with open techniques using a subscapularis-splitting approach. Concomitant capsulolabral repair is not necessary when performing a Latarjet or any other bone grafting procedure.
Early and accelerated rehab is beneficial; restoration of range and strength within the first 3 months is the goal in athletes. Thereafter sport-specific conditioning is commenced and full return to sport is possible in 6 months.

References

1. Adolfsson L. What keeps a shoulder stable—is there an ideal method for anterior stabilisation? Shoulder Elbow. 2024;16(1):4–7. https://doi.org/10.1177/17585732231224699.
2. Kim M, Haratian A, Fathi A, Kim DR, Patel N, Bolia IK, Hasan LK, Petrigliano FA, Weber AE. Can we identify why athletes fail to return to sports after arthroscopic Bankart repair? A systematic review and meta-analysis. Am J Sports Med. 2023;51(9):2480–6. https://doi.org/10.1177/03635465221089980.
3. Bhatia DN, Malviya P. How does dynamic arthroscopic tracking compare with radiologic glenoid track for identification of on- and off-track lesions in anterior shoulder instability? J Shoulder Elb Surg. 2024;33(1):23–31. https://doi.org/10.1016/j.jse.2023.05.018.
4. Wu C, Wang Y, Wang C, Chen J, Xu J, Yu W, Huang K, Ye Z, Jiang J, Tsai TY, Zhao J, Xie G. Glenoid track width is smaller under dynamic conditions: an in vivo dual-fluoroscopy imaging study. Am J Sports Med. 2022;50(14):3881–8. https://doi.org/10.1177/03635465221126650.
5. Boden SA, Charles S, Hughes JD, Miller L, Rodosky M, Popchak A, Musahl V, Lesniak BP, Lin A. Recurrent instability after arthroscopic Bankart repair in patients with hyperlaxity and near-track lesions. Orthop J Sports Med. 2023;11(9):23259671231200231. https://doi.org/10.1177/23259671231200231.
6. Bhatia DN, Kandhari V. How does anterior glenoid bone loss affect shoulder stability? A cadaveric analysis of glenoid concavity and bony shoulder stability ratio. J Shoulder Elb Surg. 2022;31(3):553–60. https://doi.org/10.1016/j.jse.2021.09.004.
7. Bhatia DN, Kandhari V. Bone defect-induced alteration in glenoid articular surface geometry and restoration with coracoid transfer procedures: a cadaveric study. J Shoulder Elb Surg. 2019;28(12):2418–26. https://doi.org/10.1016/j.jse.2019.04.050.
8. Moroder P, Damm P, Wierer G, Böhm E, Minkus M, Plachel F, Märdian S, Scheibel M, Khatamirad M. Challenging the current concept of critical glenoid bone loss in shoulder instability: does the size measurement really tell it all? Am J Sports Med. 2019;47(3):688–94. https://doi.org/10.1177/0363546518819102.
9. Park I, Shin SJ. Correlation of glenoid concavity with surgical failure after arthroscopic stabilization for recurrent anterior shoulder instability. Am J Sports Med. 2023;51(14):3845–50. https://doi.org/10.1177/03635465231203152.
10. Lau LC, Chau WW, Ng R, Ng JP, Chui EC, Ong MT, Griffith JF, Yung PS. Reconsidering "critical" bone loss in shoulder instability: 17-year follow-up study following arthroscopic Bankart repair. Adv Orthop. 2024;2024:5598107. https://doi.org/10.1155/2024/5598107.
11. Di Giacomo G, Itoi E, Burkhart SS. Evolving concept of bipolar bone loss and the hill-Sachs lesion: from "engaging/non-engaging" lesion to "on-track/off-track" lesion. Arthroscopy. 2014;30(1):90–8. https://doi.org/10.1016/j.arthro.2013.10.004.
12. Yamamoto N, Shinagawa K, Hatta T, Itoi E. Peripheral-track and central-Track Hill-Sachs lesions: a new concept of assessing an on-track lesion. Am J Sports Med. 2020;48(1):33–8. https://doi.org/10.1177/0363546519886319.
13. Wermers J, Schliemann B, Raschke MJ, Dyrna F, Heilmann LF, Michel PA, Katthagen JC. The glenolabral articular disruption lesion is a biomechanical risk factor for recurrent shoulder instability. Arthrosc Sports Med Rehabil. 2021;3(6):e1803–10. https://doi.org/10.1016/j.asmr.2021.08.007.
14. Warner JJ, Beim GM. Combined Bankart and HAGL lesion associated with anterior shoulder instability. Arthroscopy. 1997;13(6):749–52. https://doi.org/10.1016/s0749-8063(97)90012-8.
15. Arner JW, Cooper JD, Elrick BP, Rakowski DR, Ruzbarsky JJ, Horan MP, Millett PJ. Outcomes of arthroscopic anterior Labroligamentous periosteal sleeve avulsion lesions: a minimum 2-year follow-up. Am J Sports Med. 2022;50(6):1512–9. https://doi.org/10.1177/03635465221090902.
16. Tennent D, Antonios T, Arnander M, Ejindu V, Papadakos N, Rastogi A, Pearse Y. CT methods for measuring glenoid bone loss are inaccurate, and not reproducible or interchangeable. Bone Jt Open. 2023;4(7):478–89. https://doi.org/10.1302/2633-1462.47.BJO-2023-0066.R1.
17. Moroder P, Akguen D, Paksoy A, Gebauer H, Barthod-Tonnot N, Lupetti M, Markova V, Zettinig O, Parada S, Karpinski K. The global track concept for assessment of engaging Hill-Sachs defects in anterior shoulder instability. Am J Sports Med. 2024;52:1292–8. https://doi.org/10.1177/03635465241232089.
18. Rashid MS, Tsuchiya S, More KD, LeBlanc J, Bois AJ, Kwong CA, Lo IKY. Validating the glenoid track concept using dynamic arthroscopic assessment. Orthop J Sports Med. 2024;12(2):23259671241226943. https://doi.org/10.1177/23259671241226943.
19. Di Giacomo G, Peebles LA, Pugliese M, Dekker TJ, Golijanin P, Sanchez A, Provencher MT. Glenoid track instability management score: radiographic modification of the instability severity index score. Arthroscopy. 2020;36(1):56–67. https://doi.org/10.1016/j.arthro.2019.07.020.
20. Nakagawa S, Hirose T, Tachibana Y, Iuchi R, Mae T. Postoperative recurrence of instability due to new anterior glenoid rim fractures after arthroscopic Bankart repair. Am J Sports Med. 2017;45(12):2840–8. https://doi.org/10.1177/0363546517714476.
21. Dobelle E, Falguières J, Ollivier M, Argenson JN, Lami D. Infraspinatus function impairment after arthroscopic Bankart repair with Hill Sachs remplissage. Isokinetic, functional, and radiographic analysis.

Orthop Traumatol Surg Res. 2024;110:103812. https://doi.org/10.1016/j.otsr.2024.103812.
22. Gagey OJ, Gagey N. The hyperabduction test. J Bone Joint Surg Br. 2001;83(1):69–74. https://doi.org/10.1302/0301-620x.83b1.10628.
23. Beighton P, Solomon L, Soskolne CL. Articular mobility in an African population. Ann Rheum Dis. 1973;32(5):413–8. https://doi.org/10.1136/ard.32.5.413.
24. Raniga S, Arenas-Miquelez A, Bokor D. What is the most reliable method of measuring glenoid bone loss in anterior glenohumeral instability? Response. Am J Sports Med. 2022;50(13):NP58–9. https://doi.org/10.1177/03635465221121606.
25. Bhatia DN, DasGupta B. Surgical treatment of significant glenoid bone defects and associated humeral avulsions of glenohumeral ligament (HAGL) lesions in anterior shoulder instability. Knee Surg Sports Traumatol Arthrosc. 2013;21(7):1603–9. https://doi.org/10.1007/s00167-012-2119-y.
26. Calvo E, Luengo G, Morcillo D, Foruria AM, Valencia M. Revision arthroscopic Bankart repair versus arthroscopic Latarjet for failed primary arthroscopic stabilization with subcritical bone loss. Orthop J Sports Med. 2021;9(5):23259671211001809. https://doi.org/10.1177/23259671211001809.
27. Lee JH, Shin SJ. Revision arthroscopic labral repair using all-suture anchors in patients with subcritical glenoid bone loss after failed Bankart repair: clinical outcomes at 2-year follow-up. Orthop J Sports Med. 2023;11(3):23259671231151418. https://doi.org/10.1177/23259671231151418.
28. Slaven SE, Donohue MA, Tardif RA, Foley KA, LeClere LE, Cameron KL, Giuliani JR, Posner MA, Dickens JF. Revision arthroscopic Bankart repair results in high failure rates and a low return to duty rate without recurrent instability. Arthroscopy. 2023;39(4):913–8. https://doi.org/10.1016/j.arthro.2022.08.044.
29. Hong IS, Sonnenfeld JJ, Sicat CS, Hong RS, Trofa DP, Schiffern SC, Hamid N, Fleischli JE, Saltzman BM. Outcomes after arthroscopic revision Bankart repair: an updated systematic review of recent literature. Arthroscopy. 2023;39(2):438–51. https://doi.org/10.1016/j.arthro.2022.03.030.
30. Lho T, Lee J, Oh KS, Chung SW. Latarjet procedure for failed Bankart repair provides better stability and return to sports, but worse postoperative pain and external rotation limitations with more complications, compared to revision Bankart repair: a systematic review and meta-analysis. Knee Surg Sports Traumatol Arthrosc. 2023;31(8):3541–58. https://doi.org/10.1007/s00167-023-07410-2.
31. Calvo E, Dzidzishvili L, Valencia M, Calvo C. Outcomes of arthroscopic Latarjet as a revision surgery after failed arthroscopic Bankart repair. Am J Sports Med. 2024;52(1):190–200. https://doi.org/10.1177/03635465231209986.
32. Şahin K, Sarıkaş M, Çeşme DH, Topal M, Kapıcıoğlu M, Bilsel K. Does previous arthroscopic Bankart repair influence coracoid graft osteolysis in Latarjet procedure? A case-control study with computed tomography scan data. J Shoulder Elb Surg. 2024;33(4):e223–30. https://doi.org/10.1016/j.jse.2023.08.011.
33. Flinkkilä T, Knape R, Nevalainen M, Sirniö K, Ohtonen P, Leppilahti J. Previous arthroscopic Bankart repair is an independent risk factor for an inferior outcome after Latarjet procedure. Orthop Traumatol Surg Res. 2019;105(8):1481–5. https://doi.org/10.1016/j.otsr.2019.06.020.
34. Karavan MP Jr, Hurley ET, Mills FB 4th, Pasqualini I, Rossi L, Dickens JF, Anakwenze O, Mullett H, Millett PJ, Klifto CS. Primary Latarjet procedure versus Latarjet in the setting of previously failed Bankart repair: a systematic review. J ISAKOS. 2023;8(6):490–6. https://doi.org/10.1016/j.jisako.2023.08.009.

The Failed Latarjet

24

María Valencia, Mario Sayalero, and Emilio Calvo

24.1 Introduction

The Latarjet technique is particularly indicated in cases of recurrent anterior instability associated with critical glenoid bone loss [1, 2]. It is also considered the treatment of choice in patients without bone defect who may present a high risk of dislocation with soft tissue procedures, like those practicing collision sports or certain activities that need a very stable shoulder [2, 3]. Unacceptable recurrence rates have been reported in these patients using soft tissue procedures, and satisfactory results have also been reported after the Latarjet used as revision surgery of failed soft tissue procedure. For this reason, the use of Latarjet has increased in recent years [4, 5].

Latarjet has a recurrence rate of 0–18%, which can increase to 5–26% after 10 years of follow-up [6, 7]. It is a non-anatomic technique and therefore revision surgery becomes a especially difficult. The normal tissue planes are modified by scar tissue and there is an alteration of the anatomical stabilizing structures. The coracoid, which is a key landmark for surgical shoulder approaches, is no longer in its position as well as the conjoint tendon. In addition, there are few published studies on the results of Latarjet revision surgery after failure of shoulder stabilization by this technique [8]. Considering the potential etiology, the clinical evaluation and analyzing the different surgical options for failure of anterior shoulder instability treated with Latarjet, we propose an algorithm for its management.

24.2 How to Identify the Causes of Failure?

The causes of this recurrence must be identified in order to choose the best possible treatment. Some patient's characteristics determine unavoidable factors that increase the risk of recurrence, such as the atraumatic mechanism for primary dislocation, bilateral instability and female sex [9]. Soft tissue alterations such as hyperlaxity, collagen diseases or Ehlers-Danlos syndrome may be associated with postoperative instability. Regarding epilepsy, Dzidzisvili et al. demonstrated that the risk of postoperative recurrence is due to the greater bone involvement in these patients and not to their neurological problem [10].

M. Valencia · M. Sayalero
Shoulder and Elbow Reconstructive Surgery Unit, Department of Orthopedic Surgery and Traumatology, Fundación Jiménez Diaz, Madrid, Spain
e-mail: maria.valencia@quironsalud.es; mario.sayalero@quironsalud.es

E. Calvo (✉)
Department of Orthopedic Surgery and Traumatology, Hospital Universitario Fundacion Jimenez, Universidad Autonoma, Madrid, Spain
e-mail: ecalvo@fjd.es

E. Calvo et al. (eds.), *Complex and Revision Problems in Shoulder Instability*, https://doi.org/10.1007/978-3-031-81389-4_24

24.2.1 Physical Examination

It is mandatory to perform a thorough physical examination and verify that the patient's symptoms are a true recurrence, which is usually reported as episodes of subluxation or dislocation. The mechanism of dislocation, symptom-free time and time since surgery should also be recorded. We should not only consider anterior instability, which is the most frequent, but also investigate potential patients with posterior and multidirectional instability that were wrongly categorized as suffering from anterior instability. It is possible that the iatrogenic nature of the surgery influences instability. In this sense, neurological damage, muscular fatty degeneration or atrophy or complete tendon rupture must be ruled out [11]. A complete neurological examination should be performed, corresponding scars noted and, if necessary, electromyographic studies performed. Range of motion, scapular rhythm and degree of pain should also be explored. The muscular evaluation, the condition of the anterior deltoid in cases of open primary surgery and the subscapularis in cases of previous tenotomy, prominent screws or previous stabilization interventions are of special importance. The scapular rhythm must also be assessed since certain patients with shoulder instability associate scapular dyskinesia.

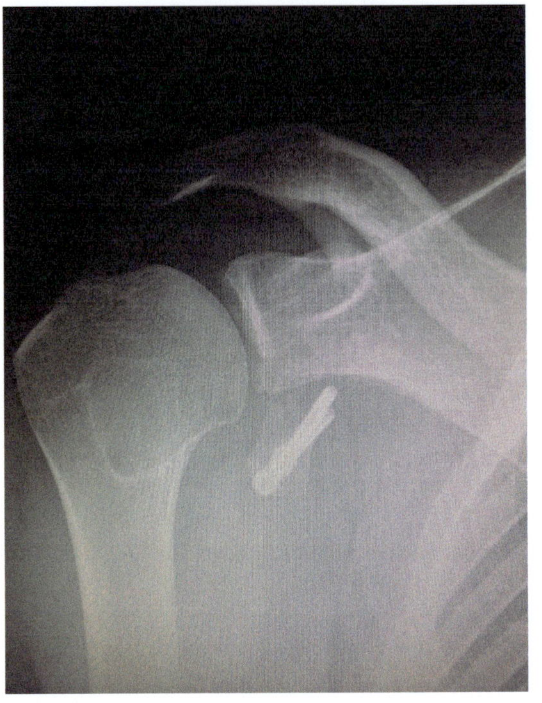

Fig. 24.1 Coracoid graft avulsion. The fragment seems viable and suitable for refixation

24.2.2 Imaging Study

Conventional shoulder radiographs can help to rule out clear causes of Latarjet failure such screw breakage or macroscopic malposition, but computed tomography (CT) is the key tool to evaluate the status and position of the coracoid graft as well as to estimate bone defects and to calculate the glenoid track (Fig. 24.1). CT gives more precise information about the position, degree of consolidation and the presence of osteolysis in the graft [12, 13] Technical errors, such as medial or inferior placement of the graft, should also be considered to identify the cause of recurrence. Most of the graft should be subequatorial, specifically at 3–6 h [4]. Regarding the glenoid surface, it will be assessed in the axial plane. The ideal coracoid graft position is flush with the articular surface [7]. Kany et al. consider that the graft is in good position when it is medialized less than 5 mm and lateralized less than 3 mm in relation to the glenoid subarticular bone [13]. It should be noted that the CT underestimates the depth of the cartilage.

Graft osteolysis should be investigated [14, 15]. Samim et al. described the calculation of the percentage of bone union of the coracoid graft [16]. According to the technique, sagittal multiplanar images of 2 mm thickness are used, subtracting the percentage of the screw. The density of ossification across the glenoid graft is defined as fusion. Fibrous union of the graft is associated with a worse recurrence rate and a lower rate of return to sporting activity [17], although it is not clear whether it is related to a higher rate of complications. Tobacco use is related to graft non-union [11]. Other causes are the scarce contact surface between the graft and the glenoid due to the shape of the glenoid neck or cases without glenoid bone defect [18]. According to Wolff's law, the bone structure of the graft is maintained by the contact pressure of the humeral head on the graft and the shear forces. Osteolysis of the graft, caused by the abscense of mechanical stimuli is especially relevant in the superior part. In cases of severe osteolysis, infection should be ruled out.

In the case of bipolar bone lesions, CT is also necessary to calculate the glenoid track prior to primary surgery and after recurrence since there are cases in which the recurrence is not due to incorrect surgery but to the fact that the width of the coracoid graft is not sufficient to restore the glenoid track. Calvo et al. found a significantly higher failure rate in those cases were coracoid transfer was insufficient to turn an off-track Hill-Sachs lesion into on-track [14]. Adding a *remplissage* to the Latarjet procedure [19] or to increase the glenoid surface with a free bone graft [12, 20–26] are the options to address these patients with a failed Latarjet in whom glenoid track has not been reconstructed.

Finally, magnetic resonance arthrography gives information about the state of the soft tissues, the glenoid track, the cartilage and signs of muscle degeneration or atrophy.

24.3 Treatment Options and Results

In certain patients with a single episode of postoperative instability, conservative treatment may be preferred [17]. These infrequent cases require a great patient's commitment to reduce high-contact activities and to perform strengthening and proprioception exercises. However, surgical treatment will show more predictable results after Latarjet recurrence in most cases. Despite being the gold standard, we must keep in mind the technical difficulty of the procedure since it is a non-anatomic technique in which the coracoid has been transposed, the axillary nerve stays medial and posterior to the conjoint tendon, while the musculocutaneous nerve is transposed medially and inferiorly [27]. Technically, for revision surgery it is very useful to identify the conjoint tendon and to follow it proximally until the subscapularis split and coracoid graft are encountered. Subsequently, the subscapularis is released, the screws are removed and the anterior glenoid neck and previous coracoid can be prepared if present. Neurolysis is not routinely recommended [28].

24.3.1 Coracoid Graft Repositioning

Coracoid graft repositioning is suggested in cases in which the Latarjet has failed due to a suboptimal position of the graft. It can also be used when the graft is avulsed but its condition is viable. It should be confirmed that the size of the graft is sufficient to reconstruct the glenoid bone defect (Fig. 24.2). Willemot et al. [29] reported satisfactory results with coracoid graft repositioning in 6 patients out of a case series of 26 who underwent Latarjet revision.

24.3.2 Free Bone Grafting Techniques

One of the main objectives of the Latarjet procedure is to increase the glenoid articular surface. Therefore, free bone autograft or allograft techniques have been the most used in Latarjet revision surgery. Buda et al. concluded through a systematic review that iliac crest autograft (ie, Eden-Hybinette procedure) with or without plication or capsular reinforcement techniques is the safest and most frequently used technique and in Latarjet revision surgery, and good or excellent results in 67–89% of the patients. They report an overall complication rate of 17.2% and a recurrence rate of 8.6%, concluding that the number of complications is not higher than in primary surgery. Fifty-one percent of the patients returned to their previous sporting level [8].

Bone grafting techniques allow to adapt the bone graft's size and shape techniques to the patient's defect, and are mainly used in cases where the glenoid bone defect has not been sufficiently reconstructed due to coracoid graft osteolysis or fragmentation or in shoulders with very

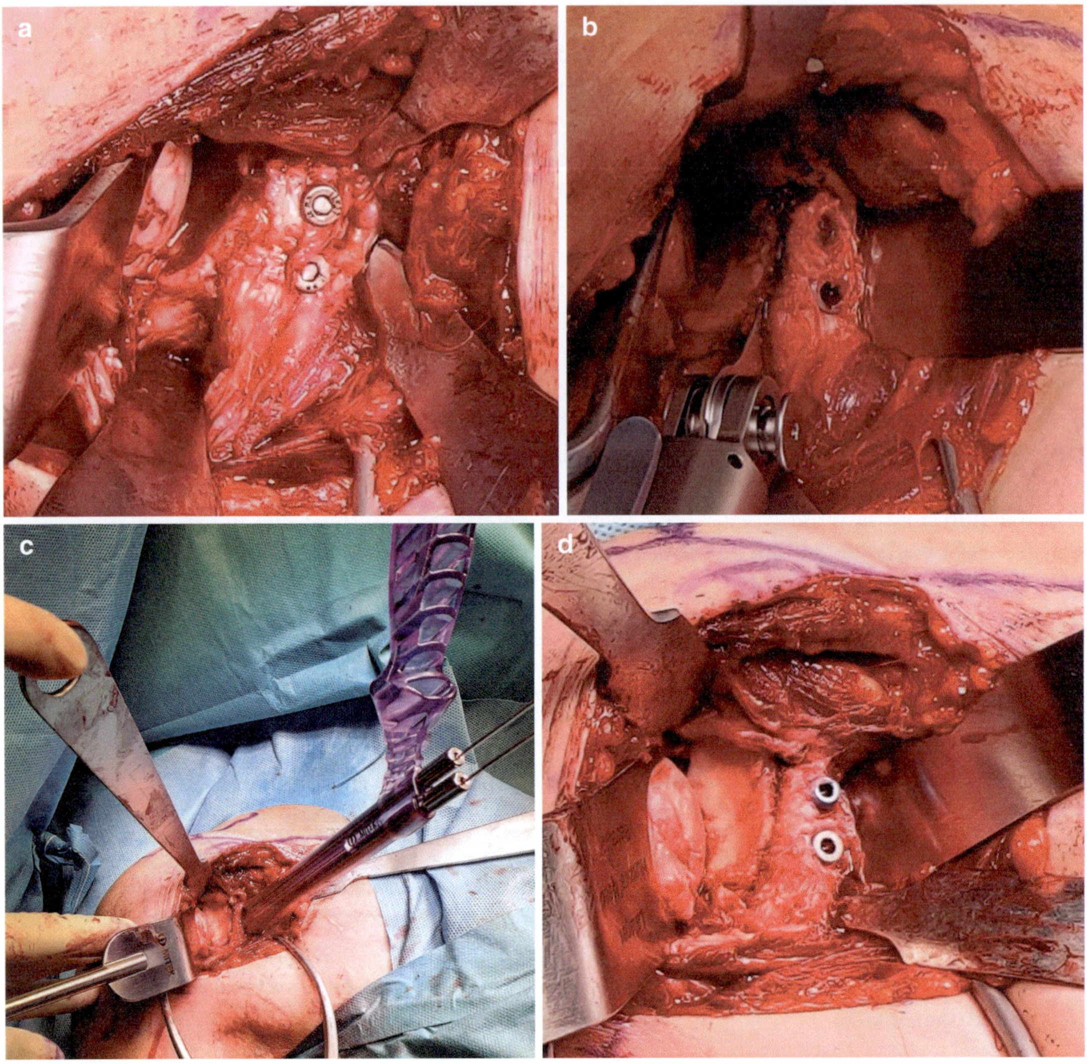

Fig. 24.2 Reconstructed by iliac crest bone graft. (**a**) Patient with postoperative instability after failed Latarjet. Note the medial position of the coracoid graft. (**b**) Graft osteotomy. (**c**) Graft repositioning using the instruments of arthroscopic Latarjet (DePuy Synthes, Rynham, MA, USA). (**d**) Final graft position flush with the glenoid articular surface

large Hill-Sachs off-track lesions that cannot be converted into on-track in spite of a well-positioned and healed coracoid graft. By means of arthroscopy or open surgery, the new graft is fixed with screws, buttons or sutures (Fig. 24.3).

Lunn et al. reported satisfactory long-term results in terms of recurrence rate (11%) and return to sport (68%) in the first series of patients with failed Latarjet treated using the Eden-Hybinette technique. However, the rate of complications was substantial, including subscapularis rupture and osteoarthritis rates of 17.4% and 11.8%, respectively [20]. Flurin et al. published a multicenter series of 46 patients with a failed Latarjet treated also with iliac crest autograft. After an average follow-up

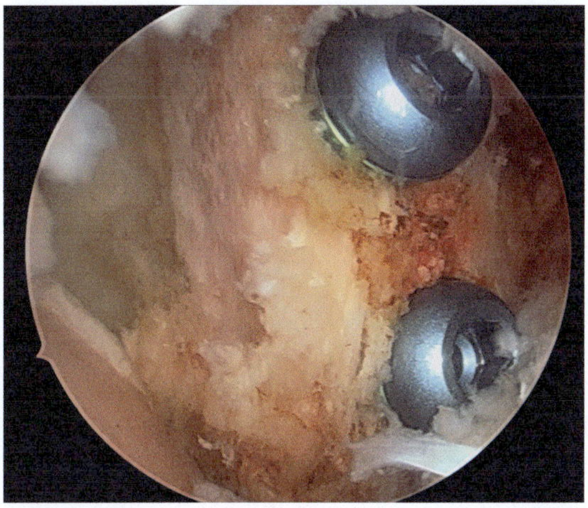

Fig. 24.3 Final arthroscopic image of a free iliac crest bone graft used to treat a failed Latarjet with severe coracoid graft osteolysis

of 3 years, they reported satisfactory results in 80% of patients, with 86% of stable shoulders and low postoperative osteoarthritis rate (11%) [24]. They related the return to sport with age and the time elapsed between primary surgery and revision.

Giannakos et al. [22] reported for the first time satisfactory results of arthroscopic Eden-Hybinette technique for failed Latarjet using screws to fix the bone graft. Boileau et al. demonstrated in a small series of patients that suture and buttons is a reliable method of fixation and achieves optimal positioning and predictable graft healing [23]. In addition, the suture button is recommended in cases in which it is impossible to remove the broken hardware. Martínez-Catalán et al. [26] reported results with good glenoid reconstruction in which the iliac crest bone graft was integrated by double suture button fixation in 17 shoulders with critical defects.

The glenoid defect can also be reconstructed using distal clavicle autograft [30] or allografts of the humeral or femoral head [23], glenoid [31] and distal tibia [12]. The distal tibia, despite its high cost and low availability, allows restoration of the anatomy since it has a radius of curvature like that of the glenoid. As it is a weight-bearing surface, it has a high bone quality and, therefore, excellent screw fixation, with an overall graft union rate of 92% according to Provencher et al. [12] in a series of 31 patients with a minimum follow-up of 3 years.

24.3.3 Soft Tissue Procedures

There is a small population of patients in whom the primary Latarjet surgery was performed correctly, the graft is in place and has healed in the correct position reconstructing the bone defects yet fails. In these cases, we should consider the possibility of a probable hyperlaxity, which should be addressed by procedures aimed at reinforcing the soft tissues.

24.3.4 Capsulolabral Reconstruction

Repair of the Bankart lesion is increasingly used in association with primary Latarjet surgery as it helps stabilize the shoulder, maintains the extra-articular graft and thus prevents the possible future development of arthritis [1]. Considering that the glenoid track was successfully restored, in those patients in whom the labrum was not properly repaired and the anterior glenoid rim does not present significant damage, the capsulolabral complex can be reattached with suture anchors [1, 32]. Cuellar et al. [32] reviewed 12 patients with Latarjet recurrence associated with capsular hyperlaxity in whom arthroscopic capsular plication was performed. The patients had a bone defect of less than 25% and were not involved in high-contact sports activities. The results were satisfactory, even with two cases of loose or broken screws and two cases of non-union of the graft.

24.3.5 Extra-articular Capsular Reinforcement

In patients with generalized hyperlaxity or whose soft tissues do not allow capsular repair, the use of tendon allograft to reinforce the anteroinferior glenohumeral ligament has been described [33]. The most recommended option is the use of iliotibial band allograft stretched in abduction and external rotation, a modification of the technique of Sanchez et al. [33], reinforcing the native anterior capsule in an extra-articular manner. This graft, passed through the subscapularis, is anchored at the inferior border of the humeral subscapularis insertion and at 3 o'clock on the glenoid. The allograft increases the containment of the anteroinferior glenohumeral ligament, blocking dislocation and subluxation. Similarly, suspension of the long head of the biceps can be used to achieve dynamic anteroinferior stabilization [34, 35].

24.3.5.1 Remplissage

Reinforcing a Latarjet by a *remplissage* procedure allows to address recurrences in shoulders that remain off-track due to a large or very medialized Hill-Sachs. A retrospective series of 41 patients with recurrence of coracoid bone stop techniques studied by Lavoué et al. [19] showed 19 cases with bipolar bone lesions treated by Bankart and *remplissage* with satisfactory results.

24.3.6 Salvage Procedures

Patients with extensive subscapularis involvement may require a pectoralis major transfer associated with a bony cap [36]. In cases of persistent instability or severe osteoarthritis, we may opt for shoulder arthroplasty [37]. The indication for arthrodesis is limited to situations of pain and persistent subluxation associated with neurological damage or severe hyperlaxity [38]. The target position would be 25° abduction, 25° antepulsion and 35° internal rotation.

24.4 Conclusion and Proposed Algorithm

The increased performance of Latarjet surgery leads to an increase in cases of recurrence and therefore revision procedures. Conservative treatment is rarely used and limited to cases with a degree of instability that does not interfere with patient's life, but surgical treatment is necessary in most cases.

Revision Latarjet surgery is a challenging surgical situation, with modified native anatomy and extense scar tissue. It is essential to find the cause of instability and the state of the coracoid graft. CT provides information about the position, degree of osteolysis and consolidation of the coracoid graft, in addition to allowing quantification of the glenoid track. The authors propose the following algorithm is proposed for the treatment of failed Latarjet (Fig. 24.4) [39]. If the coracoid graft is considered inadequate, a free bone graft is the preferred revision technique. The graft can be repositioned if it is viable and adequate in size, but avulsed or poorly positioned, and osteotomy of the graft is necessary if healed but mispositioned. If the coracoid graft is insufficient to covert the on-track Hill-Sachs lesion into on-track spite well positioned and healed, adding a *remplissage* is recommended. Finally, a properly performed primary Latarjet surgery can recur due to hyperlaxity or poor-quality soft tissue, which we will address by extra-articular capsular reinforcement.

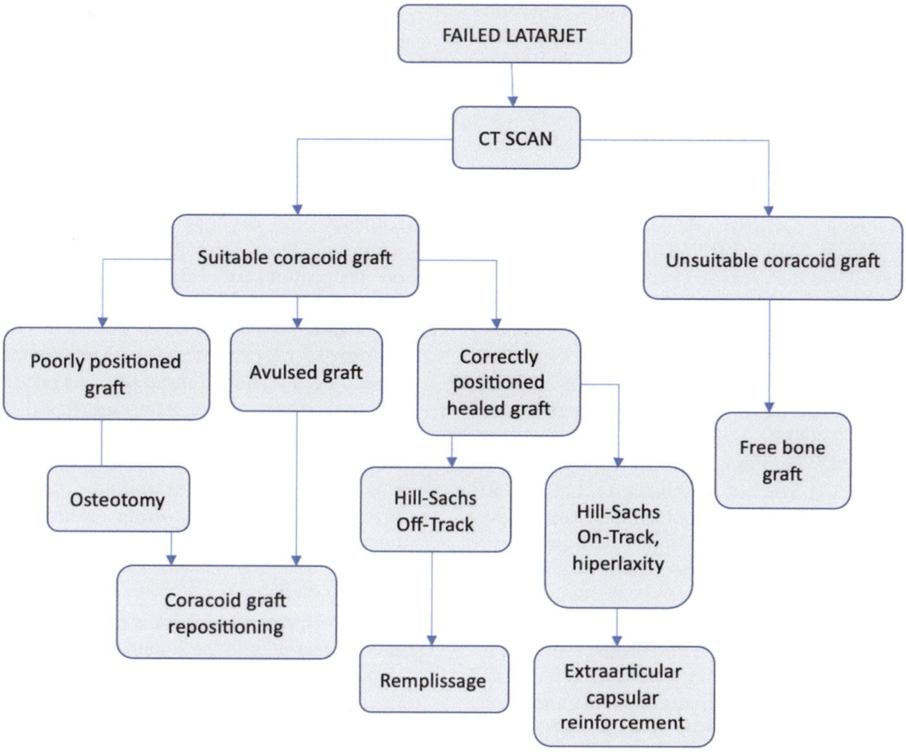

Fig. 24.4 Suggested algorithm for treating a patient with a failed Latarjet. *The coracoid graft is considered adequate if it preserves the insertion of the conjoint tendon, shows no osteolysis, and is large enough to reconstruct the glenoid surface as well as convert any off-track Hill-Sachs lesion into on-frack

References

1. Boileau P, Thélu CÉ, Mercier N, Ohl X, Houghton-Clemmey R, Carles M, Trojani C. Arthroscopic Bristow-Latarjet combined with Bankart repair restores shoulder stability in patients with glenoid bone loss. Clin Orthop Relat Res. 2014;472:2413–24. https://doi.org/10.1007/s11999-014-3691-x.
2. Calvo E, Granizo JJ, Fernández-Yruegas D. Criteria for arthroscopic treatment of anterior instability of the shoulder: a prospective study. J Bone Joint Surg Br Vol. 2005;87:677–83. https://doi.org/10.1302/0301-620X.87B5.15794.
3. Calvo E, Luengo G, Morcillo D, Foruria AM, Valencia M. Revision arthroscopic Bankart repair versus arthroscopic Latarjet for failed primary arthroscopic stabilization with subcritical bone loss. Orthop J Sports Med. 2021;9:23259671211001809. https://doi.org/10.1177/23259671211001809.
4. Calvo E, Itoi E, Landreau P, Arce G, Yamamoto N, Ma J, Sparavalo S, Wong I. Anterior and posterior glenoid bone augmentation options for shoulder instability: state of the art. J ISAKOS. 2021;6:308–17. https://doi.org/10.1136/jisakos-2019-000413.
5. Paoli AR, Pickell M, Mahure SA, McAllister D, Mai DH, Alaia MJ, et al. Trends and risk factors for 1-year revision of the Latarjet procedure: the New York State experience during the past decade. Orthopedics. 2018;41(3):e389–94. https://doi.org/10.3928/01477447-20180320-07.
6. Calvo E, Ávila C, Morcillo D. Arthroscopic Latarjet procedure: my learning curve. In: Boileau P, editor. Shoulder concepts: arthroscopy, arthroplasty & fractures. Sauramps Medical; 2014. p. 6.
7. Gilat R, Lavoie-Gagne O, Haunschild ED, Knapik DM, Parvaresh KC, Fu MC, Forsythe B, Verma N, Cole BJ. Outcomes of the Latarjet procedure with minimum 5- and 10-year follow-up: a systematic review. Should Elb. 2020;12:315–29. https://doi.org/10.1177/1758573220945318.
8. Buda M, D'Ambrosi R, Bellato E, Blonna D, Cappellari A, Delle Rose G, Merolla G, SICSeG (Italian Society of Shoulder, Elbow Surgery) Research Committee. Failed Latarjet procedure: a systematic review of surgery revision options. J Orthop Traumatol. 2021;22:24. https://doi.org/10.1186/s10195-021-00587-7.
9. Di Giacomo G, Peebles LA, Midtgaard KS, de Gasperis N, Scarso P, Provencher CMT. Risk fac-

tors for recurrent anterior glenohumeral instability and clinical failure following primary Latarjet procedures: an analysis of 344 patients. J Bone Joint Surg Am Vol. 2020;102:1665–71. https://doi.org/10.2106/JBJS.19.01235.

10. Dzidzishvili L, Calvo C, Valencia M, Calvo E. Outcomes of arthroscopic Latarjet procedure for anterior glenohumeral instability in patients with epilepsy. A case-control study. Am J Sports Med. 2022;50:708–16. https://doi.org/10.1177/03635465211067531.
11. Dalmas Y, Thélu CE, Laumonerie P, Girard M, Faruch M, Bonnevialle N. Arthroscopic double-button Latarjet: two-thirds of bone block healed at 90 days. Knee Surg Sports Traumatol Arthrosc. 2021;29:136–42. https://doi.org/10.1007/s00167-019-05830-7.
12. Provencher MT, Peebles LA, Aman ZS, Bernhardson AS, Murphy CP, Sanchez A, Dekker TJ, LaPrade RF, Di Giacomo G. Management of the failed Latarjet procedure: outcomes of revision surgery with fresh distal tibial allograft. Am J Sports Med. 2019;47:2795–802. https://doi.org/10.1177/0363546519871896.
13. Kany J, Flamand O, Grimberg J, Guinand R, Croutzet P, Amaravathi R, Sekaran P. Arthroscopic Latarjet procedure: is optimal positioning of the bone block and screws possible? A prospective computed tomography scan analysis. J Shoulder Elb Surg. 2016;25:69–77. https://doi.org/10.1016/j.jse.2015.06.010.
14. Calvo C, Calvo J, Rojas D, Valencia M, Calvo E. Clinical relevance of persistent off-track Hill-Sachs lesion after arthroscopic Latarjet procedure. Am J Sports Med. 2021;49:2006–12. https://doi.org/10.1177/03635465211019979.
15. Di Giacomo G, de Gasperis N, Costantini A, De Vita A, Beccaglia MAR, Pouliart N. Does the presence of glenoid bone loss influence coracoid bone graft osteolysis after the Latarjet procedure? A computed tomography scan study in 2 groups of patients with and without glenoid bone loss. J Shoulder Elb Surg. 2014;23:514–8. https://doi.org/10.1016/j.jse.2013.10.005.
16. Samim M, Small KM, Higgins LD. Coracoid graft union: a quantitative assessment by computed tomography in primary and revision Latarjet procedure. J Shoulder Elb Surg. 2018;27:1475–82. https://doi.org/10.1016/j.jse.2018.01.008.
17. Valencia M, Fernández-Bermejo G, Martín-Ríos MD, Fernández-Jara J, Morcillo-Barrenechea D, Coifman-Lucena I, Foruria AM, Calvo E. Subscapularis structural integrity and function after arthroscopic Latarjet procedure at a minimum 2-year follow-up. J Shoulder Elb Surg. 2020;29:104–12. https://doi.org/10.1016/j.jse.2019.05.027.
18. Kibler WB, Sciascia A, Wilkes T, Sciascia A, Wilkes T. Scapular dyskinesis and its relation to shoulder injury. J Am Acad Orthop Surg. 2012;20:364–72. https://doi.org/10.5435/JAAOS-20-06-364.
19. Lavoué V, Gendre P, Saliken D, Brassac A, Boileau P. The role of arthroscopic soft tissue reconstruction for failed Bristow-Latarjet procedure. Arthroscopy. 2019;35:2581–8. https://doi.org/10.1016/j.arthro.2019.05.010.
20. Lunn JV, Castellano-Rosa J, Walch G. Recurrent anterior dislocation after the Latarjet procedure: outcome after revision using a modified Eden-Hybinette operation. J Shoulder Elb Surg. 2008;17:744–50. https://doi.org/10.1016/j.jse.2008.03.002.
21. Weng PW, Shen HC, Lee HH, Wu SS, Lee CH. Open reconstruction of large bony glenoid erosion with allogeneic bone graft for recurrent anterior shoulder dislocation. Am J Sports Med. 2009;37:1792–7. https://doi.org/10.1177/0363546509334590.
22. Giannakos A, Vezeridis PS, Schwartz DG, Jany R, Lafosse L. All-arthroscopic revision Eden-Hybinette procedure for failed instability surgery: technique and preliminary results. Arthroscopy. 2017;33:39–48. https://doi.org/10.1016/j.arthro.2016.05.021.
23. Boileau P, Duysens C, Saliken D, Lemmex DB, Bonnevialle N. All-arthroscopic, guided Eden-Hybbinette procedure using suture-button fixation for revision of failed Latarjet. J Shoulder Elb Surg. 2019;28:e377–88. https://doi.org/10.1016/j.jse.2019.03.022.
24. Flurin P-H, Antoni M, Métais P, Aswad R. Revision of failed Latarjet with the Eden-Hybinette surgical technique. Orthop Traumatol. 2020;106:223–7. https://doi.org/10.1016/j.otsr.2019.12.009.
25. Ernstbrunner L, Pastor T, Waltenspül M, Gerber C, Wieser K. Salvage iliac crest bone grafting for a failed Latarjet procedure: analysis of failed and successful procedures. Am J Sports Med. 2021;49:3620–7. https://doi.org/10.1177/03635465211040468.
26. Martinez-Catalan N, Werthel JD, Kazum E, Valenti P. Failed Latarjet treated with full arthroscopic Eden-Hybinette procedure using two cortical suture buttons leads to satisfactory clinical outcomes and low recurrence rate. Arthroscopy. 2022;38:1126–33. https://doi.org/10.1016/j.arthro.2021.10.026.
27. Freehill MT, Srikumaran U, Archer KR, McFarland EG, Petersen SA. The Latarjet coracoid process transfer procedure: alterations in the neurovascular structures. J Shoulder Elb Surg. 2013;22:695–700. https://doi.org/10.1016/j.jse.2012.06.003.
28. LaPrade CM, Bernhardson AS, Aman ZS, Moatshe G, Chahla J, Dornan GJ, LaPrade RF, Provencher MT. Changes in the neurovascular anatomy of the shoulder after an open Latarjet procedure: defining a surgical safe zone. Am J Sports Med. 2018;46:2185–91. https://doi.org/10.1177/0363546518773309.
29. Willemot L, De Boey S, Van Tongel A, Declercq G, De Wilde L, Verborgt O. Analysis of failures after the Bristow-Latarjet procedure for recurrent shoulder instability. Int Orthop. 2019;43:1899–907. https://doi.org/10.1007/s00264-018-4105-6.
30. Tokish JM, Fitzpatrick K, Cook JB, Mallon WJ. Arthroscopic distal clavicular autograft for treating shoulder instability with glenoid bone loss. Arthrosc Tech. 2014;3:e475–81. https://doi.org/10.1016/j.eats.2014.05.006.

31. Tjoumakaris FP, Humble B, Sekiya JK. Combined glenoid and humeral head allograft reconstruction for recurrent anterior glenohumeral instability. Orthopedics. 2008;31:497. https://doi.org/10.3928/01477447-20080501-28.
32. Cuéllar A, Cuéllar R, de Heredia PB. Arthroscopic revision surgery for failure of open Latarjet technique. Arthroscopy. 2017;33:910–7. https://doi.org/10.1016/j.arthro.2016.09.017.
33. Sanchez M, Cuellar R, Garcia A, Albillos J, Azofra J. Anterior stabilization of the shoulder by means of an artificial capsular reinforcement and arthroscopy—Part II: results. J Long-Term Eff Med Implants. 2000;10:11. https://doi.org/10.1615/JLongTermEffMedImplants.v10.i3.50.
34. Kohan EM, Wong J, Stroh M, Syed UAM, Namdari S, Lazarus M. Outcome of biceps suspensionplasty for recurrent multidirectional shoulder instability. J Orthop. 2020;22:473–7. https://doi.org/10.1016/j.jor.2020.10.009.
35. Collin P, Nabergoj M, Denard PJ, Wang S, Bothorel H, Lädermann A. Arthroscopic biceps transfer to the glenoid with Bankart repair grants satisfactory 2-year results for recurrent anteroinferior glenohumeral instability in subcritical bone loss. Arthroscopy. 2022;38:1766–71. https://doi.org/10.1016/j.arthro.2021.11.043.
36. Li X, Cusano A, Eichinger J. Eden-Hybinette and pectoralis major transfer for recurrent shoulder instability due to failed Latarjet and chronic subscapularis rupture. Orthopedics. 2017;40:e182–7. https://doi.org/10.3928/01477447-20161006-02.
37. Willemot LB, Elhassan BT, Sperling JW, Cofield RH, Sánchez-Sotelo J. Arthroplasty for glenohumeral arthritis in shoulders with a previous Bristow or Latarjet procedure. J Shoulder Elb Surg. 2018;27:1607–13. https://doi.org/10.1016/j.jse.2018.02.062.
38. Diaz JA, Cohen SB, Warren RF, Craig EV, Allen AA. Arthrodesis as a salvage procedure for recurrent instability of the shoulder. J Shoulder Elb Surg. 2003;12:237–41. https://doi.org/10.1016/s1058-2746(02)86883-5.
39. Calvo E, Valencia M, Foruria AM, Gonzalez JA. Recurrence of instability after Latarjet procedure: causes, results and treatment algorithm. EFORT Open Rev. 2022;7(12):800–7. https://doi.org/10.1530/EOR-22-0095.

25 The Failed Free Bone Graft

Taverna Ettore, Albizzini Ohin Caterina, Perfetti Carlo, and Guarrella Vincenzo

25.1 Understanding Arthroscopic Bone Block: An Overview

The gold standard for surgical treatment of shoulder instability is arthroscopic Bankart repair, which focuses on repairing the torn labrum and stabilizing the shoulder capsuloligamentous complex. Arthroscopic procedures have become the preferred approach for surgical stabilization of the shoulder due to their numerous benefits, including smaller incisions, less soft tissue dissection, better visualization of the joint, improved repair accessibility, and good clinical outcomes [1]. However, arthroscopic procedures have their limitations when it comes to treating glenoid bone loss in shoulder instability. The role of glenohumeral bone loss in shoulder instability and its impact on the success of soft tissue repairs. Glenoid bone loss reduces the ability of the glenoid to resist axial forces, making it difficult for a soft tissue repair alone to maintain stability. Glenoid bone loss is a common finding in cases of recurrent shoulder instability. It has been recognized as a risk factor for failure of standard soft tissue stabilization procedures. Biomechanical studies have shown that glenoid bone loss shortens the safe arc through which the glenoid can resist axial forces. This creates a destabilizing effect on the shoulder joint, increasing the risk of recurrent instability [1]. To overcome this problem, arthroscopic bone block procedure has been developed in order to allow arthroscopic bone grafting and concomitant soft tissue repair [2, 3] to restore stability in cases of glenoid bone loss. The arthroscopic bone block procedure involves the placement of a tricortical bone graft on the anterior glenoid rim, followed by soft tissue fixation on the anteroinferior glenoid rim. The aim of the arthroscopic bone block procedure is to achieve anatomic reconstruction of the unstable shoulder by fixing both bony and soft tissue lesions. Clinical and radiological results of this procedure show promise, but complications or failure can occur.

25.2 Analyzing the Causes of Failure in Bone Block Procedures

It is considered a failure of the bone block procedure an episode of recurrent instability of postoperative shoulder pain. If recurrent instability occurs, other surgical techniques such as a Latarjet procedure are typically performed to sta-

T. Ettore (✉)
Department of Shoulder Surgery, IRCCS OGSA—Ospedale Galeazzi Sant'Ambrogio, Milan, Italy
e-mail: Ettore.Taverna@eoc.ch; taverna@shoulder.it

A. O. Caterina
International Society of Arthroscopy, Knee Surgery and Orthopaedic Sports Medicine, Milan, Italy

P. Carlo · G. Vincenzo
IRCCS Istituto Ortopedico Galeazzi, Milan, Italy

E. Calvo et al. (eds.), *Complex and Revision Problems in Shoulder Instability*,
https://doi.org/10.1007/978-3-031-81389-4_25

bilize the shoulder. Failure of arthroscopic bone block procedures for shoulder instability can occur due to various reasons. As with any other surgical procedure, accurate indication and post-operative rehabilitation are crucial. Other common causes of failure are inadequate sizing and positioning of the bone graft. If the bone graft is not properly sized and positioned, it may not provide sufficient stability to the glenoid, leading to recurrent instability. Another cause of failure is improper fixation of the bone graft. If the graft is not securely fixed to the glenoid rim, it may dislodge or fail heal and provide adequate stability. Moreover, failure can also occur if there is inadequate soft tissue repair concomitant with the bone block procedure. Insufficient soft tissue repair may result in recurrent instability, even if the bone block is successfully placed [1]. Additionally, complications such as infection, graft resorption, graft nonunion, and hardware failure can determine the failure of arthroscopic bone block procedures.

25.2.1 Surgical Indication

It is important to carefully consider the indications for arthroscopic bone block procedures in cases of glenoid bone loss. Not every patient with glenoid bone loss will benefit from an arthroscopic bone block procedure. The arthroscopic bone block procedure is specifically designed for patients with recurrent anterior shoulder instability, young age, sportive activities, and bone defects. Indications for the bone block procedure include an ISIS score greater than 3, up to five shoulder dislocation episodes, glenoid bone loss exceeding 15% or over 10% with a concurrent Hill Sachs lesion, and the first dislocation occurring within 3 years [3]. Contraindications for the procedure include a history of failed previous surgery for shoulder instability, experiencing more than five episodes of shoulder dislocation, having above 20% glenoid bone loss, and chronic instability persisting for more than 3 years since the first episode. A glenoid bone defect greater than 20% is considered a contraindication for the arthroscopic bone block procedure because it may not be adequately covered by the size of the graft that can be introduced inside the joint using an arthroscopic approach. Good soft tissue quality is indicated by a limited duration of the pathology, a small number of dislocation episodes, and no history of failed soft tissue procedures.

25.2.2 Graft Sizing

The size of the bone defect and the size of the bone graft are significant factors in the success or failure of arthroscopic bone block procedures. If the bone defect is too large and the bone graft is not adequately sized to fill the defect, there may be instability and inadequate support for the joint. The size of the graft introduced arthroscopically is usually limited to about 2 cm in length and 1 cm in high and width this is usually sufficient to fill glenoid bone defect up to 20%. Larger defects may require open procedures or alternative techniques [2].

25.2.3 Graft Positioning

Graft positioning is also crucial for successful outcomes. The bone graft should be accurately positioned on the anterior inferior glenoid rim to provide optimal stability and support. The use of an arthroscopic guide to ensure precise placement of the bone graft can help in achieving the desired positioning on the horizontal plane and on the sagittal plane. Ideally the bone graft should be positioned so that it is flush with the glenoid surface and provides a smooth and stable transition for the humeral head during movement (Fig. 25.1a, b). On the sagittal plane, the graft should be positioned under the equator of the glenoid to provide optimal bone support and prevent excessive anterior inferior translation of the humeral head. Improper graft positioning—whether too high, too low, or too medial—is associated with a higher risk of shoulder instability recurrence. This can be attributed to the fact that incorrect positioning may not adequately address the underlying glenoid bone loss and

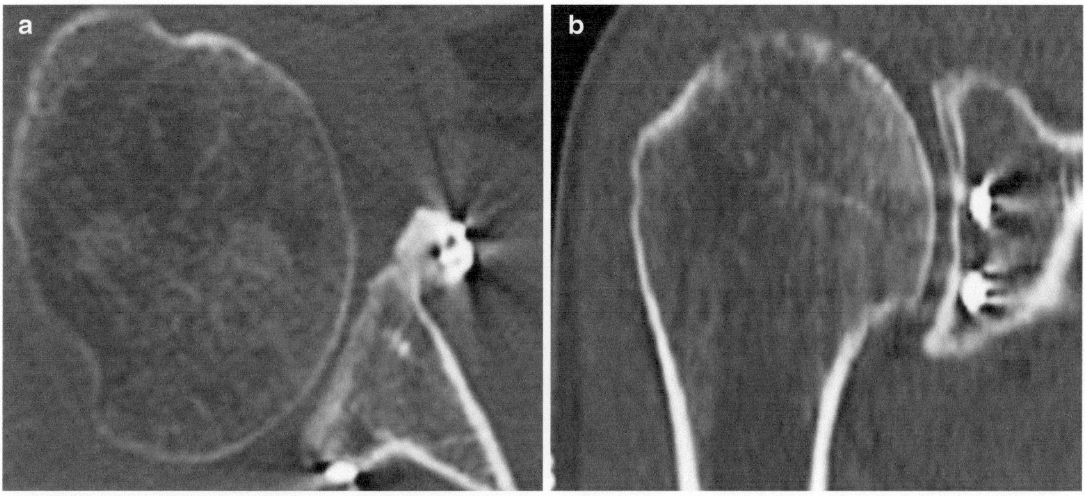

Fig. 25.1 (**a, b**) Bone graft correct position on the glenoid surface

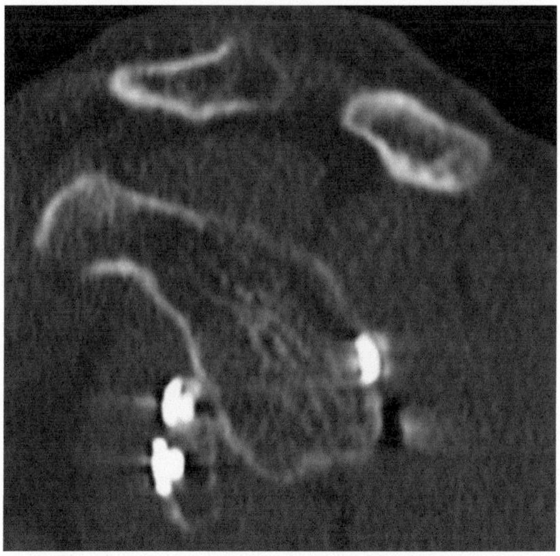

Fig. 25.2 Example of bone graft malpositioning

restore stability to the joint (Fig. 25.2). Residual pain and long-term degenerative arthritis of the glenohumeral joint are instead related to lateral positioning.

25.2.4 Fixation

In addition to positioning, fixation of the bone graft is essential for successful outcomes [4]. Improper fixation, such as inadequate tensioning or failure to secure the graft flush with the anterior glenoid rim, can lead to graft dislodgement or poor healing, resulting in failure or complications. Screw fixation can be used to secure the bone graft in place but are related to hardware complications. These complications can include graft fracture, nerve injury, vascular injury, and screw-related issues such as malpositioning or lysis around the screws leading to instability of the graft. Therefore, it is crucial for surgeons to choose a fixation technique that provides stability and promotes proper healing without compromising the integrity of the graft or risking complications (Fig. 25.3). Using arthroscopic Endobuttons fixation systems to secure the bone graft, tensioned with a tensioner device, can provide adequate tension for achieving graft healing while minimizing complications associated with screw fixation.

25.2.5 Graft Fracture

One of the potential complications associated with arthroscopic bone block procedures is graft fracture. Graft fracture can occur intraoperatively or postoperatively. Intraoperative graft fractures are primarily associated with improper surgical technique. To prevent this, it is crucial to create a flat glenoid graft surface and avoid excessive tension on the graft. A flat glenoid surface can be

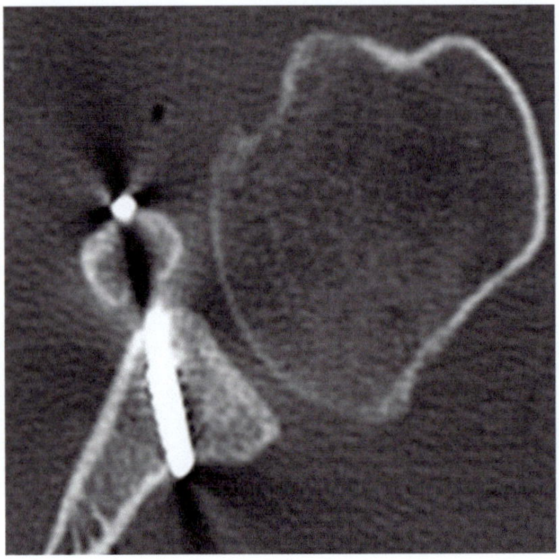

Fig. 25.3 Bone graft nonunion in Latarjet procedure with screw fixation

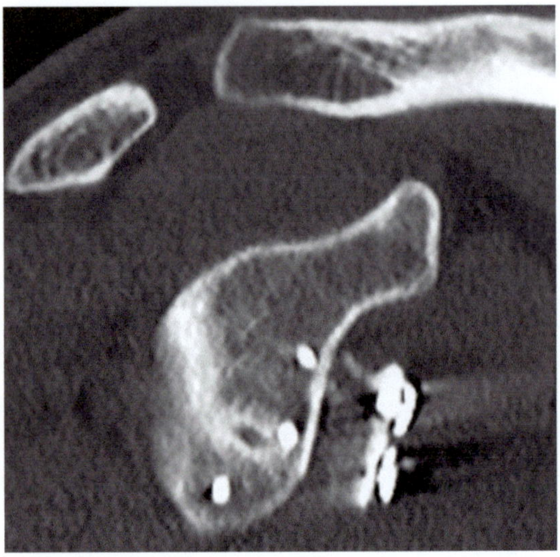

Fig. 25.4 Example of allograft nonunion

surgically achieved using a motorized shaver or bur to flatten the glenoid bone lesion. Additionally, a graduated tensioner device can help in preventing excessive tensioning (typically below 100 N/n). Postoperative graft fractures can be related to factors such as increased stress on the graft, poor bone quality, or inadequate fixation. Avoiding excessive stress on the graft during rehabilitation and ensuring proper bone healing can help minimize the risk of postoperative graft fractures.

25.2.6 Graft Healing (Nonunion)

Graft healing is also related to fixation, position, and to the type of graft implanted. Autografts, allografts, or xenografts are commonly used in arthroscopic bone block procedures [2, 5]. There is still debate over which type of graft provides the best outcomes. Some sources suggest that autografts, which involve using the patient's own bone tissue, may have better graft healing and incorporation compared to allografts or xenografts (Fig. 25.4). This is because autografts have a higher potential for osteogenic and osteoinductive properties, promoting faster and more efficient bone healing. Other sources argue that allografts and xenografts can be just as effective, if not more so, in promoting graft healing. There are advantages and disadvantages to each type of graft, and the choice ultimately depends on the surgeon's preference and the patient's individual factors such as bone quality, donor availability, and risk of complications [6].

25.2.7 Graft Resorption

Graft resorption is another complication that can lead to recurrent instability on a longer-term. Graft resorption is also related to graft positioning and fixation. If the graft is positioned in a wrong position, there is an increased risk of graft resorption (Fig. 25.5) [5] as it is not mechanically stimulated. Additionally, inadequate fixation of the graft can result in micromotion and increased resorption over time. The use of an arthroscopic guide and button fixation under tension can help minimize the risk of graft resorption by ensuring proper positioning and secure fixation of the graft. Graft type also influences the risk of graft resorption, as some studies have shown that autografts may have a lower risk of resorption compared to allografts or xenografts.

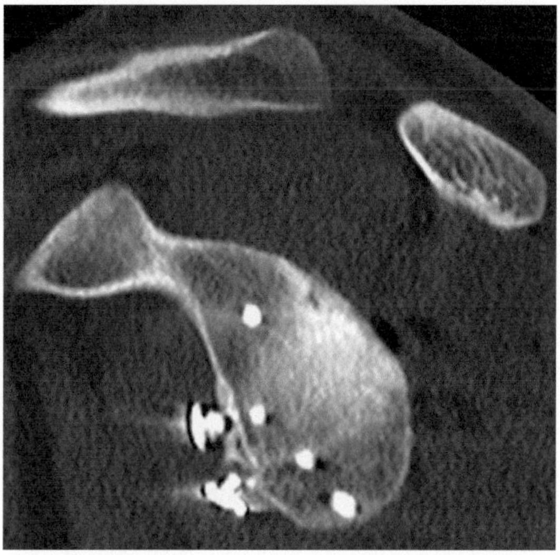

Fig. 25.5 Example of bone graft resorption

25.2.8 Soft Tissue Repair

In addition to bone graft healing, soft tissue repair plays a crucial role in achieving successful outcomes. Soft tissue repair involves reattaching and reinforcing the torn ligaments and capsule surrounding the shoulder joint. This helps to restore stability and prevent further dislocations or subluxations. The bone block procedure does not have the sling effect of the conjoint tendon, as seen in the Latarjet procedure. Therefore, an optimal soft tissue repair is recommended. The soft tissue repair also aims to leave the bone graft extra-articularly in order to minimize cartilage damage and reduce osteoarthritic changes.

25.2.9 Hardware-Related Complications

Hardware failure is another potential complication associated with bone block procedures for shoulder instability. This can occur due to factors such as improper screw placement, poor quality of screws or fixation devices, or excessive stress placed on the hardware. Screw placement can lead to suprascapular nerve injury or increased risk of osteoarthritis if the screws are angled too laterally and impinge on the articular surface of the glenoid. While screw breakage can occur due to various reasons, such as material fatigue or improper placement, it can significantly compromise the stability of the graft and increase the risk of recurrent instability. Furthermore, in case of graft resorption, screws can become uncovered by bone and lead to screw prominence, causing cartilage damage and discomfort and potentially requiring additional surgery for screw removal. Arthroscopic endobutton failures are mainly caused by technical mistakes, such as improper knotting of the sutures, insufficient tensioning of the sutures, or breakage of the sutures. This last complication can occur if the suture anchor drilling is performed after the metallic sleeves are removed from the glenoid tunnels. It is crucial to drill the holes for suture anchors while metallic sleeves are still in place [3].

25.2.10 Postoperative Rehabilitation

Postoperative rehabilitation plays a critical role in the success of bone block procedures for shoulder instability. Following surgery, the shoulder is typically immobilized in a sling for about 3 weeks. During this initial immobilization period, passive movement is allowed to prevent stiffness and promote healing. After the immobilization period, patients gradually regain full active range of motion. Strengthening exercises, especially focused on the rotator cuff muscles, are initiated after 8 weeks to improve stability and prevent re-dislocation. Patients are typically able to return to light daily activities within 6 weeks, return to sports or high-demand activities is allowed at 6 months. A trauma or early strengthening exercises can potentially compromise the healing process and result in graft failure or recurrent instability, especially if performed before complete passive range of movement is achieved.

25.3 Future Research

In order to improve the outcomes of arthroscopic bone block procedures for shoulder instability, it is important to continue researching and developing techniques that minimize complications and improve long-term stability. Areas of focus for future research include improving surgical techniques to easier arthroscopic bone grafting of the shoulder and developing new materials or graft options that promote bone integration and reduce bone resorption with sustainable costs.

References

1. Bauer S, Collin P, Zumstein MA, Neyton L, Blakeney WG. Current concepts in chronic traumatic anterior shoulder instability. EFORT Open Rev. 2023;8(6):468–81. https://doi.org/10.1530/eor-22-0084.
2. Taverna E, Golanó P, Pascale V, Battistella F. An arthroscopic bone graft procedure for treating anterior–inferior glenohumeral instability. Knee Surg Sports Traumatol Arthrosc. 2008;16(9):872–5. https://doi.org/10.1007/s00167-008-0541-y.
3. Taverna E, Garavaglia G, Perfetti C, Ufenast H, Sconfienza LM, Guarrella V. An arthroscopic bone block procedure is effective in restoring stability, allowing return to sports in cases of glenohumeral instability with glenoid bone deficiency. Knee Surg Sports Traumatol Arthrosc. 2018;26(12):3780–7. https://doi.org/10.1007/s00167-018-4921-7.
4. Jeon Y, Jeong HY, Lee DK, Rhee YG. Borderline glenoid bone defect in anterior shoulder instability: Latarjet procedure versus Bankart repair. Am J Sports Med. 2018;46(9):2170–6. https://doi.org/10.1177/0363546518776978.
5. Albizzini Ohin C, Guarrella V, Perfetti C, Larghi MM, Messina C, Sconfienza LM, Taverna E. CT-scan evaluation of osteointegration and osteolysis in different graft types and surgical techniques for the treatment of shoulder instability. Arch Bone Jt Surg. 2023;11(2):117–23.
6. Falbo R, Moore A, Singleton A, Steffenson A, Levine J, Miller RJ. Glenoid bone augmentation: a contemporary and comprehensive systematic review of open procedures. Orthop Rev (Pavia). 2022;14(3):37834. https://doi.org/10.52965/001c.37834.

26 The Failed Posterior Shoulder Stabilization

Gregory Hoy, Michael Blaser,
and Lukas Ernstbrunner

26.1 Introduction

The challenge in patients with posterior shoulder instability is recognizing the pathology and identifying the underlying cause resulting in an unstable glenohumeral joint. This is because clinical presentation is less obvious as compared to anterior instability and often includes only subtle signs of instability and or a painful shoulder [1, 2]. The other challenge is that posterior instability is often multifactorial, which can range from isolated postero-inferior labral tear, over postero-inferior glenoid and or antero-medial humeral head bone loss (reverse Hill-Sachs lesion), to a spectrum of capsular deficiency and developmental postero-inferior glenoid bony deficiency with or without excessive glenoid retroversion [3–5]. More recently abnormal acromial morphology has also been linked to posterior instability [6].

Arthroscopic stabilization is the considered gold-standard surgical treatment for symptomatic posterior instability and plays a role in both traumatic and atraumatic instability [7, 8]. Its popularity stems from its relative technical simplicity, reliable outcome in patients without significant bony pathology, and the relative complexity of bony surgery performed in the setting of posterior shoulder instability [9]. However, in those with underlying capsular deficiency or glenoid bone loss/dysplasia, failure rates of posterior stabilization are increased [10–14].

When encountering patients with failed posterior arthroscopic stabilization a thorough work-up is required to understand the underlying pathology leading to recurrent instability and ultimately guide surgical management. Besides ruling out known risk factors for failure such as female sex, younger age, and dominant shoulder involvement [11, 15, 16], 3D CT or MRI scans are effective in ruling out relevant glenoid-sided pathology [17]. Contrast MRI can be considered if there are concerns of capsular deficiency, and routine radiographs can be utilized to rule out abnormal acromial morphology [6, 18].

Surgical treatment of failed posterior shoulder stabilization can be challenging and is attempted to prevent further instability events, pain and secondary osteoarthritis. Revision arthroscopic stabilization is commonly performed if there is recurrent trauma with re-injury to the postero-inferior capsulolabral complex without underlying bony pathology [12, 19]. In the setting of capsular deficiency, multi-directional instability needs to be ruled out and surgical management

G. Hoy (✉)
Melbourne Orthopaedic Group, Monash University, Melbourne, VIC, Australia
e-mail: gahoy@mog.com.au

M. Blaser
Austin Hospital, Melbourne, VIC, Australia

L. Ernstbrunner
Reconstructive Orthopaedics Melbourne (ROM) & Box Hill Hospital, Eastern Health & University of Melbourne, Melbourne, VIC, Australia

E. Calvo et al. (eds.), *Complex and Revision Problems in Shoulder Instability*,
https://doi.org/10.1007/978-3-031-81389-4_26

may require 270° capsulolabral repair or even posterior capsular reconstruction [13, 19]. In those with bony abnormalities, ideally each of the pathology should be addressed individually; however, this can be technically challenging [5, 20–23]. Furthermore, certain techniques lack long-term results, therefore reliably predicting outcome can be difficult [24].

This book chapter aims to outline the importance of a thorough understanding of factors associated with failure of posterior shoulder stabilization, as well as the treatment options in this revision setting.

26.2 Work-Up

Arthroscopic posterior shoulder stabilization is a reliable treatment option for patients with posterior instability with a postoperative satisfaction rate of 90%, recurrence rate of less than 10% and revision rate of 5% [8]. However, these rates change dramatically at long-term follow-up, especially when concomitant pathologies such as capsular deficiency, glenoid- or humeral-sided bone loss, or glenoid dysplasia are missed in first place leading to failure rates around 45% [9, 10, 14, 25].

It remains a challenge defining reasons for failure following posterior shoulder stabilization. Utilizing clinical outcome scores is not useful, as they do not directly correlate with clinical failure [9, 11]. Therefore, pre-revision work-up should start with ruling out known risk factors for failure such as female sex, younger age, or involvement of the dominant shoulder [11, 15, 16]. Furthermore, technical factors have been identified to be associated with failure of posterior shoulder stabilization such as usage of less than three anchors [11].

Most consistently, glenoid bone loss has been linked to failure of posterior shoulder stabilization [10–12, 14]. With higher degrees of postero-inferior glenoid bone loss the higher the likelihood of repair failure. Biomechanical studies revealed that posterior shoulder stabilization in the setting of glenoid bone loss more than 20% will result in ongoing instability [26]. However, clinical data suggests that this threshold of critical glenoid bone loss is much lower: With 11% posterior glenoid bone loss failure of posterior shoulder stabilization is 10 times higher and with 15% bone loss it is 24 times higher [10]. In other words, there is a 44% failure rate of posterior shoulder stabilization when posterior glenoid bone loss exceeds 14% [14]. Three-dimensional CT or MRI scans are effective in ruling out relevant bony pathology and should therefore be part of a routine work-up [17].

Another factor to consider is excessive glenoid retroversion. It is known that soft tissue procedures are associated with inferior outcome when alterations of glenoid bony anatomy are present [3, 27, 28]. More specifically, there is biomechanical proof that posterior shoulder stabilization fails as soon as glenoid retroversion exceeds 10° [25].

Further comprehensive evaluation of advanced imaging should include analysis of posterior humeral head subluxation and glenoid dysplasia, a spectrum of developmental bony abnormality often associated with atraumatic posterior instability [3, 29]. Its spectrum includes deficiency of the postero-inferior bony glenoid, increased glenoid retroversion, increased capsular volume/deficiency and hyperplasia of the posterior labrum and cartilage [3, 30, 31]. While posterior humeral head subluxation, glenoid retroversion as well as deficiency of the postero-inferior bony glenoid can be assessed on 2D or 3D CT scans [31, 32], if there there are concerns of capsular deficiency contrast MRI might be required [18].

More recently, posterior shoulder instability has been linked to abnormal acromial morphology [6]. Posterior acromial morphology can be assessed on plain X-rays and should focus on excluding an acromion that is high-riding and flat in the sagittal plane, thus lacking osseous restraint against posterior humeral head translation. Further research is needed to determine whether surgical intervention in order to correct such abnormal acromial morphology is warranted.

26.3 Treatment Options

26.3.1 Non-operative Management

While physiotherapy focusing on scapular control and subscapularis-predominant strengthening exercises may be beneficial in the primary setting of posterior shoulder instability [33], there is little evidence that physiotherapy is useful in the setting of a failed posterior shoulder stabilization procedure.

26.3.2 Revision Arthroscopic Shoulder Stabilization

Revision arthroscopic shoulder stabilization has become more popular over the last years. However, there is limited evidence suggesting that this procedure reliably restores shoulder stability and reduces pain, albeit patients with failed posterior shoulder stabilization start with a poor functional and painful baseline thus representing a surgical challenge. Most recently pooled data suggests that persistent pain and recurrent instability after revision arthroscopic posterior shoulder stabilization are common and many patients are dissatisfied with their clinical outcome [12]. In 26 included patients, the failure rate for arthroscopic revision posterior shoulder stabilization was 30%, mainly due to recurrent instability or persistent pain, yet only 1 out of the 26 included patients required an additional surgical intervention. The poor outcomes associated with revision arthroscopic posterior shoulder stabilization pose a significant risk for high-functioning patients such as athletes. As such, only 68% of throwing and contact athletes reached their pre-injury level of sport [34]. As with any other orthopaedic stabilization procedure, the best way to avoid poor outcome is indicating the correct procedure at index presentation. It is therefore crucial to identify risk factors for failure as outlined above. Another key aspect is presence of preoperative symptoms. Similar to what has been observed with anterior instability patients [35], presence of preoperative disability was significantly linked to experiencing clinical failure postoperatively compared to those with instability alone [36]. This information is essential for patient selection, optimal treatment techniques, and patient education.

26.3.3 Posterior Capsular Surgery

A patulous or deficient capsule is often encountered in patients undergoing revision posterior shoulder stabilization [19, 37, 38]. May it be in isolation or as part of occult multi-directional instability primarily manifesting in the posterior direction, it appears that combined capsulolabral repair might be more appropriate than isolated labral repair for patients with risk factors for recurrent posterior instability.

Historically, the outcomes of open posterior capsular plication have been modest, with 31% reporting ongoing discomfort in their shoulder, 23% experiencing recurrent instability, and 21% had to change their profession because of the shouler [39]. With the advancement of arthroscopic shoulder surgery, results have improved and in those without bony pathology but persistent labral pathology and capsular deficiency arthroscopic posterior capsular plication in combination with labral repair became a powerful treatment modality, even in the revision setting [19]. Ideally, capsulolabral repair should include a 180–270° repair with four or more suture anchors.

Allograft capsular reconstruction is another option in the setting of failed posterior shoulder stabilization and might be considered in the setting of patulous or deficient capsule, ligamentous laxity or connective tissue disorder, or poor prognostic factors for failure [13, 40, 41]. Due to the significant variability in the clinical outcomes reported thus far, further research is necessary to clearly define the clinical outcomes in revision arthroscopic posterior stabilization.

26.3.4 Posterior Glenoid Bone Grafting

Bony procedures such as posterior glenoid bone grafting should be considered in those patients with posterior glenoid bone loss. It can be performed open or arthroscopically assisted, with allo- or auto-graft, and each of the described technique aims to widen the glenoid articular surface and increase the contact area for the humeral head [20, 23, 42–44].

Over the last decades, the difficulty with posterior glenoid bone grafting techniques has been defining its role within the complex spectrum of posterior shoulder instability. Outcome is usually predictable when used in traumatic posterior shoulder instability associated with glenoid bone loss and or a reverse Hill-Sachs lesion. Glenoid bone loss is also a known risk factor for failure of arthroscopic posterior shoulder stabilization [11, 45]. However, the role of posterior glenoid bone grafting in the revision setting is unclear and failure rates can be over 50% if not indicated correctly [23, 46].

26.3.5 Glenoid Osteotomy

Excessive glenoid retroversion is frequently observed in patients with posterior shoulder instability and soft-tissue procedures are associated with inferior outcome when alterations of glenoid bony anatomy are present [3, 27, 28]. Biomechanical studies suggest that posterior labral repair is insufficient to stabilize the humeral head when glenoid retroversion exceeds 10° [25].

Correcting glenoid retroversion can be done with an opening-wedge osteotomy as originally described by Scott [22]. The issue with the 'Scott-osteotomy' is that there is only limited follow-up and numbers, and those who described long-term results observed that instability persisted in 86% with similar pain levels as preoperatively, and glenohumeral degeneration was established in all patients included [5].

The author's preferred technique in the setting of excessive glenoid retroversion is therefore a recently introduced surgical technique which combines a posterior opening-wedge osteotomy with glenoid concavity reconstruction using an implant-free, J-shaped autograft iliac crest bone graft [21, 24]. The preliminary short-term results were promising; however, its role in general and specifically in the revision setting is yet to be established.

References

1. Boileau P, Zumstein M, Balg F, Penington S, Bicknell RT. The unstable painful shoulder (UPS) as a cause of pain from unrecognized anteroinferior instability in the young athlete. J Shoulder Elb Surg. 2011;20(1):98–106.
2. Fronek J, Warren RF, Bowen M. Posterior subluxation of the glenohumeral joint. J Bone Joint Surg Am. 1989;71(2):205–16.
3. Eichinger JK, Galvin JW, Grassbaugh JA, Parada SA, Li X. Glenoid dysplasia: pathophysiology, diagnosis, and management. J Bone Joint Surg Am. 2016;98(11):958–68.
4. Galvin JW, Morte DR, Grassbaugh JA, et al. Arthroscopic treatment of posterior shoulder instability in patients with and without glenoid dysplasia: a comparative outcomes analysis. J Shoulder Elb Surg. 2017;26(12):2103–9.
5. Waltenspul M, Haller T, Ernstbrunner L, et al. Long-term outcome after posterior opening glenoid wedge osteotomy for posterior shoulder instability associated with excessive glenoid retroversion. J Shoulder Elb Surg. 2022;31(1):81–9.
6. Meyer DC, Ernstbrunner L, Boyce G, et al. Posterior acromial morphology is significantly associated with posterior shoulder instability. J Bone Joint Surg Am. 2019;101(14):1253–60.
7. Arner JW, McClincy MP, Bradley JP. Arthroscopic stabilization of posterior shoulder instability is successful in American football players. Arthroscopy. 2015;31(8):1466–71.
8. Ralph J, Hurley E, Lunn K, et al. Outcomes of arthroscopic stabilization for posterior shoulder instability—a systematic review. J Shoulder Elb Surg. 2024;33(11):2530–8.
9. DeLong JM, Jiang K, Bradley JP. Posterior instability of the shoulder: a systematic review and meta-analysis of clinical outcomes. Am J Sports Med. 2015;43(7):1805–17.
10. Arner JW, Ruzbarsky JJ, Midtgaard K, et al. Defining critical glenoid bone loss in posterior shoulder capsulolabral repair. Am J Sports Med. 2021;49(8):2013–9.
11. Bradley JP, Arner JW, Jayakumar S, Vyas D. Risk factors and outcomes of revision arthroscopic posterior shoulder capsulolabral repair. Am J Sports Med. 2018;46(10):2457–65.
12. Jewett CA, Reardon P, Cox C, et al. Outcomes of revision arthroscopic posterior labral repair and capsulor-

rhaphy: a systematic review. Orthop J Sports Med. 2023;11(6):23259671231174474.
13. Karpyshyn J, Gordey EE, Coady CM, Wong IH. Posterior glenohumeral capsular reconstruction using an acellular dermal allograft. Arthrosc Tech. 2018;7(7):e739–45.
14. Wolfe JA, Elsenbeck M, Nappo K, et al. Effect of posterior glenoid bone loss and retroversion on arthroscopic posterior glenohumeral stabilization. Am J Sports Med. 2020;48(11):2621–7.
15. Asturias AM, Bastrom TP, Pennock AT, Edmonds EW. Posterior shoulder instability: surgical outcomes and risk of failure in adolescence. Am J Sports Med. 2020;48(5):1200–6.
16. Vaswani R, Arner J, Freiman H, Bradley JP. Risk factors for revision posterior shoulder stabilization in throwing athletes. Orthop J Sports Med. 2020;8(12):2325967120967652.
17. Dekker TJ, Peebles LA, Goldenberg BT, et al. Location of the glenoid defect in shoulders with recurrent posterior Glenohumeral instability. Am J Sports Med. 2019;47(13):3051–6.
18. Galvin JW, Parada SA, Li X, Eichinger JK. Critical findings on magnetic resonance arthrograms in posterior shoulder instability compared with an age-matched controlled cohort. Am J Sports Med. 2016;44(12):3222–9.
19. Chalmers PN, Hammond J, Juhan T, Romeo AA. Revision posterior shoulder stabilization. J Shoulder Elb Surg. 2013;22(9):1209–20.
20. Camenzind RS, Gossing L, Martin Becerra J, et al. Restoration of the posterior glenoid in recurrent posterior shoulder instability using an arthroscopically placed iliac crest bone graft: a computed tomography-based analysis. Orthop J Sports Med. 2021;9(1):2325967120976378.
21. Ernstbrunner L, Borbas P, Ker AM, et al. Biomechanical analysis of posterior open-wedge osteotomy and glenoid concavity reconstruction using an implant-free, J-shaped iliac crest bone graft. Am J Sports Med. 2022;50(14):3889–96.
22. Scott DJ Jr. Treatment of recurrent posterior dislocations of the shoulder by glenoplasty. Report of three cases. J Bone Joint Surg Am. 1967;49(3):471–6.
23. Villefort C, Stern C, Gerber C, et al. Mid-term to long-term results of open posterior bone block grafting in recurrent posterior shoulder instability: a clinical and CT-based analysis. JSES Int. 2023;7(2):211–7.
24. Ernstbrunner L, Haller T, Waltenspul M, Wieser K, Gerber C. Posterior open-wedge osteotomy and glenoid concavity reconstruction using an implant-free, J-shaped iliac crest bone graft in atraumatic posterior instability with pathologic glenoid retroversion and dysplasia: a preliminary report. Clin Orthop Relat Res. 2021;479(9):1995–2005.
25. Imhoff FB, Camenzind RS, Obopilwe E, et al. Glenoid retroversion is an important factor for humeral head centration and the biomechanics of posterior shoulder stability. Knee Surg Sports Traumatol Arthrosc. 2019;27(12):3952–61.
26. Nacca C, Gil JA, Badida R, Crisco JJ, Owens BD. Critical glenoid bone loss in posterior shoulder instability. Am J Sports Med. 2018;46(5):1058–63.
27. Gottschalk MB, Ghasem A, Todd D, et al. Posterior shoulder instability: does glenoid retroversion predict recurrence and contralateral instability? Arthroscopy. 2015;31(3):488–93.
28. Hurley JA, Anderson TE, Dear W, et al. Posterior shoulder instability. Surgical versus conservative results with evaluation of glenoid version. Am J Sports Med. 1992;20(4):396–400.
29. Landau JP, Hoenecke HR. Genetic and biomechanical determinants of glenoid version: implications for glenoid implant placement in shoulder arthroplasty. J Shoulder Elb Surg. 2009;18(4):661–7.
30. Harper KW, Helms CA, Haystead CM, Higgins LD. Glenoid dysplasia: incidence and association with posterior labral tears as evaluated on MRI. AJR Am J Roentgenol. 2005;184(3):984–8.
31. Weishaupt D, Zanetti M, Nyffeler RW, Gerber C, Hodler J. Posterior glenoid rim deficiency in recurrent (atraumatic) posterior shoulder instability. Skeletal Radiol. 2000;29(4):204–10.
32. Walch G, Boulahia A, Boileau P, Kempf JF. Primary glenohumeral osteoarthritis: clinical and radiographic classification. The Aequalis Group. Acta Orthop Belg. 1998;64(Suppl 2):46–52.
33. Watson L, Balster S, Lenssen R, Hoy G, Pizzari T. The effects of a conservative rehabilitation program for multidirectional instability of the shoulder. J Shoulder Elb Surg. 2018;27(1):104–11.
34. Gouveia K, Kay J, Memon M, et al. Return to sport after surgical management of posterior shoulder instability: a systematic review and meta-analysis. Am J Sports Med. 2022;50(3):845–57.
35. Zimmermann SM, Scheyerer MJ, Farshad M, et al. Long-term restoration of anterior shoulder stability: a retrospective analysis of arthroscopic Bankart repair versus open Latarjet procedure. J Bone Joint Surg Am. 2016;98(23):1954–61.
36. Chan S, O'Brien LK, Waterman BR, et al. Low risk of recurrence after posterior labral repair of the shoulder in a high-risk United States military population. Arthrosc Sports Med Rehabil. 2020;2(1):e47–52.
37. Bradley JP, Baker CL 3rd, Kline AJ, Armfield DR, Chhabra A. Arthroscopic capsulolabral reconstruction for posterior instability of the shoulder: a prospective study of 100 shoulders. Am J Sports Med. 2006;34(7):1061–71.
38. Provencher MT, LeClere LE, King S, et al. Posterior instability of the shoulder: diagnosis and management. Am J Sports Med. 2011;39(4):874–86.
39. Fuchs B, Jost B, Gerber C. Posterior-inferior capsular shift for the treatment of recurrent, voluntary posterior subluxation of the shoulder. J Bone Joint Surg Am. 2000;82(1):16–25.
40. Maloney MD, Schaffer JC, Kenney RJ. Arthroscopic posterior glenohumeral capsular augmentation with gracilis tendon allograft. Arthrosc Tech. 2019;8(11):e1277–82.

41. Sanders B, Norton C. Arthroscopic posterior capsulolabral reconstruction with gracilis allograft. Arthrosc Tech. 2022;11(7):e1261–7.
42. Frank RM, Shin J, Saccomanno MF, et al. Comparison of glenohumeral contact pressures and contact areas after posterior glenoid reconstruction with an iliac crest bone graft or distal tibial osteochondral allograft. Am J Sports Med. 2014;42(11):2574–82.
43. Nacca C, Gil JA, DeFroda SF, Badida R, Owens BD. Comparison of a distal tibial allograft and scapular spinal autograft for posterior shoulder instability with glenoid bone loss. Orthop J Sports Med. 2018;6(7):2325967118786697.
44. Wellmann M, Pastor MF, Ettinger M, Koester K, Smith T. Arthroscopic posterior bone block stabilization-early results of an effective procedure for the recurrent posterior instability. Knee Surg Sports Traumatol Arthrosc. 2018;26(1):292–8.
45. Bradley JP, Arner JW, Jayakumar S, Vyas D. Revision arthroscopic posterior shoulder capsulolabral repair in contact athletes: risk factors and outcomes. Arthroscopy. 2020;36(3):660–5.
46. Cognetti DJ, Hughes JD, Kay J, et al. Bone block augmentation of the posterior glenoid for recurrent posterior shoulder instability is associated with high rates of clinical failure: a systematic review. Arthroscopy. 2022;38(2):551–63.e555.

27 Neurovascular Complications, Stiffness, and Infection After Shoulder Stabilization

Miguel Angel Ruiz Iban,
Cristina Victoria Asenjo Gismero,
and Pablo Narbona

27.1 Introduction

Surgery for shoulder instability is generally considered as safe and effective. Most patients are young, active, and healthy, thus being less prone to complications. Furthermore, the surgical procedures (either arthroscopic or open) are considered to be reliable and safe. In general, major postoperative complication rates are well below 1% [1].

Despite of this, complications do arise after these procedures. The most frequent being recurrence of dislocation, subluxation, and residual apprehension. In patients undergoing bony procedures, complications related to the hardware used and bony complications might arise. To finish, chondral damage and degenerative changes often develop, not only in relation to the surgical procedures but also due to the natural history of the unstable shoulder. All these, relatively frequent complications, have been addressed in previous chapters.

The objective of this chapter is to review complications such as infection, stiffness, and neurovascular injury that, ranging in incidence from very uncommon to exotic, are a cause of significant concern to the surgeon. The physiopathology, etiology, epidemiology (Table 27.1), diagnosis, prevention (Table 27.2), and management of these complications will be discussed. Most of the information presented of these complications come from anterior instability literature. Being those infrequent complications, the information on its epidemiology and management in posterior instability or multidirectional instability is extraordinarily limited. Notwithstanding that, the information provided could probably be extrapolated to these specific cases. Furthermore, most of these complications have very low incidences, and most data presented below comes from systematic reviews and meta-analysis, which usually mix data from studies of very different quality, limiting the quality of the data presented.

M. A. Ruiz Iban (✉)
Unidad de Cirugía de Hombro y Codo, Madrid, Spain

Departamento de Cirugía, Ciencias Sanitarias Y Medicosociales, Universidad de Alcalá de Henares, Alcalá de Henares, Madrid, Spain

C. V. Asenjo Gismero
Hospital Beata Maria Ana, Madrid, Spain

P. Narbona
Sanatorio Allende, Cordoba, Argentina

E. Calvo et al. (eds.), *Complex and Revision Problems in Shoulder Instability*,
https://doi.org/10.1007/978-3-031-81389-4_27

Table 27.1 Incidence of complications after shoulder instability surgery

	Latarjet (%)	Arthroscopic Bankart (%)
Direct nerve injuries	0.7–0.9	0.014–0.2
Vascular complications	0.3	0
Stiffness	0.2–0.6	0.21
Infection	0.1–1.2	0

Table 27.2 Ten easy strategies to prevent complications in shoulder instability surgery

1. Develop anterior portals in an outside-in fashion (arthroscopic surgery)
2. Identify and protect the axillary nerve (open procedures and arthroscopic Latarjet)
3. Get proper training in complex procedures (using cadaveric specimens preferably)
4. Get appropriate help (or supervision) in initial cases
5. Use antibiotic prophylaxis
6. Use intraoperative cerebral oximetry monitoring with near-infrared spectroscopy (beach chair procedures)
7. Use mechanical prophylaxis for thromboembolic events
8. Consider chemical prophylaxis for thromboembolic events (procedures longer than 2 h and subjects with risk factors)
9. Use warming blankets
10. Consider warming of irrigation liquids (arthroscopic procedures longer than 2 h)

27.2 Neurological Complications

Perioperative nerve injuries are feared complications that have a low incidence. As the structures treated during shoulder instability surgery are in close contact to the brachial plexus and the axillary nerve, injuries at that level are not completely uncommon. There are many reasons for the development of a neurological symptom after a shoulder instability procedure: sometimes nerve damage is caused by the direct action of the surgeon in the surgical field, causing nerve damage by direct injury of the neural structure; in other cases the nerve lesion occurs in relation to the positioning of the patient or the traction applied to the upper extremity during surgery. In addition, if a nerve block is used as part of the anesthetic procedure, damage of the brachial plexus can develop. Finally, some patients will develop a distal neuropathy in relation to the surgical procedure.

The diagnostic approach to all these injuries, no matter the etiology, is similar: a thorough neurological assessment of the upper extremity is mandatory in the initial postoperative period [2]. This should include sensitive evaluation of all the major branches of the brachial plexus and motor assessment of the axillary, ulnar, radial, median, and musculocutaneous nerve. Immediate postoperative evaluation is often incomplete due to transient paresis or anesthesia related to the anesthetic procedures and might not be feasible before the patient is discharged; in these cases, discharge should not be delayed, but special attention must be taken to ensure that the exam is performed in the first outpatient visit.

If any clinical neurological deficit is present, it should be registered exhaustively in the clinical notes and a detailed assessment of the possible etiology should be made. When there is a reasonable suspicion that an acute intraoperative nerve injury occurred and the motor-sensory defect suggest a complete transection of a major nerve branch, or progressive changes are developing, advanced imaging procedures (MRI or CT scan) to identify compression hematomas or hardware problems are warranted; then the case for acute surgical exploration must be made. For partial or minor neurological deficits, repeated clinical assessment at the third week is necessary. At that time, if symptoms are not improving, electromyography and nerve conduction studies (NCS) allow for precise documentation the severity of the injury and help in determining the recovery prognosis.

27.2.1 Direct Intraoperative Nerve Injuries

Direct injury to nerve branches during shoulder instability surgery is relatively common. The axillary nerve courses form the brachial plexus posteriorly below the subscapularis in close vicinity to the inferior capsule and can be damaged during anterior bone bock procedures and during arthroscopic surgery that involves the inferior capsule, when sutures are placed in the inferior capsule, or when repairing capsular tears [3]. The suprascapular nerve, as it runs over the suprascapular notch and the posterior-superior glenoid neck can be damaged by hardware such as screws and buttons used in bony procedures. The musculocutaneous nerve is in close relation to the cojoined tendon and can be damaged during the Latarjet procedure. To finish, the complete brachial plexus is in relative proximity to the surgical field and can be inadvertently damaged by a stray medial portal or a misplaced medial retractor. The particular injuries caused and the incidence seem to be quite dependent on the specific surgical procedure so this needs to be analyzed specifically.

The transition from open Bankart repair to all-arthroscopic procedures has been associated with a significant reduction of the neurological complications. Owens et al. reported in an analysis of the data from the American Board of Orthopaedic Surgery certification examination a nerve injury rate of 0.3% after arthroscopic repair, significantly lower than open repair where an incidence of 2.2% was found [4]. This difference was also detected by Williams et al. in a systematic review, with open Bankart procedures having higher incidence of temporary nerve injury (0.5%) when compared to arthroscopic Bankart procedures (0.2%) [5]. This incidence of nerve damage after arthroscopic Bankart repair might be even lower as reported by Rodriguez et al. in an extensive systematic review on 14,000 procedures from 197 studies. They found a single case of musculocutaneous nerve injure (probably due to traction) and an isolated case of axillary nerve injury after arthroscopic Bankart repair (incidence of 0.014%).

Nerve injuries have seldom been reported after arthroscopic HAGL repair, Only one case of transient musculocutaneous nerve palsy was found by Grundstein et al. [6] in a comprehensive systematic review. Despite of this, the axillary nerve is in clear danger during repair, especially when dealing with the aIGHL in the beach chair position [7]. Careful positioning, particularly for the anterior-inferior 5 o'clock portal and posterior-inferior 7 o'clock portal, is necessary to prevent injuries of the axillary nerve and medial circumflex artery anteriorly or suprascapular and axillary nerve posteriorly.

The *remplissage* procedure is widely considered to be safe and void of neurological complications. In particular, direct nerve damage attributed to the *remplissage* technique has never been reported. A recent systematic review by Lazarides et al. of 570 remplissage procedures from seven studies showed only one case of transient ulnar neuritis (probably due to traction and solved conservatively) [8].

The Latarjet procedure, either arthroscopic or open, brings the surgeon in closer proximity to the musculocutaneous and axillary nerves. The suprascapular nerve can also be affected by the anterior screws if they are placed in an upward position [9].

There is no apparent difference in the risk of complications between the open Latarjet and the arthroscopic Latarjet: Hurley et al. in a systematic review on the topic found incidences of nerve injuries of 0.9% and 0.7% respectively [10]. Injuries affect more often the musculocutaneous nerve (30%) and the axillary nerve (13%), with suprascapular nerve injury developing only in arthroscopic procedures.

There are no reported cases of nerve injury in posterior instability procedures. However, a cadaver study alerts of the possibility of axillary nerve injury during posterior bone block surgery, particularly at the exit point of the K-wires [11]. To reduce the risk, wire and screw insertion should be parallel to the glenoid articular surface, while increased medial angulation with respect to the glenoid surface may heighten the risk.

Once a nerve injury is identified in the postoperative period, the management should be guided by the severity of the damage and the mechanism of injury [2]. A careful retrospective evaluation of the surgical procedure should be done and critical analysis of the surgical notes and video, if available, are warranted. Imaging studies might help in defining hardware related problems such as suprascapular nerve impingement. For most nerve injuries a "wait and see" strategy is best as most injuries are either compression or partial injuries and most will improve over time. However, if a complete transection of a major branch (mostly the axillary nerve during a Latarjet procedure) is suspected, or there is progression of symptoms, the case for surgical exploration, followed by direct repair with or without grafting should be made.

Prevention of these injuries should focus on improving the surgical technique. For arthroscopic procedures anterior portals should be made using an outside-in technique, paying utmost attention to medialmost portals [12]. Capsular repair should be done carefully and understanding the expected position of the axillary nerve (at least 10 mm away from the capsule, but often not much farther than that). During a Latarjet procedure, either arthroscopic or open, the axillary nerve should be identified and protected. The importance of proper training in complex procedures using cadaveric specimens preferably and appropriate supervision in the initial cases cannot be overemphasized.

27.2.2 Nerve Injuries Related to Patient Positioning and Traction

Both the lateral decubitus and the beach chair position are associated to intraoperative neurological complications associated to the position of the patient and the traction performed over the arm of the patient. Lateral femoral cutaneous nerve palsy can develop in up to 1.5% of patients operated in beach chair position [13]. It usually develops in subjects with high BMI, preexisting comorbidities and longer procedures. It is related to the flexion of the hip and the retraining straps used during positioning of the patient. It is often transient and usually resolves in less than 6 months. Brachial plexus injury associated with traction to the upper extremity is rare and often transient but affects between 0.2% and 2.5% of subject operated in lateral decubitus. Most reported injuries are transient musculocutaneous or ulnar nerve neuropraxia but one of the authors of this chapter (MRI) had an (unreported) case of a complete transient brachial plexus paresis [14].

27.2.3 Neurological Complications Related to the Anesthetic Procedure

Regional anesthesia techniques are increasingly used as part of the anesthetic procedure during shoulder instability surgery. These procedures, that apply anesthetic on the direct vicinity of major neurological structures, have an intrinsic risk of nerve injury that is often overlooked [15]. Postoperative paresthesia, sensory or motor deficit, and dyspnea are the usual symptoms and seem to develop in up to 10% of subjects when the nerve block procedure is performed under ultrasound guidance [16]. In most cases, symptoms resolve in the first postoperative month without lasting disability, suggesting milder cases of neuropraxia, but persistent nerve injury is present in 0.5% of shoulder procedures; these are consistent with structural injuries, axonotmesis, or neurotmesis, and can have more complex consequences [16]. The use of a suprascapular nerve block (as opposed to an interscalene nerve block) seems to reduce drastically the incidence of these events without major disadvantages regarding postoperative pain [17].

27.2.4 Distal Peripheral Neuropathies

The development of distal peripheral nerve injury remote to the surgical site is not terribly uncommon after shoulder surgery. The patients develop median or ulnar, or more rarely axillary, neuropathy in the following weeks or months after shoulder surgery. This is believed to be due to different reasons: prolonged sling immobilization, traction during surgery, use of compression sleeves or gravity-dependent edema due to arthroscopic fluid. Smith et al. identified in a systematic review four cases that developed after an arthroscopic labral repair. Most of these neuropathies resolve spontaneously but 17% might require a surgical release [15].

27.3 Vascular Complications

Two main vessels are at risk during either arthroscopic or open procedures during shoulder instability surgery: the cephalic vein and the axillary artery. The vascular safety of the arthroscopic portals was investigated by Meyer et al. [12] and found that anterior portals placed the cephalic vein at risk but were reasonably away from the axillary artery; they recommended an outside-in approach to establish them. More recently the development of the arthroscopic Latarjet technique has made common the use of anterior portals developed medially to the conjoint tendon; the transpectoral portal can damage the neurovascular structures, so care should be taken to place it in an outside-in fashion; with a relatively superficial trajectory at 45° toward the tip of the coracoid; and under visual control of the subdeltoid space [18]. During open surgery for instability the deltopectoral approach is commonly used and the cephalic vein is also at risk.

The incidence of vascular injuries during instability surgery is very low. Injury to the cephalic vein is seldom reported but is probably underreporting both in arthroscopic and open surgery. Injury to the axillary artery has never been reported during arthroscopic instability surgery and a recent systematic review including data from more than 14,000 shoulders from 194 studies failed to find any case of vascular complication [19]. There are some isolated descriptions of axillary artery damage during the Latarjet procedure: Griesser et al. in a systematic review of 1900 shoulders from 45 studies found five axillary pseudoaneurysms and one acute axillary artery laceration, for an incidence of 0.3% [20].

Acute intraoperative injuries of the cephalic vein are easily diagnosed during the procedure due to apparent bleeding in the surgical field or through the portal. These are easily solved with direct ligation of the cephalic vein. Inadvertent injuries might be a cause of postoperative hematoma formation, a complication that develops in 0.01% of Bankart procedures [19] and 0.7% of Latarjet procedures [21].

Axillary artery injuries can be identified during surgery, allowing for primary repair of the laceration or in cases with more severe injuries, interposition grafting. But more often, axillary artery injuries are identified in a delayed fashion, days to months after the index procedure, as pseudoaneurysms that can be properly diagnosed with the help of ultrasound and angiography [20]. Management usually required resection of the pseudoaneurysm, although endovascular repair is increasingly used.

27.4 Stiffness

Patients who undergo procedures for shoulder instability rarely have postoperative issues regarding symptomatic loss of range of motion. This is due to the association of two different factors: first, many unstable patients present some degree of hypermobility in the context of hyperlaxity, and mild loss of range of motion might go unnoticed or be better tolerated; second: loss of active external rotation is highly prevalent preoperatively in patients with symptomatic instability due to apprehension and postoperatively these patients are satisfied even if they do not regain full range of motion.

Despite of this, some shoulder instability procedures are, by design, looking for some restriction of the range of movement: the traditional open procedures that included a subscapularis plication, although now out of fashion, associated a restriction in external rotation and of the final range of motion in flexion and abduction. But contemporary soft tissue procedures, even when performed arthroscopically, do not only aim to correct the labral injury but associate some degree of capsular plication to correct for the plastic deformity of the inferior capsule. It is difficult to assess properly the degree of plication needed to avoid redislocation without causing secondary stiffness. The repair of humeral avulsions of the glenohumeral ligaments and the *remplissage* procedures also deal with the capsule and might cause stiffness. On the other hand. The bony procedures, particularly the Latarjet procedure, should not be associated with significant loss of range of motion but anterior scarring can reduce range of motion.

Patients undergoing arthroscopic Bankart capsule-labral repair might be at risk of increased postoperative stiffness, and Rodriguez et al. in a systematic review of the complications of Bankart repair that included data of 14,000 procedures from 197 studies, found a relatively low incidence of 0.21% [19]. Interestingly, different systematic reviews on the complications of the Latarjet find a variable incidence of postoperative stiffness: Cho et al. found an incidence of 0.6% in 2560 procedures from 35 studies [22]; but Arner found an incidence of 0.2% in 2831 cases coming from 72 studies [21]. To finish, arthroscopic Latarjet might reduce the incidence of this complication as Hurley et al., in a systematic review comparing open and arthroscopic Latarjet procedures, did not find any case of postoperative stiffness after 2140 arthroscopic Latarjet procedures [10].

There has been significant concern on the use of the *remplissage* procedure, as it might be associated with reduction of the range of motion in external rotation. The available biomechanical evidence is controversial (as recently summarized by Lazarides et al. [8]): Of the eight biomechanical studies analyzing the effect on external rotation of the *remplissage* procedure, only two found any relevant defects: Grimberg et al. analyzed the effect of the *remplissage* procedure in seven cadaveric shoulders and found a loss of a mean of 10° of external rotation compared to the intact shoulder [23]; Werner et al. found similar results [24]. The other six studies [8] did not find biomechanical evidence of loss of external rotation. In the clinical setting, Gouveia et al. performed a systematic review and found data on external rotation deficit in nine studies, analyzing 395 subjects; they found external rotation deficits that ranged from 4.5° to 14° [25]. Davis et al. meta-analyzed the data of six studies on external rotation deficit and found a mean defect of 3° in 0° of abduction and of 5° in 90° of abduction [26]. These defects do not seem to affect patient satisfaction or return to sport rates [25, 26], but might be relevant to subjects with specific sport related requirements such as goal keepers and baseball players. On the other hand, the reported external rotation deficit might be temporary as MacDonald et al. found that external rotation deficits present in subjects with remplissage performed in addition to a Bankart repair at 1 year follow-up seemed to disappear at 2 years follow-up [27].

The management of the postoperative stiff shoulder after shoulder instability procedures is especially difficult, and there is no relevant information on the literature to guide a specific treatment protocol. The authors prefer a very conservative approach with the focus placed on assisted self-applied physical therapy with appropriate pain management, adding intraarticular steroid injections if needed. Most patients evolve satisfactorily with time, improving even after the first postoperative year [27] and some degree of adaptation to the limitation can be expected. Surgery should be limited to very specific cases and delayed until after at least 9–12 months after surgery.

27.5 Infection

Infection is one of the most feared complications by shoulder surgeons as it presents significant diagnostic and therapeutic challenges. Although hematogenic dissemination is possible in delayed infections, in the context of postoperative infection, the surrounding skin is the habitual origin of the microorganism [28, 29]. As with other postoperative shoulder infections, the most common pathogens isolated are *Cutibacterium acnes* and coagulase-negative Staphylococci, accounting for more than 80% the infections [30]. These are normal commensal flora inhabiting the hair follicles and sebaceous glands of the shoulder and axilla, and they can be isolated from the shoulder skin in 40–74% of healthy individuals [28]. Known risk factors for postoperative infection of the shoulder are obesity, older age, male sex, and previous shoulder injections in the 3 months before surgery. Duration of surgery also seems to have a clear effect, as procedures lasting more than 45 min have a threefold risk of infection, and those lasting >90 min have a fourfold risk of infection compared to shorter procedures [31].

The incidence of postoperative infection seems to be heavily influenced by the type of procedure. The general incidence of infection after shoulder arthroscopy is believed to be around 0.2–1% but instability procedures seem to have a lower incidence. Furthermore, arthroscopic procedures have a very low infection rate: Williams et al. found, in a systematic review, that open Bankart procedures had a higher incidence of infection (1.4%) when compared to arthroscopic Bankart procedures (0.3%) [5], being this latter data in line with the results obtained by Rodriguez et al. who, in an extensive systematic review of the complications of Bankart repair that included data on 14,000 procedures from 197 studies, found a single case of superficial infection and no deep infections after arthroscopic Bankart repair.

The reported infection rate of the open Latarjet procedure varies between studies: two systematic reviews have found incidences of deep infection in this procedure to be between 0.1% [10] and 1.2% [22]. Performing this technique arthroscopically does not seem to affect the infection rate [32]. Anyway, it does seem that the risk of infection after open procedures is higher than that of arthroscopic Bankart repair as found by Goodloe et al. in an analysis of a large surgical database including almost 6000 arthroscopic Bankart procedures, 798 open Bankart procedures and 471 Latarjet procedures found that the infection risk was 7 times higher for open Bankart and 25 times higher for Latarjet procedure [1].

The main challenge of the management of this complication is obtaining an early diagnosis. Although sometimes the typical signs of infection (swelling, inflammation, pain fever or drainage) are present, these are not always evident: swelling is found in 68% of cases, wound secretion is found in 50% of cases and fever in only 32% of cases [33]; most of the time the only clinical signs of infection are pain and loss of range of motion. Both these symptoms are frequent after shoulder surgery and discriminating between a normal postoperative course that presents with higher than usual inflammation and pain, and an infectious complication, is often difficult. Thus, the threshold for obtaining blood tests, performing further imaging and doing aspiration studies should be low [28]. Anyway, the diagnosis is often delayed, and Athwal et al. performed the initial debridement in his case series of infections after rotator cuff repair a mean of 49 days after the index procedure [34].

The blood workup should include a white blood cell count (that increases only in 12% of infections), erythrocyte sedimentation rate (elevated in 50% of cases), and C reactive protein (elevated in 50% of cases [34]). Computed tomogram scans and magnetic resonance imaging might play a role in identifying nonevident collections (Fig. 27.1), but ultrasound in this setting is especially useful as it is readily available and allows for guided aspiration of any collection found. Aspiration is essential if clinical and analytic findings support the diagnosis of infection as cell count and gram staining of the obtained liquid can help in the diagnosis: a white cell count greater than 20,000/μL, indicates a high probability of an infectious event [29]. Gram staining has a relative low yield but should always be performed, as it can quickly guide antibiotic therapy.

Once the diagnosis of periarticular infection is stablished, treatment should be started as soon as possible. For subjects with superficial infections, oral antibiotics might be enough; but, if a deep infection is suspected, surgical debridement with copious lavage and wide spectrum antibiotic therapy is mandatory. Antibiotic treatment can be delayed until the surgical procedure is performed and more samples for culture are obtained. If the initial procedure was arthroscopic, an arthroscopic lavage with careful assessment and lavage of both the glenohumeral and subacromial space is a good alternative, but an open procedure is also an option. A key step in this procedure is to obtain proper samples for microbiological and pathologic assessment: at least three to five samples should be sent for culture and some samples should be sent also for pathology. Care should be taken to obtain the microbiology samples avoiding possible skin contamination using a new unused instrument to pick each sample and avoiding skin contact with the help of a cannula. After instability surgery, the quandary is to decide on hardware removal as this will clearly compro-

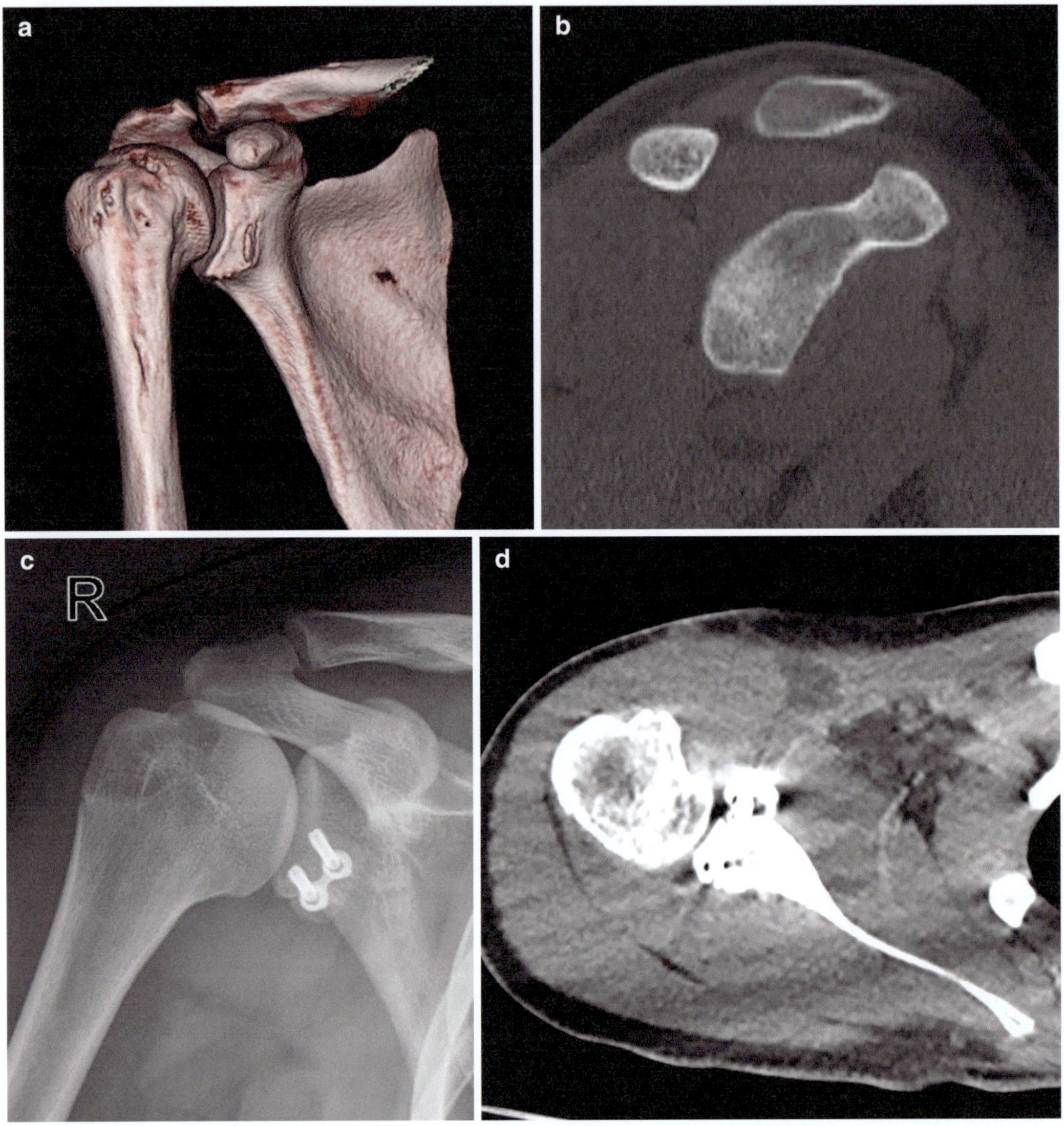

Fig. 27.1 A 15-year-old high-level athlete presented with recurrent anterior shoulder dislocation and a large anterior bone defect (**a, b**). HE underwent an initially successful open Latarjet procedure (**c**). Local inflammation and fever developed 4 weeks after the initial surgery. The scan shows a clear collection in direct relation to the coracoid graft (**d**)

mise the outcome of the initial procedure. There is no clear guidance in the literature [29–30, 34], but the current practice of the authors of this chapter is to retain the hardware in the initial debridement and lavage and consider removal of these if the initial debridement is not successful and the pathogens identified are multiresistant.

After surgical debridement and lavage, empirical antibiotic therapy should be started immediately after samples are obtained. The empiric antibiotic regime should be aggressive. A combination of two wide spectrum antibiotics, one effective against gram-positive microorganisms (such as vancomycin or daptomycin) and another effective against gram-negative pathogens (usually a third-generation cephalosporin such as ceftazidime or cefotaxime), is recommended, but consultation with a musculoskeletal infection disease specialist would be ideal. Once culture information is retrieved, the antibiotic protocol can be adjusted and oral alternatives are often available, as antibiotic treatment should be kept for at least 6–8 weeks, in particular if hardware removal was not performed. A high alert should be kept during the first 4 weeks, and frequent analytic workups should be done to confirm reduction of acute reactant levels. A low threshold should be kept for repeating surgical exploration as it is often needed: Athwal et al. found that in their cases series of infected rotator cuff repairs, a mean of three procedures were needed to eradicate infection.

Infection management should start with prevention. Antibiotic prophylaxis is common practice around the world and has shown to be effective in reducing postoperative infection after arthroscopic shoulder surgery: Randelli et al. in a survey of Italian surgeons found that it reduced infection rates from 0.6% to 0.01%. The habitual antibiotics used for prophylaxis (cephazolin or amoxicillin-clavulanic acid) are usually effective against *C. acnes* and coagulase-negative Staphylococci, so there is no need to stray away from the standard protocol. Controversy exists on the usefulness of preoperative topical decolonization of the skin: different studies have shown efficacy of topical disinfectant in reducing colonization, but no studies have shown efficacy in reducing infection rates [28, 29].

27.6 Postage Stamp Fracture

Anterior glenoid rim fractures (the so-called postage stamp fractures, Fig. 27.2) are a potential complication after suture anchor technique during arthroscopic Bankart repair. The fracture develops after a recurrence of the anterior instability, the fracture line propagating through the previous anchor sites, producing a serrated edge that resembles a postage stamp [35]. Technical factors such as anchor positioning, distance between anchors, angle placement and material have been suggested to create a stress riser that may precipitate a postage stamp fracture [36]. The material composition of the anchors used for Bankart repair can affect the incidence of this complication, as the use of bioabsorbable anchors might cause cyst formation or osteolysis (anchor hole enlargement) causing a weakness in the anterior margin of the glenoid; but these postage stamp fractures have been shown to develop also in subjects treated with titanium anchors; furthermore, all-suture anchors can an cause tunnel

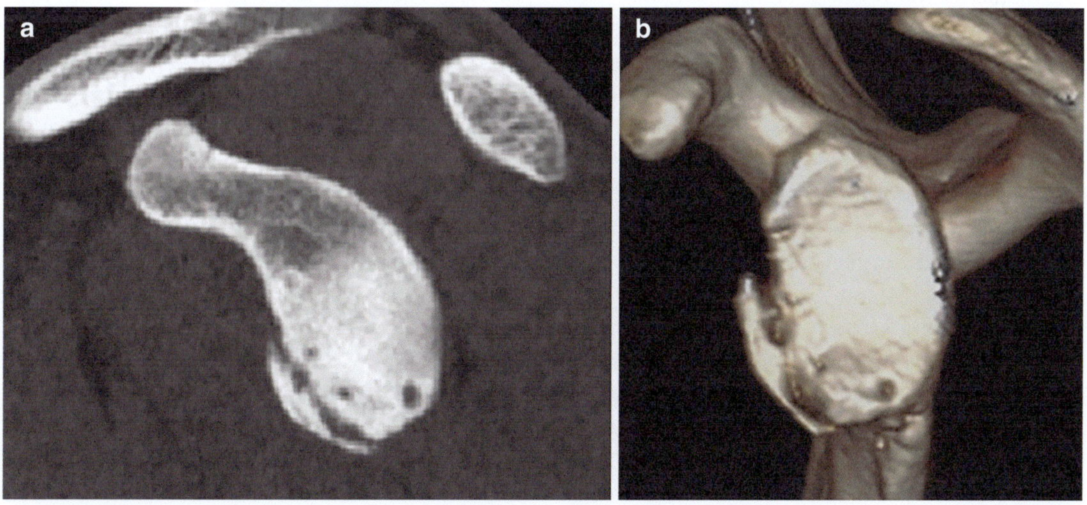

Fig. 27.2 Computed tomogram scan (**a**) and three-dimensional reconstruction (**b**) of a subject who sustained a postage-stamp fracture of the anterior glenoid rim after a minor trauma 12 months after an arthroscopic Bankart procedure with bioabsorbable anchors

enlargement [37].A larger number of anchors used to repair the Bankart lesion can increase the chances of fracture development as if the anchors cause holes in close proximity, the stress may be concentrated along the line of weakness, causing a fracture, this has shown to be true in a recent biomechanical study by Lobao et al. that also showed that larger diameter anchors lowered the mechanical threshold for fracture [38]. Woolnough et al. performed a systematic review on the characteristics of subjects that suffered a postage stamp fracture after a Bankart stabilization, including 43 subjects from six different studies. The fractures were reported more frequently in younger male patients, involved in sporting activities and in which the Bankart repair was performed with three or more anchors; osteolysis at the anchor sites was also a risk factor and fractures usually developed in the first 2 years after surgery [39].

The incidence of this complication is unknown, but it seems to be relatively rare: in a comprehensive systematic review on the complications of Bankart repair that included 14,000 shoulders from 196 studies, Rodriguez et al. found only five cases coming from a single study, for a incidence of 0.04% [19]. In contrast, in a retrospective (unpublished) case series by one of the authors of this chapter (PN) the incidence of postage stamp fractures was 2.1% (eight cases in 379 patients had undergone primary isolated arthroscopic Bankart repair). In all cases, the fracture was associated to a traumatic incident. In six patients, bioabsorbable anchors were used during primary surgery while titanium knotted anchors were used in the remaining two patients. The delay between initial surgery and the fracture was between 9 months and 7.5 years.

To diagnose a glenoid rim fracture, the gold standard is a computed tomogram with three-dimensional reconstruction (3D CT scan); while MRI might give important information about the healing of the initial Bankart repair. The 3D CT allows precise measurement of the fracture fragment and allows for the assessment of the viability of a potential fracture reconstruction technique or a bone supplementation procedure.

There are many alternatives to manage an anterior glenoid rim fracture after a failed Bankart repair. A Latarjet procedure with resection of the fractured rim seems to yield good results and was used successfully in three competitive athletes treated by Banerjee atlt al [35]; this was also the treatment of choice in 26% of cases in the systematic review of Woolnough et al. This is the treatment of choice when there is significant glenoid bone loss and the rim fracture is deemed irreparable. Other alternatives include repair of the fracture with anchors, using an arthroscopic Bankart Bridge repair technique as described by Millet et al. [40], which was the treatment of choice of 41% of cases in the systematic review of Woolnough et al. Other less common options, include fragment resection followed by Bankart repair or fracture fixation with percutaneous screws [41].

27.7 Other Complications

27.7.1 Cerebrovascular Events

Catastrophic neurological injuries related to cerebral hypoperfusion (stroke, blindness, brain death, and even death) are extremely rare conditions that are often associated to the beach chair position. These events have dramatic social, economic, professional, and medicolegal implications. Positioning the patient in beach chair position is associated with the development of hypotensive episodes and frequently hypotensive anesthesia is required to lower bleeding and improve visibility during arthroscopic procedures. Furthermore, even when peripheral blood pressure is maintained, the beach chair position is associated with cerebral hypoperfusion related to different, not completely understood mechanisms [42, 43].

The incidence of these complications is very low. Friedman et al. performed a survey among 93 members of the American Shoulder and Elbow Surgeons and found only eight cases, all occurred during surgery in beach chair position, in an estimated 200.000 shoulder procedures in this position, an incidence of 0.004% [44]. A systematic review produced a similar figure of 0.004% incidence [45].

Thc focus in this casc should bc placed in prevention: for most subjects undergoing instability surgery in the beach chair position, the use of intraoperative cerebral oximetry monitoring using near-infrared spectroscopy should be considered. Although its true efficacy is disputed [42], it is used extensively as it is noninvasive, easy to use, has relatively low cost, and is widely available, furthermore the current literature suggests that its use may improve patient safety [43].

27.7.2 Venous Thromboembolic Events

Venous thromboembolic events are rare after surgery for shoulder instability. The general incidence of venous thromboembolism for shoulder arthroplasty and arthroscopy is 0.65% and 0.01%, respectively [46]. A recent systematic review including more than 30,000 subjects undergoing shoulder arthroscopy found a incidence for venous thromboembolism and pulmonary embolism of 0.15% and 0.08% [47], but these rates are probably lower for instability arthroscopic surgery as the type of patients operated on rarely have the risk factors associated with thromboembolic disease (older age, comorbidities, obesity, and previous thromboembolic events). For the Latarjet procedure, Hurley et al. found a thromboembolic event incidence of 0.06% after open Latarjet procedure in a systematic review that included data on more than 5000 cases from 74 studies [10]. It seems that the risk of this complication is increased in the Latarjet procedure when compared to arthroscopic Bankart repair: Goodloe et al. studied a database of more than 7000 subjects undergoing shoulder stabilization procedures and found that the incidence of deep venous thrombosis was 0.1% for arthroscopic Bankart repair and 0.8% for Latarjet-Bristow [1].

The focus in this case should be placed again in prevention: for most subjects undergoing instability surgery mechanical prophylaxis (early mobilization and compression stockings) will be enough, but chemical prophylaxis might be needed for longer procedures (>2 h) and subjects with the abovementioned risk factors [47].

27.7.3 Hypothermia

Perioperative hypothermia (defined as a drop of core temperature below 35°) develops often in shoulder surgical procedures, with incidences around 50% after arthroscopic surgery and arthroplasty [48, 49]. Hypothermia has well known deleterious effects such as increasing infection rates, cardiac events, coagulopathy, and bleeding. It also prolongs hospital stay and full recovery time. Most often the only symptom observed is patient shivering, which is an extremely unpleasant sensation and is a leading cause of postoperative discomfort [50]. Prevention of hypothermia is essential and is based on active warming of the subject with air blankets but might not be enough; warming of the irrigation liquids is an effective intervention and the use of nerve blocks instead of general anesthesia can also be of help.

27.7.4 Heterotopic Ossifications

Heterotopic ossification is rarely a problem after shoulder surgery, although it can develop after shoulder arthroplasty. After arthroscopic surgery, the rare case reports and small series presented in the literature refer to subjects treated for subacromial problems and acromioclavicular joint injuries [51], but no cases of heterotopic ossification are presented in the larger, most recent, systematics reviews after open or arthroscopic stabilization [19, 22].

27.8 Conclusions

Infection, neurovascular injury, and other general complications are rare after shoulder instability surgery. The precise incidence depends on the specific procedure performed, but, in general, the transition from open to arthroscopic Bankart repair has lowered the complications rate. The

Latarjet procedure seems to be slightly riskier regarding the abovementioned complications.

Nerve injuries develop in relation to direct nerve injury, due to improper positioning or traction, or in relation with the anesthetic procedure. A careful postoperative neurological assessment is necessary to identify these injuries soon and define the ethiology, this will guide further management.

Infection is specially challenging as diagnosis can often be difficult and the success of treatment is time sensitive. A diagnostic work-up, including blood tests and imaging can help distinguish between a rocky postoperative course and a deep infection and the threshold to perform those should be low. If deep infection is suspected, surgical treatment should be considered immediately, and the antibiotic treatment, started after proper sampling of the infected tissue, should be based in the habitual flora present in these infections.

General complications such as thromboembolic or cerebrovascular events and hypothermia can also develop in shoulder instability subjects. For these problems, the focus should be placed in prevention.

References

1. Goodloe JB, Traven SA, Johnson CA, Woolf SK, Nutting JT, Slone HS. Increased risk of short-term complications and venous thromboembolism in Latarjet-Bristow procedures compared with Bankart repairs. Arthroscopy. 2021;37(3):806–13. https://doi.org/10.1016/j.arthro.2020.10.039.
2. Leland DP, Pareek A, Therrien E, Wilbur RR, Stuart MJ, Krych AJ, et al. Neurological complications following arthroscopic and related sports surgery: prevention, work-up, and treatment. Sports Med Arthrosc Rev. 2022;30(1):e1–8. https://doi.org/10.1097/JSA.0000000000000322.
3. Matsuki K, Sugaya H. Complications after arthroscopic labral repair for shoulder instability. Curr Rev Musculoskelet Med. 2015;8(1):53–8. https://doi.org/10.1007/s12178-014-9248-5.
4. Owens BD, Harrast JJ, Hurwitz SR, Thompson TL, Wolf JM. Surgical trends in Bankart repair: an analysis of data from the American Board of Orthopaedic Surgery certification examination. Am J Sports Med. 2011;39(9):1865–9. https://doi.org/10.1177/0363546511406869.
5. Williams HLM, Evans JP, Furness ND, Smith CD. It's not all about redislocation: a systematic review of complications after anterior shoulder stabilization surgery. Am J Sports Med. 2019;47(13):3277–83. https://doi.org/10.1177/0363546518810711.
6. Grundshtein A, Kazum E, Chechik O, Dolkart O, Rath E, Bivas A, et al. Arthroscopic repair of humeral avulsion of glenohumeral ligament lesions: outcomes at 2-year follow-up. Orthop J Sports Med. 2021;9(6):23259671211004968. https://doi.org/10.1177/23259671211004968.
7. Cuellar A, Cuellar R, Jorge DH, Cuellar A, Ruiz-Iban MA. Effect of patient positioning in axillary nerve safety during arthroscopic inferior glenohumeral ligament plication. Knee Surg Sports Traumatol Arthrosc. 2017;25(10):3279–84. https://doi.org/10.1007/s00167-016-4193-z.
8. Lazarides AL, Duchman KR, Ledbetter L, Riboh JC, Garrigues GE. Arthroscopic remplissage for anterior shoulder instability: a systematic review of clinical and biomechanical studies. Arthroscopy. 2019;35(2):617–28. https://doi.org/10.1016/j.arthro.2018.09.029.
9. Sastre S, Peidro L, Mendez A, Calvo E. Suprascapular nerve palsy after arthroscopic Latarjet procedure: a case report and review of literature. Knee Surg Sports Traumatol Arthrosc. 2016;24(2):601–3. https://doi.org/10.1007/s00167-014-3075-5.
10. Hurley ET, Schwartz LB, Mojica ES, Campbell KA, Matache BA, Meislin RJ, et al. Short-term complications of the Latarjet procedure: a systematic review. J Shoulder Elb Surg. 2021;30(7):1693–9. https://doi.org/10.1016/j.jse.2021.01.024.
11. Valencia Mora M, Martinez Menduina A, Hernandez Galera C, Perez Exposito R, Aramberri GM. Risk of neurological injury in posterior bone block surgery for recurrent glenohumeral instability: a cadaveric study. Arch Orthop Trauma Surg. 2018;138(12):1719–24. https://doi.org/10.1007/s00402-018-2986-x.
12. Meyer M, Graveleau N, Hardy P, Landreau P. Anatomic risks of shoulder arthroscopy portals: anatomic cadaveric study of 12 portals. Arthroscopy. 2007;23(5):529–36. https://doi.org/10.1016/j.arthro.2006.12.022.
13. Holtzman AJ, Glezos CD, Feit EJ, Gruson KI. Prevalence and risk factors for lateral femoral cutaneous nerve palsy in the beach chair position. Arthroscopy. 2017;33(11):1958–62. https://doi.org/10.1016/j.arthro.2017.06.050.
14. Li X, Eichinger JK, Hartshorn T, Zhou H, Matzkin EG, Warner JP. A comparison of the lateral decubitus and beach-chair positions for shoulder surgery: advantages and complications. J Am Acad Orthop Surg. 2015;23(1):18–28. https://doi.org/10.5435/jaaos-23-01-18.
15. Smith RDJ, Wright CL, Shaw B, Bhai S, Bhashyam AR, O'Donnell EA. Peripheral neuropathies after shoulder arthroscopy: a systematic review. JSES Rev Rep Tech. 2023;3(4):454–60. https://doi.org/10.1016/j.xrrt.2023.07.001.

16. Silverstein ML, Tevlin R, Higgins KE, Pedreira R, Curtin C. Peripheral nerve injury after upper-extremity surgery performed under regional Anesthesia: a systematic review. J Hand Surg Glob Online. 2022;4(4):201–7. https://doi.org/10.1016/j.jhsg.2022.04.011.
17. Hussain N, Goldar G, Ragina N, Banfield L, Laffey JG, Abdallah FW. Suprascapular and Interscalene nerve block for shoulder surgery: a systematic review and meta-analysis. Anesthesiology. 2017;127(6):998–1013. https://doi.org/10.1097/ALN.0000000000001894.
18. Boileau P, Lemmex DB. Editorial commentary: the shoulder transpectoralis portal for arthroscopic Latarjet: medial to the coracoid can also be a safe side! Arthroscopy. 2021;37(2):477–9. https://doi.org/10.1016/j.arthro.2020.12.177.
19. Rodriguez K, Hurley ET, Park CN, Bulleit C, Levin JM, Klifto CS, et al. Complications following arthroscopic Bankart repair: a systematic review. J Shoulder Elb Surg. 2024;33(2):435–40. https://doi.org/10.1016/j.jse.2023.08.013.
20. Griesser MJ, Harris JD, McCoy BW, Hussain WM, Jones MH, Bishop JY, et al. Complications and re-operations after Bristow-Latarjet shoulder stabilization: a systematic review. J Shoulder Elb Surg. 2013;22(2):286–92. https://doi.org/10.1016/j.jse.2012.09.009.
21. Arner JW, Tanghe K, Shields T, Abdelaziz A, Lee S, Peebles L, et al. Shoulder Latarjet surgery shows wide variation in reported indications, techniques, perioperative treatment, and definition of outcomes, complications, and failure: a systematic review. Arthroscopy. 2022;38(2):522–38. https://doi.org/10.1016/j.arthro.2021.09.020.
22. Cho CH, Na SS, Choi BC, Kim DH. Complications related to Latarjet shoulder stabilization: a systematic review. Am J Sports Med. 2023;51(1):263–70. https://doi.org/10.1177/03635465211042314.
23. Grimberg J, Diop A, Bou Ghosn R, Lanari D, Canonne A, Maurel N. Bankart repair versus Bankart repair plus remplissage: an in vitro biomechanical comparative study. Knee Surg Sports Traumatol Arthrosc. 2016;24(2):374–80. https://doi.org/10.1007/s00167-014-3052-z.
24. Werner BC, Chen X, Camp CL, Kontaxis A, Dines JS, Gulotta LV. Medial posterior capsular plication reduces anterior shoulder instability similar to remplissage without restricting motion in the setting of an engaging Hill-Sachs defect. Am J Sports Med. 2017;45(9):1982–9. https://doi.org/10.1177/0363546517700860.
25. Gouveia K, Harbour E, Athwal GS, Khan M. Return to sport after arthroscopic Bankart repair with remplissage: a systematic review. Arthroscopy. 2023;39(4):1046–59.e3. https://doi.org/10.1016/j.arthro.2022.12.032.
26. Davis WH, DiPasquale JA, Patel RK, Sandler AB, Scanaliato JP, Dunn JC, et al. Arthroscopic remplissage combined with Bankart repair results in a higher rate of return to sport in athletes compared with Bankart repair alone or the Latarjet procedure: a systematic review and meta-analysis. Am J Sports Med. 2023;51(12):3304–12. https://doi.org/10.1177/03635465221138559.
27. MacDonald P, McRae S, Old J, Marsh J, Dubberley J, Stranges G, et al. Arthroscopic Bankart repair with and without arthroscopic infraspinatus remplissage in anterior shoulder instability with a hill-Sachs defect: a randomized controlled trial. J Shoulder Elb Surg. 2021;30(6):1288–98. https://doi.org/10.1016/j.jse.2020.11.013.
28. Sircana G, Passiatore M, Capasso L, Saccomanno MF, Maccauro G. Infections in arthroscopy. Eur Rev Med Pharmacol Sci. 2019;23(2 Suppl):279–87. https://doi.org/10.26355/eurrev_201904_17502.
29. Voss A, Pfeifer CG, Kerschbaum M, Rupp M, Angele P, Alt V. Post-operative septic arthritis after arthroscopy: modern diagnostic and therapeutic concepts. Knee Surg Sports Traumatol Arthrosc. 2021;29(10):3149–58. https://doi.org/10.1007/s00167-021-06525-8.
30. Atesok K, MacDonald P, Leiter J, McRae S, Stranges G, Old J. Postoperative deep shoulder infections following rotator cuff repair. World J Orthop. 2017;8(8):612–8. https://doi.org/10.5312/wjo.v8.i8.612.
31. Yeranosian MG, Arshi A, Terrell RD, Wang JC, McAllister DR, Petrigliano FA. Incidence of acute postoperative infections requiring reoperation after arthroscopic shoulder surgery. Am J Sports Med. 2014;42(2):437–41. https://doi.org/10.1177/0363546513510686.
32. Deng Z, Zheng Y, Su J, Chen S, Deng Z, Zhu W, et al. Open versus arthroscopic Latarjet for recurrent anterior shoulder instability: a systematic review and meta-analysis. Orthop J Sports Med. 2023;11(5):23259671231174476. https://doi.org/10.1177/23259671231174476.
33. Pauzenberger L, Grieb A, Hexel M, Laky B, Anderl W, Heuberer P. Infections following arthroscopic rotator cuff repair: incidence, risk factors, and prophylaxis. Knee Surg Sports Traumatol Arthrosc. 2017;25(2):595–601. https://doi.org/10.1007/s00167-016-4202-2.
34. Athwal GS, Sperling JW, Rispoli DM, Cofield RH. Deep infection after rotator cuff repair. J Shoulder Elb Surg. 2007;16(3):306–11. https://doi.org/10.1016/j.jse.2006.05.013.
35. Banerjee S, Weiser L, Connell D, Wallace AL. Glenoid rim fracture in contact athletes with absorbable suture anchor reconstruction. Arthroscopy. 2009;25(5):560–2. https://doi.org/10.1016/j.arthro.2008.10.027.
36. Park JY, Lee SJ, Oh SK, Oh K, Noh Y, Suh KT. Glenoid rim fracture through anchor points after arthroscopic Bankart repair for shoulder instability. Int Orthop. 2015;39(2):241–8. https://doi.org/10.1007/s00264-014-2604-7.

37. Ruiz Iban MA, Vega Rodriguez R, Diaz Heredia J, Perez Exposito R, Zarcos Paredes I, Ruiz DR. Arthroscopic Bankart repair with all-suture anchors does not cause important glenoid bone osteolysis: a volumetric CT study of 143 anchors. Knee Surg Sports Traumatol Arthrosc. 2021;29(7):2152–8. https://doi.org/10.1007/s00167-020-06192-1.
38. Lobao MH, Abbasi P, Svoboda SJ. How many anchors to use in arthroscopic Bankart repairs? A biomechanical study of postage-stamp glenoid fractures. J Shoulder Elb Surg. 2023;32(12):2541–9. https://doi.org/10.1016/j.jse.2023.05.022.
39. Woolnough T, Shah A, Sheean AJ, Lesniak BP, Wong I, de Sa D. "Postage stamp" fractures: a systematic review of patient and suture anchor profiles causing anterior glenoid rim fractures after Bankart repair. Arthroscopy. 2019;35(8):2501–8.e2. https://doi.org/10.1016/j.arthro.2019.02.047.
40. Millett PJ, Braun S. The "bony Bankart bridge" procedure: a new arthroscopic technique for reduction and internal fixation of a bony Bankart lesion. Arthroscopy. 2009;25(1):102–5. https://doi.org/10.1016/j.arthro.2008.07.005.
41. Yildirim K, Beyzadeoglu T. Arthroscopic assisted percutaneous screw fixation of a postage stamp anterior glenoid fracture. Acta Chir Orthop Traumatol Cechoslov. 2021;88(6):456–60.
42. Murphy GS, Greenberg SB, Szokol JW. Safety of beach chair position shoulder surgery: a review of the current literature. Anesth Analg. 2019;129(1):101–18. https://doi.org/10.1213/ANE.0000000000004133.
43. Salazar DH, Davis WJ, Ziroglu N, Garbis NG. Cerebral desaturation events during shoulder arthroscopy in the beach chair position. J Am Acad Orthop Surg Glob Res Rev. 2019;3(8):e007. https://doi.org/10.5435/JAAOSGlobal-D-19-00007.
44. Friedman DJ, Parnes NZ, Zimmer Z, Higgins LD, Warner JJ. Prevalence of cerebrovascular events during shoulder surgery and association with patient position. Orthopedics. 2009;32(4):256–61.
45. Salazar D, Hazel A, Tauchen AJ, Sears BW, Marra G. Neurocognitive deficits and cerebral desaturation during shoulder arthroscopy with patient in beach-chair position: a review of the current literature. Am J Orthop (Belle Mead NJ). 2016;45(3):E63–8.
46. Mancini MR, LeVasseur MR, Hawthorne BC, Marrero DE, Mazzocca AD. Venous thromboembolism complications in shoulder surgery: current concepts. J ISAKOS. 2021;6(5):283–9. https://doi.org/10.1136/jisakos-2020-000538.
47. Triplet JJ, Schuette HB, Cheema AN, Marigi EM, Hassett LC, Barlow JD, et al. Venothromboembolism following shoulder arthroscopy: a systematic review. JSES Rev Rep Tech. 2022;2(4):464–8. https://doi.org/10.1016/j.xrrt.2022.05.003.
48. Heo H, Kim YY, Lee JH, Kim G, Kwon D. Comparison of the incidence of inadvertent perioperative hypothermia between general anesthesia and interscalene brachial plexus block in shoulder arthroscopy: a randomized prospective study. Medicine (Baltimore). 2024;103(2):e36855. https://doi.org/10.1097/MD.0000000000036855.
49. Jildeh TR, Okoroha KR, Marshall NE, Amato C, Trafton H, Muh SJ, et al. The effect of intraoperative hypothermia on shoulder arthroplasty. Orthopedics. 2018;41(4):e523–8. https://doi.org/10.3928/01477447-20180511-02.
50. Steelman VM, Chae S, Duff J, Anderson MJ, Zaidi A. Warming of irrigation fluids for prevention of perioperative hypothermia during arthroscopy: a systematic review and meta-analysis. Arthroscopy. 2018;34(3):930–42.e2. https://doi.org/10.1016/j.arthro.2017.09.024.
51. Zhou L, Gee SM, Hansen JA, Posner MA. Heterotopic ossification after arthroscopic procedures: a scoping review of the literature. Orthop J Sports Med. 2022;10(1):23259671211060040. https://doi.org/10.1177/23259671211060040.

Dislocation Arthropathy: Shoulder Arthritis After Instability Surgery—A Growing Problem

28

Guillermo Arce and Marcos Deimundo

28.1 Introduction

When treating patients with shoulder instability, the primary objective of surgical intervention is to restore joint stability and enable patients to resume an active lifestyle and sports activities without experiencing dislocations or subluxations. Most medical literature emphasizes preventing dislocation recurrence as the critical treatment endpoint [1–6].

There are two types of techniques to achieve joint stability: anatomic repairs, such as labrum repair and Arthroscopic Bankart Repair (ABR), and nonanatomic repairs, such as remplissage, free bone blocks, and the Latarjet procedure. It is generally believed that ABR produces less or no shoulder arthritis, while the bone blocks, including the Latarjet, can lead to more joint deterioration [2–11]. However, these outcomes are only some of the problematic situations. After a relatively long follow-up, shoulder osteoarthritis (OA) is common in patients suffering from shoulder instability with or without surgical treatment. This is a devastating complication in young or middle-aged patients [12–14].

This scenario poses a significant challenge for the physicians and surgeons in charge. They are often faced with several dilemmas, such as the reason behind the degenerative changes in this young patient, how they occurred, what measures can be taken to alleviate the patient's symptoms, and whether there is any way to prevent this joint deterioration from happening again.

This chapter aims to accomplish three main objectives. First, we strive to examine the possible causes or risk factors of unstable shoulder osteoarthritis. Second, we plan to describe the impact of different surgical treatments on this problem. Finally, with the agreement of the ISAKOS Shoulder Committee, we will provide guidelines or best practices to reduce the incidence of this severe complication.

28.2 Dislocation Arthropathy without Surgery

The correlation between shoulder instability and joint deterioration is well-known. Multiple dislocation episodes can significantly damage the shoulder cartilage. Subluxations and abnormal biomechanics can also contribute to joint deterioration.

In cases where the first-time dislocation occurs due to high-energy trauma, such as in collision sports, the impact can cause labrum avulsions with glenoid bony fragments and a posterior-superior impaction fracture at the humeral head. These injuries, called bony Bankart and Hill Sachs lesions, are treated with

G. Arce (✉) · M. Deimundo
Instituto Argentino de Diagnóstico y Tratamiento
IADT, Buenos Aires, Argentina

E. Calvo et al. (eds.), *Complex and Revision Problems in Shoulder Instability*,
https://doi.org/10.1007/978-3-031-81389-4_28

Table 28.1 Reported data about osteoarthritis after shoulder instability with conservative treatment without surgery [18–21, 23, 24]

Author and publications	OA without surgery	Follow-up in years
Hovelius L, et al. JBJS 1996	Mild 11%	10
	Moderate 9%	
	Total: 20%	
Hovelius L, et al. J Shoulder Elb Surg 2009	39%	25
Novakofski K J Shoulder Elb Surg 2020	58% pain	17
	12.2% OA	
Kruckeberg B OJSM 2020	17% OA	15.2

OA osteoarthritis

different surgical techniques; however, the associated damage to the articular cartilage is rarely evaluated [15, 16].

The "dislocation arthropathy" is defined as cartilage deterioration, joint narrowing, and osteophyte formation after symptomatic shoulder instability with or without shoulder stabilization procedures [17–23].

The progression of joint degeneration leads to a decreased range of motion and increased joint stability but heightened pain and stiffness over time [24–26].

The Samilson and Prieto Classification is commonly used to determine the grade of articular damage and surgical treatment options for shoulder arthritis [17, 27].

According to Hovelius et al., when left untreated, dislocation arthropathy has a natural history that includes 29% mild, 9% moderate, and 17% severe cases, which totals 56% after 25 years of follow-up in patients who have experienced at least one dislocation [18–21].

Novakofski and his colleagues recently published a study that followed a group of 254 patients (73% male) for at least 10 years, with a mean follow-up of 17 years. The patients were experiencing symptomatic instability and dislocations. The study found that 58% of the patients reported experiencing pain, and 12.2% of the patients had symptoms of OA [23].

Table 28.1 below summarizes the findings of nonsurgically treated shoulder instability patients with OA (Table 28.1).

According to the published data, approximately 50% of patients with symptomatic shoulder instability who are not treated surgically may experience pain, and 30% may develop some degree of shoulder arthritis in the long run [18–27].

28.3 Shoulder Arthritis After Arthroscopic Bankart Repair (ABR)

Facing symptomatic shoulder instability with multiple dislocation episodes, the patient is already at risk of developing arthritis. If they undergo an ABR, they can expect a good outcome regarding the recurrences. However, it is essential to note that cartilage deterioration and osteoarthritis changes will continue after the surgery and may even worsen in some cases [24, 28–30].

Table 28.2 summarizes the occurrence of osteoarthritis following Arthroscopic Bankart Repair.

After reviewing the reported data presented in Tables 28.1 and 28.2, we may conclude the following:

1. Many patients already have mild or moderate OA before the ABR procedure.
2. The OA either appears or worsens after the ABR and during the extended follow-up period.
3. It is difficult to determine whether the operation triggers the high postoperative OA grade or is simply a consequence of the previous instability and a long sequel.

Table 28.2 Reported data about shoulder osteoarthritis after arthroscopic Bankart repair [1–3, 27–35]

Authors	OA Before surgery	After surgery	Total	Procedure	Mean follow-up: years
Buscayet F, et al. AJSM 2004	9.2%	19.7%		ABR	6.5
Francheschi F, et al. AJSM 2011		4% mild 14% moderate 4% severe	22%	ABR	8
Larsen Van Gestel M, et al. KSSTA 2019	9.8%	49% mild 7.3% moderate 3.6% severe	60%	ABR	13.1
Plath J, et al. AJSM 2015		41% mild 16% moderate 12% severe	69%	ABR	13
Castagna A, et al. AJSM 2010		29% mild 10% moderate	39%	ABR	10.9
Murphy A, et al. JSES 2019		35.4% mild 8.8% moderate 1.7% severe	59.4%	ABR	10
Pivitera D, et al. AJSM 2012		20% mild 25% moderate 15% severe	60%	ABR	13.5
Aboalata M, et al. AJSM 2016		12%		ABR	13
Emlund et al. KSSTA 2012		24% mild 18% moderate	42%	ABR	7.9
Zaffagnini S, et al. KSSTA 2012		37%		ABR	14.7
Kruckeberg B, et al. OJSM 2020		28%		ABR	15.2
Rosenberg B, et al. AJSM 1995		42% mild 9% moderate 3% severe	54%	BR	15
Ono Y, et al. JSES 2019		36.8% moderate to severe		ABR	10
Verweij L, et al. KSSTA 2021		65%	65%	ABR	12

28.4 Contributing Risk Factors to Develop Osteoarthritis After ABR

During the Bankart repair, certain operative factors can increase stability and reduce the recurrence rate. However, these factors may also produce arthritis, which is a negative outcome. These factors include rigid body anchors, knots, and postoperative stiffness [31, 33]. Apart from these, several other risk factors contribute to the development of arthritis after the surgery. These include older age at the first episode, glenoid rim fractures, and the number of preoperative dislocations [27, 36].

Table 28.3 summarizes the risk factors that may increase the chances of developing osteoarthritis after ABR.

Table 28.3 Risk and contributing factors to develop osteoarthritis after ABR [27, 36]

Risk factors in developing shoulder arthritis after ABR
1. Osseous glenoid rim lesions
2. Older age at the first episode, >23 years old
3. The number of dislocations. Delayed surgery
4. The number of anchors and knots
5. Hard body anchors below the cartilage level but not inside the bone
6. Postoperative decrease in external rotation

To recover the labrum bumper effect, some authors recommended placing the anchors on the glenoid face about 2 mm from the glenoid edge. Even though this location may positively impact stability, it could negatively affect the articular cartilage. Hirose T. et al. recently reported less glenoid rim erosion locating the anchors at the glenoid edge [37].

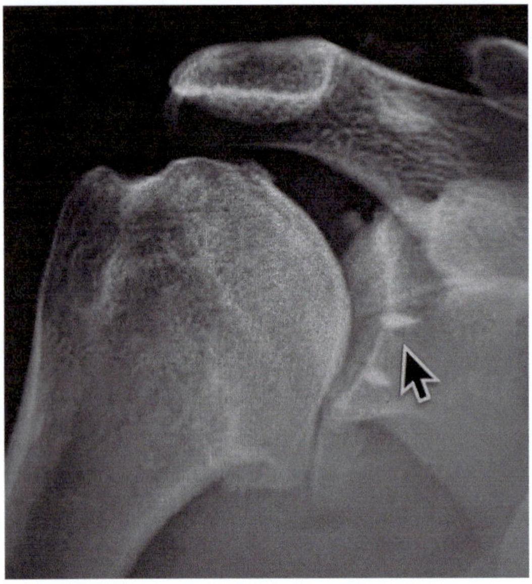

Fig. 28.1 Right shoulder. Advanced osteoarthritis 10 years after Arthroscopic Bankart Repair. X-ray evaluation of degenerative changes and anchor placement

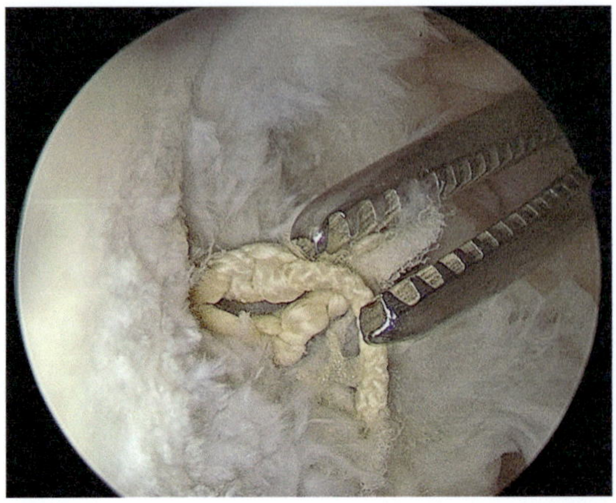

Fig. 28.2 Arthroscopic findings at second-look arthroscopy after Bankart Repair. Nonabsorbable sutures and big knots produce cartilage damage

The quantity and positioning of anchors and knots play a crucial role in maintaining or harming the articular cartilage. Anchors placed below the cartilage level but protruding from the bone can cause severe joint damage. Therefore, it is essential to thoroughly assess the position of the anchors for all patients who experience pain after undergoing ABR (Fig. 28.1). The rigid body anchors may be positioned below the cartilage level, but it is essential to steer them into the bone for better placement. If not properly anchored, the cartilage may thin out over the years, and the anchors may become prominent, leading to joint scratches and damage.

Nonabsorbable sutures and large knots are commonly found in shoulders with arthritis after ABR. These knots scratch the cartilage during shoulder motion and contribute to the development of OA (Fig. 28.2).

The humeral head articulates with the glenoid and the capsule. This means that knots over the glenoid face can cause cartilage damage, and significant, nonabsorbable knots at the capsule can also scuff the humeral head.

Another risk factor for developing OA is shoulder stiffness. The so-called anatomic repairs reduce the labrum to its original native location to regain shoulder stability. However, when the capsule is plicated, they can partially restrict the range of motion after the index procedure.

The plastic elongation of the shoulder capsule caused by dislocation episodes or the patient's natural looseness is challenging to measure accurately. To treat unstable shoulders, the surgeon must repair the labrum and adjust the capsule's tightness or amount of pleating. Reducing the volume of the capsule is essential for successful treatment, but it can also cause biomechanical changes and joint overloading. This increase in shearing forces on the cartilage can lead to arthritis [13–16].

The humeral head typically has an average retroversion of 30°. Following surgery and postoperative rehabilitation for anterior shoulder instability, patients must recover at least 30° of external rotation. Failure to do so can lead to the humeral head not being centered at the glenoid, resulting in stiffness. This stiffness can cause a posterior translation of the center of rotation and secondary articular damage [27, 29].

Also, the "remplissage" is indicated to treat the humeral head bone defect. This French term means "filling." A part of the posterior capsule and the infraspinatus tendon is introduced into the posterior humeral head bone defect (Hill Sachs lesion) to prevent engaging and dislocations. This procedure is often used to improve shoulder stability during an ABR, but it can also alter shoulder biomechanics and limit the range of motion, leading to osteoarthritis [38, 39].

28.5 Shoulder Arthritis After Glenoid Bone Reconstructions: Bone Blocks and Latarjet

Dislocation episodes produce labrum tears and considerable glenoid fractures. The so-called bony Bankart lesions are pieces of bone detached from the glenoid, increasing the instability. In other cases, bone loss appears after many dislocations or subluxation episodes. This "attritional bone loss" must be reconstructed with bony procedures [40, 41].

When the glenoid bone loss exceeds 13.5%, surgeons recommend a bony reconstruction procedure using allograft or autograft. Free bone blocks or the Latarjet technique is commonly used. These bone blocks help restore stability and the glenoid track, but most do not have the native glenoid cartilage, which may lead to the development of osteoarthritis in the long term [7, 9–11, 42].

In addition, the precise position of the Latarjet coracoid graft or bone blocks is critical. Any glenoid bone graft slightly lateral and prominent from the glenoid articular surface will result in early degeneration of the joint (Fig. 28.3).

Lalanne et al., with a mean follow-up of 22 years, described significant differences in developing OA regarding the Latarjet graft position. When the bone block was located laterally overhanging the glenoid face level, OA was 71.4%. Otherwise, the OA findings were only 16.6% when the graft was well positioned [42].

Gilat compared the recurrences and outcomes of the Latarjet and free bone graft options. The "non-Latarjet" auto and allografts have similar results regarding instability recurrence and arthritis changes to the original coracoid transfer [43, 44].

Lukas Verweij reported the evolution of the degenerative changes of the unstable shoulder with or without bony procedures. The conservative treatment increased the OA changes more than Latarjet (60% and 34%, respectively). The only techniques that deteriorated the joint more than the conservative approach were the derotation humeral osteotomy (85%) and the Eden-Hybinette original technique (65%) [45].

Bouju et al., with a mean of 13 years follow-up study, also demonstrated the excellent outcomes of the Latarjet, reporting only 8.5% OA after the glenoid grafting when the technique is performed precisely [46].

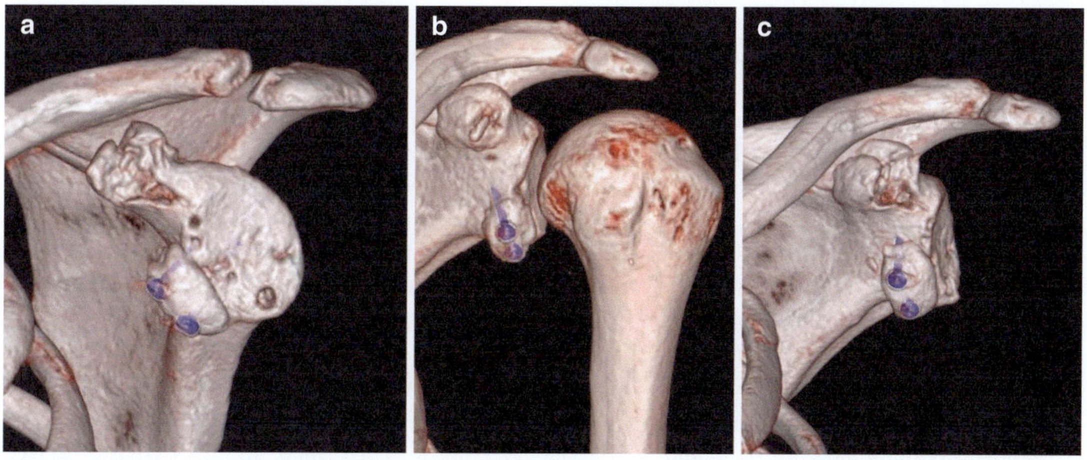

Fig. 28.3 Left shoulder. 3D postoperative CT scan. (**a–c**) The graft position is checked at the sagittal, coronal, and axial planes. The graft was positioned correctly

Table 28.4 Reported data on the development of osteoarthritis after free bone blocks auto or allografts and Latarjet [7, 42–50]

Author	OA %	Procedure	Mean follow-up years
Verweij L, et al. KSSTA 2021	40%	Latarjet	16
Verweij L, et al. KSSTA 2021	60%	Iliac crest autograft	24
Bouju Y, et al. Orthop and T SR 2014	8.5%	Latarjet	13
Ernstbrunner L, et al. AJSM 2019	Severe 37% Progresive 45%	Latarjet	11
Lalanne C, et al. Orthop and T SR 2021	71% lateral graft 17% medial graft	Latarjet	22
Gilat R, et al. AJSM 2020	12% 4%	Latarjet Free bone block	7
Menon A, et al. KSSTA 2022	26%	Latarjet	17
Chillemi C, et al. Arch Orthop Trau Surg	53%	Latarjet	26
Wang L, et al. J Orthop Surg Res	13%	Latarjet	4
Davey M, et al. Shoulder Elbow 2024	41%	Latarjet	23
Hurley E, et al. J Shoulder Elb Surg 2019	39%	Latarjet	17
Gilat R, et al. KSSTA 2021	11% 1%	Autograft Allograft	8 5
Flurin PH, et al. Orthop Traum Surg Res	11%	Iliac crest auto	3

Table 28.4 summarizes the most recent information on osteoarthritis following glenoid bone reconstruction procedures, as presented in Table 28.4.

28.6 Arthroscopic Treatment of Early Stages of Dislocation Arthropathy

Patients complaining about pain and stiffness after ABR or bone block procedures should be deeply evaluated. Good quality X-rays, 2-D or 3-D CT scans, and an MRI should be obtained to recognize the origin of the pain and the loss of external rotation. The anchors' placement should be determined when osteoarthritis changes appear early after the index procedure.

Six months after the ABR, the patients should be almost asymptomatic. If pain and stiffness persist, a second-look arthroscopy is warranted to rule out intra-articular problems that can damage the cartilage. In this setting, all causes of pain and stiffness are checked. Any anchor at the articular cartilage and knots contacting the joint surfaces must be removed. Bone block or implant impingement needs to be removed or smoothed.

In situations where the external rotation loss is critical, a conservative capsular release can be done by pie-crusting the capsule to increase the range of motion without compromising the previous labrum repair [36].

The Comprehensive Arthroscopic Management (CAM) procedure described by Mook and Millet et al. is indicated in patients with mild to moderate OA changes (Samilson y Prieto grade A to C) with more than 2 mm joint space and an inferior osteophyte at the humeral head [51].

A joint debridement, loose body removal, long head of the biceps tenotomy or tenodesis, capsular releases, chondroplasty, and osteophyte removal are performed. In cases where the free bone block or the Latarjet graft is lateral to the glenoid rim, removing the excessive bone and repairing the capsule can alleviate symptoms caused by impingement.

After surgery, a complete rehabilitation program is recommended to increase the range of motion, strength, and scapula control.

28.7 ISAKOS Shoulder Com-Suggested Measures to Decrease Arthritis after Shoulder Instability Surgery

During its Consensus Meeting in Milano in May 2024, the ISAKOS Shoulder Committee extensively discussed the reported causes of Dislocation Arthropathy.

After reviewing the published data, the level V experts' experience was added to consent about the best practices to prevent shoulder OA before and after surgery.

Table 28.5 outlines the consent recommendations for preventing shoulder osteoarthritis that may result from instability surgery.

The development of osteoarticular damage and osteoarthritis is a severe complication that can occur before and after arthroscopic Bankart repair or Bone Blocks. Sometimes, this complication can be worse than the recurrence of dislocations. Surgeons should explain these potential complications to patients and their families before the operation. Surgeons must perform the best technique possible to avoid instability while minimizing degenerative changes.

We expect this chapter to raise awareness of critical complications, improve decision-making, and utilize superior techniques to achieve better long-term results for patients with shoulder instability.

Table 28.5 ISAKOS good practices suggestions to prevent dislocation arthropathy

1.	Decrease the number of preoperative dislocations. Early surgical repairs
2.	Assessment of osteoarticular damage and osteoarthritis before shoulder instability surgery. Patients' information and education
3.	Place the anchors at the glenoid rim—Anchors' eyelets inside the bone—Knots and sutures at the capsule side, not near the cartilage
4.	Knotless and all suture anchors inside the bone
5.	Tailored capsular plication to avoid postoperative stiffness
6.	All patients with pain or decreased external rotation after ABR warrant detailed X-rays, CT scans, and MRI evaluations
7.	Patients with pain and stiffness 6 months after surgery justify a second look arthroscopy to prevent cartilage damage by anchors or knots
8.	Free bone blocks and the Latarjet coracoid graft must be located at the edge or medial to the glenoid rim

References

1. Larsen van Gastel M, Willigenburg N, Dijksman L, Lindeboom R, van den Bekerom M, van der Hulst V, et al. Ten percent re-dislocation rate 13 years after the arthroscopic Bankart procedure. Knee Surg Sports Traumatol Arthrosc. 2019;27(12):3929–36.
2. Murphy A, Hurley E, Hurley D, Pauzenberger L, Mullett H. Long-term outcomes of the arthroscopic Bankart repair: a systematic review of studies at 10-year follow-up. J Shoulder Elb Surg. 2019;28(11):2084–9.
3. Aboalata M, Plath J, Seppel G, Juretzko J, Vogt S, Imhoff A. Results of arthroscopic Bankart repair for anterior-inferior shoulder instability at 13-year follow-up. Am J Sports Med. 2016;45(4):782–7.
4. Harris J, Gupta A, Mall N, Abrams G, McCormick F, Cole B, et al. Long-term outcomes after Bankart shoulder stabilization. Arthroscopy. 2013;29(5):920–33.
5. Bottoni C, Johnson J, Zhou L, Raybin S, Shaha J, Cruz C, et al. Arthroscopic versus open anterior shoulder stabilization: a prospective randomized clinical trial with 15-year follow-up with an assessment of the glenoid being "on-track" and "off-track" as a predictor of failure. Am J Sports Med. 2021;49(8):1999–2005.
6. Berendes TD, Wolterbeek R, Pilot P, Verburg H, Slaa RL. The open modified Bankart procedure: outcome at follow-up of 10 to 15 years. J Bone Joint Surg. 2007;89:1064–8.
7. Menon A, Fossati C, Magnani M, Boveri S, Compagnoni R, Randelli P. Low grade of osteoarthritis development after Latarjet procedure with a minimum 5 years of follow-up: a systematic review and pooled analysis. Knee Surg Sports Traumatol Arthrosc. 2021;30:2074–83.
8. Kavaja L, Pajarinen J, Sinisaari I, Savolainen V, Björkenheim J, Haapamäki V, et al. Arthrosis of the glenohumeral joint after arthroscopic Bankart repair: a long-term follow-up of 13 years. J Shoulder Elb Surg. 2012;21(3):350–5.
9. Rollick N, Ono Y, Kurji H, Nelson A, Boorman R, Thornton G, et al. Long-term outcomes of the Bankart and Latarjet repairs: a systematic review. Open Access J Sports Med. 2017;8:97–105.
10. Zimmermann S, Scheyerer M, Farshad M, Catanzaro S, Rahm S, Gerber C. Long-term restoration of anterior shoulder stability: a retrospective analysis of arthroscopic Bankart repair versus open Latarjet procedure. J Bone Joint Surg. 2016;98(23):1954–61.
11. Ernstbrunner L, De Nard B, Olthof M, Beeler S, Bouaicha S, Gerber C, et al. Long-term results of the arthroscopic Bankart repair for recurrent anterior shoulder instability in patients older than 40 years: a comparison with the open Latarjet procedure. Am J Sports Med. 2020;48(9):2090–6.
12. Komnos G, Banios K, Liantsis A, Alexiou K, Varitimidis S, Bareka M, et al. Results of arthroscopic Bankart repair in recreational athletes and Laborers: a retrospective study with 5 to 14 years of follow-up. Orthop J Sports Med. 2019;7(11):2325967119881648.
13. Zink S, Pfeiffenberger T, Müller A, Krisam R, Unglaub F, Pötzl W. The arthroscopic Bankart operation: a 10-year follow-up study. Arch Orthop Trauma Surg. 2022;142(11):3367–77.
14. Bock J, Buckup J, Reinig Y, Zimmermann E, Colcuc C, Hoffmann R, et al. The arthroscopic Bankart repair procedure enables complete quantitative labrum restoration in long-term assessments. Knee Surg Sports Traumatol Arthrosc. 2018;26(12):3788–96.
15. Cameron M, Kocher M, Briggs K, Horan M, Hawkins R. The prevalence of glenohumeral osteoarthrosis in unstable shoulders. Am J Sports Med. 2003;31(1):53–5.
16. Lu Y, Pareek A, Wilbur R, et al. Understanding anterior shoulder instability through machine learning. New models that predict recurrence, progression or surgery, and development of arthritis. Orthop J Sports Med. 2021;9(11):23259671211053326.
17. Samilson R, Prieto V. Dislocation arthropathy of the shoulder. J Bone Jt Surg Am. 1983;65:456–60.
18. Hovelius L, Augustini BG, Fredin H, et al. Primary anterior dislocation of the shoulder in young patients: a ten-year prospective study. J Bone Joint Surg. 1996;78:1677–84.
19. Hovelius LK, Sandström BC, Rösmark DL, et al. Long-term results with the Bankart and Bristow-Latarjet procedures: recurrent shoulder instability and arthropathy. J Shoulder Elb Surg. 2001;10:445–52.
20. Hovelius L, Sandström B, Saebö M. One hundred eighteen Bristow-Latarjet repairs for recurrent anterior dislocation of the shoulder prospectively followed for fifteen years: study II-the evolution of dislocation arthropathy. J Shoulder Elb Surg. 2006;15:279–89.
21. Hovelius L, Saeboe M. Arthropathy after primary anterior shoulder dislocation; 223 shoulders prospectively followed up for twenty-five years. J Shoulder Elb Surg. 2009;18(3):339–47.
22. Brophy R, Marx R. Osteoarthritis following shoulder instability. Clin Sports Med. 2005;24(1):47–56.
23. Novakofski K, Melugin H, Leland D, Bernard C, Krych A, Camp C. Nonoperative management of anterior shoulder instability can result in high rates of recurrent instability and pain at long-term follow-up. J Shoulder Elb Surg. 2022;31(2):352–8.
24. Kruckeberg BM, Leland DP, Bernard CD, Krych AJ, Dahm DL, Sanchez-Sotelo J, Camp CL. Incidence of and risk factors for glenohumeral osteoarthritis after anterior shoulder instability: a US population-based study with average 15-year follow-up. Orthop J Sports Med. 2020;8(11):2325967120962515.
25. Coifman I, Brunner UH, Scheibel M. Dislocation arthropathy of the shoulder. J Clin Med. 2022;11(7):2019–20.
26. Cerciello S, Corona K, Morris B, et al. Shoulder arthroplasty to address the sequelae of anterior instability arthropathy and stabilization procedures: systematic review and meta-analysis. Arch Orthop Trauma Surg. 2020;140(12):1891–900.

27. Buscayret F, Bradley T, Szabo I, Adeleine P, Coudane H, Walch G. Glenohumeral arthrosis in anterior instability before and after surgical treatment incidence and contributing factors. Am J Sports Med. 2004;32(5):1165–72.
28. Plath J, Aboalata M, Seppel G, Juretzko J, Waldt S, Vogt S, et al. Prevalence of and risk factors for dislocation arthropathy. Am J Sports Med. 2015;43(5):1084–90.
29. Franceschi F, Papalia R, Del Buono A, Vasta S, et al. Glenohumeral osteoarthritis after arthroscopic Bankart repair for anterior instability. Am J Sports Med. 2011;39:1654–9.
30. Castagna A, Markopoulos N, Conti M, Rose GD, Papadakou E, Garofalo R. Arthroscopic Bankart suture anchor repair: radiological and clinical outcomes at minimum 10 years of follow-up. Am J Sports Med. 2010;38:2012–6.
31. Privitera DM, Bisson LJ, Marzo JM. Minimum 10-year follow-up of arthroscopic intra-articular Bankart repair using bioabsorbable tacks. Am J Sports Med. 2012;40:100–7.
32. Elmlund AO, Ejerhed L, Sernert N, Rostgard LC, Kartus J. Dislocation arthropathy and drill hole appearance in a mid- to long-term follow-up study after arthroscopic Bankart repair. Knee Surg Sports Traumatol Arthrosc. 2012;20:2156–62.
33. Zaffagnini S, Marcheggiani Muccioli GM, Giordano G, et al. Long-term outcomes after repair of recurrent posttraumatic anterior shoulder instability: comparison of arthroscopic transglenoid suture and open Bankart reconstruction. Knee Surg Sports Traumatol Arthrosc. 2012;20:816–21.
34. Rosenberg B, Richmond J, Levine W. Long-term followup of Bankart reconstruction. Am J Sports Med. 1995;23(5):538–44.
35. Ono Y, Dávalos Herrera D, Woodmass J, Lemmex D, Carroll M, Yamashita S, et al. Long-term outcomes following isolated arthroscopic Bankart repair: a 9- to 12-year follow-up. JSES Open Access. 2019;3(3):189–93.
36. Vezeridis P, Ishmael C, Jones K, Petrigliano F. Glenohumeral dislocation arthropathy: etiology, diagnosis and management. J Am Acad Orthop Surg. 2018;29:e51–61.
37. Hirose T, Nakagawa S, Uchida R, et al. On-the-edge anchor placement may be protective against glenoid rim erosion after arthroscopic Bankart repair compared to on-the-face anchor placement. Arthroscopy. 2022;38(4):1099–107.
38. Ding Z, Cong S, Xie Y, Feng S, Chen S, Chen J. Location of the suture anchor in Hill-Sachs lesion could influence glenohumeral cartilage quality and limit range of motion after arthroscopic Bankart repair and remplissage. Am J Sports Med. 2020;48(11):2628–37.
39. Argintar E, Heckmann N, Wang L, Tibone JE, Lee TQ. The biomechanical effect of shoulder remplissage combined with Bankart repair for the treatment of engaging Hill-Sachs lesions. Knee Surg Sports Traumatol Arthrosc. 2016;24(2):585–92.
40. Flurin P-H, Antoni M, Métais P, Aswad R. Revision of failed Latarjet with the Eden-Hybinette surgical technique. Orthop Traumatol Surg Res. 2020;106(2):223–7. https://doi.org/10.1016/j.otsr.2019.12.009.
41. Wang L, He S, Wu X, Lv X, Wang T, Tan H. Efficacy and safety of the Latarjet procedure for the treatment of athletes with glenoid bone defects ≥ 20%: a single-arm meta-analysis. J Orthop Surg Res. 2024;19(1):159. https://doi.org/10.1186/s13018-024-04641-y.
42. Lalanne C, Vervoort T, Cassagnaud X, Szymanski C, Bourgault C, Pougès C, et al. Long-term prevalence and impact of glenohumeral osteoarthritis after Latarjet-Patte procedure for anterior instability. Orthop Traumatol Surg Res. 2023;109(4):103050. https://doi.org/10.1016/j.otsr.2021.103050.
43. Gilat R, Wong SE, Lavoie-Gagne O, Haunschild ED, Knapik DM, Fu MC, et al. Outcomes are comparable using free bone block autografts versus allografts for the management of anterior shoulder instability with glenoid bone loss: a systematic review and meta-analysis of "the non-Latarjet". Knee Surg Sports Traumatol Arthrosc. 2020;29(7):2159–74. https://doi.org/10.1007/s00167-020-06194-z.
44. Gilat R, Haunschild ED, Lavoie-Gagne OZ, Tauro TM, Knapik DM, Fu MC, et al. Outcomes of the Latarjet procedure versus free bone block procedures for anterior shoulder instability: a systematic review and meta-analysis. Am J Sports Med. 2020;49(3):805–16. https://doi.org/10.1177/0363546520925833.
45. Verweij LP, Pruijssen EC, Kerkhoffs GM, Blankevoort L, Sierevelt IN, van Deurzen DF, et al. Treatment type may influence the degree of post-dislocation shoulder osteoarthritis: a systematic review and meta-analysis. Knee Surg Sports Traumatol Arthrosc. 2020;29(7):2312–24. https://doi.org/10.1007/s00167-020-06263-3.
46. Bouju Y, Gadéa F, Stanovici J, Moubarak H, Favard L. Shoulder stabilization by modified Latarjet-Patte procedure: results at a minimum 10years' follow-up, and role in the prevention of osteoarthritis. Orthop Traumatol Surg Res. 2014;100(4):S213–8. https://doi.org/10.1016/j.otsr.2014.03.010.
47. Hurley ET, Jamal MS, Ali ZS, Montgomery C, Pauzenberger L, Mullett H. Long-term outcomes of the Latarjet procedure for anterior shoulder instability: a systematic review of studies at 10-year follow-up. J Shoulder Elb Surg. 2019;28(2):e33–9. https://doi.org/10.1016/j.jse.2018.08.028.
48. Ernstbrunner L, Wartmann L, Zimmermann SM, Schenk P, Gerber C, Wieser K. Long-term results of the open latarjet procedure for recurrent anterior shoulder instability in patients older than 40 years. Am J Sports Med. 2019;47(13):3057–64. https://doi.org/10.1177/0363546519872501.
49. Chillemi C, Guerrisi M, Paglialunga C, Salate Santone F, Osimani M. Latarjet procedure for anterior

shoulder instability: a 24-year follow-up study. Arch Orthop Trauma Surg. 2020;141(2):189–96. https://doi.org/10.1007/s00402-020-03426-2.
50. Davey MS, Hurley ET, Kilkenny C, Anakwenze OA, Klifto CS, Mullett H. Long-term outcomes of anterior shoulder instability treated with open Latarjet procedure—a systematic review of outcomes at a minimum 15-year follow-up. Shoulder Elbow. 2022;16(1):8–14. https://doi.org/10.1177/17585732221141062.
51. Mook W, Petri M, Greenspoon J, Millett P. The comprehensive arthroscopic management procedure for treatment of glenohumeral osteoarthritis. Arthrosc Tech. 2015;4(5):435–41.

MIX
Papier aus verantwortungsvollen Quellen
Paper from responsible sources
FSC® C105338

If you have any concerns about our products,
you can contact us on
ProductSafety@springernature.com

In case Publisher is established outside the EU,
the EU authorized representative is:
Springer Nature Customer Service Center GmbH
Europaplatz 3, 69115 Heidelberg, Germany

Printed by Libri Plureos GmbH
in Hamburg, Germany